Psychosomatic Medicine

A Clinical Study

of Psychophysiologic Reactions

Edward Weiss, M.D.

Professor of Clinical Medicine
Temple University Medical Center, Philadelphia

O. Spurgeon English, M.D.

Professor and Head of Department of Psychiatry
Temple University Medical Center, Philadelphia

Third Edition

W. B. Saunders Company

Philadelphia   London   1957

*"For this is the great error of our day. . .
that physicians separate the soul from the body."*

PLATO

Preface to the Third Edition

Since the publication of the first edition of this book the psychosomatic concept has been widely accepted. The medical experiences of World War II were largely responsible. Physicians who served in the military forces returned to civilian practice with a healthy respect for the psyche as a factor in producing illness and a genuine desire to learn more about the subject. For the first time in half a century a familiar pattern of medical education has been infused with new ideas and subjected to bold experimentation. The social-psychiatric point of view has gained wide acceptance in medical education and the doctor-patient relationship has been subjected to scientific scrutiny. The fragmented, "organic-disease" approach has given way to the patient as a person so that one might question whether a book on psychosomatic medicine is any longer necessary. However, until textbooks of medicine incorporate this point of view in a wholly integrated text we believe that such a book as this one can fill an important need in the practice of medicine as well as in all phases of medical education—undergraduate, graduate and postgraduate.

The chapters have been rearranged so that the material of a general nature makes up Part I while the applications to special problems occur in Part II. Much has been rewritten and considerable new clinical material has been added. New charts and tables summarizing diagnostic points and treatment suggestions are included.

Even more strongly than before, we believe that the psychosomatic concept has an important contribution to make, especially in relation to chronic illness and disease which remain the greatest challenge to medical science.

We continue to be indebted to our colleagues for their assistance. Dr. Morris Kleinbart and Dr. H. Keith Fischer have been unfailingly helpful. Dr. Barney Dlin, Vancouver, B.C., Dr. Isador Forman, Dr. Max Katz, Dr. Norman Learner, the late Dr. J. E. Meyer, Columbus, Nebraska, Dr. Ruben R. Pottash, Dr. William A. Steiger, Dr. Harry H. Wagenheim, Dr. Francis Hoffman, Carol Scholz, as well as many others have been helpful in making suggestions for revision and Jeanne Speiser has been a great help in editorial work and seeing the book through press.

June, 1957   Edward Weiss
                                               O. Spurgeon English

Preface to the First Edition

Understanding illness and treating sick people consists of something more than a knowledge of disease. This the senior author learned quite forcibly some twenty years ago shortly after he had entered clinical medicine through the doors of pathology. At that time he was consulted by a young woman whose headaches were of obscure origin. With pathological knowledge and scientific zeal, he vigorously proceeded to investigate, by means of physical examination and laboratory studies, her various organs and tissues. In the course of the "complete investigation" lumbar puncture was done. Following this she became worse than ever; she developed even more severe headaches, pain in her back, and various intestinal disturbances. She remained bedridden for nine months. During this period still more physical investigations were made. While the diagnosis, despite all these efforts, puzzled him at that time, the fact that the family continued to employ him remains a mystery to this day. At long last, however, the family's patience was exhausted and they decided to dispense with such services. They then asked an old physician, who had looked after the patient during her childhood, to take care of her. He knew what the young "scientist" had not attempted to discover: that the patient's only brother, to whom she was closely attached and who acted in the capacity of head of the family, was interested in a young woman whom he would probably marry. The patient's illness was her infantile way of expressing disapproval of her brother's marriage and, when the meaning of the illness was made clear to her, she promptly recovered.

It was a valuable lesson for the young doctor. It brought the realization that his training in medical school and hospital, supplemented by a study of diseased organs and tissues, had not fitted him for the practice of medicine. He has been trying to remedy that deficiency since, and in the course of that re-education he has been fortunate enough to associate himself with the psychiatrist-author of this book.

He has discovered that cases similar to the above are by no means the exception in the practice of medicine. On the contrary, many authorities agree that they constitute about a third of all cases, and that still another third of all patients have emotional factors which complicate and add to the burden of their physical disease. These are the problems dealt with in this book.

For many years the authors have been working together on clinical problems and teaching at the Temple University Medical School. A particular part of that teaching has been known as a "psychosomatic conference," a teaching exercise for senior medical students. It consists of the presentation of patients from the general medical wards, who have been studied psychologically as well as medically. The idea and the case material for this book grew out of those conferences. We are indebted to Dr. C. L. Brown, Professor of Medicine, for his encouragement and support of that teaching and for his kind permission to use the clinical material.

In January, 1939, a new periodical appeared under the title of Psychosomatic Medicine. Commenting upon this publication, an editorial in the Journal of the American Medical Association paid tribute to the dynamic psychology of Sigmund Freud in its fundamental application to this new synthesis in medicine. No work on psychosomatic medicine could have been attempted without the biologically oriented psychology of Freud. Following his discoveries, Ferenczi, Abraham, Jones, Jelliffe, and more recently, Felix Deutsch, Wittkower, Menninger, Alexander and his associates at the Chicago Institute of Psychoanalysis, and Flanders Dunbar and her associates at the Presbyterian Hospital in New York, by their important researches, have added materially to our knowledge of this subject. In 1935 Dunbar, in addition to her valuable studies, collected the widely scattered literature in this field in what must have been a tremendous task, and published it under the title "Emotions and Bodily Changes."

The epochal discoveries of Freud, the researches mentioned and the compilation of literature by Dunbar, made the present work possible. Accordingly we have borrowed freely from these sources, as well as from numerous other contributors, to whom references will be made.

With this latest development in research, all medicine tends to become psychosomatic medicine. We believe, therefore, that future textbooks of medicine will have to embody this approach.

Few illustrations such as are found in the usual medical book could be used in the present work. In dealing with the emotional life the only picture which can be reproduced is a verbal one in the form of an illustrative case. This requires more time from the reader than it takes to glance at a photograph, but we feel sure that he will be rewarded for his effort by a better understanding of the psychic forces that produce illness.

The book is constructed so that the busy practitioner can read the first two chapters and the last four and get a general idea of the subject. If he is encouraged to read more we will consider our work well done. For the specialist we recommend that he do the same basic reading and, in addition, the section devoted to his subject. For the reader whose interest runs deeper, we suggest the liberal use of the index, which has been fashioned so that the material on a given subject is indicated from the standpoint of general discussion and as it applies to specific cases.

We are indebted to many of our colleagues for their support in this undertaking and wish especially to express our gratitude to Dr. Paul Sloane, Dr. Morris Brody and Dr. Hugo Roesler for their studies and notes on special cases, and to the many other consultants whose advice had to be sought in the psychosomatic approach to medical problems.

EDWARD WEISS
O. SPURGEON ENGLISH

Contents

Part One. General Aspects of Psychosomatic Medicine

A Family History Which Suggests a Background for Psychological Difficulties. Evidences for a Childhood Neurosis. Sensitivity to Specific Emotional Factors. A Specific Personality Structure. Demonstration of Specific Behavior. Hyposensitization by Psychotherapy or by the Avoidance of Provocative Situations.

Part Two.   Special Applications to General Medicine and the Specialties

Contents

xiii

Part One

General Aspects of
Psychosomatic Medicine

Chapter I

Psychosomatic Medicine

Although the term psychosomatic was first used more than one hundred years ago* it did not come into common usage until Dunbar introduced it into American medicine about 1935. Following World War II its adoption was rapid. For the first time a term was available that made sense to the general physician in relating the emotions to bodily illness. However, many objections have arisen to its use (chiefly that it perpetuates the dichotomy of body and mind which it was supposed to eliminate) but it seems to us to have served a useful purpose.

As used in this book, the term psychosomatic indicates a method of approach to general medical problems, that is, the simultaneous application of physiological and psychological techniques to the study of illness in an effort to make a definitive diagnosis and in preparation for comprehensive medical care. We also apply the term in a more limited sense to a specific affection, indicating that the disorder is one which can be understood only when psychological as well as physiological factors are taken into consideration (Halliday).

Psychosomatic describes an approach to medicine as old as the art of healing itself. It is not a specialty but rather a point of view which applies to all aspects of medicine and surgery. It does not mean to study the soma less; it only means to study the psyche more. It is reaffirmation of the ancient principle that the mind and the body are one, that they function as interactive and interdependent organs—a principle which has always guided the intelligent general practitioner. As a science psychosomatic medicine aims at discovering the precise nature of the relationship of the emotions and bodily function. Research in the subject is founded on the confluence of modern physiological investigation, as developed by laboratory science and animal experimentation and by the discoveries of psychoanalysis, both representing dynamic outgrowths of medicine. These modern streams of thought and investigation are in the process of integration and the combination gives promise of establishing real progress in medicine. The whole subject was given a great impetus as a result of World War II. Indeed it may be said that psychiatry was established on a

* Margetts credits Heinroth, a German psychiatrist, with the first use of the term in 1818 in a discussion of insomnia.

firmer scientific basis in World War I and saw a substantial integration into general medicine in World War II. This, then, is psychosomatic medicine. When the integration is complete we may not have to use the term, for good medicine will be psychosomatic.

Physicians have always known that the *emotional life* had something to do with illness, but the structural concepts introduced by Virchow led to the separation of illness from the psyche of man and a consideration of disease as only a disorder of organs and cells. With this separation of diseases into many different ailments came the development of specialists to attend to all of these distinct diseases. With the specialists came the introduction of instruments of precision and the mechanization of medicine began. This was a logical outcome of the development of general science. As noted in the Merck Report, January, 1951, the laws of the movement of the planet, the laws of motion, the law of gravity, the laws of gases, the laws of hydraulics—all of these, following the domination by physics and chemistry of 17th century science, were to be applied practically, and would result in the world of wheels, and steam power and clocks and vehicles—in a word, machinery. Seventeenth century science also developed calculus as an instrument for measuring the physical world, so there came both the desire to explore the physical world and the desire to measure it. The new science had a profound influence on all disciplines. Medicine could not escape the philosophy that the material universe behaved like a machine which obeyed regularly defined and discoverable laws. Was it not logical to conclude that life itself was nothing but a series of complex physical-chemical reactions and that all one had to do was discover the laws governing such reactions? Medicine, influenced by mechanism, began to apply the tools of physical science to the study of the human body in health and disease. The heart was a pump, the lungs a bellows, the arms and legs obeyed the laws of leverage. If the body was a machine, then sickness was a malfunctioning of the machinery, and healing was akin to "fixing" the machine. Medicine now contented itself with the study of the organism as a physiological mechanism, impressed by blood chemistry, electrocardiography, and other methods of investigation, but unimpressed by and, indeed, often holding in contempt the psychological background of the patient, which was not considered so scientific as the results of laboratory studies. This period may, in truth, be referred to as the "machine age in medicine." It is not to be denied that remarkable developments occurred during this period of laboratory ascendancy, but it also must be admitted that the emotional side of illness was almost entirely neglected.

PSYCHOSOMATIC PROBLEMS IN THE PRACTICE OF MEDICINE

Between the small number of obviously psychotic persons whom a physician sees and the larger number of patients who are sick solely because of physical disease are a vast number of sick people who are not "out of their minds" and yet who *do not have any definite bodily disease to account for their illness*. Psychosomatic medicine is chiefly concerned with them. We have estimated that about *a third* of the patients with chronic illness who consult a physician fall into this group. These are the so-called purely "functional" problems of medical practice.

Approximately *another third* of the patients with chronic illness have symptoms that are *in part dependent upon emotional factors,* even though organic findings are present. This second group is even more important than the first from the standpoint of diagnosis and treatment. These psychosomatic problems are often very complicated and, because serious organic disease may be present, the psychic factor is capable of doing more damage than in the first group. This phase of the subject will be referred to especially in the discussion of organic heart disease.

A third group of disorders, generally considered wholly within the realm of "physical disease," have to do with the vegetative nervous system, such as *migraine, asthma,* and *essential hypertension.* Psychosomatic medicine is much interested in these disorders because it believes that the psychic factor may be of great importance in their etiology and, even more importantly, in their management.

Of course, the percentages stated depend upon the bias and training of the observer. In a similar investigation of 1000 general medical cases from the Lahey Clinic, 534 had physical disorders only, 272 were of nervous origin, and 134 had physical and mental disorders combined. These were unselected ambulatory patients who had come to the Clinic for a general medical examination. The observers (Allan and Kaufman) admit that their evaluation of nervous factors might differ from that of other investigators.

A more recent and more detailed survey from the private outpatient clinic at Johns Hopkins Hospital by Lewis showed that of 163 carefully studied consecutive patients, 49 per cent had psychogenic disorders alone and 27 per cent represented a combination of psychic and somatic processes. Thus 76 per cent of the patients were suffering wholly or in part from emotionally determined disease. The majority of these patients were in the third to sixth decades of life and were from the upper and middle class. The medical problems were predominantly chronic in nature and usually not severe enough to require hospital care, in other words, the kind of problems with which the average internist deals every day. We regard this study as one of the most trustworthy from the standpoint of the training and objectivity of the observer as well as the sampling of the clinical material. Lewis summarized his findings and other material in the table on page 6.

Roberts and Norton studied patients in a medical out-patient clinic of a general hospital and found that the total incidence of "psychopathy" was almost the same in a patient group that came from a distinctly different socio-economic level. This confirms what we have always believed—that psychic factors are as prevalent and important in the medical out-patient clinic of a general hospital as in a private diagnostic center.

But similar studies have been done elsewhere than in the United States. From Denmark (Foreign Letters, J.A.M.A., 1955) it was reported that an investigation of occupants of the medical wards of two general hospitals to ascertain the amount and nature of the psychiatric problems

Table 1.   Incidence of Psychic Disorders in Medical Patients Noted by
Various Observers

Author	No. of Patients	Psychogenic %*	Mixed %†	Total %
Hamman, L.	500	23	11	34
Allan, F. N., and Kaufman, M.	1,000	27	13	40
Lewis, B. I.‡	163	49	27	76
Roberts, B. H., and Norton, N. M.	50	58	22	80
Lewis, B. I.§	151	20	41	61
Robinson, G. C.	174	36	30	66
Combined Totals	2,038	29 (590)	18 (359)	47 (949)

* Illnesses due in their entirety to psychological factors.
† Illnesses due to both psychic and somatic factors.
‡ First series.
§ Second series.
From Lewis, B. I.: J.A.M.A. *150:*776–780, October 25, 1952.

showed that of 264 consecutive patients admitted to each hospital who
were examined by a psychiatrist, 5.3 per cent were found to have psychoses, 25.4 per cent neuroses or psychopathy, and 2.5 per cent mental
deficiency. Another investigation by the same committee was undertaken
of 21 medical practices comprising a total of 17,000 doctor-patient contacts. Psychiatric problems were involved in 22 per cent of those contacts,
which probably occupied between 30 and 50 per cent of the working
hours of the practitioners.

And now we must touch upon a fourth problem, that is, the possible
relationship of psychological disturbances to *structural alteration.* The
viewpoint of disease bequeathed to us from the nineteenth century could
be indicated in the following formula:

Cellular disease→Structural alteration→Physiological (or functional)
disturbance.

In the twentieth century this formula underwent alteration in some
situations. For example, in essential hypertension and vascular disease
the formula was altered to read:

Functional disturbance→Cellular disease→Structural alteration.

We are still in the dark as to what may precede the functional disturbance, as in the example just cited of essential hypertension and the
resulting vascular disease. It seems possible that future investigations
will permit us to say that it is possible for a psychological disturbance to
antedate the functional alteration. Then the formula would read:

Psychological   disturbance→Functional   impairment→Cellular   dis-
ease→Structural alteration.

With the last problem, however, this book is not greatly concerned.

We restrict ourselves, for the most part, to known psychosomatic relationships; in other words, we discuss *clinical problems* for which there are immediate, practical applications.

THE MANAGEMENT OF PSYCHOSOMATIC PROBLEMS

The Illness Is "Functional." How has modern medicine handled the above groups of patients? When we review this subject we find that the patients in Group I were commonly told that no organic disease was present and that the whole thing was "functional." They were often dismissed without further care, only to land eventually in the hands of some irregular practitioner or quack healer. Certainly in dealing with many of these patients it is necessary to do more than assure the patient of the absence of physical disease. Nor does it do to dismiss a patient with the statement that his illness is functional.

To the physician this term usually means "psychogenic," although he does not always admit it, even to himself. To the patient the term may mean anything from obscure illness of physical origin to "imagination," depending on the attitude and manner of the physician. Certainly if the physician is not clear in his own mind as to the nature of these problems he cannot give a satisfactory explanation to his patient. Slapping the patient on the back, with the statement, "It's all in your mind; forget it," is surely to be resented. The patient either says or thinks "You mean I'm going crazy?"—a thought which already may be disturbing him greatly—or he suspects that the doctor is suggesting that the trouble is "imaginary," which is resented more than anything else, and justifiably so. We will discuss the problem again but here it may be stated that once we are straight as to the nature of the problem and know that the emotions are involved, we must tell the patient so in terms which he can understand. There will be more respect for the psyche as a force producing illness when we deal honestly with it. Physicians have taken all kinds of twists and turns to avoid the use of the hated term, psychogenic. Often "neurogenic" replaces it and thus the physician is permitted to hold on to the notion that somehow there is a physical answer to the problem. We shall discuss this point shortly.

Suspicion of Physical Disease. Sometimes the patient was told that the physician did not think that anything was the matter, but suspicion was cast upon some organ or system which needed watching and care. For example, the patient with symptoms referred to the heart region was told that his heart was all right. Nevertheless he was cautioned to rest, medicine was given, and each time that he visited the physician his heart was examined again, or his blood pressure was taken. It was impossible to eradicate the suspicion of organic disease under such circumstances. We will consider this point later, but here it may be emphasized that in dealing with the majority of functional problems we must examine thoroughly, satisfy ourselves as to the *absence of organic disease* and then stop examining with the firm statement, "You have no organic disease."

Pathologic Curiosities. Very frequently, following "thorough study" by means of the usual medical history, physical examination and laboratory investigation, some "pathologic curiosity"* was discovered which really had nothing to do with the illness, and the patient was then treated as though organically diseased, and subjected to unnecessary medical or surgical treatment, which in many instances intensified the neurotic condition.

In other words the attitude of modern medicine has not been so very different toward these patients from that described in 1884 by Clifford Allbutt, the great English clinician, who said in speaking of the visceral neuroses: "A neuralgic woman seems thus to be peculiarly unfortunate. However bitter and repeated may be her visceral neuralgias, she is told either that she is hysterical or that it is all uterus. In the first place she is comparatively fortunate, for she is only slighted; in the second case she is entangled in the net of the gynecologist, who finds her uterus, like her nose, is a little on one side, or again, like that organ, is running a little, or it is as flabby as her biceps so that the unhappy viscus is impaled upon a stem, or perched upon a prop, or is painted with carbolic acid every week in the year except during the long vacation when the gynecologist is grouse-shooting, or salmon-catching, or leading the fashion in the Upper Engadine. Her mind thus fastened to a more or less nasty mystery becomes newly apprehensive and physically introspective and the morbid chains are riveted more strongly than ever. Arraign the uterus, and you fix in the woman the arrow of hypochondria, it may be for life."

DIAGNOSTIC PROBLEMS IN PSYCHOSOMATIC MEDICINE

More specifically then, what are some of the diagnostic and therapeutic problems of psychosomatic medicine and how are they to be approached?

For example, there is the *failure to recognize neurosis* and treatment of the patient as organically diseased. This has happened most frequently because of the attempt to establish the diagnosis of "functional" disease by ruling out organic disease through medical history, physical examinations and laboratory investigation. The point that we particularly wish to make is that *the diagnosis of "functional" illness must be established not simply by exclusion of organic disease, but on its own characteristics as well.* In other words neurosis has its own distinctive features to be discovered by psychosomatic study, for only in this way can serious errors in diagnosis and treatment be avoided. If the above statements are admitted, it must naturally follow that personality study is just as important in the problems of illness as laboratory investigation.

This kind of approach will do a great deal to relieve the fear of the physician that he is missing something organic because it will supply him with additional information to confirm his diagnosis of functional disease. It is perfectly true, of course, that organic disease can be overlooked and the patient treated as a neurotic, which is the reverse of the situation above mentioned. Later on we shall cite such cases. Physicians are constantly harassed by this fear of overlooking organic disease. They are of

---

* By "pathologic curiosity" is meant some congenital or acquired lesion that has no significance from the standpoint of health. Slight deviations of the nasal septum and calcified primary tuberculous lesions in the lung are examples.

the opinion when dealing with this class of patients that the structural disease is hidden and will come to light with the passage of time. Again this may be true but in the majority of instances it is not.

A study from the Mayo Clinic was illuminating in this regard: Macy and Allen studied the records of 235 patients approximately six years after the diagnosis of chronic nervous exhaustion had been made, with the idea that if the clinical picture at the first examination was due to unrecognized organic disease, such organic disease should be detected by subsequent examinations over a period of years. The accuracy of the diagnosis proved to be 94 per cent, which seems to indicate that this kind of functional illness, at any rate, is not due to organic disease. It is interesting to note in passing that 289 separate operations had been performed on 200 patients of the group that they studied.

In an excellent study of psychoneurotic patients encountered in the general medical clinic of the New York Hospital, who were examined at the end of five years, Friess and Nelson found that of 269 consecutive patients only 8 per cent had been incorrectly diagnosed as psychoneurotic. They, too, called attention to the errors which can be avoided if the physician is aware that positive evidence of neurotic personality traits and neurotic behavior is essential for a diagnosis of psychoneurosis. The diagnosis should never be established, they say, solely on the basis of exclusion of organic disease, for this common practice frequently results in postponement of the correct diagnosis until such time as therapy may be of no avail. They suggest that it is far more prudent to confess ignorance of the diagnosis rather than to make a diagnosis of psychoneurosis in a patient with unexplained complaints but no evidence of neurotic personality traits.

Bennett undertook a detailed analysis of 150 patients from the psychiatric department of a general hospital, who had been treated previously for "organic disease." Two hundred forty-four surgical operations had been performed upon these 150 patients, to say nothing of the many expensive laboratory investigations and unnecessary medical treatments. When the patients finally were treated by psychotherapy full recovery occurred in 80 and improvement in 28. The study once more demonstrates how an illness basically psychic is not recognized as such until it develops into a frank psychiatric syndrome.

The "Either-Or" Concept.   When emotional factors are associated with actual organic disease too little attention is paid to the emotional factors. The feeling exists and the statement is made that "the physical findings are sufficient to account for the illness." In this connection let us again emphasize that just as we cannot limit ourselves simply to the exclusion of organic disease in dealing with the purely functional group, so even more importantly in the second group is there the necessity for not resting content with the finding of an organic lesion. *The day is near at hand for the final outmoding of the "either-or" concept (either functional or organic) in diagnosis and to place in its stead the idea of how much of one and how much of the other, that is, how much of the problem is emotional and how much is physical* and what is the relationship between them. This is truly the psychosomatic concept in medicine.

In a consideration of the "cause" of illness, Halliday indicates the approach to this complicated problem with a simple illustration.

"Let us take," says Halliday, "a fragment of conversation which may be overheard when a toddler begins to howl in the street:

"Onlooker to mother—'Why is he crying?'

"Mother—'Oh, he cries at anything; he is just a baby.'

"Small brother—'He saw a cat and it frightened him.'

"Onlooker—'Well, he has a fine pair of lungs anyway.'

"These remarks provide an explanation of the child's mode of behavior in terms of the three fields of etiological discourse. In the field of the *individual* the cause is announced to be the characteristic of 'being a baby'; in the field of *environment,* the encounter with a cat; in the field of *mechanism,* the lungs in their instrumental perfection. It will be noted that if any mode of behavior is to take place, 'cause' must operate in all three fields at a particular point in time. In the example quoted, we may assume that the behavior called 'crying' would not have appeared in the absence of (*a*) the characteristic of being a baby, or (*b*) the environmental factor of the cat, or (*c*) the mechanismic integrity of the respiratory organs."

Halliday then explains that when the findings as to cause in each of the three fields of "etiological discourse" can be related to one another, we may say that the illness is explained. Thus in diphtheria "the cause in the first field is the characteristic summarized by the phrase 'being Schick-positive'; cause in the second field is an encounter with the diphtheria bacillus; cause in the third field is the toxin produced on the fauces . . ."

When we think in terms of the psychosomatic point of view we must employ the same approach. In peptic ulcer, for example, we must think of (1) the individual: What kind of person is he? (predisposition, physical and psychological); (2) the environment: What has he met? (tobacco, food, social and psychological problems); and (3) mechanism: What happened? (vascular supply, hyperacidity, hypermotility, et cetera) .

Here the psychic element is an integral part of the study, one of many and diverse etiological factors emerging at various levels of the personality development.

Functional and Organic.   At this point it may not be amiss to quote further from Halliday in regard to that long-confused subject "Functional versus Organic Disease":

"Another source of obscurity is to confuse the technique of approach with the object of study. A common example is the mysterious phrase 'mind and body.' This seems to indicate that an individual is composed of two distinct and contrasted entities, a mind entity and a body entity. If the phrase has any meaning, it is this: The individual may be studied by a psychological approach and the individual may be studied by a structural or physical approach. It is our techniques or methods of investigation which are diverse and multiple, not the individual, who is a unity."

THE NATURE OF EMOTIONAL PROBLEMS

These patients are suffering from disturbances in their emotional lives; that is, the illness is wholly or in part of *psychological* origin and can be satisfactorily studied and treated only if this factor is adequately dealt with. It is true that the ill health may arise in a predisposed individual from longstanding dissatisfactions in business, social or home life. (Why he is predisposed will be discussed in the next chapter, which deals with personality development.) Here we may state that the experiences of military psychiatry have demonstrated that everyone has his "breaking point" and that illness is determined by the impact of an upsetting event on a sensitized individual. If the environmental factor is powerful enough the staunchest personality may break down; conversely if the personality is sensitive enough, because of neurotic predisposition, a comparatively minor episode may be the precipitating factor for a psychotic, psychoneurotic or psychosomatic illness. Failure of adjustment to environment is manifested by a disturbance in some part of the personality, either as bodily symptoms of various kinds or as affections of the spirit resulting in attacks of anxiety, obsessions, phobias, depression, and other disturbances of mood.

What is not so generally realized is that the mere discovery of the so-called dissatisfactions or unpleasant occurrences in the life situation of the individual is not a sufficient explanation or even an adequate indication of the psychic background of the illness. In other words, besides excluding physical disease in the one case and correctly evaluating the part it plays in another, it is of the greatest importance to know *the patient's ability to adjust to certain life situations, his pattern of reacting to them, the degree of anxiety in his make-up and the nature and seriousness of his conflicts.* Psychosomatic study is necessary if we are to establish a specific relationship of the psychic situation to the personality of the individual. Just as the typhoid bacillus, specific for typhoid fever, depends upon the susceptibility of the individual, so does specificity of the psychic event depend upon personality structure of the person. To make such studies one must have some training in psychopathology. When psychopathology is given an equal place with tissue pathology in our medical curriculum and is as well taught, we will finally realize that psychotherapy is an integral part of our medical discipline. If, as these studies seem to indicate, one half to two thirds of all patients with chronic illness have problems in which the psyche is implicated—and in one third to one half the psyche is chiefly responsible for the difficulty—then it would seem that our traditional medical teaching has been faulty in neglecting to prepare the medical student for the problems that he will have to meet when he begins to practice.

PSYCHOSOMATIC STUDY IN ILLNESS

Can any advice be given as to how to proceed with this kind of study? Although this will be developed in a subsequent chapter, in a general way it may be stated now that, in addition to the physical study, it consists simply in getting to know the patient as a *human being* rather than as a mere medical case. Too often, as already stated, the patient is looked upon as a physiological mechanism and is studied by means of medical history and physical examination aided by "instruments of precision" and chemical tests. Tape measure and test tubes carry the erroneous notion of exactness and thoroughness—erroneous because the emotional life of the individual, which may hold the key to the solution of the problem, is not investigated or, at best, inadequately so.

PSYCHOTHERAPY

And now to come to one of the questions frequently raised by physicians regarding these matters, "Suppose you *do* find something of importance in the emotional life of a patient, some conflict that is causing illness—What good does it do the patient to know? What can you do about it?"

First of all, it is often a great help to the patient to know that the ailment is not organic in origin but is due to a disturbance in his emotional life. *When a neurotic symptom is divorced from a fear of organic disease—cancer, for example—it loses its force, whereupon the slogan, "carry on in spite of symptoms," often helps the patient a great deal.* This is especially true if the psychological approach which we have discussed is combined with the study and the emotional background of the illness is made clear to the patient.

What Is Psychotherapy?   What, indeed, *is* psychotherapy? Too often it is assumed to be something vaguely referred to as "the application of the art of medicine." This defies analysis but seems to represent a combination of the experience and common sense of the seasoned practitioner, an intuitive knowledge of people, the cultivation of a charming bedside manner, such trifles as serving food in attractive dishes, and the generous use of reassurance. The psychological approach in medicine, essential for psychotherapy, consists of something more. It is a *medical discipline* to an equal degree with internal medicine itself. It is an effort to understand the personality structure of patients, the mental mechanisms which are at work, and the specific relationships of psychological situations in the precipitation of the illness. We try to utilize this knowledge to promote the patient's emotional development so that no longer does he have to find the answer to his problems through illness. Thus, instead of treating symptoms we try to improve the patient's emotional adjustment in order that his symptoms will no longer be necessary to him. What the physician, nurse, and social worker may mean to the patient in terms of emotional significance is an integral part of this procedure to which we shall later devote some attention.

Reassurance, in the majority of instances, unless combined with an analysis of the illness from the standpoint of the behavior, gives only temporary help and, depending upon the degree of anxiety, has to be constantly repeated, like a dose of digitalis in a failing heart. Closely allied to reassurance is another superficial treatment which rarely results in more than temporary help, *i.e., environmental manipulation* without any attempt to give the patient insight into his conflicts.

Real psychotherapy, which is directly the opposite of simple reassurance, tries to make the patient understand the meaning of his symptoms and the nature of his conflicts. It is a reeducational process and when properly done leads to sufficient emotional development so that the necessity for symptom formation is abolished. It may be defined as a process which utilizes psychodynamic principles to bring about emotional growth, thus permitting greater development of the individual's capacities and better social adjustment.

The best example of psychotherapy is psychoanalysis, but for various reasons this method cannot be applied directly to the majority of patients. Nevertheless, psychoanalytic insight and guidance in management combined with reeducation and reassurance prove adequate to handle the emotional factor in the majority of psychosomatic disturbances. Between simple reassurance at one end of the scale and adequate psychoanalysis at the other, there are all degrees of psychotherapy which can be applied depending upon the degree of illness and the circumstances of the patient.

Major and Minor Psychotherapy.   A considerable number of patients whom we have been seeing cannot be sent to psychiatrists, nor is it even necessary. Not that there is anything reprehensible about consulting a psychiatrist—this too is a problem of education—but there are not enough psychiatrists to take care of the thousands of such patients; moreover, as we have tried to show, a great part of this work lies in the field of general medicine.

Now, many general practitioners feel themselves capable of doing minor surgery but only a few have the skill to attempt major operations. They would not permit themselves to attempt something for which they are not prepared. This is just as true of psychotherapy. The general physician must be able to treat minor ailments but he must also be able to recognize when the problem is beyond him, and in such cases refer the patient elsewhere for major psychotherapy. Such knowledge and such an approach frequently will save the patient from unnecessary, troublesome, and expensive medical or surgical treatment with a resulting further degree of invalidism. So much for some of the more obvious benefits to be obtained through the psychosomatic approach. An inescapable part of any practical introduction to psychosomatic medicine, however, is the cost of psychotherapy.

Cost of Psychotherapy.   What of the question of the time, effort and expense of psychotherapy? True it is that all of this takes time and effort, and it must be paid for, yet when we look into the time, effort and expense consumed by many patients or by institutions taking care of these patients in the traditional medical approach, we realize that an hour or two well spent in a discussion of the life situation of such patients might have obviated a great deal of this expenditure. It is really amazing what the total expense of a great many of these needless studies amounts to, so far as the institution is concerned, and of course the same thing is true in the case of private patients. The day is close at hand when we shall regard some of these thick-chart patients, this *polyphysical approach,* with the same amusement and disdain with which we now regard the polypharmacy of a bygone age in medicine. In our own studies of "thick-chart" cases—patients from the out-patient department selected solely on the basis of having a chart an inch thick—we found a new phrase to replace "the high cost of psychiatry." It was "the high cost of no psychiatry." The patients who had accumulated thick charts, often representing dozens of visits with numerous referrals to specialty clinics, hundreds of dollars worth of laboratory work, innumerable prescriptions for placebos and barbiturates, and often unnecessary surgery as well, could frequently be better understood by an hour's interview conducted along psychosomatic lines (Chapter III).

EMOTIONAL ILLNESS AND PUBLIC HEALTH

From the standpoint of the neglect of the psychosomatic approach, hospitals are beginning to understand that it is not only intelligent but economical to command the services of a psychiatrist in the general medical division, and the same question has applied in the past to the pensioning and disability ratings of veterans. Besides, we are aware of the great cost in terms of money and wastage of human resources in the problems of insurance and total disability. Taken together, these three problems—the unnecessary cost of private and public medical care, pension payments to veterans, and total disability benefits paid by insurance companies—constitute a staggering burden to the economy of America. And there is one important common denominator that applies to all of them: the unrecognized or inadequately dealt with *emotional component of illness.*

In addition to what has been said, in view of the proposals for health insurance and socialized medicine that are confronting us nowadays, the public health program faces a real need for attention to the psychic component in illness. The major weakness of all such systems has been the lack of knowledge concerning the emotional factor in illness. It is chronic illness in which the psychic component is of the greatest importance from the standpoint of diagnosis and treatment.

Admittedly the evaluation of the emotional component is a very difficult problem. It enters in such subtle ways and makes for such complications that it challenges evaluation under even the best of circumstances; when there is added, as it sometimes must be, the conscious effort to deceive, the problem is multiplied. How disabled is the patient with hypertensive vascular disease, how disabled the patient who has suffered a coronary occlusion? One personality refuses to give in to his illness, fights hard, and makes an excellent recovery; another with the seeds of passivity and dependency within him succumbs to chronic invalidism, and his unconscious desire to remain sick is nurtured by disability payments.

Understanding such problems really depends on a knowledge of psychopathology and the personality structure of the patient. Perhaps personality tests will be helpful, especially the Rorschach (described and evaluated in Chapter III), an objective test which is often useful in the evaluation of the personality. Nothing, however, will take the place of a skillful interview for which the examining physician has been firmly grounded in both disciplines, tissue pathology and psychopathology, so that he may use both approaches simultaneously in his study of the patient. Psychotherapy can help patients, who would otherwise be anxious to obtain total disability, to understand that it would be better for them from the standpoint of their health and their character to continue to work, even part time, accepting income for which they themselves are responsible. The insurance examiner, identified with the company, is in a difficult position to make this evaluation, but the outside physician trained in the psychosomatic approach should not find it difficult to determine just what part the somatic aspect plays in the disability and how much of the condition can be attributed to emotional factors, and deal with his patient accordingly.

SUMMARY

The main point of this discussion can be stated briefly: The study and treatment of illness constitutes much more than the investigation and eradication of disease. Yet there is nothing new or startling in this viewpoint. We have heard a great deal in recent years about the study of the organism-as-a-whole, but for the greater part we have only been paying lip service to the concept. We have been led to believe that the art of the physician, having to do with his common sense or intuition, as opposed to his "science," is sufficient to grasp the problems which we have been considering here. It is not enough. A real understanding of psychodynamics is necessary in order properly to study the emotional life in relation to ill health. In other words, the physician must be able to define the specific mental factors producing an illness, rather than be satisfied with vague generalizations about "neurogenic background." Just as we would criticize the physician of today who would call all fevers malaria, so must we criticize the physician who hints obscurely at "nervous" factors in the background of an illness and makes no real effort to understand the psychic situation.

It is our hope that every physician will be so trained that he may be able to understand and manage the many emotional problems that are presented to him daily. At the postgraduate level we need short orientation courses in centers that are properly staffed. At the graduate level better training facilities should be developed for residents in medicine, and the other medical specialties, to acquire the psychosomatic approach to medical problems. At the undergraduate level, we need, not more and more hours of psychiatry inserted into the curriculum, but a real integration of the psychosomatic point of view in every department, preclinical as well as clinical. As Margolin has said, we need homogenization instead of stratification. This of course must wait until teachers are available in these various departments who have a real understanding of psychodynamics. Beyond this, or rather before this, our students must come to us prepared in the social sciences as well as in the physical sciences. And the social sciences must include a psychology that gives a better explanation of human behavior than is now furnished in most colleges. All of this, unfortunately, is a long way off, and yet we are moving swiftly. Military medicine gave a great impetus to this development and the pressure is coming from the people themselves. We would be wise to anticipate them. Therein lies our hope for an important development in medicine. As a part of this process and essential for its development, general hospitals must establish divisions for the observation and treatment of psychoneurotic and psychosomatic problems (Bennett et al.). The time has passed for psychiatry to lead an isolated existence. Until it is brought into physical proximity with general medicine it cannot achieve final integration into the body of medical knowledge.

Veterans Administration hospitals have led the way in regard to this integration of psychiatry and medicine. Psychiatric facilities are an important part of such general hospitals; consultations and cooperative studies between psychiatrists and the other medical specialists are accepted procedures that have found their way into the practice of civilian medicine.

In his *History of Medicine* Garrison stated that the fundamental error of medieval medical science, as originally pointed out by Guy de Chauliac and later elucidated by Allbutt, was in the divorce of medicine from surgery. He might have added that the fundamental error of modern medical science has been in the divorce of both from psychiatry.

References

Allan, F. N., and Kaufman, J.: J.A.M.A., *16:* 1135, 1948.
Allbutt, T. C.: Visceral Neuroses. p. 17. P. Blakiston's Son and Co., Philadelphia, 1884.
Bennett, A. E.: J.A.M.A., *130:* 1203, 1936.
Bennett, A. E., Hargrove, E. A., and Engle, B.: J.A.M.A., *147:* 1019, 1951.
Dunbar, F.: Psychosomatic Diagnosis, pp. 696–697. Paul B. Hoeber, Inc., New York, 1943.
Foreign Letters, J.A.M.A., *158:* 1386, 1955.
Friess, C., and Nelson, M. J.: Am. J. M. Sc., *203:* 539, 1942.
Halliday, J. L.: Brit. J. M. Psychol., *19:* 367, 1934.
Lewis, B. I.: Am. J. Med., *14:* 586, 1953.
Macy, J. W., and Allen, E. V.: Ann. Int. Med., *7:* 861, 1934.
Margetts, E. L.: Canadian M. A. J., *63:* 402, 1950.
The Merck Report, Jan. 1951.
Roberts, B. H., and Norton, N. M.: New England J. Med., *246:* 82, 1952.
Stern, K., Bonlanger, J. B., and Cleghorn, S.: Am. J. Psychiat., *106:* 851, 1950.

Chapter II

Personality Development and Psychopathology*

PERSONALITY DEVELOPMENT

To understand the problems of psychosomatic medicine it is necessary to have a knowledge of psychopathology as well as of tissue pathology. Pathology of the psyche or, as some would prefer to say, pathology of the personality, develops early in life but may go unnoticed for many years. The onset is insidious and detection is not easy because our methods of measurement are still not precise and the public has not been educated to recognize the early manifestations of personality disturbance. Just as we have had campaigns to focus public attention upon the early evidences of tuberculosis, cancer and appendicitis, so do we need further education regarding the early manifestations of psychopathology.

If one is to deal with the whole field of psychiatry he must command a very extensive knowledge of psychopathology. In this chapter we shall try to limit ourselves to the psychopathology most pertinent to the problems of general medicine.

The psyche or personality is a functioning unit which has many parts and many functions. It acts as a coordinating center to achieve such immediate physical and emotional satisfactions as are socially permissible and at the same time makes plans for those which are best reserved for the future. The parts of the personality have to work together harmoniously in order to gain the emotional rewards which maintain satisfaction and adequate self-esteem. A marked and prolonged fall in self-esteem may be as devastating to the functioning of the organism as a marked and prolonged reduction in the blood count. The personality must have an optimum number of sound, logical ideas well related to environmental activities, for a *poverty of ideas* may be as disastrous as a poverty of red or white blood cells. The personality must have a sufficient quantity of

---

* Although few direct references are made in this chapter, the material is derived from the fundamental contributions of Freud, his associates and students. References for the chapter and to the subject of psychosomatic medicine as a whole will be found at the end of the chapter.

good will in relation to other human beings (society) to serve as an energy reservoir in the carrying out of good ideas. A serious defect in the quantity of good will is as unfortunate as a serious defect in a vital organ. During its development the personality must avoid the acquisition of too much *hate*, because this pathological emotion may be as obstructive to good functioning of the person socially and economically as an accumulation of scar tissue in a heart valve would be obstructive to the normal circulation of the blood.

GROWTH PROCESS

There is a greater tendency for psychopathology to begin early in personality growth than for tissue pathology to begin early in physical growth. It is not difficult to see why this should be so. At birth, with few exceptions, the structure of the body organs and organ systems is complete. Expansion in size of the structure follows but the structure is complete when extra-uterine life begins. Such is not the case with personality structure and growth. At birth the child has only the faintest rudiments of personality structure. The brain, which serves as the area of the body in which the personality gradually takes shape, is like a clean slate ready to be written upon by experience, or, viewed in a three-dimensional way, a bare plot of ground upon which an edifice will be constructed.

We must recognize that there are varying degrees of capacity in the nervous system, as well as in other systems of the body, to deal with stimuli both from within and without the organism. However, there are two points to be kept clearly in mind when trying to evaluate the importance of heredity versus environment in personality formation. First, the *constitution* is a relatively fixed and unchanging factor and therefore can usually be regarded as only of theoretical importance in the individual case. Second, constitution is in most cases a small component in personality formation when compared with the importance of the impact of *experiences* on the individual.

The system of scientific observation which has told us most about the growth of personality is psychoanalysis. The psychology of Freud is unusually well suited to be a medical psychology because it relates mental processes to biological processes.

Disturbances in Parents

To understand personality growth we must understand the importance of parental relationships. There are parents whose personality one hesitates to call neurotic, and yet who act as "carriers" to produce neuroses in their offspring. Examples of such persons are the "cold" parent, the overindulgent parent and the sexually frustrated parent, among other types.

The "Cold" Parent.   Let us consider the rather grim, affectively cold parent, who has perhaps been successful socially and economically, who may have a fairly satisfactory relationship with certain adult friends, and who supplies every material luxury for his family, but who emotionally can never come down to the level of his children and can never give them the warmth of affection which their developing personalities need. The compulsion of such parents for material success has arisen out of their own childhood disappointments which have been successfully repressed. They may be devoting much time and money to public or community welfare; indeed, they may be considered full of human kindness, but as far as their own family is concerned they are cold and exacting. The lack of friendship and the inability to show affection may seriously impair the personality development of the children in such a home. Neurosis and personality anomalies may develop in the children of such parents, depending upon the interaction of other persons in the home setting.

The Overindulgent Parent.   Parents with tendencies quite opposite to the above, seldom considered abnormal by the general public, shower affection upon the child, overprotect him from all dangers, disappointments and frustrations, and thereby leave him ill-prepared to fight the unavoidable battles of later life. Not only is such a child protected, lest the "evil" of sexuality permeate his consciousness, but he is prevented from achieving a sense of values in other spheres. Because the parent cannot bear the child's ill will no pleasure is denied him. Since no effort is demanded, there is no incentive or capacity for effort fostered in the child's personality. How then can he compete when he has never been allowed to find out what life is about? Education to meet the responsibilities, the denials and the dangers of life is essential for proper emotional development and must be begun early.

This type of parent personally may have made a fair adjustment to life, but he lacks the insight to see that the *good* parent is not only a *giving* parent. He has never learned that a parent who restricts and gives in proportion to effort is in the end the best parent, because such an attitude prepares the child for a life in which one's success *is* dependent upon effort.

The Sexually Frustrated Parent.   The parent whose love life is not being gratified with the marital partner will often obtain his emotional satisfaction by a bond with the child. He courts the child's attentions but excludes the marital partner and in subtle ways prevents the child from growing up emotionally. Frequently this pathological emotional bond later results in a spoiled marriage or ruined career. The responsible parent would be shocked to be told of the unconscious trends that make such a state of affairs possible, but sometimes such a shock may mean rescuing some child from later neurosis or personality anomaly.

The Parent with Unconscious Hatred for the Child.   Lastly, there are parents who actually have a deep unconscious hatred for a child. Their care of the child consists of a compulsive insistence on certain behavior standards, which is not at all for the child's "good," but is a defense against that parent's own unconscious personality trends. For instance, the mother who as a girl had to combat sexual tension, may insist upon such restricted conduct on the part of her daughter that it ruins her social adaptation. Some mothers cannot help but feel that a daughter is a serious rival, especially when the father shows her greater devotion. The mother may envy the girl's chances for enjoying pleasures that she missed and, as a result, unconsciously hamper the child's chances for happiness. Occasionally, but less often, does the father by similar methods hurt the personality development of a son.

The Effect on the Child.   Unhappiness, moodiness, resentment, defiance, ill manners, asocial conduct or neurosis may result from the effect of such parental personalities upon the child. To repeat, these parents are not thought of as neurotic, and yet they have a subtle disturbance in their capacity to love. The fact that they are often regarded as model parents who, inexplicably, are cursed with problem children, has led to a rejection of the theory that parental attitudes have much to do with neuroses. Those who overlook the subtle mechanisms of personality formation say, "How can that child have such a nasty disposition? His mother gave him everything. It must be glandular." Or one hears, "How can that boy be so disinterested in worthwhile things? His father has such high ideals and is so interested in public matters." Many neuroses and personality disturbances, as well as psychoses, come out of such homes. But the parent, like the public, does not understand how the child could acquire this fault in personality, and resents having the defect pointed out.

The Components of Anxiety

As we study the growth processes, the first and most important psychopathological phenomenon to be considered is anxiety. *Anxiety is a specific unpleasurable state of tension which indicates the presence of some danger to the organism.* When danger is real we speak of fear; when it is fancied, we call it anxiety (conscious or unconscious ideas of a frightening nature). Anxiety lies at the root of all psychopathology and for that matter plays an important part in normal behavior.

There are two basic causes of anxiety: *fear of physical harm* and *fear of loss of love.* Later in life secondary causes of anxiety are situations which threaten to bring about either of these conditions, such as battle experience or loss of money or loss of social prestige.

Anxiety has two elements: a *psychic* and a *somatic* (or physiological) component. The psychic component of anxiety is the sensory cortical registration of displeasure and apprehension, the instinctual awareness that something is wrong; and the somatic component is the motor response of rapid heart action, rapid or embarrassed respiration, flushing and perspiration, and even a disturbance in the function of the gastrointestinal tract. Anxiety can make its effects felt in every tissue of the body, although in many cases it seems to limit its expression predominantly to those organs and tissues supplied by the autonomic nervous system.

The Feeding Process

The human being from birth onward has a need for optimum conditions of comfort as the growth processes advance. During the first months of life the body needs food and warmth not only because of their importance for physical growth but also for the tactile pleasure derived therefrom. The world of the infant is small and events which would seem to be of little consequence to the adult may have the greatest significance for the infant, in regard to both his immediate and his later responses.

The sensual pleasure derived from the feeding process is an example. The total nutritional process will leave a pleasant memory impression upon the mind if the good will and esteem of those who take care of the child are added to the feeding process. A sufficiency of food of the right kind, given at regular intervals and administered by one who loves the child, does much to lay the groundwork for a relaxed personality which regards the world as a friendly place. Thus the nutritional process, a feeling of security and the capacity to love are harmoniously combined.

If, on the other hand, there is insufficient food or a sudden change in the type of food or method of feeding, or if there is impatience or hostility on the part of the one who feeds the child, then the distress of hunger or of cold, or the lack of emotional warmth, permits anxiety to appear. There seems to be a blind sense (which we may be permitted to call instinct) that if such conditions continue long enough death will ensue. In the beginning, this apprehension that something threatens the integrity of the self is a reflex pattern and, as a matter of fact, much of it remains reflex throughout life. An important part of the therapeutic educational process is the effort to help the individual to understand the *source* of his anxiety and to teach him *what he must do to relieve it*. It is fundamental to our understanding of personality development to realize how much basic insecurity and resulting anxiety may occur through deprivation of food, warmth or love, or through misunderstanding of the physiological rhythms, during the early weeks and months of life, and that such difficult situations in the life of a child will produce anxiety through a definite physiological mechanism.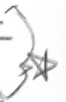

Parents unaware of the serious effects which trauma and deprivation have upon the personality of the child may permit much psychopathology in the form of anxiety to develop during the first year of life. Children are often neglected and fed carelessly as to rhythm or improperly as to the type of food; or they are weaned forcibly and without regard for the limited adaptive powers of the infant to a new experience. Depending upon the constitution of the infant such treatment is very apt to cause anxiety. Memory impressions are made and psychological reflexes are built up. These patterns are "forgotten" with the passing of time, but if numerous or highly charged with anxiety they may form the nucleus of illness later on. Each event is registered on the brain as a memory with varying degrees of intensity and what cannot readily be recalled is referred to as unconscious. That part of the mental mechanism which holds these memories and their accompanying charges of emotion is called *the unconscious* (commonly referred to as the *unconscious mind*). The process whereby these painful events are pushed into the area of the unconscious and held there is called *repression*. The more pain, shame, disgust, or other painful effect that occurs during development, the more likely that repression will occur, and the more difficult it will be to recall the traumatic event in later life. The emotions combined with the memories and ideas accumulated during growth make the unconscious a dynamic center of psychic energy rather than a static storehouse of innocuous impressions. Much of what can be done in the therapy of psychosomatic illness depends upon the ability to work with and modify the unconscious.

Anxiety and the Gastrointestinal Tract.   The digestive processes form the most important phase of the infant's life during the first year. If this function has been exposed to and associated with too much strife, deprivation or ill will, they become associated in the mind of the infant. One is "conditioned" to the other. The memories of unpleasant experiences associated with the gastrointestinal function exist in that part of the mind we call the unconscious. As the child grows older life conditions often improve, but a revival of the same situation of deprivation at the hands of fate or ill will from classmates, business associates or spouse may reactivate anxiety. Now if this anxiety and its cause are recognized and can be dealt with through escape or compromise, or through sharing the experiences and their effects with some stronger person, thus gaining reassurance and new strength, a solution is found. If the anxiety is not recognized and is not adequately discharged it finds no release and must exert its force upon the body itself. Then some organ or organ system is very apt to bear the brunt of this potent force and will function badly as a result. If during the years when the swallowing and digestive processes are of paramount importance in the life of the child there were anxiety-producing experiences, then similar experiences, later in life, are likely to reproduce symptoms of the upper gastrointestinal tract.

Preventing Anxiety.   Already one thing is clear which we must emphasize in respect to preventive medicine and that is, that mothers who feed their children calmly, adequately, gently, warmly and affectionately can do much to prevent the formation of anxiety in the early months of life. It is quite generally agreed that breast feeding has some advantage over bottle feeding in providing this reassuring warmth, intimacy and security so valuable in keeping anxiety at a minimum. But if this is not expedient the one who cares for the infant will do better if she realizes that intimacy, proximity, patience and serenity associated with food intake can aid greatly in stabilizing and strengthening the physiological rhythm of the gastrointestinal tract.

Management of Feeding Problems.   The physician who deals with a feeding problem often feels that he must do something "scientific" such as changing the formula or suggesting a new procedure. Often he doesn't care to run the risk of the ill will of the mother by discussing her responsibility for the child's anxiety. Nevertheless, the cause of many feeding problems lies in the attitude of the mother or nurse and the treatment of such problems is *the management of the one caring for the child.* The physician would learn much if, instead of concentrating on the discussion of symptoms, he would ask, "Are you enjoying the care of this baby? Does he worry you? What are the things you concern yourself about regarding him?" When the child's care assumes too great an importance and becomes too much of a "problem" to the mother, then the mother becomes too big a problem to the child and symptoms result.

High-strung mothers have created many lifelong gastrointestinal invalids. *Psychotherapy for the mother rather than a new formula for the baby is the proper answer.* In this connection, it may be said that if the atmosphere of the home is not right it is impossible to keep the child from absorbing it, no matter how many books on child care and child psychology the mother may read. On the other hand, if the parents love each other and love their children they may break a few rules of psychology without harming their children.

To *summarize,* in cases of vomiting, diarrhea, or refusal to take food in children:

1. Examine for physical disease but always have in mind the fact that the gastrointestinal tract may be disturbed by unpleasant emotional stimuli which the child cannot "swallow," "digest" or "assimilate."

2. The mind of the child is just as much in need of emotional nourishment as the body is in need of physical nourishment. This emotional nurture should begin just as early in life and be supervised every bit as carefully.

3. The meaning of weaning to the child's emotional life should be explained to the mother. The following can be emphasized:

(*a*) Breast feeding of the infant should be a mutually enjoyable experience to mother and child.

(*b*) Be flexible in nursing schedule.

(*c*) Indigestion (colic) will occur in fretful, insecure babies just as in fretful, insecure adults.

(*d*) Do not make the weaning process too rapid. Some babies take longer than others. Think of what your particular baby seems to need rather than worrying about whether he conforms to the book.

(*e*) Make new foods palatable, of the right temperature, and attractive.

(*f*) Do not let your interest become so seriously focused on the weaning process that you forget to play with the baby. The baby needs more mothering and more play at this time. It will help him to accept weaning.

Thumb-Sucking

Sucking the thumb or the fingers is a habit which has aroused considerable controversy. Once this behavior is understood there is no further cause for alarm on the part of either mother or physician. We have explained that the infant derives pleasure and relieves tension by sucking. When the child is hungry, tense, lonely or tired, and no one feeds him, plays with him or otherwise pleasantly distracts him he will comfort himself by sucking his thumb. Any child, even the most well adjusted, will occasionally resort to the practice but it will not become persistent or excessive if the child is well fed, weaned carefully and slowly, and if he is played with enough. When thumb-sucking is encountered as a persistent habit the following points should be kept in mind in advising the parent:

1. Do not forget that the activity of sucking is normal. In the first year to eighteen months of life, sucking is one of the chief pleasures.

2. If thumb-sucking is excessive do not interfere directly with the

activity. Avoid scolding and pulling the thumb out of the mouth, avoid mechanical restraints, avoid foul-tasting applications and above all, avoid shame, criticism and ridicule.

3. Play with the child more often and use play materials suitable to his age. Encourage him to play with other children.

4. See that he has opportunity (space) to be active and to explore.

5. If the home atmosphere is not one of happiness, ease and friendliness the adults should strive to make it so rather than to concern themselves only with the baby's problem.

Toilet Training

Pressure of Social Demands.   The early weeks and months of the life of the child are those in which he receives food, warmth, love and affection. There comes a time, however, toward the end of the first year when the pressure of certain social demands is made upon our young human being. He is asked to change his pattern of voiding his excretions at will and to accept the pattern of depositing them in a specified place at a specified time. In the beginning this is by no means easy but with a repetition of the request in a friendly manner over a period of time the aim is accomplished, and no conflict is engendered. Some children have the good fortune to receive their training in these important tasks in such an environment. Let no one believe that this is not a very important time in the education of the child and the development of the personality. We glibly speak of the friendly manner necessary in carrying out this educational process. But in the weeks and months necessary for toilet training there is opportunity for many unfortunate incidents to occur. There are many mothers, nursemaids and others who come in contact with the child, who themselves have great anxiety surrounding the idea that the human being must rid himself of the waste products of metabolism with ritualistic timing and manner. They dislike the odor, the "uncleanliness" of the untrained child, and show anxiety, anger and disgust when the child does not learn the appointed task quickly enough. They make such an issue of rapid conformity to an established toilet routine that the child can be made most tense and apprehensive lest he displease. The mother or nurse may be so insistent upon the importance of rapid learning of sphincter control that she forgets the influence of relaxed play in a friendly environment; thus, many other aspects of the child's life also become entirely secondary to his mastery of toilet training. He is forced to concentrate so much psychic energy (libido) upon duty and responsibility that he is pushed in the direction of becoming a cheerless automaton, living with the single concept of doing his duty—and such a person he may remain all of his life.

Overconformity.   To the unreasonable demands mentioned above there are two other broad general lines of reaction—*conformity* and *rebellion*. If either departs from a reasonable norm it is difficult to say which is the more disastrous. In the child who is forced to be too compliant out of fear of punishment, temporary disapproval or permanent loss of love, there are many possibilities for the development of psycho-pathology. He may become excessively docile and obedient with an inordinate urge for order and punctuality in every activity with which he is connected. He becomes anxious and tends to live too much for the approval of others or the approval of his own overstrict conscience. He may develop symptoms, such as a fear of going out socially—parties, sports events, and the like—lest he have the need to go to the toilet and either none would be available or he would be ashamed to release the stool when the opportunity came. We speak here of the bowel being "too well trained" when, of course, we mean a personality that during childhood was made too anxious over a mishap in bowel control. This "fear of the upbringer" gradually becomes one of those memory impressions lodged in that great reservoir for registering past events—the unconscious. In later life it may manifest itself as a fear of society or at least as a disinclination to participate in social activities.

Rebellion.   The other pathological direction taken by emotions and ideas stirred up during this period of toilet training is toward rebellion. Some children are able to resent and fight back at the parent or nurse whose demands are too great or made too unsympathetically. They react with soiling or later with enuresis, and may even insist on being incontinent during the day. They ignore requests to use the toilet or demands to keep their clothing clean. They may even smear the walls with excreta partly because children are attracted to their own excretions, but partly because they resent the manner of training or the lack of love interest in the trainer and act as if to say: "I ignore your wishes. I'll have my own way. Since you treat me unkindly I'll make it unpleasant for you." It is not always easy to see why one child conforms too well while another takes the other extreme. Undoubtedly the more rebellious has been made to feel a little more secure during his early months of life so that he can better endure the displeasure of those around him over his failure to conform. Moreover, it is not to be assumed that the first reaction of apparent docility does not have its element of resentment also. But by swallowing his fear and resentment at being treated so strictly he often does more harm to his personality development than that which occurs in the more rebellious child.

Compulsiveness.   The overobedient child often turns out to be overserious, lacking in buoyancy and ease of manner, overmeticulous and disapproving of others who are not so fastidious. Having been given little love or tolerance such people are apt to be stingy both with love and material things. They tend to worship duty and do not learn to participate fully in life's pleasures. Their attention has been focused unduly upon the relatively unimportant problem of early and complete mastery of their excretions and they remain slaves to the correct management of the material details of life. They may be unable to understand or decide bigger and more human issues. Such individuals are called the compulsive type of personality.

Nonconformity.   The nonconformist or rebellious child may show his hostility to his overstrict and unfriendly upbringer by a series of "dirty tricks." He uses the bowel and bladder to express something he wants to say because he has neither the words nor the courage to do so directly. After a period of struggle with his superiors he usually ends by giving in and accepting the wishes of those who would have him control himself. But during this time an attitude and a pattern of organ function have been associated and remain stored in the unconscious mind. Later in life it may happen that when hostility is felt toward someone, or in regard to some situation, and the emotion cannot adequately express itself, it may seek expression by resorting to this old childish pattern, that is, with a return of urinary urgency or bowel frequency. In such cases the rebellion of childhood is at work and forces which have been repressed in the unconscious express themselves through the body physiology, producing a symptom.

Management of Toilet Training.   The achievement of bowel and bladder control is a very important phase of human personality development. Instead of being recognized as such it is usually regarded as an unpleasant stage of childhood to be hurried through as quickly as possible and without regard for the child's feelings.

Moving the bowels and bladder at will is normal for the child. He cares nothing for cleanliness. Society is doing itself a favor, as far as he is concerned, when it asks him to assume the difficult responsibility of controlling his excretions. Even under the most favorable circumstances he is thrown into conflict. He is forced to choose between two pleasures. He cannot have the comfort of evacuation at will and still retain the friendship of his mother or nurse. He must endure the distress of bowel and bladder control in order to have the love and good will of his parent. Under the best circumstances (a good relationship between mother and child) this should take considerable time. If the mother scolds and punishes instead of understanding that time, patience, kindness and praise are necessary, the child may be trained quickly but at great cost to his emotional development. Moreover, such early training is very apt to be broken later on. Since the motor tracts of the spinal cord are not completely myelinated until the child is one year old, the futility of attempting toilet training much before this time is evident. Some ambitious mothers, eager to have a clean child, will begin toilet training long before one year. Normally complete cleanliness and dryness is not achieved until between the ages of two and two and a half. Therefore, it is apparent how much patience and tolerance must be exercised in order that the child should not get the unfortunate opinion of himself that he is dirty, stupid, bad and inferior.

The ability to control bowels and bladder increases gradually with the child's ability to talk and express his feelings in regard to toilet needs, and also on his corresponding ability to understand the speech of parents and what they expect of him. The mother will notice at what time of day the bowels usually move and begin placing the child on the toilet at these times. If after five to ten minutes no results are obtained he should be taken off. There is no point in keeping him there for long periods of time. Give praise freely if evacuation is accomplished. Often the child will move the bowels just after being taken off the toilet. Probably it is deliberate and for a short time he may do the same thing. He is merely getting used to the method and making his own decision about whether to accept it. If he is a little slow to accept it the mother should be patient and kind, and if she does not make too much fuss, it will take care of itself. Such behavior in the beginning does not necessarily mean stubbornness or indifference. But stubbornness can be aroused if the mother is too impatient for quick results. Many constipation, colitis, and even personality problems in adults can be traced to the mistakes in training of this period of life. If more women knew these simple facts and trained children accordingly instead of trying to regulate toilet habits in relation to their own prejudices against dirt, there would be fewer anxious, inhibited and rebellious children. The truth of the matter is that a well adjusted, intelligent child will quickly become clean, with little training, once the proper time has arrived.

Enuresis.   Enuresis is the term applied to bed-wetting and inadequate bladder control beyond the age when bladder control is usual in the average child. While occasionally there are physical reasons, in the majority of cases this represents a defect in personality development. It means that the child has not formed an emotional bond to his mother of sufficient strength to enable him to exert the necessary control. If he loves the mother enough—which means the mother must have loved him enough—usually he can accept this responsibility. His resolve to please the mother permeates into the deeper layers of the mind, and leads to an acceptance of the mother's desire, whereupon control of the nervous mechanism of the bladder is maintained. If insufficient desire to please the mother (nurse or other person) has not been awakened, the child concerns himself only with his own comfort and empties the bladder when tension causes the slightest discomfort.

In the months when control is being established (around the age of two or even later) *the arrival of a new baby* in the home may cause a return of enuresis. This comes about because the child is envious of the attention the new baby gets and he resorts to this earlier means of drawing attention to himself. Of course, it may mean more than a simple bid for attention. It may also express resentment toward the new baby or resentment toward lack of attention for any other reason. Enuresis may persist to the age of puberty, sometimes into adolescence, and rarely into adulthood.

MANAGEMENT OF ENURESIS.   It is bad medical advice to assure the parents that the enuretic child "will grow out of it." It is true that in time most enuresis disappears. But this may be after years of bed-wetting, shame, embarrassing situations and painful scenes, each leading to further crippling of the personality.

1. Enuresis, aside from some rare physical disease, means a personality defect.

2. Explain the nature of the defect to the parent.

3. Point out that scolding and shaming are not only useless but actually harmful.

4. Advise the mother to make consistent efforts to win the child'•

goodwill. Make bladder control a by-product of friendly cooperation between mother and child.

5. Give approval when the bed is dry. Do not disapprove when it is not.

6. Rewards (candy, trips, etc.) are not contraindicated but such bribery should not be necessary or, at least, should not be in the foreground of the picture. Consistent goodwill and pleasant day-to-day living between mother and child with a simple explanation of what is expected should be enough to solve the problem.

7. Care should be taken not to make the enuretic child feel that he is dirty. First, it contributes to a feeling of inferiority and secondly, since the child cannot distinguish between the organs of sex and of excretion, in later years he may find it difficult to avoid transferring the idea of dirt to the natural sexual functions.

Organ Language

If the reader up to this point has been able to project himself into the life of the young child he has had evidence of the value of Freud's insistence on the role of the environment in the development of control of the physiological functions. Control of the physiological functions in a socially acceptable manner makes a lasting imprint upon the mind and becomes part of the mental processes. As we learn to control our bodies and their functions we build up our psychic structure. The mind is not created independently of the body but is very definitely linked with it. The function of the mind is to promote the control of ourselves and our relations to other people. When feelings and thoughts exist which cannot be expressed by word or action, they may find expression through some organ or organ system. The result is a "language of the organs" which may express itself in illness if the personality is not sufficiently developed to solve its problems through other channels (see p. 85). The organ which "speaks" is most likely to be the organ whose function was in the ascendancy when environmental conditions were bad and produced pain (anxiety) in the mind. But constitutional predisposition, identification with a parent, or other factors, may also determine the "choice of organ."

Much work remains to be done in respect to the choice of organ for the expression of neurosis. Very often an organ or system which is diseased quite naturally continues to engage the neurotic interest of the individual. It is obvious why this should be so. But the site of selection in the organ or system which is apparently free of disease is not so obvious. Why should it become the focal point for an organ neurosis? It has been proposed, for example, that bronchial asthma occurs in the person predisposed by heredity plus frequent or prolonged respiratory illness, such as whooping cough in early childhood, but definite proof is lacking. Explanations are offered elsewhere (Alexander) regarding the role of vector influences in certain organ systems. The gastrointestinal tract, for example, a system adapted to the physiological functions of intaking, retaining and eliminating, may lend itself readily to the expression of similar psychological trends within the individual.

Sexuality in Personality Development

Having solved the problem of bowel and bladder control, the child is nearing the age of three. By this time his interest in himself and the outside world has increased. He wants to know the why and wherefore of things with an ever-expanding curiosity. Most of his questions are answered except in one sphere, that of sexuality. Grown-ups often regard this as something about which the child must not have information. When these same grown-ups are questioned as to why the child should not be enlightened they are rather vague. They say it is "dangerous" or that it "just isn't done" but when pressed for a good reason as to why it is dangerous they have difficulty finding an answer, showing that they have been blindly following tradition and not thinking about the real cause for their stand. Now it is true that young children are bewildered, excited, and often made anxious by witnessing the sexual act itself before having any facts about its meaning or before they have reached an age to appreciate its significance. And of course it repeatedly happens, especially with large families occupying small quarters, that a young child does witness the sexual act. However, there is a great difference between a sudden unwarranted exposure to the sexual act and the gradual education of the child by giving factual information about love and reproduction as the child asks for such information. No child of any age can assimilate all the information about sex at once. When such information is given gradually the knowledge is incorporated into the rest of the personality in a healthy way. Thus children learn to control that aspect of their personality just as they control other wishes and impulses.

Some adults feel that there are certain aspects of life against which the impressionable minds of children must always be guarded, for example, birth, sexuality, bodily injury and death. But it must be remembered that these are all events which have to be met some day and there is a proper time to begin acquaintance with them. About as good a guide as any as to the best time for imparting this information is when the child asks to have it. If circumstances force him prematurely into contact with these events the child is likely to start his questioning at that time and if he does not we should wonder why and help him to understand the meaning of the event. Some recent experiments have shown how wise animals and children can be in choosing a correct diet for themselves. Giving children an opportunity to choose their own ideational diet we believe is equally safe. When their curiosity in these matters is satisfied and any necessary reassurance given, no psychopathology should arise. However, there are many homes where any interest on the part of the children in sexual matters is met with disapproval followed by threats, punishment or misinformation. Such an attitude results only in anxiety due to fear of loss of love or to fear of physical harm.

Masturbation. Karl Menninger states, "All psychiatric experience confirms the view that the boy who refrains from masturbation out of fear and guilt is more unstable, more subject to physical and 'nervous' breakdown, more likely to develop character disturbances than is the boy who is able to masturbate without feelings of guilt or to control such guilt feelings as masturbation arouses in him."

THREATS OF INJURY.   As the child learns about the world in general he wants to know where he comes from. As he inquires about the use of things he naturally questions the use of his genital organ. As he touches himself and finds this part of the body unusually sensitive to pleasure he has a desire to handle it more; this we call masturbation. This "playing with the self" is regarded as reprehensible by many adults and the child is told of the dire consequences supposed to follow in its wake. It is said to make one feebleminded, it "dries up the brain and causes it to run out through the spinal cord," it "weakens the lungs, the heart," it "makes one anemic, causes cancer, tuberculosis, syphilis; it causes pimples on the face and produces an effect on the posture *that anyone can detect,*" and so on! This misinformation may remain a fairly fixed belief in the minds of some adults. It may produce or influence many symptoms because these persons feel that they have been guilty of doing a bad thing and *deserve* to be punished by heart disease, cancer, syphilis, etc. The morbid fixation of a patient's attention to some organ of the body and its functions usually has its roots early in childhood experience. The fears instilled, or the threats of injury to the genitals or other punishment, may so impede the development of the sexual impulse as to contribute to impotence, frigidity or sexual perversion.

MASTURBATION A NORMAL PHENOMENON.   Masturbation is regarded by most psychiatrists, psychologists and educators as a normal phenomenon for all ages from birth until marriage. It may occur in children less than a year old and then be present off and on until in adult life a better sexual adjustment is established. At about the age of five years there may be some increase in the tendency to masturbate. This coincides with an increase in the feeling of rivalry with the parent of the same sex. Growing out of this conflict there is an increase in the need for love in order to quell the consequent tension. If this fear of loss of love is met with added attentions and the play life is normal, no serious conflict need be engendered; nor is there any prolonging of the urge to self-gratification through masturbation which the child in his loneliness uses as a substitute gratification for love. There is usually an increased tendency to masturbation at the time of puberty due to the increased activity of the sex glands and to the closer contact with the opposite sex which occurs at this age.

Tantrums

Rage reactions in children are common and, within certain limits, are not abnormal. They may be simple reactions to a feeling of helplessness, for example, when the child is learning to manage new toys. This fact should be kept mind by parents who have the urge to buy toys which may be beyond the child's power to use. If the toy is right for him and he merely gets angry once in a while no attention need be paid to this burst of rage. However, these rages may relate themselves to his discipline, and if he has rages too frequently over trivial matters, or if he tries to force those around him to yield to his whims in this way, he may need special management.

Management of Tantrums. If the rage (or *negativism*) is prolonged and does not respond to kind reasoning the child may have to be ignored while the rage spends itself. He may be reasoned with afterward. Try to inject understanding into the discussion, a sense of humor if possible, and help the child to save face. Avoid lecturing and moralizing but instead try to encourage better control by understanding and friendliness. Here, as in so many other problems of child training, it is most important that the parent does not get side-tracked into intellectual discussion of what is "good" and "bad" to do. Just as children gradually win control over their bodies so do they over their minds and the parent must convey to the child that he (the parent) understands selfish, egoistic behavior. Such a parent is better able to retain a friendly feeling between the child and himself, which will enable the child to give up selfish emotional releases. The parents should concern themselves more about what the child feels regarding them and the world in general than how *they* (the parents) feel about the child's "bad" habits.

Nightmares

A common problem of childhood and one not to be taken lightly is the matter of night terrors. Probably no child escapes having an occasional nightmare. He cries out in his sleep, usually wakes up crying, reports his frightening dreams and with a little reassurance goes to sleep again. However, this phenomenon of growth may become too frequent and the intensity of the anxiety too great. The anxiety and the terrifying dreams grow out of fears and threats of punishment which have been exaggerated. Fear of punishment is usually the result of the child's own aggressive or sexual impulses. He fears that he cannot control these impulses, that they may break loose and then bring punishment. It is especially during sleep that the forbidden impulses are permitted free play. Games which involve ideas of war, destruction or other catastrophe, sex play, motion pictures depicting cruelty, fairy stories of the same content or exciting television programs may stir up the impulses of hostility or sexual fantasies which result in guilty feelings, and these, in turn, produce fantasies of punishment. Hostility toward a parent or sibling may create an anxiety dream. The children may be afraid to sleep alone or in the dark or their fears may be expressed during the day as fantasies of harm coming to themselves or someone close to them.

Management of Nightmares. Anxiety of this degree requires attention. How often we meet the statement regarding the child, "He will grow out of it." It is true that in time the behavior pattern changes, but unless the basic cause of the fear has been removed the anxiety merely becomes repressed, *i.e.*, stored up in the unconscious mind, ready to cause some future trouble—a real phobia or a disturbance in organ function. Anxiety, expressed in nightmares, may be as dangerous to future health and efficiency as a focus of pulmonary tuberculosis—probably more so. Therefore, if night terrors are frequent and intense, the physician should (1) not ignore them or allow the patient to ignore them, (2) make an effort to elicit the content of the dream. Is it robbers, war, a threatening parent, an animal, a fear of murder, or other catastrophe? To the boy the threatening figure will often resemble the father and this may be obvious to him. This occurs when the father has been too severe or when the mother has portrayed him too often in this role. To the girl the threatening figure will more often be the mother. (3) Try to help the child link up the "scary picture" of the dream with the actual events which have stimulated the dream. Help the child to understand what he is afraid of. If the mother is a strict person explain to her the necessity for less discipline. If the anxiety is growing out of horror stories remove their source and give the child more friendship and reassurance. (4) Help the child to feel safe and loved during the day and, in most cases, he will rest more comfortably at night.

Other Problems of Childhood

During infancy and childhood there are many other problems such as truancy, lying, stealing, cruelty, indifference to studies, the basis for which lie in the same factors which have been discussed so far. These likewise are to a degree normal reactions of childhood. When, or perhaps before, they become disturbing to parents or school authorities advice from the physician is needed. However, since this volume is not primarily devoted to childhood problems we have briefly discussed only some of the most important. One cannot stress too much the necessity for study of the early years of emotional development in order to understand the psychopathological trends which produce neuroses and psychosomatic disorders.

Adolescence

Puberty, with its sudden increase in activity of the glands of internal secretion, marks the beginning of adolescence. This extra impetus to the psychic sexual organization may precipitate *anxiety attacks.* Those occurring at night take the form of frightening dreams in which the dreamer is falling from a high place, or is being pursued, shot at, pinioned and held down, or the like. Daytime anxiety may take the form of unpleasant bodily sensations, a feeling of faintness, fear of being ill, fears of developing cancer, tuberculosis, heart trouble, venereal disease, and so on. Youngsters may remain at home because they fear for their own safety or for the safety of some member of the family.

Treatment should be in the form of factual enlightenment on the causes of anxiety and reassurance and friendliness on the part of the parents or other adults with whom the young person is in contact. This has been discussed. But we can repeat that the anxiety attack means, "I fear that I cannot control my sex impulses or my aggression" and the pursuing, threatening figure in the dream or the fear of disease in the waking state means, "I should be or I am being punished or attacked." Explain to the adolescent that his impulses do not differ from those of others; discuss them with him and assure him that all will be well if he will trust himself and carry on his usual activities. He may have to be seen frequently for further reassurance and further discussion before the anxiety is brought under control.

While clumsy psychotherapy can be especially harmful at this period the tactful physician will know how to cultivate in the patient an understanding of his anxiety about sexual impulses. Such feelings that are poorly understood or sexual drives which are inadequately harnessed to wholesome ideas are generally the basis of anxiety attacks during adolescence. It is important for the physician to know what to look for in these cases just as he knows what to look for in the urine of a patient with symptoms of kidney disease. One need not fear "putting sexual thoughts" into the mind of a young boy or girl. They are already there, often unrelated to healthy social thinking and conduct, and it is the job of the physician to relate them. If they are not the cause of the difficulty no harm has been done. Every child of this age should have a knowledge of healthy sexual functioning, and if the parent has been unable to impart it the physician should be able to take over the role of the parent in this regard.

Masturbation in Adolescence.   Adolescents frequently are openly or secretly distressed about their masturbation activities. They may come to a physician to discuss the matter directly or they may come under the pretext of some other complaint to see if the interview will make it easy for them to introduce the subject. In fact, symptoms of fatigue, indigestion or headaches may occur following a sudden breaking off of the habit of masturbation. The physician should be able to lead up to the question tactfully by taking a personal as well as a medical history. If masturbation is a matter of anxiety the physician should stress (1) that masturbation is a normal phenomenon, (2) that in itself it has no bad effects upon health, either physical or mental, (3) that to reduce its frequency the young person must strive to live a healthy and well-rounded social life, that (4) if anxiety and guilt persist after these efforts a serious neurosis may be the underlying factor and this will require psychiatric care.

Prestige.   Adolescents are often unhappy over their lack of popularity either with their own or the opposite sex, or both. When this is the case to a serious degree it usually is the result of shyness and timidity (anxiety) dating back to early childhood. It may mean that the adolescent was never taught to play with other children or never had the opportunity to do so. It may mean that he was shamed, frowned upon or punished for manifesting sexual interest. It should be realized that the social life of adolescence requires the manifestation of a certain amount of sexual interest. The boy who goes to dancing school and is supposed to ask girls to dance with him, perhaps after he has previously been shamed for his interest in girls, and the girl who is nagged by her mother because she is not more popular with boys but who had always been told that boys were dangerous (sexually aggressive) creatures, are both under a considerable handicap.

Social Anxiety.   Parents who want their adolescent children to mingle socially in a happy way must begin early in the child's life to make him comfortable with other children. If the adolescent is afraid of the opinion of other boys or girls he must have the opportunity to discuss his fears about himself and then be helped to enter social situations and prove that his fears are groundless. Adolescents often worry about their appearance—that their nose is too long, their eyes not the right color, their legs not symmetrical enough, their hair unattractive, their teeth not straight. If an obvious defect is present and can be corrected it may be done. If it is not an obvious defect then it is likely the necessary help is in the realm of emotional acceptance of one's self and suggestions for more normal activities toward socialization.

The presence of *acne* upon the face or back may be a real source of emotional distress to the adolescent. Its relation to the emotions is not well understood but psychotherapy is part of its management. It is frequent in emotionally disturbed adolescents and, by its very presence, adds to the emotional problem.

The aim in management must be to help the adolescent with his struggles of this difficult life period. He can be neither child nor adult. The physician may be a very important person in whom he is to find security and counsel and the physician who can be a wise counsellor at this period may be doing a very good job in preventive medicine.

Emancipation from Parents.   Adolescents often develop a strong resentment against parental restrictions of any kind. They resent being advised to come in at a certain hour, they resent having to account for their spending money, and so on. Any real difficulty of this kind is usually due to a failure on the part of the parents to give the child a proper perspective upon living. The child has not been made to feel that the time spent with his parents was a preparation for living apart from them, or he has not been made to feel that supervision was aimed at making him able to discipline himself. If this philosophy is carried out with goodwill the adolescent will usually accept it. If trouble arises it is generally because the child has been disciplined too much according to the parents' own whims rather than according to a consistent pattern.

Prohibitions.   It is probably safe to say that in the home where comradeship and generosity of spirit have existed between parents and children there is no special resentment of authority or impatience for emancipation. The frequent cry of the adolescent is, "They do not trust me." Too often his protest is justified. The parents do not trust him especially in relation to sex. They often suspect the worst when the adolescent's conduct is on a higher plane than they realize. The parent fears and prohibits rather than shares something of the young person's activities by a friendlier, accepting manner.

Of course, even in the best of homes the adolescent swings between a feeling that he is completely ready for the world one day and a fear that he is still quite young and dependent the next. Parents must understand this vacillation and be flexible enough to deal with it.

Struggle with Religious and Ethical Concepts.   Some adolescents come into conflict with their religious teaching and the prevailing codes of behavior. They become concerned about the actual difficulties that human beings have in being kind and just. They wonder if they have not been misled by an impractical philosophy of life or if they are not too weak within themselves to combat the world as they find it. They have misgivings as to how they are to hold the ideal relationship with God and still maintain a satisfactory working relationship with man. Such conflicts are usually not serious. If the adolescent has an opportunity to discuss his concern now and then with an older person who understands his dilemma, the problem will usually take care of itself. An overconcern or constant rumination about the nature of God and the place of religion, however, to the exclusion of a normal interest in adolescent activities, may mean compulsion neurosis or early schizophrenia and calls for psychiatric advice.

Codes for Sexual Behavior.   Some adolescents are relatively untroubled by sexual fantasy and sexual desire while others have great preoccupation and much emotional unrest in this sphere.

The adolescent with a strong sex drive usually has some psychological problem superimposed upon his normal sexual desire, for example, a need for reassurance that he is loved. He seeks for comfort and reassurance on this score much as a child does when it asks to be taken in its mother's arms. The sexual relationship in the adolescent, therefore, may serve an excessive need for this kind of reassurance—the proof that he or she is attractive and lovable can only be attained by a sexual relationship. Of course, there are many other motives, such as the necessity for proving himself potent or sophisticated. The usual advice offered is that work and physical exercise will diminish sexual desire. To explain that sexual desire has other motives capable of satisfaction, without the sexual act itself, may help some. A boy who insists on sexual intercourse as "proof of affection" can often be shown that such affection exists without the necessity for his indulging in sexual play. Modern adolescents are not much impressed by arguments that sexual relations are contrary to religious teachings, dangerous to health, or harmful to social prestige. Relating their thinking on the subject with responsibility to society as a whole is probably more effective.

Cautious Management Needed.   We have suggested that adolescence needs a guiding hand, and here and there a friendly suggestion. But we must not disturb the adolescent with clumsy psychotherapeutic endeavors. In general we do not try to probe too deeply; we do not try to settle all of his affairs at once. We must understand his needs, be his friend, give him the proper perspective and often he will work out his own destiny satisfactorily. Patience, tact and time are important. If, after a reasonable period of friendly supervision, he becomes *more* involved with somatic symptoms, fears, obsessive ruminations and failure to adapt socially, then referral to a psychiatrist is indicated.

We must remember that adolescence is the period when habits in thinking and behavior are formed which may lead to mental disease, particularly schizophrenia. An adolescent does not have to be too withdrawn or too "queer" to be thought of as a potential schizophrenic. He may be going through the motions of living and yet be very lonely and unhappy. The physician is often in a position to have something to say on these matters. His advice is often asked by parents, or by adolescents themselves, and even if his advice is not sought he may still, as a friend, be able to drop a useful hint. The physician must be aware of these emotional problems because crucial time may be lost if the assumption "he'll snap out of it" is the only attitude adapted toward these problems.

It not infrequently happens that an individual in middle life, particularly a woman, becomes distressed at the behavior of her adolescent children. Up to this point she has kept them well dominated as "her babies" and they have not shown any inclination to get out from under control. However, as the adolescent comes in contact with the ideas and opinions of others he may not remain as passive and yielding as before. Then it is that his parents become concerned over the late hours, the company he keeps, the interest he shows in dancing, dates, or foolish and time-wasting hobbies. He, on the other hand, remains unconcerned; he seems to have no interest in any future occupation and is quite indifferent to the opinion of his elders. He may be irritable, moody, truculent, and even though he lives under the parental roof he shares nothing of himself with the parents and comes and goes as a stranger. They do not know what he is thinking and often feel they have "lost" their child. The youngster may even insist upon an early marriage as one means of getting away from home. Or he may form what parents regard as very undesirable friendships and social connections, and may even go so far as to become involved in delinquent behavior.

Parents as Friends.   We have discussed the necessity for the parents to begin making friends of their children at an early age and to try to keep up the friendship. If this is done with understanding no insurmountable problems should arise. However, when an adolescent does become a real problem to himself or to others it is a pretty safe assumption that in some manner the parents are to blame. The parents may have acted with good intent but their good intentions have disregarded the feelings and wishes of the young person and hence misunderstanding grows through the years. The adolescent may quite frankly state that it is not he but his parents who need advice and he will often be right. Whatever the problem is, the management does not consist in dealing with the adolescent alone but the parents must be taught to understand the adolescent just as he is brought to understand them. The adolescent who is merely "lectured to" by the physician is not likely to show much change. He has already been lectured to, too much, and having developed a lack of respect for authority he is not likely to pay much attention to a physician unless the latter really tries to understand his point of view. The physician should try to act as an intermediary between him and his parents and an honest effort should be made on the part of everyone concerned to understand and remedy grievances.

THE NORMAL PERSONALITY

We have described the growth of personality from birth through adolescence. What then is a "normal" personality? There are no set standards for personality. There are wide variations in the kind of personality which will make a successful social adaptation. However, for our purposes we should attempt some standard even though it is crude. People have good mental health, say leading authorities, when they are *(1) free of symptoms, (2) unhampered by mental conflict, (3) have a satisfactory working capacity and (4) are able to love someone other than themselves.*

As to the first criterion of the normal personality, we have already referred to the way in which symptoms may register a complaint or act out an attitude by means of "body language." In the presence of anxiety the eye may refuse to see unpleasant sights or the ear to hear unpleasant words. The stomach may become "sick" because of an unsatisfactory life situation, or the same situation may cause a headache or a pain in the neck. Symptoms may be regarded as an evidence of physical disease by the family and the physician too, but when finally proved to be "functional" are looked upon, often with ill concealed contempt, as the mark of an inadequate personality.

Regarding the second criterion, "unhampered by mental conflict," obviously much hangs upon the word *unhampered.* Everyone has a certain amount of mental conflict. There are always decisions to be made but the well adjusted person makes his choices with a minimum of conflict, after weighing all factors. An example of hampering conflict is the girl who cannot make a choice of marriage between two suitors or who cannot make a choice of leaving her parents to marry some man whose work requires her to live in a distant city. She is miserably torn in her loyalties and either makes a choice and is not happy or postpones her decision until chances for marriage no longer exist. The girl unhampered by conflict makes her choice and once having made it is no longer tormented by regrets.

To have a *satisfactory working capacity* is most important in a well-adjusted personality. In the preceding paragraphs we have discussed its value to the individual as a means of livelihood, and as a source of pleasure, prestige, and a sense of usefulness.

All efforts in shaping the personality should lead toward what is termed *maturity.* The characteristics of maturity have been defined by Saul (1947) as follows:

1. predominance of independence and responsibility, with little need to regress;
2. predominance of giving and productivity, although with the capacity to receive normally;
3. lack of egotism and competitiveness;
4. a well integrated conscience which furthers development;
5. sexuality free and integrated with mating and responsible, productive activity;
6. hostility toward self and others minimal but freely available for defense and constructive use;
7. grasp of reality unimpaired by persisting childhood reactions, and
8. freedom from childhood patterns of reaction and hence full capacity for discrimination and adaptability.

Saul admits that such a concept may be somewhat ideal at the present stage of our development. But this list of attributes gives us a certain yardstick by which to measure the degrees of immaturity found in those people met in daily practice of medicine. The physician in his daily work needs a concept of maturity just as he needs a measure of healthy thyroid or liver functioning.

Normal Personality

Emotional Features	Behavior
A minimum of mental conflict	Ability to reach a decision without too much stress or delay.
Satisfactory work capacity	Enjoys work. No undue fatigue. No need for frequent change. Maintains optimum efficiency.
Ability to love someone other than self	Takes pleasure in social relationships, marital relationships, parental relationships. Understands the emotional needs and point of view of others and makes appropriate response.

Physical Status
  Absence of symptoms (of neurotic origin)

THE ABNORMAL PERSONALITY

Psychopathology

Deviations from the mature, well functioning personality are gradual in development, but by the time they have produced symptoms, mental, physical or both, they become classifiable under various general categories. The first and mildest of these deviations are the psychoneurotic disorders. The chief characteristic of these disorders is the presence of anxiety which may be felt as such, or may be unconscious and present itself in such phenomena as conversion, displacement, or depression of spirits, without gross or bizarre distortions in personality reaction.

PSYCHONEUROTIC DISORDERS

Anxiety Reaction.   Some degree of anxiety is present in the daily life of almost everyone. Its formation in infancy has been discussed and no one escapes its presence. In fact, since no one is completely motivated by love we can say that a certain dread of what will happen if we do not meet the expectations of others motivates more or less all of our daily activity. Some individuals have all the ingredients for security in their environment—a job, good friends, family, etc.—but are tortured by the fear that all is not well, that something threatening is about to happen to them or to those they love. This dread of the catastrophic may be attached to thoughts of driving a car, going into crowds, staying alone in the house at night. In such instances, the sufferer fears that he cannot control himself, or cannot control the environment. He is not clear as to whether the danger is going to come from outside himself or from within, from some failure of his psychic or physiological apparatus.

Sometimes anxiety attacks (a sudden sense of painful sensations) convince the patient that he is physically ill. These sensations consist of such things as difficulty in breathing, palpitation of the heart, weakness in the extremities, nausea and "all gone" feelings combined with great physical tension and a psychic sense of doom. These may occur either in the daytime or at night, the latter usually being termed nightmares. Whether or not anxiety attacks are a prominent feature of the anxiety state, the patient tends to focus considerable attention upon his body and health generally. He finds his happiness and efficiency curtailed by the fact that there is always something he must "worry" about rather than being able to go about his daily routine with a buoyant spirit and a mind free of morbid thoughts.

ETIOLOGY. The cause of these anxiety states has already been described in the discussion on the origins of anxiety in childhood. Anxiety is ubiquitous and omnipresent owing to the inability of parents to understand the importance of emotional relatedness and acceptance of children in early life. Children are not made to feel that they belong and they do not have satisfactory interests outside of themselves. Without this they are unable either to identify with a warm, capable female figure or to feel comfortable with men. Later, therefore, when anxiety develops it appears in personalities that are empty, cold and unable to feel deeply and satisfyingly about other humans. Such individuals fear that their own hostilities, dependencies and sexual impulses will bring disaster. They are not able to trust people or believe what is told them about their own health, strength and virtue. As a result the mechanism of the anxiety attack plunges them into an exaggerated syndrome of stage fright. They are prone to draw personal morbid conclusions to the effect that they are very ill physically, and their anxiety, dependence and inability to think logically and rationally lead them into a chronic state of discomfort which they feel is inevitable and disastrous and which they are helpless to combat.

Patients with anxiety states rarely seek psychiatric help immediately. The sufferer feels uncomfortable and repeatedly tries to search out a possible diagnosis for himself from all the disease entities he has already heard of. In this he is often aided by friends and relatives. It is in this phase of his illness that he is usually seen by the general practitioner or the specialist in some other field than psychiatry.

PROGNOSIS. This condition once present does not undergo self-cure. The patient may undergo changes and develop defenses against the stress of anxiety by the formation of phobias. If he does not develop a phobic formation he may remain a chronic invalid going from physician to physician, from hospital to hospital, in search of relief. Or he may become disillusioned and, in despair, remain at home lost as one of the thousands of chronic nervous invalids that abound in this country. Such persons rarely, if ever, become mental hospital cases. Their behavior does not become bizarre or uncontrolled enough to warrant mental hospital care but they can become absolutely dependent and useless as contributing members of society.

MANAGEMENT. The management of anxiety reactions should be

psychotherapeutic. Nothing else has been found to be of any permanent value. Drug treatment in the form of vitamins, sedatives and tranquilizers is only palliative and accomplishes little more than temporary improvement. Psychotherapeutic help to be effective can be given by a psychiatrist, if there is one available, who may (*a*) treat the patient five times weekly by psychoanalysis (ambulatory), (*b*) treat the patient by psychotherapy once weekly (ambulatory) or, if the illness is severe enough, (*c*) treat him in a hospital. On the other hand, the patient may be treated by a physician, a general practitioner or a specialist utilizing the principles of psychotherapy as outlined here.

1. Take history.
2. Make necessary laboratory examinations.
3. Explain cause of symptoms.
4. Ascertain areas of faulty thinking regarding symptom formation.
5. Ascertain areas of immature or socially inadequate behavior.
6. Show how these have produced symptoms and are keeping them active.

Case 1.   Anxiety Reaction

Mrs. C. Age 31. Housewife, high school graduate. Catholic. Symptoms: "Spells" of weakness, shakiness, hazy vision, tension in head, tightness in skin of one year's duration with fatigue and fear of staying alone or going shopping alone. Patient had worrisome, overemotional parents who restricted her activity and whose only way of showing love was to overprotect her instead of enjoying her.

At age 15 she began to complain of bodily discomforts and was told to "rest." An "exploratory" appendectomy was done at age 21 for gastrointestinal distress. After working as a clerk for three and a half years she married. She has a child now seven and a half years old. When pregnant with this child she was told she had "fractures of the spine." She wore a brace and "felt sorry for herself." With a second pregnancy she was not happy and when a miscarriage occurred she felt guilty and believed her negative thoughts may have helped to bring it about. "God was punishing me." She soon began to experience anxiety attacks and feared being alone or going shopping alone.

In psychotherapy it was explained that she had not only been thinking morbidly but also was not aware of her need for attention and affection. It was further explained that her morbid thinking kept her sick and that achieving her needs for affection would be the medicine that would make her well. What she needed was friendly, warm, reassuring relationships. Guilt and other emotions, she was told, were acting as barriers between her and this medicine.

On her second visit to her therapist she talked of her menstrual period as a cause of symptoms. The physiology and psychology of the menstrual period was explained. She worried about a return of her "sick feeling" (anxiety attack) and she was again told the reason for its occurrence and urged to carry on in spite of it. She discussed her sexual adjustment and indicated that in this as in other areas of her activity she had a diminished capacity for enjoyment. This she related to her fear of pregnancy and guilt over not being more active in the maternal role.

On her third visit she had no physical symptoms but said that she had felt depressed for three days because of an innocuous remark made by her sister-in-law. Because of this she was afraid that the therapist would "disapprove" of her progress. She was reassured about this and told that she must expect "emotional" problems such as depression as she relinquished her symptoms.

On her fourth visit she had more to discuss about her early life with her worrisome mother and physically ill father. She saw her tendency to think morbidly and to fail to find something wholesome in each day's existence. In the sessions following the third visit she was willing to talk of her personal problems and their solution. She had given up her

Lincocin®

Oral
500 mg. capsules
Pediatric capsules, 250 mg.
Available in 24's and 100's

Injectable
10 cc. multiple-dose vial
2 cc. ampoule—600 mg./2 cc.

many physical complaints. In all she was seen nine times and felt well enough to discontinue therapy.

Let us try to describe what happened in therapy to bring about relief of symptoms and better social functioning. (1) The therapist gave her a dramatic but succinct picture of the cause of her illness. (2) Her need for affection was emphasized. (3) It was made clear that the type of medicine she needed was in terms of relating to people in her environment.

In one session, for instance, the therapist had an opportunity to demonstrate her regressive tendency (the tendency to talk of symptoms and invite attention and sympathy). She had been denied that prop by both her family and by the therapist. It was pointed out that by nursing her symptoms and by failing to play the proper role in her family she was inviting more guilt and self-criticism.

On one of her visits the therapist tried to point out what happens when symptoms are reconverted. That is, he explained that when the somatic distress leaves there is an emotional problem waiting which clamors for solution. The concern that was exercised to make her understand the cause of her discomfort as well as giving her an opportunity to talk about her personal problems made it possible for her to give up offering her symptoms in place of her feelings. To offer symptoms is much safer for such persons than to offer "self." To reverse this, they need help. The discerning psychiatrist makes it possible for them to understand how to put themselves into the life they live rather than offer aches, pains, complaints and fears as a substitute.

Anxiety Reactions

Emotional Features	Physical Disability
Fear—apprehension—nameless dread	Anxiety attacks
Anxiety in attacks with cardiac palpitation— or general anxiety over social acceptance	Sudden weakness
	Cardiac palpitation
Nightmares—irritability	"All gone feeling"—tension—feeling of "going to pieces"
Moodiness—depression of spirits—tendency to seclusion. Fear of losing mind—fear of fainting or falling in street—fear of dying or being victim of some disease—fear of violence to self or others. Fear of jumping from heights	"Jittery"—dizziness—visual disturbance— feeling of "tightness" in body
	Nausea—belching—vomiting
	Urinary urgency—diarrhea
	Chest pain—back pain

Some impairment in the sexual function

Dissociative Reaction. This type of response to emotional conflict is not a common one. It is seen as sharply delineated periods of amnesia, fugue state, depersonalization, stupor or sleepwalking. It is not sufficiently common to warrant more than passing mention in a book on psychosomatic affections and the reader is referred to a textbook of psychiatry for further information.

Conversion Reaction. This type of reaction is quite commonly seen in general practice and is the condition which, possibly more than any other over the centuries, has led physicians to regard the psyche as an etiological agent in symptom production. The mechanism of symptom formation in this syndrome is that the psychic energy (anxiety) resulting from conflict is not experienced consciously in the mind as pain but is "converted," *i.e.,* displaced into a physical symptom. The emotional charges find their way into some organ or organ system giving a symptom or set of symptoms. The symptom often symbolizes fairly clearly the underlying conflict—so much so that some of our everyday expressions portray the fact that conflict can produce symptoms. Examples of these are: "He makes me sick," "This job gives me a headache," "She gives me a pain."

An effort has been made to differentiate conversion reactions from psychophysiological disorders, the former being a more direct leap from the unconscious to a part of the body which symbolizes the conflict, the latter being the result of chronic tensions expressing themselves continuously over a long period by way of the vegetative nervous system. We cannot make too arbitrary a distinction since it seems logical that there is some symbolization process in psychophysiologic disorders. At any rate, while there is a tendency for the voluntary musculature to be involved in conversion reactions, they are by no means limited to these areas. Among the symptoms described are paralyses of limbs or of one whole side of the body, inability to speak, tremors, anesthesias, dysthesias, visceral manifestations of vomiting, diarrhea, localized intestinal hyper or hypotonus resulting in gaseous distention (pseudocyesis), cardiospasm or colic, blindness, deafness and disturbances of smell, as well as localized vasomotor reactions.

ETIOLOGY.   The etiology, as we have already stated, is an attempted somatic compliance to an idea repressed in the unconscious because it conflicts with the ideals of the patient. But the repression is only partly successful. The idea escapes and gains expression in the symptoms, giving partial alleviation to the tension underlying the conflict as well as partly alleviating the guilt that is also present.

PSYCHOPATHOLOGY.   Patients with a conversion reaction are often sensitive and imaginative. Typically it is found they have been reared in the midst of austerity but at the same time allowed to wish for much more. As children, many of their emotional needs are ungratified and instead of being prepared for sturdy, dutiful living, circumstances permit them to daydream solutions to their emotional needs which lie beyond the bounds of reality. One of the parents may unwittingly further this fanciful dream living. The result is an imaginative, volatile, restless, urgent longing, pressing for gratification in a personality trying to be dutiful, altruistic and conforming. A conversion reaction results. These reactions often appear at a period of heightened emotional stress or strain.

Case 2.   Conversion Reaction

A woman of 46, married and the mother of three children, suffered from urticaria. This urticaria occurred whenever she came in contact with her father. It mattered not whether she visited him in his home or whether he came to hers. They always affected each other adversely and as a result of the tension which arose between them the patient would develop itching welts on her skin. History revealed that the father had been jealous of his daughter's attractive femininity when she was a growing girl. He had criticized her severely for her boldness and what he regarded as her lack of modesty. She had had spirit and defiance and while she loved her father she would not yield to his domination. Their arguments often terminated in his beating her with a strap. She had been both resentful and humiliated yet somehow gratified by this evidence of his interest and concern.

With the background of such an emotionally charged relation to the first man in her life, the patient married a man who reminded her in various ways of her father. Naturally, erotic and romantic frustration continued and this added to her resentment. When she came in contact with her father, the source of so much of her difficulty, she uncon-sciously reenacted the beating episodes. The urticaria served to reinstate at the same time the situation which gave vent to her defiance and gratification.

This patient was distressed to discover that she retained such a twisted lover-like rela-tion to her father, but when she understood it and endured what she called "shame and disgust" over the idea, the urticaria disappeared.

How can we explain what happened to bring about the removal of symptoms? In the first place, urticaria lends itself to many symbolic interpretations. It itches, it burns, it stands out, it is "white with fury," and "red with indignation." It blushes, it is hot with excitement. It is tumescent. In this case, the patient demonstrated over and over in her discussions about her father the fact that she was alternately highly resentful and yet sensually very attracted to him, and sometimes these feelings did not alternate. They were present at one and the same time. By means of psychotherapy she came to under-stand these things and expend through abreaction much of the emotional charge in these memories, relieving the "toxic" effect of the memories upon her skin. Here it can be said that the urticaria did symbolize sexuality but it had to have assistance from the autonomic nervous system for its appearance.

Conversion Reactions

Emotional Features	Physical Disability
Emotionally unstable and capricious—ambivalent feelings clearly shown	Motor: Tics—convulsions—paralysis—astasia—abasia
Emotionally immature	Sensory: Anesthesias—paresthesias—in body or in organs of special sense
Tendency to react emotionally rather than logically	Visceral: Esophageal spasm—cramps—vomiting—diarrhea
Vivid imagination and active fantasy life	Vasomotor: Blushing
Amnesia. Dual or multiple personality	

Some impairment in the sexual function

Phobic Reaction. The phobic reaction is an "avoidance" reaction and is simply the behavior pattern of an individual who has discovered that contact with places or situations arouses large quantities of anxiety. He naturally avoids them. This includes such situations as riding in cars, buses, trolleys, being in high places, closed places, open spaces, subways, tunnels, crowds, and so on. Some of these situations may be bearable if the patient is accompanied by a trusted person, usually a close relative, but even this, in some instances, is not enough. This aspect tends to confirm the fact that the pathology here is a great insecurity and fear on the part of the patient of how he will control himself. The psychopathology and treatment are the same as for the anxiety reaction.

Obsessive Compulsive Reaction. In this neurosis there is a con-tinued appearance of unwelcome ideas in the mind or an urge to re-peatedly carry out certain acts. A common example is that of the person who must go back several times after leaving the house to make sure that the gas has been turned off or the door locked. The repetitive nature of these continued thoughts or acts testify to the patient's problem of overconscientiousness in which he seems to keep saying, "I must remem-ber or I will be punished. I must be obedient. I must be good. I must keep my attention fixed on this thought or my instinctual desires will get out of hand."

The *compulsive* individual is doing or undoing through physical measures such as washing, touching, rearranging, rather than by worrying or doubting. The _obsessive_ patient tries to _think_ his way through to comfort by excessive preoccupation with ideas such as "Does God exist?" while the compulsive patient _acts_ his way through the expiation. Sometimes obsessive thinking and compulsive acting exist together.

ETIOLOGY AND PSYCHOPATHOLOGY.   The obsessive compulsive personality reaction is seen in people who are overconscientious, overscrupulous, slaves to duty and bent upon correctness, precision, punctuality and meeting obligations. To a great extent the joy of living and cooperating has been squeezed out of their lives. As children they probably derived pleasure only from a concern about overcoming the dangers of instinctual expression. This particular mental outlook has been found to stem largely, although not exclusively, from the period of toilet training when duty, punctuality, regularity and self-control are stressed. Other factors are the lack of affection from the earlier oral phase of development and the continued strictness carried over into the genital phase. There are many compulsive individuals who are cold, meticulous, pedantic, bossy, overattentive to detail, impersonal and abrupt in their dealings with others, yet who, it must be admitted, are often efficient people. However, this efficiency is vitiated by the number of people around them whom they irritate and alienate.

Case 3.   Obsessive Compulsive Reaction

A man of 38, married and a teacher, suffered various compulsions which were not actually problems to him but became great problems to his sensitive and freedom-loving wife. All bills had to be paid exactly on time. He was more than scrupulous in making sure that all house doors were locked. Moreover, he could not bear to have the garage door open unless a car was on the way in or out. He was extremely punctual about appointments and train schedules and if his wife ever kept him waiting or did not plan her schedule to be ahead of time, he would become angry and scold her. He was forever trying to reform her so as to conform with his overscrupulousness. As a result he was never satisfied with her and they quarreled and were on the verge of divorce. It was difficult to get him to see the nature of the woman he married and become able to accept and admire her as a _different_ but nevertheless acceptable and lovable human being.

His case shows what happens when children are overtrained to love order, schedules, routine, and abstract qualities such as punctuality, instead of people. Moreover, such individuals show a retaliative form of sadism which says, "I was made to do it—I was made to put all my interest in these things—you must do it also. I obtained love only through adopting these ways. Now you must do the same or I will not love you." Such people have a great anxiety about accepting easygoingness in themselves or others. They are convinced that such behavior will lead to bad conduct. They work for love by doing their "duty." First they learn this from their parents and later come to introject the parents as their own conscience and work for their own approval. These are not easy people to live and work with, and any thoroughgoing change needs a long period of psychoanalysis. They need an intensive retraining in values and thinking of the kind which psychoanalysis offers. The man referred to softened under psychiatric treatment and became much easier to live with when he began to see that he provided most of the problems in the marriage. The compulsive patient rarely sees anything wrong with his own point of view or behavior. In fact he feels more virtuous than others.

In treatment such a patient must be confronted again and again with his cold and sadistic attitudes both toward himself and others. He needs to understand the childhood experiences which caused them to develop. He needs to be sensitized to identify with the feelings of others. He needs to modify his harsh super-ego so that he can be easier on himself and dispense with his protective rituals.

Obsessive Compulsive Reactions

Emotional Features	Physical Disability
Need to dwell upon an idea or carry out an act repetitiously, accompanied by inability to concentrate on the main issue of life	Theoretically there is none, but actually the amount of anxiety present is usually sufficient to cause fatigue and gastrointestinal tract symptoms and to interfere with adequate sex function
Serious personality, little sense of humor, intolerant of human foibles	
Difficulty in identifying with others	
Doubts about sincerity of others	
Limited capacity to enjoy life	
Temper outbursts. Efforts to control behavior of others	

Some impairment in the sexual function

Depressive Reaction.   This psychoneurosis is one that is frequently encountered. It is not always easily isolated from an anxiety reaction or an obsessive compulsive reaction, since patients often display some depression in the presence of anxiety reactions and since they possess some of the grimness and lack of joy in living that is seen in the obsessive compulsive reaction.

ETIOLOGY AND PSYCHOPATHOLOGY.   Here, as in related neuroses, there have been childhood deprivations resulting in guilt, feelings of inferiority, love inhibitions, ambivalence, overscrupulousness and an unsatisfactory formula for living which prohibits happiness, a sense of ease and pleasure in human relations. As a result, frustration and resentment complicated by guilt and self-criticism result in a slowing up of efficiency.

SYMPTOMATOLOGY.   The patient usually puts his distress predominantly in physical terms. He "doesn't feel up to par." He sleeps poorly, suffers from poor appetite, fatigue, impaired initiative, "doesn't enjoy things the way he used to." Zest is lacking in sex activity, often with complaints of tension in the head or in body musculature. Patients complain that they do not have their former interest in anything.

Case 4.   Depressive Reaction

A man of 47 came to his family physician complaining of low energy, poor concentration, insomnia, jittery spells, tension in his skin, a lack of enjoyment in work, friends, and family life, accompanied by some loss in sexual desire. Sedation, Thorazine and testosterone were tried without benefit, and psychotherapy was advised. Psychiatric diagnosis showed that his deficits were not in the realm of the glands but in the realm of emotions. First, it was elicited that his mother had died of cancer when he was 10. He could not remember her as a healthy woman giving him affection and encouragement. Following her death he and his father moved in with his grandparents. There he was lost in the family group and he could not remember much except that he went to school and "everything was all right." He went into business without a college education and did well, but in spite of a good marriage, children and many friends he did not prosper emotionally. When his employer advanced him he concluded it was "because there was no one else." He was given responsibilities but instead of feeling honored he thought of them as "part of the grind."

His children did well in school but "So what," he said, "so did a lot of others." Never having received acceptance and encouragement he could never feel that anything he did mattered. He advanced to a prominent place in his firm but envied men who had their own businesses and felt that they looked down upon him when they met in social circles. This man had been building, over the years, a large and thick wall between himself and happiness, partly because he was unable to appreciate the value of his efforts to others, and partly because his excessive need for recognition kept him from being as aggressive as he wished lest he be rebuffed and rejected. So he repressed his aggression, did not ask for appreciation. With his deprivation his self-esteem gradually grew lower with the passing years, and because of the repression of his aggression he was unable to obtain from life what he wanted and needed. When he came to understand these mechanisms within himself and began to push out for recognition and "get back into life again," his depression disappeared.

PSYCHOTIC DISORDERS

Affective Reactions.   MANIC DEPRESSIVE REACTIONS.   No physician practices long without having contact with the phenomenon of mental depression, i.e., depression of spirits. All victims of neuroses suffer from feelings of inferiority, lowered self-esteem, fatigue, lack of energy and difficulty in concentrating. However, in the neuroses these symptoms are mild or fleeting compared with the same phenomena in the manic depressive psychoses. In the latter there is a more clear-cut and definite beginning to the period of depression and the degree of incapacity is more marked. Because of lack of interest and lack of will power the patient is nearly or completely paralyzed in carrying on his usual occupation. He may sleep poorly and lose appetite, lose weight, have an extremely pessimistic attitude toward the future, and be very derogatory toward himself and his abilities. He may falsely believe that he has sinned and harmed others in so doing. All this may lead to thoughts of or even attempts at suicide. If such a state is encountered after 40, the history may reveal similar attacks that have occurred within the previous twenty years. Persons subject to attacks of depression may also have cyclic phenomena of exalted spirits, a feeling of well-being, overconfidence and overactivity, resulting in acts displaying bad judgment and even delusions of grandeur.

Affective Reactions
(Manic Depressive Reactions)

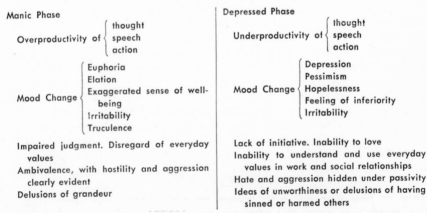

Manic Phase

Overproductivity of
- thought
- speech
- action

Mood Change
- Euphoria
- Elation
- Exaggerated sense of well-being
- Irritability
- Truculence

Impaired judgment. Disregard of everyday values
Ambivalence, with hostility and aggression clearly evident
Delusions of grandeur

Depressed Phase

Underproductivity of
- thought
- speech
- action

Mood Change
- Depression
- Pessimism
- Hopelessness
- Feeling of inferiority
- Irritability

Lack of initiative. Inability to love
Inability to understand and use everyday values in work and social relationships
Hate and aggression hidden under passivity
Ideas of unworthiness or delusions of having sinned or harmed others

Suicide.   The lack of emotional and ideational control character-izes either phase of this state as a *psychosis* rather than a neurosis. How-ever, a depressed patient in the early stages of development may come to the general physician complaining primarily of physical symptoms, and if the physician is thinking in terms of physical disease and has a blind spot for the emotional side of the illness he may find himself treating a severe emotional illness along physical lines. A sudden suicide may shock him into a realization that he has made a serious diagnostic error. General medical men must learn to recognize the early signs of suicidal tendencies just as we recognize the early evidences of pulmonary tuberculosis. The best way to discover whether a patient is thinking of suicide is to ask him. This need not frighten or distress him; if done calmly and kindly it is reassuring.

All those who have suicidal thoughts are not suicidal. Many such people are relieved to discuss their suicidal thoughts with a physician, knowing and declaring that they would never carry them out. But if the patient is evasive and not sure that he can be trusted to control his suicidal impulses then he should be hospitalized—with his cooperation if possible. If not, the physician and family should put him in the hos-pital for his own protection.

Psychopathology.   What psychotherapy accomplishes is to make these patients aware of how they have unconsciously suppressed their demands from life and how hostile they have become for doing so. They seem to radiate a slow burning resentment as if to say, "I refuse to join you in any enjoyment of life." Psychotherapy has to free the libido so that the patient can reinvest it in his work, his family and friends.

We believe the difference between the depressive reaction and the depressive phase of the affective psychosis to be one of degree rather than kind. The psychodynamics is essentially the same, with the differ-ence being in the greater amount of original emotional deprivation in psychotic patients. They are more distrustful and so rapport is harder to obtain for therapeutic purposes. Furthermore, amounts of hostility generated are greater, using up more of the healthy libido to keep the patient from destructive outbursts. In the manic phase of the illness the pent-up aggression expends itself in expansive, erotic and aggressive behavior. In the depressed phase this is kept within bounds but at great expense to the total functioning of the personality.

Etiology.   The etiology, then, of the manic depressive reactions we consider to lie in a defective personality development. The love needs of childhood have not been met and healthy satisfying outlets for ag-gression and prestige have not been provided. As a result the libido turns in upon the self and in the depressive phase of the illness healthy per-sonality is used up in controlling the ungratified impulses, resulting in the slowing up, the loss of interest, the self-criticism and the refusal to participate. At the height of futility and rage, suicide may be at-tempted. The manic phase represents an abortive unsatisfactory attempt to repair past difficulties by a hectic, overactive preoccupation with new ideas or new schemes, with hollow humor or truculent irritability if the poorly laid plans and ideas are not agreed to.

Prognosis.   The manic depressive reactions always end in a matter of months even if untreated, and the patient is merely given nursing care and prevented from harming himself. The average duration of the untreated case is six to eighteen months although prior to the use of shock treatment depression sometimes lasted two years or more.

Management.   The treatment of choice for a manic depressive reaction should be enough psychotherapy to bring about a repair of the patient's damaged personality, the treatment being carried out when he is mentally accessible for psychotherapy. Since this is time-consuming and it is practically necessary to get most of these patients back on the job as soon as possible, electroshock treatment is used extensively in these conditions both in the depressed and manic phases. Results are better in the depressed phase.

Shock Therapy.   In the treatment of the manic depressive reactions electroshock therapy should not be utilized without being combined with and followed up by psychotherapy. In 80 per cent of the cases electroshock therapy reverses the depressive reaction but it does nothing to help the patient understand the underlying psychopathology and he remains vulnerable to future attacks.

Duration of depressions has been significantly shortened by electroshock therapy. Apparently depressive episodes are shortened only when there is sufficient excitation of the brain cells to produce a massive discharge. Prominent mental and physical expressions of this are: unconsciousness, a tonic-clonic spasm of the body musculature, increased arterial and venous pressures, laryngospasm, tachycardia, apnea, vagal heart slowing, disorientation, amnesia and, occasionally, post-treatment hyperactivity. Usually from six to twelve treatments are required. The most frequent complication is fracture, usually of dorsal or lumbar vertebral bodies. Approximately one patient in 1000 dies, usually from cardiac failure when there is preexisting cardiac disease, which may or may not be detectable.

The main attempts to minimize the effects of this massive discharge take the direction of an alteration in the form, amount, duration and area of application of the electric current, supposing that side effects result from excessive amounts of electricity.

Succinylcholine, a muscle relaxant, attenuates the muscular contraction. Decreasing the Valsalva phenomenon reduces the sudden strain of an increased return of blood to the heart. Since there is a respiratory paralysis, respiration must be supported for a 3 to 5 minute period. Oxygen is given to decrease the possibility of brain damage from asphyxia. Short-acting barbiturates like Pentothal sodium are given: to reduce anxiety caused by the treatment, to prevent the feelings of suffocation and pain from the fasciculatory muscle contraction due to the depolarizing action of the muscle relaxant, and to lessen post-treatment hyperactivity. Atropine blocks the vagal slowing of the heart.

Convulsive therapy has been given preferably in hospitals by experienced operators and assistants. When treatment is given to out-patients, supervision is important as there is often a memory deficit after treatments which may culminate in a temporary amnesia, despite spacing of treatments.

How the convulsion works to bring about a better integration of the psychic structure is not known. Speculation includes occurrence of a total reorganization or retrenchment in the face of the severe stress of treatment; this psychotic pattern has the least fixed and most easily disrupted synaptic brain pattern. The convulsion may be linked with unconscious fantasies of punishment to the self and aggression toward others. Treatment may at once be punishment for these fantasies and also give reassurance that the individual's aggression can be countered and controlled by the environment, hence guilt or hostility is more quickly dissipated. But so far as we know, no patient has remembered and it seems impossible to prove what takes place psychologically.

SCHIZOPHRENIC REACTION.   We now come to the most serious psychotic disturbance of all—schizophrenia. Since more than 20,000 schizophrenics are entering our mental institutions yearly, *the practicing physician is seeing many such cases in his practice during the early course of their development.* Schizophrenia is a mental illness which does not break out suddenly but has a long incubation period. In the course of development many of these cases pass through a stage in which physical complaints are in the foreground. Many of them come to physicians with vague or bizarre complaints during what may be called the hypochondriacal stage. A careful history which touches on the personality will often elicit delusional beliefs about the body or about some outside influence which is affecting them such as electricity, poisoned food, or the like.

Failure in Adaptation.   The history of these people's lives shows that they attempt adaption somewhat as follows: They are sensitive in all human relations from infancy onward. They are lacking in those early life "feeling experiences" and ideas which would enable them to draw emotional sustenance from others, be they relatives or friends. This leaves them walled off emotionally from others. They are particularly unable to accept and utilize the sexual experience for its emotional value. They fit poorly into the social scene at all ages. They do not establish close and satisfying personal relationships. They have great emotional investment in fantasy. As they come in contact with other people they are hurt or ignored and at the same time frustrate themselves by their own inadequacies. There occurs disorganization in thinking so that they cease to be logical in both thought and action. There comes to be a splitting apart of ideas and feelings appropriate to the ideas. There is gradual social and economic failure. Anxiety and conflict are settled through false beliefs and false conclusions which lead to hallucinated punishment or gratification. Because of hypochondriacal pain they may conclude that cancer is present. Because of great loneliness the schizophrenic, for example, may believe that he can talk through the air to celebrated personages. From repressed sexual desire a woman may conclude that she is sought after by rich and important admirers who wish to marry her. A progressive lack of interest in the activities in the patient's environment both near and remote is the rule. The extension of the conflict *beyond* somatic distress to a relatively complete loss of emotional and ideational control shows the much greater seriousness of psychosis over neurosis.

Treatment.   If seen early many schizophrenic patients are amenable to psychological treatment, but only in the hands of a trained psychiatrist. For the more advanced cases, hospitalization and insulin shock therapy may be helpful. But the physician ought to recognize the schizophrenic patient early, before he is too fixed in bad habits of thinking, feeling and acting. Medical practitioners usually have the first opportunity to see schizophrenics. Perhaps if their condition were recognized early and treated more effectively we would not have such a tremendous number occupying beds in mental hospitals.

The schizophrenic, like the manic-depressive, has a great love of self. He has often been hurt and he does not trust himself to confide in many people. The one he trusts must be able to think and feel with him and must never disappoint him. The schizophrenic is willing, reluctantly so, but nevertheless willing to be led back to reality provided the leading is done slowly, kindly, patiently, and provided the real world and its values can be made more pleasant and attractive than his world of fantasy.

Schizophrenic Reaction

1. Sensitive to impersonal stimuli and in personal relations from infancy onward.
2. Lacking in the early warm life relationships and ideas of sharing.
3. Particularly unable to accept and utilize sexual experiences for constructive emotional value.
4. Fit poorly into social scene at all ages.
5. As growth continues do not establish close and satisfying personal relationships.
6. Great emotional investment in fantasy.
7. Frustrate themselves as well as being easily hurt by others.
8. Disorganization in thinking.
9. Splitting apart of idea and appropriate affect.
10. Gradual social and economic failure.
11. Gradual rejection of real world.
12. Regression to childish thinking and behavior.
13. Anxiety and conflicts settled through false conclusion and belief (delusion) and through hallucinated punishment or gratification.
14. Very little spontaneous tendency or conscious desire to leave this adaptation for normal world and its values.

PARANOID REACTIONS.   There is a special type of psychotic reaction called paranoia. It is characterized by a slowly developing system of false beliefs without the sufferer having passed through the outward manifestations of personality disorganization seen in most schizophrenias and manic depressive psychoses. These persons have been deeply hurt and much anxiety is present. Their psychosexual development has encountered many frustrations and they are thought to have dealt poorly with unconscious homosexual conflicts. While much is unknown about the development of the paranoid personality, the end result is that the sensitive spots in the psyche are healed to some extent by false conclusions about these persons themselves or the world about them. If they have failed economically they may acquire the belief that they are fabulously rich. If they have not succeeded socially they either compensate for this by believing that they are important and sought after or project the blame onto someone else and censure that person for their failure or unhappiness. Aside from sharply localized false beliefs the personality functions are intact. In some cases the amount of feeling accompanying the belief is quite intense and, in contrast to the situation in schizophrenia (where there is little cohesion between belief and appropriate feelings to the belief), there is considerable emotion corresponding with the idea. The result may be that the one believing himself an important religious personage must deliver impassioned sermons, and the one who believes his career has been interfered with by jealous persons seeks justice and in his zeal to see justice done may take the law into his own hands and be homicidal.

Paranoid Reaction

1. Sensitive to psychic as well as more impersonal stimuli from childhood onward but limited in emotional and ideational capacities.
2. Limited capacity to identify with others and accept and correlate other points of view.
3. Psychosexually immature with tendency toward latent homosexuality.
4. Not pliable in adaptations and hence frustrate themselves and are hurt by others.
5. Social and economic adjustment is poor and relief from painful realization of this fact has to be false belief (delusion) through mechanism of overcompensation or projection. This occurs without passing through the personality disorganization of schizophrenia or manic depressive psychoses.

Projection.   Between the fixed delusions of the true paranoiac and the average individual there are many degrees of *compensatory and projection mechanisms.* The sensitive, frustrated wife who has paranoid tendencies may feel that her husband or husband's relatives have ruined her conjugal happiness whereas the fault has been her own inability to make a good adjustment in life. The husband may feel that his lack of business success has been due to favoritism shown to his colleagues by the boss. The belief in such cases is not absolute—it varies from day to day, and when challenged the holder will admit some doubt as to the truth of his assertions—while the delusions of true paranoia are constant and unchangeable. Nevertheless, these so-called "paranoid" personalities are not easy to live with or to work with. Their friendliness will not stretch to the point of permitting insight into their "nearly false" beliefs. They lack the flexibility which is necessary for a correction of personality inadequacies. They can bring neither a sense of humor nor a sense of fairness to bear upon their shortcomings when the latter are pointed out and this makes for difficulties in their personal relationships. Much anxiety in the neurosis of a husband or wife may be stimulated by a paranoid spouse. The sense of righteousness which the paranoid person shows, combined with his cold unwillingness to try to put himself in the other fellow's place—to try to sense his feelings or see his point of view—, can be quite disturbing to the husband, wife or child dependent upon such a person for affection and understanding.

Normal Personality		Neuroses	Psychoses
Emotional Features Unhampered by mental conflict	Ability to reach a decision without too much stress or delay	Hampering mental conflicts Mild mood disturbances Capacity for decision impaired	Mental conflicts Severe mood disturbances Capacity for decision impaired
Satisfactory work capacity	Enjoys work No undue fatigue No need for frequent change Maintains optimum efficiency	Work not enjoyed Fatigue a frequent and pronounced symptom Impairment of work efficiency	Severe disturbances in efficiency; concentration upon or participation in work may be totally impossible
Ability to love someone other than self	Takes pleasure in social relationships, marital relationships, parental relationships. Can understand the emotional needs and point of view of others and make appropriate response	Disturbances in ability to enjoy social relations, i.e., inability to relate themselves to others in such a way as to gain security and emotional response. Limited capacity to give emotionally yet some conventional relation to others is maintained even though imperfect and at the cost of anxiety	Severe disturbances in ability to relate themselves to others; in fact, they tend to renounce their relations to others more or less completely
Physical Status Absence of symptoms (of neurotic origin)		Conversion of emotional stress (anxiety) into somatic symptoms in one or many parts of body	Somatic symptom formation during onset of illness but eventually symptoms are in sphere or control of emotion, thought, speech, action
			Varying amount of loss in control of well integrated thought, emotion and speech, and regressions to childish levels — and/or solution of anxiety through false beliefs or false sensory perception

PERSONALITY DISORDERS

One often encounters an individual who cannot be classified as psychotic, psychoneurotic, or even as psychophysiologically ill. Yet he does have a disorder which manifests itself by a lifelong pattern of peculiar action or misbehavior rather than by mental or emotional symptoms. Behavior is often unusual, unconventional, eccentric or troublesome in some way and yet causes the individual minimal subjective anxiety and little or no sense of distress. Such a disorder is called a personality disorder. Personality disorders are divided into three main groups on the basis of the dynamics of personality development.

1. **Personality Pattern Disturbances.**   Personality pattern disturbances are regarded as deep-seated disturbances with little room for regression or much improvement with the passage of time. In this category falls the **inadequate personality,** so called because the individual with such a disturbance is neither physically nor mentally deficient but shows an inability to adapt, poor judgment, ineptness, lack of physical and emotional stamina, and social incompatibility.

The **schizoid personality** is found in the individual who avoids close relationships with others and who cannot be emotionally expressive in a direct way. He is inclined toward daydreaming, aloofness, emotional detachment. He avoids competition and his daydreams revolve around being a person of remarkable attractiveness or great prowess. He is often unsociable and eccentric and, in general, makes a very unsatisfactory social contribution.

Illustrative of the **cyclothymic personality** is the individual who seems to have an outgoing personality with surface warmth and generosity. He reaches out to others and has an enthusiasm for competition. However, he is inclined to have moods of mild depression and his geniality is usually reserved for outsiders. He is apt to be indifferent to and sometimes actually cruel to his family or to others whom he knows well. Such an individual, with an extreme sensitivity in his interpersonal relationships, may show envy, extreme jealousy, suspiciousness and stubbornness and is prone to feel himself exploited by the environment.

The prognosis for change in individuals with these disturbances is in general rather poor. First, they practically never become cured or changed when left to themselves. If they change at all it is through a long period of intensive psychotherapy in the form of psychoanalysis. The inherent traits referred to often prevent them from obtaining a very good result from such intensive psychotherapeutic treatment. However, if there exists within such a person a fairly strong desire to change and if there are strong family supports, such a patient might derive some help from intensive psychotherapy. It should be emphasized that these patients are not regarded as being hereditarily mentally ill. It is felt that their personality difficulties are the result of a certain type of environment—an environment showing little warmth or concern—an environment in which the patient, in early childhood, was forced to the conclusion that he was unwanted by his family.

2. **Personality Trait Disturbances.**   This classification applies to individuals with personality difficulties which are prone to become exaggerated under stress. They may show mild personality changes.

The **emotionally unstable personality** reacts with excitability when confronted by minor stress. Under such circumstances his judgment may be poor and, in his dealings with people, harmony is always being threatened by latent hostility, guilt and anxiety.

The **passive-aggressive personality** is classified into three types. The **passive-dependent type** is characterized by helplessness, indecisiveness and a tendency to cling to others. The **passive-aggressive type** exhibits pouting, stubbornness, procrastination, inefficiency and passive obstructionism. And finally, the **aggressive type** is the individual who reacts with irritability, resentment, temper tantrums and destructive behavior. The term does not apply to cases more accurately classified as antisocial reaction.

The **compulsive personality** adheres to strict standards of conscience or of conformity. He is overinhibited, overconscientious but often has an inordinate capacity for work.

3. **Sociopathic Personality Disturbance.**   This characterization is applied to those who are ill in terms of a deficiency in conformity to conventional cultural codes. When allowed to do as they please they suffer no personal discomfort. However, their behavior may represent an underlying personality disorder of considerable severity even up to and including a masked psychosis.

Antisocial reaction is a term applied to those who are frequently in trouble and who do not profit by experience or punishment. They maintain no real loyalty to any person, group or code. They are usually callous, self-centered, and are greatly concerned with their own gratification and insensitive to the feeling and needs of others. They lack a sense of responsibility, have poor judgment and are very good at excusing their own behavior.

The **dyssocial reaction** is a term applied to people who disregard the usual social codes and come in conflict with them as a result of having lived all their lives in an abnormal home environment. They may be quite loyal and adhere to codes within their own group but feel no compunction whatever about exploiting society as a whole. Nomadic groups such as gypsies fall into this category.

Sexual deviations of various sorts should be classified under the sociopathic personality disturbances. These include homosexuality, tranvestism (wearing clothes of the opposite sex), pedophilia (preying upon and seducing children by adults), fetishism (sexual excitement obtained by the ownership of some piece of clothing or other symbol of the opposite sex) and sexual sadism (rape, sexual assault and mutilation).

In recent years an effort has been made to subdivide a group of cases formerly called "psychopathic personality" or "constitutional psychopathic inferior." These terms are no longer being used but specific reactions are referred to under any one of the three groupings just named.

Psychopathology of the Personality Disorders.   As already stated, these disorders do not seem to be hereditary. It is believed that they are the result of environmental disturbances—that is, a failure during childhood to meet the emotional needs of the growing child. When needs are not met and frustration occurs, when cruelty and disregard are practiced, personalities must develop self-centeredly. Distorted thinking seems to occur as follows, "Nobody cares for me, I must care for myself. Since no one has shown me kindness, I do not need to show any in return—in fact, if I do, I will only get hurt."

It is said that people with personality disorders are hard, that they have no conscience. It is true that they have not been sensitized to an awareness of the feelings and needs of others and they have not been helped to relate themselves to others in a helpful, friendly way. As a result they become cold, self-centered, distrustful. Some actively and aggressively behave as if they wish to take revenge upon someone for the lacks in their own early life. Others misbehave more passively in subtle ways and seem to expect society to understand, absorb and pay for their personality deficiencies.

Prognosis.   The prognosis in all of these personality disorders is not good. First, the patient rarely wants treatment. Second, even if he should undertake treatment, he has little incentive to undergo the pain and distress of change. And finally, by the time he has become a social problem, the family and society are so angry with him that they are unlikely to have the patience for an intensive treatment program with its heavy cost and time-consuming effort. Further, it must be remembered that such patients are devoid of a feeling of wanting to change or working for love so that successful treatment would have to take place in an institution where freedom would be held out as a goal while attempts at therapy were being made.

Treatment.   Treatment of these cases should progress, we believe, along psychotherapeutic lines. With enforced institutionalization to serve as a lever, appropriate affects might be aroused and the patient helped to understand himself, abreact some of his distressing emotions and be able to make attachment to, identify with and try to emulate some healthy member of society—usually someone in the therapeutic setting.

Undoubtedly considerable experimentation will have to be made with treatment of these patients. They are difficult problems and new treatment techniques will have to be developed. More education will be necessary to make the public in general and the families in particular aware that the treatment of these patients is slow and tedious, and requires highly skilled professional and personal help.

Addiction.   Many narcissistic persons are unable to find enough emotional satisfaction and so resort to alcohol or drugs, which dull the pain of reality and give them gratification in fantasy. All alcoholics and drug addicts have some form of neurotic personality disturbance. They have a longing for affection which they cannot gratify. They have social anxiety and often live a solitary emotional life. They cannot love altruistically, so that they derive little real satisfaction from heterosexual activity. Consequently, they may renounce sex entirely, and find happiness and satisfaction only in overindulgence in alcohol or drugs. When they are under its influence their self-esteem is raised to a tolerable level. Then they can be friendly, especially with those of their own sex, but because of their unusual sensitivity, irritability is likely to break through on slight provocation.

ALCOHOLISM.   The personality problem of the alcoholic is such that he is one of the most difficult treatment problems encountered in medicine today. Family and friends may consult the clergyman and the family physician as to what to do while the patient himself may be indifferent to his plight. As has been so often stated, the problem drinker has a lack of concern about the feelings of others which is crucial in regard to treatment. When he wants to drink, he does not care what his family thinks, what his employer thinks, what his fellow workmen think. He becomes completely absorbed in trying to improve his sense of well-being—temporarily at least—with alcohol. This lack of concern which he shows for family, friends, employer and others holds equally true for the physician. The family physician and even the psychiatrist find it difficult to hold the alcoholic's interest and concern.

Usually, the problem drinker does far better in Alcoholics Anonymous, an organization founded about two decades ago which is conducted on the local level by abstinent alcoholics. They meet regularly each week for inspiration and sociability and for exchange of ideas. They give personal help to the alcoholic who sincerely wishes to gain release from his drinking habit. This organization has done wonders for many thousands of alcoholics. Some people are reluctant to identify themselves with Alcoholics Anonymous and, if they take treatment at all, they insist upon more personal attention than the group form of therapy. Few psychiatrists of experience are willing to attempt to treat the alcoholic by psychotherapy in an ambulatory way since he does not bring his neurosis for treatment in the serious, consistent manner of other psychiatric cases. Many problem drinkers have to enter an institution for a period of time where they have the security of the institution and the personnel to take them away from alcohol and where they get a new perspective on their drinking problem.

During the last decade a drug has been developed that helps the alcoholic abstain from drinking. Antabuse, given in doses from 0.5 to 1.5 grams daily, will produce unpleasant physiological symptoms if the patient reverts to drinking. However, the patient must be in good physical condition to undertake the Antabuse therapy and he must be fairly cooperative in order to remain on this drug. If the drug is discontinued, drinking may be resumed within a few days.

The management of alcoholism is really not very satisfactory in any treatment situation. The family physician who sets out to try to help alcoholics must reckon with an uneven treatment record. Some patients will respond fairly well and others will be most resistant to therapy. Alcoholics are time-consuming patients, capricious and unpredictable, and the physician should make a special study of treatment or, if possible, link himself with a colleague who specializes in the care of this illness.

DRUG ADDICTION.   In spite of increased concern, drug addiction has not lessened in the past decade. The medical profession still needs to exercise caution in prescribing drugs even though few drug addictions are brought about in this way. Not only is there a growing problem with the narcotic drugs but the abuse of barbiturates is increasing rapidly. More and more people are depending upon their "sleeping pill" at night. Such individuals are highly indulgent and refuse to do their resting at night without being anesthetized. Not infrequently the barbiturates are taken as "anxiety relievers" before a meeting or conference, or some taxing social situation. Dependency upon them grows.

There is also an increasing tendency to use stimulating drugs to increase alertness while studying, driving a car or for a "pickup" in the morning. Some of our many automobile accidents are due to the fact that these drugs have been utilized to excess so that judgment has become impaired. Needless to say this indiscriminate use of drugs should be discouraged by physicians.

There are also addictions resulting from morphine substitutes. It stands to reason that any drug which functions as well as morphine to relieve pain and reduce tension and enhance the sense of well-being will be repeatedly resorted to by patients as well as others.

Psychopathology.   It seems possible that any person can become addicted to the use of narcotics. Living in accordance with the pleasure principle would doubtless assume the ascendancy if drugs were administered over a sufficiently long period under the proper circumstances. Such an assumption cannot be proved, of course, but a study of the psychopathology of addicts indicates that it is the ego's inability to deal with reality in a way that brings adequate instinctual gratification through the conventional routes that causes one to fall prey to the very inadequate adaptation to life through drug addiction. The drug user demands that his sense of well-being be fed by something taken within the body rather than by an altruistic activity of some kind through his own mental efforts. This equates with the state of affairs in infancy when he demanded comfort without being capable of any socially useful effort of his own. The drug addict regresses to this level.

It should be said that psychiatric formulations of addiction do not satisfy the neurophysiologist and pharmacologist. The discovery of the "tranquilizing drugs" and the development of the hallucinogenic drug, the diethylamide of lysergic acid (LSD-25), have led to an investigation of mental disease in terms other than psychological, to seek for evidence of chemical defects at cellular levels. Pharmacologists are using electrophysiological techniques in studying drugs at the same time that psychological techniques for assessing behavioral changes induced by drugs in both man and animals are being utilized. Within the last few years growth in the borderline fields of psychopharmacology and neuropharmacology have been astonishing and may yield important information not only in regard to addiction but in the whole realm of mental illness (Isbell).

Management.   Management of the addict involves several principles. First, he must be hospitalized while under treatment since his self-control is never adequate to meet the distress of withdrawal without the aid of enforced abstinence. Next, the use of one of the ataraxic drugs has been found to be of great value in minimizing the withdrawal symptoms. And lastly, an intensive social and psychotherapeutic rehabilitation must go on following withdrawal of the drug to bring about both insight and ego growth so that the patient can live a successful life—a satisfying and useful life which will be adequately gratifying without the use of drugs. A modern psychiatric institution or one devoted to the treatment of addicts is necessary for this program.

THE MECHANISM OF PSYCHOSOMATIC DISORDERS

We have tried to indicate that the psychopathology of psychophysiologic disorders does not differ essentially from that of the neuroses and psychoses. Freud's theory of the libido and his concept of anxiety prove just as useful in this as in the latter field. The psychopathology of psychosomatic disorders is merely an extension or a fuller utilization of what we have learned. It is a further application of our knowledge that disturbed emotions may disturb bodily functions, not only temporarily but permanently, so that finally even structural changes may occur.

The study of the total reaction of the organism in contrast to the study of isolated functions has received a new impetus from animal psychology. Taking their departure from the school of Pavlov, which dealt mainly with circumscribed conditioned reflexes, a vigorous group of animal experimenters in this country have succeeded in producing neurotic symptoms in animals by increasing the difficulties of certain tasks with which the animals were confronted if they were to satisfy their hunger. In these studies the investigator's interest was directed toward the behavior of the whole animal.

Such observers as Masserman, Gantt, and Liddell by their important researches have thrown interesting light on this subject. It is difficult to predict what such observations will prove in regard to human behavior and human illness but it does offer a technique for studying psychological reactions in which the factors involved are few in number and therefore lend themselves to manipulation and exact observation.

Physiological Responses to Emotions.   Alexander, who has made notable contributions to this subject, develops the concept somewhat after the following fashion:

The classic experiments of Cannon on the physiological effects of fear, hunger, pain and rage laid the basis for many of the psychosomatic studies of today. It is well known from everyday experience that emotions such as fear, anger, resentment, guilt or embarrassment have definite physiological effects. We are well aware that weeping, laughing, blushing, and even disturbances in bowel and bladder control occur under the influence of strong emotions. These, however, are all transitory processes occurring in the everyday life of healthy persons. Systematic psychosomatic studies have shown not only that transitory physiological changes may be caused by the emotions but that sustained emotional strain may lead to chronic disturbances of physiological functions. These in turn may be responsible for certain bodily diseases.

Alexander continues by stating that these ideas introduced a cleavage in medical thinking because the emotions as a cause of illness and disease were not so tangible as germs or allergens. Moreover, the medical man took refuge in the fact that these physiological processes did after all have to originate in the body. For example, that such an emotion as embarrassment may cause *blushing* was answered by the medical scientist thus:

"Well, blushing can be explained physiologically. The dilatation of the blood vessels in the cheek is caused by nerve impulses conducted from higher brain centers via the autonomic nervous system. What the psychologist or psychoanalyst calls embarrassment, in the last analysis, is *nothing but some physiological process in the brain.* This physiological process in the brain which is conducted through the nervous system to the blood vessels of the cheek is the only thing which merits scientific consideration."

"This response," Alexander goes on, "is correct except for the statement 'embarrassment is nothing but a process in the brain.' Embarrassment certainly is a distinct process in the brain, but at the same time it is a subjective sensation which can be described in psychological terms and which also merits scientific consideration. In fact, at the present state of our knowledge it can be described only in psychological terms. We do not know much about the nature of that assumed physiological process which takes place in the brain when a person feels embarrassment. However, embarrassment as a psychological phenomenon can be most precisely described by the person who blushes. The person can tell us—of course, only if he wants to—whether he was embarrassed because he lied, or because he was praised, or because he suddenly heard the voice of his sweetheart.

"It is obvious, therefore, that at present if we want to study scientifically the phenomenon of blushing, we do better if we examine its causes in psychological terms. We may hope that some time in the future we shall also know the concomitant physiological processes, but even then it is an open question whether we shall dispense with our psychological understanding of embarrassment. For example: One person blushes when praised by the teacher in the presence of others because in childhood he had competed with his brother for parental approval and, remembering the illicit means by which he often obtained this approval, he now feels guilty and ashamed. Could the most minute physiological description explain as much as does this psychological one? Even so common a process as blushing from embarrassment can be understood fully only in the light of the life history of the individual. The same is true for weeping or laughter. Only when we know what makes Smith so sensitive to certain human events can we understand why his eyes fill with tears over a sentimental scene in the movies, whereas Jones in the same situation remains completely composed. Only the history of Mr. Smith and Mr. Jones will explain to us how and why the one became highly sensitized to seeing an old, helpless man peering through a window at a happy family on a Christmas Eve and why the other found the same scene trite and boring. Whether the most advanced brain physiology will ever be able to substitute for this type of knowledge is certainly an open question. It is difficult to imagine that it will.

"Certain it is, however, that at the present state of our knowledge the factors which cause weeping, laughing, or blushing cannot be properly described without using both psychological and physiological methods. The innervation of the tear gland in weeping or the dilatation of the blood vessels in blushing, the conduction of the nerve influences from the brain cortex to the eyes and the cheek can only be described in physiological terms, whereas the causative emotions are definable only in psychological terms. Similarly the local processes which immediately cause the ulceration of the stomach or an asthmatic attack must be described in strictly physiological terms; the causative emotional tensions, on the other hand, must be described and understood in psychological terms. Omitting this psychological part of the whole process does not increase the scientific nature of our description. On the contrary, understanding the local mechanisms involved in the development of an ulcer or asthma is only half of the story. Omitting the other half, the part which requires at our present state of knowledge psychological descriptions, would be to give up the most important aim of medicine, the understanding of causes. An appropriate use of psychological and physiological methods of description—each in its proper place—is the essence of the psychosomatic approach."

Alexander concludes that the interrelation of biochemical changes and emotions is today beyond question. Emotional tensions through the autonomic nervous system do influence the body chemistry and the changed body chemistry in turn reacts upon the emotional life. With the clear recognition of such mutual influences the cleavage between emotional and organic factors can be relegated to the past. Body chemistry and emotions do not represent two different sets of facts, one physical, the other mental. When we speak of emotions we refer always to definite physical processes in the brain which, however, can be studied psychologically because these brain processes are perceived subjectively as emotions and can be communicated to others by the use of language. The combined biochemical and psychological approach is now only in its beginnings but will undoubtedly become the main trend of future research and therapy.

The Adaptation Syndrome.   Of importance in any consideration of the role of the emotions in physiological integrations are the studies of Selye which culminated in his description of the "General Adaptation Syndrome." With this concept, Selye attempts to integrate a number of seemingly unrelated observations into a single unified biologic system. The keynote of unification is the tenet that all living organisms can respond to stress as such and that in this respect the basic reaction pattern is always the same, irrespective of the agent which produces the stress. This response is called the general adaptation syndrome—its derailments, the diseases of adaptation. Anything that causes stress endangers life, unless it is met by adequate adaptive responses; conversely, anything that endangers life causes stress and adaptive responses. Adaptability and resistance to stress are fundamental prerequisites for life, and every vital organ and function participates in them.

Selye postulates that exposure of the organism to stress (any nonspecific noxious stimulus of sufficient intensity) will cause the liberation of toxic metabolites in the tissues and the production of the first stage of the syndrome, viz., the alarm reaction. This stage is divisible into two distinct phases. The first or shock phase is characterized by tachycardia, decrease in muscle tone and body temperature, formation of gastric and intestinal ulcers, hemoconcentration, anuria, edema, hypochlorhydria, leukopenia followed by leukocytosis, acidosis, a transitory hyperglycemia followed by a decrease in blood sugar, and a discharge of epinephrine from the adrenal medulla.

Mirsky, interested in the endocrine as well as emotional aspects of the adaptation syndrome, summarizes Selye's studies as follows:

"If the damage is not too severe and permits survival, the toxic metabolites stimulate the anterior lobe of the pituitary to discharge adrenocorticotropic hormone which, in turn, stimulates the secretion of adrenal cortical hormones, and thereby raises the resistance of the body. This results in the second phase of the alarm reaction, viz., the counter-shock phase. This phase is characterized by an enlarged and hyperactive adrenal cortex, rapid involution of the thymus and other lymphatic organs and a reversal of most of the signs characteristic of the shock phase.

"If the noxious stimulus is continued, the counter-shock phase gives way to the second stage of the general adaptation syndrome, the stage of resistance, at which time there is a regression of most of the morphological lesions observed in the first stage; and resistance to the continued stimulus reaches a minimum. This stage is attributed to the continued secretion of cortical hormones. The third and final stage of the syndrome appears after prolonged exposure to the noxious stimuli and is called the stage of exhaustion and is attributed to a failure in the adaptive mechanisms. When this occurs, the lesions characteristic of the alarm reaction reappear, and death ensues.

"Under special experimental conditions, exposure to non-specific noxious agents may cause hypertension, nephrosclerosis, myocardial lesions and arthritides. These Selye attributed to the excessive amounts of pituitary and adrenal cortical hormones which are produced to increase the resistance to the action of the noxious stimuli. Selye calls these the 'diseases of adaptation.' The clinical studies of Albright, of Brown and of others lend support to Selye's concept and indicate that stress situations in man also may induce the adaptation syndrome."

The Response to Stress in Man.   Man has been able to adapt himself to the vicissitudes of life—to heat and cold, to dry and wet, to sunlight and darkness. He can mobilize defenses against invading organisms and within certain limits has the remarkable capacity to recover from physical injury. The great majority of people make satisfactory adjustments to acute and chronic emotional stress. While the mechanisms by which this is accomplished are complex and not yet understood, it is known that the pituitary-adrenal system and hypothalamus are fundamentally involved. One must subscribe to the conservative statement that in the endocrine and hypothalamic system are mechanisms which together can explain some of the interrelations between physiological and psychological function. Selye, Thorn and MacLean deserve special mention for their pioneer work in illuminating this concept.

Evaluation of the role of the adrenal cortex in the response of man to stressful situations has been a problem of major interest to medical investigators. Thorn and his associates have made many contributions to this subject employing changes in the level of circulating lymphocytes or eosinophils and in the urinary excretion of 17-ketosteroids as indicators of adrenal cortical activation. Further studies, by the same group (Hill and others), of college oarsmen before and after racing employed techniques which measured adrenal cortical activation more directly; at the same time psychiatric and psychological studies were made.

It was found that physical activity alone was not the major factor responsible for adrenal activation and the marked fall in circulating eosinophils, because during practice sessions, in which muscular effort closely approximated that which was exhibited during the varsity race, the response was minimal, whereas the added psychological stress of the race produced marked changes. Also favoring the importance of psychological factors was the observation that the coxswain and the manager displayed an eosinopenia as marked as that of the crew members.

The "Visceral Brain."   MacLean credits Papez with a theory regarding a mechanism of emotion in which the rhinencephalon and the hypothalamus are looked upon as the centers of elaborate emotions. While the rhinencephalon in higher animal forms yields more and more control over the animal's movements to the neocortex, its persistent, strong connections with the lower autonomic centers suggest that it continues to dominate in the realm of visceral activity. Consequently MacLean refers to it as "the visceral brain" to distinguish it from the neocortex which controls the body musculature and subserves the function of the intellect.

In primitive forms the visceral brain provides the highest correlation center for ordering the affective behavior of the animal in such basic drives as obtaining and assimilating food, fleeing from or orally disposing of an enemy, reproducing, and so forth. It is likely that the visceral brain continues to subserve such functions in higher forms, including man. It is probable, then, that this primitive brain would have significant implications in regard to symbolism affecting the emotional life of the individual. MacLean asserts that if the visceral brain participates in this symbolic representation of unrelated phenomena and at the same time lacks the analyzing ability of the word brain (neocortex), it is possible to conceive how it might become involved in a variety of correlations leading to symptoms of emotional origin. Lacking the control of neocortex, its impressions would be discharged without modifications into the hypothalamus and lower centers. Considered in the light of psychoanalytic observation, the visceral brain would have many of the attributes of the unconscious. Thus certain puzzling aspects of the psychological status of patients with psychosomatic disease would be more readily understood. For example, patients with superior attainment in the intellectual sphere often have evidences of an arrest of their emotional development at the infantile level. Thus there may be a great difference between what they "feel" and what they "know."

The question arises in reference to psychosomatic disease as to whether or not patterns of emotional behavior leading to excessive visceral expression are repeated so often in childhood as to become permanently ingrained in the visceral brain, with the result that they are perpetuated in later life. In the psychosomatic patient it would almost seem there is little direct connection between the visceral brain and the word brain, and that feelings, instead of being relayed to the intellect for evaluation, find immediate expression through autonomic centers. In other words, feelings, instead of finding expression and discharge in the symbolic use of words and appropriate behavior, might be conceived as being translated into a kind of "organ language." Such a concept, says MacLean, would have a bearing on some of the differences that have been noted between patients with psychoneuroses and those with psychosomatic illness. The former have reached a higher level of emotional development and have a greater facility than psychosomatic patients in giving verbal expression to, and "acting out," their feelings. Again MacLean calls attention to a psychotherapeutic point of considerable importance, namely, that in the psychosomatic disorder one would expect less benefit from words and interpretations than from the doctor-patient relationship; in other words, less benefit from an intellectual approach and more benefit from an approach utilizing the feelings (transference).

This concept of a visceral brain has far-reaching implications for psychiatry. It suggests that our intellectual functions are carried on in the newest and most highly developed part of the brain (neocortex), while our affective behavior continues to be dominated by a relatively crude and primitive system (the visceral brain). This, says MacLean, provides a clue to understanding the difference between what we "feel" and what we "know."

Relation to Mental Processes. The demonstration by Selye that the pituitary–adrenal mechanism must be intact in order for an animal to survive a shocking stimulus constituted an important discovery in biology. Although it is probably true that the reaction of this system represents only one aspect of a very complex mechanism called forth in man in response to stress, the observations have had a tremendous effect on the development of our thinking about both the physiological and psychological aspects of this problem.

Selye and Fortier called attention to the fact that important alterations in the morphology and function of the nervous system can result from hypo- or hyperactivity of the pituitary–adrenal system, the main endocrine regulator of adaptive processes, and that the coexistence of disordered endocrine mechanisms with psychoneurotic or psychotic states suggests some relationship between pituitary–adrenal and mental processes. It has been observed that stimuli of a neurogenic or psychogenic nature are particularly potent activators of the pituitary adrenocorticotropic function and produce rapid and intense alarm reactions.

From the very first observations on the treatment of chronic arthritis with cortisone and ACTH it was noted that striking changes in mood and mental outlook occurred. At first it was believed that the feeling of well-being was the natural response of a chronically ill person to the dramatic improvement brought about by these new preparations, for example, the patient with chronic deforming arthritis, leading a wheel chair existence, who was suddenly enabled to walk again. However, with further experience it was noted that certain mental effects could hardly be accounted for on this basis, and, indeed, instead of exhibiting euphoria some patients became depressed and others actually psychotic.

Clark, Bauer and Cobb reported a detailed study of 10 patients with severe arthritis who presented evidence of a mental disorder in connection with the administration of these drugs. They did not regard it as a form of toxic delirium nor were they able to draw any positive conclusions about the cause of the disturbance from their studies. Some of the early symptoms were insomnia, restlessness, delusional ideas, and a peculiar feeling in the front of the head sometimes followed by a frank psychosis. Fortunately, complete recovery occurred spontaneously in all cases. Other similar observations have been made. Rome and Braceland found severe mental reactions in 10 per cent of 100 patients treated with these drugs at the Mayo Clinic, and Brody concluded that the variety of reactions to these drugs depended upon the personality of the patient. The drugs brought out the latent emotional responses of the individual. Most patients showed some initial euphoria but this gave way to various reactions in keeping with the individual personality structure.

However, Goolker and Schein in a careful study of 80 patients encountered on the general medical wards of Mt. Sinai Hospital, New York City, in whom the major emphasis in treatment was with cortisone and ACTH, concluded that only 15 per cent showed distinctly aberrant reactions and that most of these were transient, self-limited and mild in character. They found a complete discrepancy between the dosage, the pretreatment state and the psychic outcome. They described the primary mental change as a state of cerebral excitability which occurs during the first few hours after the drug is given.

At the same symposium Fox and Gifford reported their psychological observations on 98 patients who had received ACTH or cortisone. The three most nearly constant findings were alterations in appetite, sleep and motor activity. Most of the patients felt stimulated and experienced a sense of well-being. When the drugs were discontinued, they felt a sense of emptiness and depression. ACTH and cortisone bring about an acceleration of the rate of biochemical change and promote the mobilization of energy for cellular work. The authors present the hypothesis that these metabolic changes constitute physiological sources of instinctual tension and result in an increased drive to discharge energy or an increased need to obtain instinctual satisfaction. In a discussion of this paper George Engel pointed out the necessity for caution in the evaluation of behavioral changes attributed to administered hormones. He called attention to the great difficulty involved in the interpretation of the interrelationship of biological and psychic processes.

While the evidence is far from conclusive it does suggest that there are definite behavioral aspects which must be taken into account in the administration of the steroid preparations, but the implications in regard to the theory of instincts cannot be judged at this time.

Organ Neurosis.   As we have already indicated, conversion symptoms are symbolic substitute expressions for an unbearable emotion which the individual represses and therefore cannot express through the normal channels of voluntary behavior. In addition to this conversion mechanism Alexander describes a different type of emotionally

conditioned bodily disturbance which manifests itself in the viscera and
is referred to as *vegetative neurosis.*

A simple example is the elevation of blood pressure under the influence of emotion such as rage and fear. Here the elevation of blood
pressure has no direct psychological meaning. It is not a symbolic expression of rage or fear; rather it is a physiological concomitant of the
emotional states of rage and fear. Whereas a conversion symptom is a
symbolic expression of a well defined psychological content (an attempt
at relief), a vegetative neurosis is not an attempt to express an emotion
but is the normal physiological accompaniment of constant or periodically recurring emotional states. Chronic emotional tension causes
chronic vegetative changes, and it is the chronicity of the condition
which makes it morbid. Alexander suggests that the clarification of this
issue has both theoretical and practical significance. It saves us from
erroneous and futile therapeutic attempts to "interpret" such bodily
expressions psychologically. Instead the physician who correctly understands the nature of these disturbances will try to help the patient to
overcome certain chronic unrelieved emotional states which have a disturbing influence upon the vegetative functions of the organism.

SPECIFICITY.   According to one assumption, any emotional tension
may influence any vegetative function. The choice of symptom depends
upon the history of the patient and his constitution: If he has a weak
stomach, he might have a stomach upset when he gets angry; if he has
a labile vasomotor system, he might develop high blood pressure under
the influence of unrelieved aggressions. A quite different assumption,
which may be called the theory of specificity, has guided the work of
Alexander and his associates. According to their view, "physiological
responses vary with the *quality* of the emotional state. Just as external
behavior varies according to the nature of the emotion, so responses in
the nervous control of the visceral organs vary. We know from experiments with animals that every emotional state has its specific vegetative
tonus. The vegetative reactions to rage and fear are different, for example, from those due to relaxation during the process of digestion. It
is to be expected therefore that the vegetative disturbance will vary in
correspondence with the chronic unrelieved emotional state. The question is still undecided, however, to what extent constitutional factors
or preexisting organic pathology or sensitivity influence different clinical
pictures. Further careful clinical studies will have to decide this important issue."

Thus in the chapter on gastrointestinal problems we shall again quote
from the studies of Alexander and his associates and show that in peptic
ulcer the major problem surrounds a conflict between a conscious desire
for independence and success, and strong unconscious cravings of
passivity and dependence.

PERSONALITY TRENDS.   In regard to this question Saul calls attention to the fact that it is the oral form of attachment to the mother,
consisting of a mixture of impulses, desires and feelings which become
interwoven with sucking and later the eating mechanisms, that enters
into psychosomatic gastrointestinal problems. Other biological mech-

anisms and forms of attachment to the mother seem to be important in the allergies. These are the dermal and respiratory. In other words, in many persons the form of attachment to the mother as seen in fantasies, dreams and real life is not, as in many instances of gastrointestinal disorders, strongly "oral," but consists rather in a desire for shelter. The longings are represented not by wishes to be fed and all that this can imply emotionally, but by wishes to be sheltered and protected. Such individuals often gravitate to modes of life which gratify these tendencies. Perhaps it could be said that, given a choice, they would prefer snug housing to good food. Here, too, can be points of weakness and fixation, to form a physiological pathway for the attachment to the mother and become interwoven with powerful feelings and longings.

When the relationship to the mother, with all of its significance to the child (and in later life, unconsciously, to the adult) is threatened, or when a person is under stress, the longings for help or consolation are expressed in various combinations or forms in different persons—wanting to be fed, wanting to be carried or led, wanting to be snuggled and sheltered, and so on—reflecting the oral, ambulatory, dermal, respiratory, and other mechanisms and forms of attachment to the mother. The impulses may be gratified by personal relationships, sexual or sublimated, which reestablish in some degree the relationship to the mother. Examples of sublimated forms of gratification are: oral, eating and drinking; respiratory, talking and crying; dermal, baths and massage. The impulses may be repressed so that symptoms appear when the tension disturbs organ function. Of course, oral as well as dermal and respiratory trends can exist in the same individual.

Saul concludes, "The dermal and respiratory mechanisms, trends, and relations to the mother are analogous to the oral ones. They are fundamental to an understanding of psychobiological functioning. Preliminary observations strongly suggest that they play a role in the skin and respiratory allergies similar to that of the oral trends in the gastrointestinal disorders."

EVIDENCE AGAINST SPECIFICITY.   In recent years opinion has been moving away from the concept of specific personality types and personality profiles for psychosomatic disorders. In a well reasoned discussion of this subject Kubie finds it difficult to check the correlations of the clinical observations of definite personality types with specific disorders. "Again and again, on examination of patients suffering from clinically identical disorders, e.g., from migraine, ulcerative colitis or cardiospasm, I have been impressed by the dissimilarities at least as vividly as by the similarities among the individuals in each clinical group. Indeed I could not convince myself that the similarities were greater than those which obtain among any heterogeneous group of neurotic patients. To that I add a fact that is well known to all of us: namely, that as one explores deeply in any analysis, one comes to certain common origins of the neurotic process, whereupon seemingly sharp differences in the symptoms with which the patient has presented himself appear to be relatively superficial vagaries superimposed on the more constant underlying neurotic process. Thus in the course of time most analysts come to feel that the neurotic process is remarkably constant, while the neurotic symptom is as variable as is the dream symbol. An equally wide variety, it seems, is possible for neurotic symptoms in general, and for psychosomatic disturbances in particular. This point receives further substantiation from the fact that in different phases the same patient may represent his problems in psychosomatic constellations which are wholly different from one another. In one patient an ulcerative colitis was replaced by a severe dermatitis which in turn was replaced by a severe migraine, all of them finally being replaced by a psychotic break.

"Under these circumstances it would seem that the quest for a uniform specificity in psychosomatic disorders arises out of a fallacious assumption about the specificity of the dynamic sequences in the etiology of the neuroses in general."

Kubie poses three basic questions:

1. What in general are the indivisible dynamic units in the neurotic process?

2. At what point in the chain of events do specific determinants become operative?

3. Finally, how does the psychosomatic process as such arise? Why does the effort to solve an unconscious conflict ever turn in the bodily direction?

Kubie considers that until we can answer the third question, it is unlikely that we will find specific factors for specific types of personality dysfunction.

Macalpine also feels that in the absence of basic understanding of the mechanism of psychosomatic symptom formation it is impossible to maintain that there are definite psychosomatic personality types. She insists that one must differentiate psychosomatic from psychoneurotic symptom formation. In her view, psychosomatic symptom formation is not caused by the necessity for symbolic representation. It is not a defense against psychological conflict but a disorder of physiological function which cannot be translated into psychological terms. She feels that it is more closely related to psychosis than neurosis and calls for a different kind of therapeutic approach. Instead of psychoanalytic treatment it may yield to a more superficial therapy.

Macalpine thinks that the psychosomatic symptom represents a remnant of an early anxiety state experienced by the body-mind unit in its preconceptual and preverbal stage.

The Interaction of Psyche and Soma. If we think of psychosomatic illness from the standpoint of a continuum or frequency distribution curve, the soma might be placed at one end and the psyche at the other. Then an illness, for example asthma, might be placed at any spot on this frequency distribution curve depending upon the contribution from the somatic (allergic) or psychic background. For example, in a case of seasonal asthma, occurring in connection with ragweed hay fever, the somatic contribution might be so important that one would place the case at the somatic end of the curve, whereas in another patient with perennial asthma, in which allergic factors appeared to play an unimportant role while psychological factors seemed of greater importance, one would place the case near the psychic end of the curve. However, in many instances the contribution of soma and psyche might be so nearly equal that such cases would be placed at the top of the curve. This is the way we prefer to think of psychosomatic affections (see p. 74).

However, in many instances of illness—even in the example cited of asthma—there are so many factors that enter into the problem and in so many devious ways that it is perhaps an oversimplification to try to divide them strictly into somatic and psychological forces, unless one thinks of the soma in terms of heredity as well as acquired factors and of the psyche as composed of social as well as emotional factors. Then, too, one must consider the soma as interacting with the psyche in both directions, i.e., soma affecting psyche as well as the reverse.

In this connection an important consideration in regard to psychosomatic affections is their relation to each other and to mental disorders. Halliday, working with the insured population of the Scottish health service, stated the problem in this way. He finds that "different psychosomatic affections may appear in the same individuals simultaneously, but the more usual phenomenon, as revealed in their natural history, is that of the alternation or of the sequence of different affections.

"The sequence of peptic ulcer, fibrositis, and bronchitis is not uncommon in the medical history of middle-aged persons who have been on the sick list for long periods. It is possible that the changing endocrinological setting associated with particular phases of the life cycle may be one of the factors determining such sequences. The adult, like the child, may 'grow out' of one affection, but he may grow into another."

The Relationship of Psychosomatic and Mental Disorders.   Halliday also observed that a study of the natural history of psychosomatic affections shows that neurotic or psychotic illnesses may accompany psychosomatic organic diseases or may appear as preceding, alternating or sequent disorders. During the course of psychoanalytical treatment this switching over is sometimes illustrated dramatically when, as a mental symptom becomes alleviated, a somatic manifestation takes its place.

"It has been suggested that the appearance of an idiopathic psychosis (schizophrenia, manic-depressive psychosis, paranoia) renders a psychosomatic expression unnecessary—a statement which is only partially true, since patients with these disorders often show functional disorders of the skin, as well as abnormalities in posture. There is, however, some rather loose evidence suggesting that among sufferers from the psychoses certain common psychosomatic affections such as peptic ulcer, rheumatoid arthritis and fibrositis are relatively rare. Psychosis and psychosomatic organic disease may alternate."

At the Boston State Hospital Swartz and Semrad found an incidence of psychosomatic disorders of 3.4 per cent in 518 psychotic patients as contrasted to 4.5 per cent in the nonpsychotic group. They suggest, what has often been mentioned before, that psychosomatic disorders are in a sense a defense and a protection against a psychotic break—that to a certain extent an "either (psychosomatic) —or (psychotic)" mechanism may prevail. They have the impression that psychosomatic and psychotic disorders are not only incompatible but that each is to a great extent mutually effective in excluding the other. They do not find any correlation between specific psychosomatic disorders and specific psychotic disorders.

Observations on 32 psychotic patients with bronchial asthma by Sabbath and Luce showed that asthma preceded and coexisted with psychosis in 19 patients and appeared to be antagonistic in 11, that is, there were no asthmatic symptoms during the overt psychosis. Occasionally an increase in mental symptoms was accompanied by an increase in the severity of the asthma. In several instances in the latter group there was an abrupt onset of psychosis with sudden cessation of asthmatic symptoms. In general, the patients who retained their asthma during the psychosis showed less break with reality and more nearly intact personality. Whether a patient retained or lost his asthmatic symptoms, the psychosis appeared to be related directly to the amount of the personality uninvolved in the psychotic process and related inversely to the level of psychosis.

Other observers find little evidence for this alternation of psychosis and psychosomatic disorders. Engel's studies of ulcerative colitis fail to demonstrate any reciprocal relationship between this disorder and psychosis.

We are of the opinion that in general such a relationship does exist and that just as in the neuroses physical symptoms and mental distress often alternate, so does the same thing happen with regard to certain vegetative organ disturbances and psychosis.

SUMMARY

As has been said, all illness is a problem of disturbance of psyche and soma, hence *all medicine is psychosomatic medicine.* In fact when this is thoroughly understood there will no longer be a necessity for the term psychosomatic medicine; both parts of the term will be implicit in the word medicine. However, disease has been regarded for many decades as being due to tissue pathology alone, and it is only in recent years that psychiatry, by gaining greater knowledge of the neuroses and psychoses, has shown that the first cause of certain disease pictures is psychopathology rather than tissue pathology. Therefore, psychosomatic medicine represents an extension of our knowledge of neuroses and psychoses to the psychopathology of other conditions previously thought to be in the realm of purely physical medicine. In succeeding chapters attempts will be made to demonstrate not so much that a medical problem is purely functional or purely physical but that psychological and physical factors are both present and that the question becomes: How much of the one and how much of the other is present and what is the relationship between them?

References
Abraham, K.: Selected Papers on Psychoanalysis. Hogarth Press, London, 1927.

Alexander, F.: Psychoanalysis of the Total Personality. Nervous and Mental Disease Publishing Co., New York and Washington, 1930.

Alexander, F.: Modern Attitudes in Psychiatry. Columbia University Press, New York, 1946.

Alexander, F.: Ten-Year Report, Institute for Psychoanalysis, Chicago, pp. 8, 9, 10, 1932-1942.

Alexander, F.: Psychosom. Med., *5:* 205, July, 1943.

Brody, S.: Psychosom. Med., *14:* 94, 1952.

Clark, L. D., Bauer, W., and Cobb, S.: New England J. Med., *246:* 205, 1952.

Ferenczi, S.: Further Contributions to the Theory and Technique of Psychoanalysis. Hogarth Press, London, 1926.

Fox, H. M., and Gifford, S.: Psychosom. Med., *15:* 614, 1953.

Freud, S.: Collected Papers. Vols. I–IV. Hogarth Press, London, 1934.

Freud, S.: Three Contributions to the Theory of Sex. Nervous and Mental Disease Publishing Co., New York and Washington, 1916.

Freud, S.: Psychopathology of Everyday Life. The Macmillan Co., New York, 1919.

Freud, S.: New Introductory Lectures on Psychoanalysis. W. W. Norton and Co., Inc., New York, 1932.

Freud, S.: The Problem of Anxiety. W. W. Norton and Co., Inc., New York, 1936.

Freud, S.: Civilization and Its Discontents. Jonathan Cape and Harrison Smith, New York, 1930.

Glover, E.: Brit. J. M. Psychol., *23:*152, 1932.

Goolker, P., and Schein, J.: Psychosom. Med., *15:* 589, 1953.

Hill, S. R., Jr., et al.: Arch. Int. Med., *97:* 269, 1956.

Isbell, H.: Tr. Coll. Phys., Phila., *24:* 1, 1956.

Jones, E.: Collected Papers on Psychoanalysis. Hogarth Press, London, 1923.

Kubie, L. S.: The Psychosomatic Concept in Psychoanalysis. International Universities Press, New York, 1953, pp. 63–81.

Macalpine, I.: Lancet, *1:* 278, 1952.

MacLean, P. D.: (a) Psychosom. Med., *11:* 338, 1949; (b) Proc. Council High Blood Pressure Research. American Heart Association, New York, 1956.

Menninger, K.: Bull. Menninger Clinic, *7:* 36, 1943.

Menninger, W. C.: Psychiatry in a Troubled World: Yesterday's War and Today's Challenge. The Macmillan Co., New York, 1948.

Mirsky, I. Arthur: The Biology of Diabetes Mellitus in Man, Presented at the Institute on Psychosomatics, University of Nebraska, Feb. 11, 1948.

Rome, H. P., and Braceland, F.: Am. J. Psychiat., *108:* 641, 1952.

Sabbath, J. C., and Luce, R. A.: Psychiat. Quart., *26:* 562, 1952.

Saul, L. J.: Nerv. Child, *5:* 332, 1946.

Saul, L. J.: Emotional Maturity: The Dynamics and Development of Personality, J. B. Lippincott Co., Philadelphia, 1947.

Selye, Hans: J. Clin. Endocrinol., *6:*117, 1946.

Selye, H.: Brit. M. J., *1:* 1383, 1950.

Selye, H., and Fortier, C.: Psychosom. Med., *12:*149, 1950.

Stephen, K.: Psychoanalysis and Medicine. Cambridge University Press, London, 1933.

Swartz, J., and Semrad, E. V.: Psychosom. Med., *13:* 314, 1951.

Thorn, G. W., and Laidlaw, J. C.: Tr. Am. Clin. & Climatol. A., *65:* 179, 1954.

Chapter III

Psychosomatic Diagnosis

Diagnosis depends much more upon the history than it does upon physical examination or laboratory studies. This is especially true in regard to psychosomatic affections. In the first chapter we discussed the faulty concept of functional versus organic disease and the necessity for giving up the "either-or" diagnostic approach. In other words, personality study will show that psychosomatic disorders have their own distinctive features and that diagnosis must be established by the simultaneous application of physiological and psychological techniques. The diagnosis of a "psychosomatic" affection can only be established by positive data from a psychological standpoint *in addition* to an evaluation of the part that physiological and "organic" factors play.

We frequently use the diagrams on the next page to illustrate this topic. The upper diagram illustrates the usual approach in the study of illness which will presumably lead to a diagnosis. It consists of the bare facts of the medical history, the physical examination and the various laboratory investigations. It is *diagnosis by exclusion* and fails in so many instances simply because the personality and life situation of the patient —in other words, a study of the emotional life—which may provide the key to the solution of the problem, is completely neglected or at most inadequately investigated. One of the purposes of this book is to help repair this deficiency. The *proper psychosomatic approach* is shown in the *lower* diagram.

When a person gets sick he is sick all over; that is, the body and mind are one, and he gets sick for a variety of reasons, physical and psychic. In other words, it is usually not one thing that determines illness; it is many things, multiple factors, acting together. As we pointed out in the first chapter, in our approach to illness we must ask ourselves

What kind of person are we dealing with? (inherited and acquired characteristics, physical and psychological)

What has he met? (germs, allergens, or emotionally disturbing events)

What has happened? (physiological mechanism or pathogenesis of the disorder)

Page 71

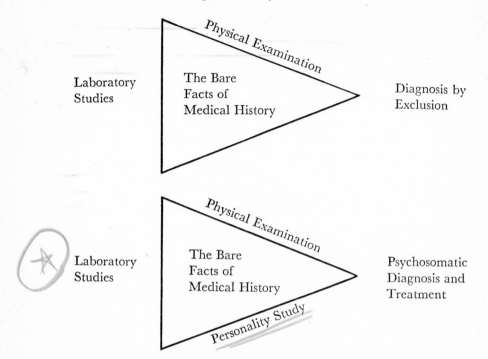

For example, allergic responses occur when a prepared organism, possessing certain physical and psychological characteristics, meets certain elements, physiological and psychological. In some allergic disorders a single preponderant factor may be largely responsible, for example, in pollen hay fever; in others, such as asthma, frequently there are multiple interrelated factors, allergens and psychic disturbances, which act in a complementary fashion to produce the disorder.

THE PSYCHOSOMATIC POINT OF VIEW

This is the psychosomatic point of view: that the psyche enters, or better, emerges as one of the several factors which acting together disturb the function of the organism. We will leave aside the great problem—how much of the illness depends upon constitutional factors and to what extent special life experiences are responsible. It is the old question of heredity and environment, nature and nurture, and we have no way of delimiting these factors with exact measurements.

Generally speaking, physicians look upon the problem of psychic factors in illness in several ways. There is a group which considers the physical factors as being all-important and indeed wholly responsible for any personality change: "Why shouldn't he be nervous after having had such a serious disease so long?" In a smaller group one finds protagonists for *psychogenesis:* "The psychic factor is fundamental and all-important in determining illness." A third group believes that physical and psychological factors are but different phases of the disordered constitution, perhaps parallel manifestations of the same basic fault, existing together and related to one another. To put it another way, psychological forces and somatic manifestations may have their roots in the same unconscious processes which discharge partly on the level of psychic representation through thoughts and feelings and partly on the physiological level through the autonomic nervous system (Kubie). This is the viewpoint which we favor, the psychosomatic viewpoint. We are not interested in proving psychogenesis, we are only interested in studying the psychic factor in illness, just as we study physical factors, and in relating them where possible. We would like the psyche to be treated with as much respect as germs or allergens.

Just as we insist on this unity regarding the nature of illness ("The body and the mind are one"), just so do we urge that the means of investigation are *two* (that is, physical and psychological) and that their simultaneous application represents psychosomatic diagnosis. And they are applied simultaneously although their application is often unconscious and unscientific. The physician in his usual approach to the patient, even when using the orthodox methods of medical history, physical examination and laboratory studies, is at the same time making many intuitive observations about the unconscious mental processes of the patient as exhibited in his language and behavior. As Halliday says, "When we meet an individual we receive certain impressions, and experience certain feelings, which provide us with a sense of the person-as-a-whole—his total characteristics—and to this we give the name of personality. Most medical men, especially perhaps those in general practice, come, as their clinical experience grows, to sense that certain kinds of disease tend to go with certain types of person. The impression of types depends on the general configuration of the patient: on his external expression (which is a matter not only of the facies but also of attitude, posture and manner of movement); on his 'internal expressions' (as revealed outwardly in pallor, flushings, throbbings, size of pupils); and also on impacts that are often indescribable but which arouse intuitions belonging to the order of 'hunches.' " What we suggest is that order be brought into this intuitive process. We now have enough understanding so that we can begin to forge a scientific instrument in the exploration of unconscious processes. In other words, we are trying to establish rules of psychological exploration as exact as those of physical investigation.

Rather than be satisfied with loose terminology—"neurogenic factors," "emotional upsets," "physical and mental fatigue," "emotional stress and strain"—we must make an effort to define the specific emotional problem and relate it to the total personality make-up of the individual.

Postulates for Psychosomatic Diagnosis

Just as we try to establish a kind of "Koch's postulates" for an allergic problem, hay fever, for example:

1. heredity,
2. seasonal history,
3. skin tests,
4. antibodies,

5. induction of an attack with pollen,

6. hyposensitization or avoidance of the offending substance in controlling attacks;

so in the psychosomatic problem we try to establish:

1. a family history which suggests a background for psychological difficulties (heredity and pseudoheredity),

2. evidences for a childhood neurosis,

3. sensitivity to specific emotional factors (temporal relationship of present illness and emotionally disturbing event) especially at epochal or crucial life periods (puberty, marriage, childbirth, climacteric, etc.),

4. a specific personality structure (other evidences of neurosis or character disturbance),

5. demonstation of specific behavior on taking the history (artificial exposure to a conflict situation),

6. hyposensitization by psychotherapy or the avoidance of the provocative situation.

Psychosomatic Diagnosis

ALLERGIC DISORDER	PSYCHONEUROSIS
1. Specific symptomatology	Suggestive symptoms
2. Heredity	Family history (heredity and pseudo-heredity)
3. Seasonal history	Crucial life periods (childhood, puberty, climacteric, senescence)
4. Antibodies	Specific personality structure
5. Skin tests	Sensitivity to specific emotional factors
6. Induction of attack	Demonstration of specific behavior during interview
7. Hyposensitization or avoidance of offending allergen	Hyposensitization by psychotherapy or avoidance of provocative situation

1. **A Family History Which Suggests a Background for Psychological Difficulties.**   It is impossible to separate constitutional and hereditary factors in the development of psychosomatic disorders. What is often attributed to heredity is in fact pseudoheredity, that is, acquired as a result of environmental influences. Later in the chapter attention is paid to the various familial factors which suggest a background for psychological difficulties. How much of this is transmitted through the germ plasm and how much may be acquired by "social contagion" is difficult to say. Unconscious identification with a sick parent or parent figure is an important cause of psychoneurotic and psychosomatic disturbances.

2. **Evidences for a Childhood Neurosis.**   Evidences for childhood neurosis will often be missing. Neither the individual nor his family can recall the indications of disturbed behavior or bodily dysfunction. Nevertheless, it is well known that almost invariably disturbed behavior or psychosomatic illness of adult life has been preceded by illness of emotional origin in childhood.

The fact that every child in his normal development shows some evidence of disturbed behavior or disorder of emotional origin makes this problem difficult to evaluate. It is a question of degree. Physicians so often say "The child will grow out of it." And so he may seem to do, but the nucleus of the disorder remains and may manifest itself later in life with a more severe illness. Apparently the adolescent period is the crucial one in which the emotional disorders of childhood may be submerged and adequately compensated or may undergo recrudescence and leave a mark which will be felt later in life.

3. **Sensitivity to Specific Emotional Factors.**   When we ask ourselves why a psychosomatic disorder begins at a particular time we must attempt to sketch a cross-section of the individual's life situation at that time in order to discover emotionally disturbing events. We know that these are apt to occur at certain epochs in life, such as puberty, marriage, childbirth, climacteric, and during the senescent period. If the person is heavily predisposed, the incident that precipitates illness may be trivial; if he is comparatively well adjusted, it may require a major event to disturb him or precipitate a psychosomatic affection. In either event the incident is related to his personality structure.

4. **A Specific Personality Structure.**   Almost never does a symptom of emotional origin exist alone. There are always other evidences of personality disturbance, either in the mental or the physical sphere. Both cross-section and longitudinal studies of the life situation, as well as the personality make-up, will show characteristic trends which indicate the predisposition to certain behavior manifestations or to a particular type of disorder.

5. **Demonstration of Specific Behavior.**   When meaningful material is touched upon in taking the history the evidence in the patient's behavior is unmistakable. We must of course allow for the stress incident to the first contact between the patient and the physician but usually there is no difficulty in determining from the patient's behavior that a specific vulnerability exists when certain subjects are broached. It is like the dentist searching for crevices with his sharp-pointed instrument. We too must search for defects in the personality but it is the experienced interviewer who discovers the defect and yet avoids causing pain.

6. **Hyposensitization by Psychotherapy or by the Avoidance of Provocative Situations.**   That a patient improves by means of psychotherapy may be much more obvious to the physician and to the family than to the patient. Indeed the patient will often deny that he is better even while members of his family attest to his improvement. One often obtains a better impression from what the patient does than from the way he says he feels. We do not ask people how they feel; we prefer to ask "What have you done?"

It is also true that manipulation of the environment can bring about improvement in a great many instances. This is the area in which the social worker can be so helpful. The failure to improve when the environment is improved is in itself an indication for psychotherapy.

A last word in regard to this topic: One must be very cautious about attributing improvement to psychotherapy. So often something in the environment has changed and the physician does not know it. The physician may take credit when it belongs elsewhere. Of course, it also may happen that the patient will give credit elsewhere when it belongs to the physician.

One special point that we would emphasize: Neurosis or psychosomatic ailment usually does not make its first appearance in middle life; one must always suspect organic disease.

In so far as allergy is concerned the fact that the removal of an allergen or a hyposensitization process "cures" the patient proves only that one factor has been removed and the morbid chain of events interrupted; and exactly the same reasoning can be applied to psychological factors.

SOME BACKGROUND FACTORS

Organ Neurosis.   Certain psychosomatic disorders have been spoken of as organ neuroses. From a psychological standpoint there are different varieties of organ neuroses depending upon the severity of the underlying disorder. There are very mild disturbances of organ functioning, psychosomatic dysfunctions, which are hysterical symptoms. They are spoken of as conversion phenomena—a substitute expression of an emotional tension which cannot find adequate outlet. The substitute expression is symbolic, *i.e.,* nervous vomiting may, as part of its meaning, express unconscious disgust. There are other disorders, however, which have been referred to as vegetative neuroses. These arise not as an attempt to express an emotion but as the physiological accompaniment of constant or recurring emotional states. Here the somatic symptoms are not so much substitute expressions of repressed emotions as they are normal physiological accompaniments of the emotional state (Alexander). They are the adjustment of the organism to definite tasks which it has to face in a danger situation. They represent a utilitarian preparation and an adaptation of the internal vegetative processes (homeostasis) to a specific type of behavior which is requested from the organism. Elevated blood pressure, *e.g.,* does not relieve anger; it appears in place of emotional tension and accompanies the emotion of rage. It may then be that the chronicity of the emotional tension (plus other factors) makes the condition morbid—psychosomatic organic disease. Any vegetative nervous system disorder deserves study of the psyche as well as the soma and often will prove to be a psychosomatic affection.

ORGAN NEUROSIS AND "ORGANIC" DISEASE.   The emotions often exploit an organic illness and thus it is that frequently, following an infectious disease or operation, convalescence lingers and invalidism sets in. The explanation so often given is that the organic disease produces the neurosis whereas the actual mechanism is that the organic process breaks down the individual's defenses, regression occurs, and the individual's predisposition, determined by the personality structure, permits the neurosis to emerge.

An example of a contrary aspect of the relation of organic disease to neurosis is the severe neurotic disorder, hypochondriasis, in which the patient is obsessed with his neurotic symptoms and inattentive to some serious organic disorder. We have repeatedly observed patients whose only concern was with the psyche while they were dying from organic disease. Recently a patient focused all of his attention upon his heart, which was normal, while an abdominal tumor, which could be readily felt, took his life.

An important subject in psychosomatic illness is the shift from mental sphere to somatic expression. Very often in the organ neuroses the improvement of a symptom because of treatment or for any other reason may lead to mental symptoms such as mood disturbances and sometimes manic and depressive states. An important therapeutic lesson comes out of this consideration because sometimes in psychosomatic illness when we get rid of symptoms by means of medicine, surgery or manipulation, without getting at the fundamental problem, which is emotional conflict, the difficulty is reflected immediately in mental symptoms. Jelliffe, in an article "What Price Healing," gave the history of a patient with contraction of the bladder of psychic origin, in whom dilatation of the bladder relieved urinary symptoms but was promptly followed by psychosis. Elsewhere we cite the example of the surgical removal of a goiter followed by psychosis. Such cases call attention to the necessity for psychological evaluation of the patient before surgery is attempted.

Pseudoheredity. Dunbar has laid emphasis on pseudoheredity as opposed to actual heredity in the determination of illness. This is a very important consideration to which too little reference has been made. Children identify with their parents and unconsciously imitate them in this way; patterns of behavior are laid down (which include illness as an aspect of behavior) so early in life that we often attribute a disorder to heredity when in fact it was acquired. This of course is a very involved question and we presume that the final answer can hardly be hoped for, that is, to separate constitutional and environmental factors with absolute precision. But unconscious identification with a sick parent or other member of the household in early childhood very often is the basis for an illness later in life which we may attribute wholly to heredity. When a young child is exposed to a sick parent the effect is often seen in psychosomatic illness in adult life. How often one hears a patient say that because she was exposed to a sick and complaining mother she learned to detest neurotic women and "made up her mind that she would never become one." Unfortunately this conscious resolution has little to do with the problem; it is the unconscious identification which determines illness. Without realizing it she is the "picture" of the mother in illness as in health.

Emotional Age. Emotional immaturity, which after all is the background of neurotic and psychosomatic illness, often reflects itself in the appearance of the patient, and people who look much younger than their years are often suspect as the kind of people who are apt to become ill from emotional causes. This problem will be discussed again, but the emotional age is a revealing index to the kind of personality that may break down from environmental stress. If the emotional age is in harmony with the physical and intellectual and chronological ages then a person is often said to be well adjusted and such people are usually free from psychosomatic illness, whereas those with immature emotional life as reflected in their appearance—those in whom the emotional age is not in keeping with the chronological, physical and intellectual age—

are the people who provide the soil for psychosomatic sickness. Thus in medical circles "How young you look" may be a dubious compliment.

HISTORY-TAKING

Physician's Qualifications.   An important element of the doctor-patient relationship enters into the taking of the history. We shall refer again to the qualifications of the physician who should interest himself in psychosomatic problems. Here it is only necessary to say that he must be so constituted that he can listen to the patient uncritically. Sympathy for patients suffering from illness of emotional origin is an essential part of the equipment of the physician who would interest himself in psychosomatic problems. It goes without saying that if he is unsympathetic it will show in his manner and will discourage the patient from revealing feelings that are essential to an understanding of the problem. But empathy, an ability to project oneself into the feelings of other people, is even more important. Sympathy alone may be the undoing of a positive doctor-patient relationship; empathy plus training is essential. Therefore a physician's ability to use the psychosomatic approach will depend upon these factors plus his knowledge of psychopathology and tissue pathology applied simultaneously. His human understanding, his sensitivity and sympathetic appreciation of emotional factors as a cause of illness, as well as his orientation and experience, are all important in determining his ability to deal with psychosomatic problems.

One of the most important elements in the psychotherapeutic relationship is transference, about which we will speak later. It has to do with the patient-physician relationship and is involved in all contacts between physicians and patients from the moment they begin.

The Social Worker and Psychosomatic Diagnosis.   We will discuss the role of the social case worker in the next chapter but here it may be said that she can be of great help in establishing a diagnosis as well as in treatment. This has long been recognized in clinic and hospital practice and was clearly demonstrated during World War II when the team of psychiatrist, psychologist and social worker was developed to such a considerable extent. We think that the same thing will happen in civil practice and that not only the psychiatrist but the internist, pediatrician and the other major specialties will discover how useful a well trained medical social case worker can be in developing the social background of illness and assisting in the management of patients and their families. Margolis has described this kind of a working relationship in regard to rheumatic disease. The terms social and psychiatric are as interrelated and interdependent as are the terms psyche and soma. Medicine has an important lesson to learn in the fine art of interviewing as developed by social case work (Garrett).

Criticism of Clinical Records.   Some years ago Kilgore criticized the standardization of hospital clinical records. His criticism, part of which follows, still stands. "The amazing epidemic of standardization that has been visited upon American institutions in this century has not permitted our clinical records to escape. In practically all hospitals with any pretensions one finds the clinical records usually in trim aluminum covers, with some variation in charts and laboratory sheets, but with the clinical history proper invariably displayed under a stereotyped system of paragraphs, with or without the guidance of printed forms. The histories are thereby given an orderliness which is pleasing to the eye and which makes tacit claim to the admirable quality of thoroughness."

STANDARIZED HISTORIES.   "And yet, these standardized histories are open to a very serious criticism. My criticism may be interpreted from the following illustration: In a medical ward of a class A teaching hospital I recently saw a Jewess, aged forty-five years. Five minutes of conversation brought out the facts that she had always been in reasonably good health until after the death of her husband a year ago; that she then looked hopefully for support from her eldest son; but that about three months ago she gradually experienced the final and crushing conviction that his talents were limited to the selling of newspapers, which yielded a profit of less than a dollar a day. She therefore, in addition to caring for her home and the younger children, took employment in a restaurant, standing eight hours a day washing dishes. Then came backache, sleepless nights of worry, anorexia, loss of 20 pounds, nervousness, utter exhaustion, hospitalization. Cursory examination revealed only the ordinary effects of such a life, including possibly some thyroid disturbance.

"Now, I ask of you sticklers for form and order, what do you suppose that woman's folder contained? Five and one-half closely written pages of matter comprised under twenty-eight captions, all neatly underlined with red ink and ruler! Figure out the time that probably took, and then ask yourselves how much time and energy remained to devote to the clinical problem of that woman. We toil through those five and one-half pages in search of useful bits of information. Here and there we find a few—fragmentary and uncorrelated. In the place for 'social condition' it is stated that she is a widow; under 'occupation' that she is a housewife; under 'marital history' that she has four children, but not a word about that fiasco of the eldest son. The paragraph on 'habits' speaks of weight loss but gives no hint of the possible cause. Breathlessly we work down to the captions 'complaint,' 'onset of illness' and 'course of present illness' and find only some sketchy references to pains in the back, palpitation, breathlessness on effort, gas in the stomach, and so on, but never a word of the restaurant or the thoughts in the poor woman's head. Then comes the sacred array of paragraphs on the various systems, with reiteration of shortness of breath under 'cardiorespiratory system,' of stomach gas under 'gastrointestinal,' etc., etc."

No INFORMATION ON PATIENT AS A PERSON.   "The writer of this history was evidently painstaking and industrious, and yet what a mess he made of it! There is not the slightest doubt that if, before he ever set foot in medical school, he had been confronted with this patient and had been asked to write down what he could find out about her condition, he would have done incomparably better. And as a commentary on the teaching of clinical history-taking is not that the height of irony? The reason for this enormity is obvious. The writer of the history has been so occupied in constructing and polishing the frame in order to meet the standard specifications that he has been unable to paint the picture; indeed, he has scarcely seen the patient and her experiences at all.

"This case, to be sure, is worse than many of our hospital clinical histories, but it is none the less a good illustration of a valid general criticism of unrestrained standardization: namely, stereotypism, perfunctoriness, mediocrity."

SPECIAL SERVICE HISTORIES.   Still another criticism of hospital histories from the standpoint of the psychosomatic approach is, that if a patient is admitted to a special ward he gets the kind of a history that the ward or service requires, namely, a history taken from the specialist's point of view, neglecting the person for the part.

It is not to be presumed that the busy physician will undeviatingly follow an outline in every case. Indeed, we realize only too well that this is an impossibility. What we rather hope is that by studying the obscure or difficult problems in his practice in this way he will gradually incorporate a psychosomatic habit into his medical thinking, and into his approach to all patients. Then, very often, only a short time will be required to understand the problem.

Experience of course is important in history-taking but if one practices medicine for fifty years he will still have to give time to the patient. In other words, there are no short cuts in history-taking. While the most experienced people will quickly grasp the situation, time must be taken because the patient cannot be hurried in his recital of what to him are important facts and he certainly cannot be hurried when it comes to an understanding of his illness in terms of behavior.

The revered family doctor of the small community utilized his knowledge of his patients' personal lives in evaluating their history. He knew everything that was going on and had a background of understanding gained from personal observation. Now in our elaborate medical institutions, with a lack of knowledge of the patient's background, we overemphasize the so-called scientific aspects of medicine and relegate to the background the social and emotional factors that may enter into illness. As a consequence our methods of history-taking have not kept pace with other methods of progress in medical science. Really our history forms and techniques are indicative of one of the basic faults in medical knowledge and medical teaching. We have advanced very little from the teachings of Osler in our traditional concept of disease. Osler's insistence on a solid pathological foundation for medical understanding and his careful clinical observations marked an epoch in the development of medicine.

Unfortunately Osler's warmth and human understanding and his intuitive appreciation of emotional factors in illness could not become a part of our medical heritage. The body was divided into many organs and systems; specialists looked upon disease from their narrow viewpoint; and the curriculum was built up by introducing more and more special points of view. As a result the comprehensive viewpoint which is so necessary to the study of illness as an aspect of behavior made little headway until comparatively recently. The medical history form which we gave to our medical students reflected this organic approach and this age of specialization, and as a consequence we often look in vain throughout a long history for some evidence of the human being who is sick. If patients were allowed to talk more and were examined less it would probably be a good thing for medicine as a whole. As one of our patients who had been through the mill of medical investigation recently remarked, she was suffering from "testitis." How numerous are the patients who have been examined again and again by means of x-rays, chemical studies, and various other expensive and complicated methods, accumulating a sheaf of papers an inch thick, with an end result hurtful rather than helpful because the diagnosis is obscured by concentration on a part rather than on the whole.

The Person in the Patient. The majority of people who consult a general physician *wish* to find some physical cause for their ailment; hence they fall readily into the system of answering specific questions about physical health but volunteering no information about themselves as persons. Moreover, people look upon the physician as an authoritarian figure who will "do something" about their illness and they are usually quite unprepared to have to do something for themselves, in other words, discuss themselves as persons as well as "medical cases." We must look for the person in the patient. We have frequently observed that the patient who insists that his illness is "physical" is apt to be suffering from a disorder of emotional origin while the patient who is eager to blame it on the psyche often has an organic disease. Many people, seriously sick with advanced organic disease, seek to delude themselves with the idea that it may be "all mental." This applies especially to the many lay persons who have now read some of the popular writings on psychosomatic medicine.

The introduction of the psychosomatic point of view does not require a different form of history-taking; it only requires an awareness of the role that emotions play in illness, and consequently more emphasis on certain aspects of history-taking. *Thus the history need not differ in form but it must differ in substance.* In accordance with what has already been said, more attention will be paid to the behavior of the patient and to the actual words that he uses in describing his complaints as well as to the asides and apparent irrelevancies that so often give important clues to the emotional factor. Other fundamental considerations are to give the patient time, allowing him to talk with as few interruptions as possible; avoiding extensive note-taking so that the patient may feel that you are more interested in him as a person than in the setting down of the history; and showing interest and sympathy for what the patient sometimes regards as trivial or silly. In addition more attention must be given to the chronological development of the life history with special emphasis on the various factors in the childhood period that may have influenced the development of the personality; with special attention to puberty and adolescence and the frequent emotional problems of that period. Interest will focus on the various epochs and crucial periods in life when psychosomatic disturbances are apt to arise, and a particular effort will be made to obtain a more complete picture of the family background.

More detailed discussion of these points and others follows.

TALKING WITH PATIENTS.   In addition to the *medical history,* which must contain more information regarding the family and social background of the patient than our present histories do, we should make a complete *physical examination* and such *laboratory tests* as are necessary to exclude physical disease or to establish the precise nature of the organic problem and the amount of disability which it in itself is capable of causing.

Having assured the patient that no physical disease is present in the first instance, or that it is present to a certain extent in the second group, but that *the disability is out of proportion to the disease,* it is usually easy by examples of psychic causes for such physiologic disturbances as blushing, gooseflesh, palpitation and diarrhea to make the patient un-derstand that *a disturbance in his emotional life may be responsible for the symptoms.* Then, important clues for this disturbance can usually be found by encouraging a discussion of problems centering around vocational, religious, marital and parent-child relationships. This is usually best accomplished *indirectly* rather than by direct questions. Often it will help to mention a similar problem, describing a case which illustrates the emotional background. The more one can persuade such a patient to talk about "his other troubles" the sooner do we come to an understanding of "the present trouble." *The greater our success in switching the conversation from symptoms to personal affairs, the sooner do we come into possession of the real problem disturbing the patient.* We are all familiar with the patient who is preoccupied with his bowel function and wants to talk about nothing else, whose whole life really seems to surround his daily bowel movement. It is the physician's duty tactfully to switch him from a discussion of his symptoms to a discussion of his personal life. Encourage him to talk about himself as a person rather than as a medical case. In adults, domestic problems and profes-sional and business relationships play a large part in functional illness. In young, unmarried people, family relationships, choice of a career, and often religious and sexual problems are important topics for discussion.

It is often taken for granted that the medical student will know how to talk to patients if we give him a history form to follow. Nothing re-quires greater skill and nothing is so important in regard to the problems of illness. It is really a question of listening rather than talking but our talking has to be able to elicit the proper information. The untutored person can talk to a patient for hours and get no information; the person trained in psychodynamics will know what subjects to discuss with the patient and will know what meaning to attach to the things that are said. Often the doctor talks too much instead of allowing the patient to talk. It has been said that most people use words either to avoid the labor of thought or to conceal the results of thinking. Sometimes the physician covers his anxiety by talking. Unconsciously he avoids some topic that is uncomfortable for him. More often it is because he is in a hurry—he cannot take the time to allow the patient to tell his story.

It is very important for us to recognize that just as the patient has unconscious feelings that interfere with his talking so does the physician have unconscious feelings that interfere with his listening. If we are not at least somewhat aware of these feelings it is almost impossible to take a good history. The patient who is always asking for advice or the patient who is too cordial or too willing to express his admiration for the physician is often covering feelings that are important to bring out if we wish to make progress in understanding the illness. Hidden feelings of anger, guilt, anxiety and distrust will often reveal themselves to the discerning physician in devious ways and unless they are recognized the history cannot be a satisfactory one.

However, making the patient aware of these feelings requires great tact, training and experience.

ALLOWING THE PATIENT TO TALK.   Although time-consuming it is important to allow the patient to tell his story with as few interruptions as possible because in this way important associations are obtained and the groundwork is laid for a good relationship with the patient. Occasionally the patient has to be led back to a discussion of the present illness but aside from such interruptions it is best to allow him to tell the story in his own way. Then one may go over the history in chronologic order with questions regarding the very first evidences of illness, which will frequently antedate the onset that the patient has first suggested. Inquiries should be made regarding the symptoms which preceded an operation because so often the history that the patient gives will begin from the time of "my operation." For example, it is important to know if the appendix was removed because it was acutely inflamed or for the so-called chronic appendicitis which often is a part of the clinical picture of psychosomatic illness. Questions regarding previous medical experiences are also important because so often the patient has picked up erroneous ideas which are harmful to him and until they are dealt with they may remain permanent obstacles to recovery.

It is usually best not to make extensive notes because then the patient feels that you are more interested in the record than you are in him. He is often vaguely irritated and thus distracted from telling his story. Often he prefers to think that some of the things he says will not be made part of a permanent record. A few notes with brief quotations of the patient's actual words will often serve as the framework on which the history later can be constructed.

The telephone, of course, is a great nuisance—to patient as well as physician. The patient rarely mentions it but he is greatly annoyed by constant telephone interruptions and the communication of feeling is often impaired. Many psychiatrists have won this battle with the telephone by refusing to take calls while interviewing a patient; the average physician cannot do this but we do suggest that with certain patients it may be essential.

In dealing with the chief complaint patients with psychosomatic illness frequently say "I hardly know where to begin." A satisfactory method is to ask the patient what is troubling him at the present time and then allow him to tell his story in his own way, observing not only what he says but how he says it, and making quotes of the statements that the patient uses. The greater the number of complaints the more likely that the illness is emotional. We often will find that the patient in his own words expresses the formula of body language to which we have already referred (p. 28).

GIVING THE PATIENT TIME.   The essence of the psychosomatic approach in history-taking is to give the patient sufficient time to tell his story. This of course is one of the great problems in the practice of medicine. Physicians are always saying, "But how can I possibly take the time to try to understand some of these problems?" And we answer, "You must take the time; there are no short cuts." Of course, in the midst of a busy practice one cannot allow an hour for every new patient, and for simple diagnostic problems, as are the majority of cases in general practice, it is not necessary. When the problem is complicated, however, as in the case of most chronic illnesses, the kind of cases that are seen so often in the practice of internal medicine, one must find time. We suggest that if time is not available during regular office hours special appointments be made for certain patients so that sufficient time may be allotted and the interview may proceed in an unhurried fashion. Once you get to know the life situation, subsequent visits need not necessarily take up a great deal of time. Often one can put his finger on the problem very quickly, as it is realized that repetition is the key note of neurotic behavior. People get into trouble over the same situation again and again; the characters may change but the situation remains the same.

Chronologic Development of the Life History.   There are two main approaches to the study of the patient with suspected psychosomatic disorder: *a cross-section study* of the life situation at the time the illness began, and *a longitudinal survey* of his personality from family background and early infancy to the present time. The first approach, the cross-sectional viewpoint, is represented by the story of the present illness; it is the traditional approach of the physician to his patient, and the only requirement so far as the psychosomatic history is concerned is to develop the social and psychological aspects in order to see if there is a relationship between the life situation and the medical illness.

When we approach the past history we must necessarily undertake the longitudinal study of the personality. This will be facilitated by charting the medical events on one side of the page and the life situation on the other, in the manner suggested by Adolf Meyer and widely employed by Cobb and his associates. (See the section on Arthritis for an example.) The presentation of the problem in this manner will often make it possible to see at a glance a very complicated illness from the standpoint of the relationship between medical and emotional events. It is best to employ both the age of the patient and the year of the calendar in charting medical events and life situation. Patients will often give age in relation to one medical experience, calendar year in relation to another, and "so many years ago" in referring to still other events in their medical histories. Adherence to a definite technique of chronological development is advisable in order not to become confused in regard to the timing of events.

The cross-sectional approach tries to relate the present illness and the precipitating emotional factor. The longitudinal study relates personality development and medical history. The latter gives a better idea of the personality structure and psychopathology because it shows the background and the development of the personality. One technique does not exclude the other; on the contrary, the data derived are complementary and help to establish a definitive psychosomatic diagnosis.

Explaining "Body Language" to Patients. The subject of body language which we introduced earlier is a very satisfactory approach to many medical problems. Sherrington suggested that the most satisfactory way to deal with tension is by action, the least satisfactory is by thought, and in between is speech. In other words, in all people with psychosomatic illness there is some impairment of total functioning and very often a great deal of energy is consumed by thought (fantasies). If we can encourage them to get their thinking onto the surface by talking about their problems we can often understand the illness better and at the same time provide some measure of relief. Thus we can compare a person to a tea kettle—if the steam can't get out the spout it tries to blow the lid off. In the same way people accumulate tension which is almost certain to explode in symptom formation or, to use a slightly more involved analogy, we often say to our patients that they are like engines with the steam up. If the wheels do not go round in productive work and the whistle is not blowing in talking about their troubles, then the steam must try to get out somehow and it makes an effort to part their seams. This is almost too pat a description of the circumstances in such a case as hypertension. It is a homely explanation which people readily grasp as they realize that this short-circuiting of energy is capable of disturbing bodily functions. Therefore we can say to patients that if they cannot express their tension by word or action—if they cannot say with their mouths what is disturbing them—then one of their organs will try to say it for them. Thus the patient with nausea, who has no evidence of organic disease, may be indicating that he cannot "stomach" certain situations; the patient with an itch often "lets things get under his skin." If we would only listen to our patients we would find that they express their body language in symbolic formulas.

ORGAN LANGUAGE. A method of helping patients to understand their symptoms which we find useful is based upon the symbolism of symptoms. Many clinical instances can be cited:

Frequently, a feeling of oppression in the chest accompanied by sighing respirations, in the absence of organic findings, indicates that the patient has a "load on his chest" that he would like to get rid of by talking about his problems. The patient who has lost his appetite and as a consequence has become severely undernourished (so-called "anorexia nervosa," which in its minor manifestations is such a common problem) is very often emotionally starved just as he is physically starved. The common symptom fatigue is frequently due to emotional conflict which uses up so much energy that little is left for other purposes. Again emotional tension of unconscious origin frequently expresses itself as muscle tension giving rise to aches and pains and sometimes these are represented by sharp pains such as atypical neuralgia. Thus, we suggest that atypical neuralgia of the arm or face may be due to focal conflict as well as "focal infection." An ache in the arm, instead of representing the response to a focus of infection, may mean that the patient would like to strike someone but is prevented from doing so by the affection or respect that is mingled with his hostility. Itching for which no physical cause is found very often represents dissatisfaction with the environment which the individual takes out upon himself; martyr-like, he scratches himself instead of someone else. "All-gone" feelings in the epigastrium, "shaky legs," and even vertigo are common physical expressions of anxiety, and the anxiety attack, so frequently called a "heart attack," a gallbladder disturbance, hyperthyroidism, neurocirculatory asthenia and hyperinsulinism, is still far from being understood in general clinical medicine in spite of the fact that Freud described it more than forty years ago.

Many more examples could be given, but they are unnecessary because these and other similar problems will be discussed in detail among the case reports that follow. Only one more point remains before concluding this part of the discussion and that is that *the gastrointestinal tract is, above all other systems, the pathway through which emotions are often expressed in behavior.* Why this is so becomes apparent in the chapter dealing with psychopathology.

An interesting study of the semantics of organ language by Stern, Boulanger and Cleghorn showed that expressions having to do with organ functions exist as close parallels in English, German and French. They found several ways in which words for organs and their function are employed. First, there are expressions which imply a conscious awareness of the autonomic concomitants of emotional reactions (e.g., "to be scared spitless," "it makes my flesh creep"). Second, there are expressions in which the word for an organ is employed as a substitute for an emotional attitude ("soft-hearted," "to have guts"). Some of these expressions have a shade of concrete physiological meaning, e.g., "spineless," "no backbone," implying a lack of muscular tone associated with lack of initiative. Third, another group of expressions has implications which have proved accurate only with recent psychoanalytic methods of investigation ("I cannot stomach him," "I have to swallow it"). Fourth, there is another group of expressions which indicate a longstanding awareness of psychosomatic relationships ("he gives me a headache"). Finally, there are expressions the scientific connotations of which are still uncertain, e.g., "splenetic" (irritable). Interestingly, an expression "Ich habe die Nase voll" (to have a full nose, that is, "to have enough") exists only in German while grammatical units having to do with the heart and stomach have a close parallel in all three languages.

The Case Illustration.   Another very satisfactory way to get people to discuss themselves in relation to their illness is to use a case illustration. Repeatedly this is effective when other methods of trying to make people see the relation between emotions and illness fail. If one can think of an apt case illustration the patient can readily identify himself and even where there are marked divergences the patient will often see a partial application which will encourage him to talk about his personal life. Sometimes he will deny the application only to go on from that point to discuss emotional factors of importance which previously he was unable to think of.

The Autobiography.   Among the techniques which can be used for diagnostic purposes is the autobiography. Certain reticent people are able to express their feelings better on paper than in the interview with the physician. With such patients it is sometimes helpful, after the first or second interview, to suggest that the patient prepare an autobiography which will enable the physician "to understand the background of the illness" more readily than by spending the time in interviewing. In connection with the autobiography it must be remembered that what the patient leaves out is often more important than what he puts in. Additional information can often be obtained from corrections that the patient has made or "slips" of the pen.

We find it best not to instruct patients as to content or length of the autobiography but simply to suggest that they write their life story, including medical experiences, so that the physician may become acquainted with them as persons as well as medical cases, in shorter time than interviewing would permit. The autobiography is then used as a basis for further interviews. A slight variation which is often useful is to suggest that the patient write down any thoughts that he may have after the interview and bring them along the next time. This often produces material stimulated by the interview which ordinarily would be repressed before the next visit. Patients sometimes seem a little reluctant to place a written record of their intimate lives in any one's hands and when we sense this we suggest that we will be glad to return the record once we have had the opportunity to read it.

The Associative Anamnesis.   Even when using the history form it is always advisable to allow the patient, insofar as is possible, to tell his story in his own way. This technique of letting the patient tell his own story has been developed to a fine art by Felix Deutsch, in what he calls "the associative anamnesis." He encourages the patient to talk about himself, guiding him skillfully with a question or remark formed by some of the patient's own words. This stimulates the patient to bring up material which has the most important emotional value. Deutsch notes the time and circumstances of the onset of symptoms—a correlation which cannot be emphasized too often. Physicians regularly neglect to elicit what was going on in the patient's environment when his symptoms began.

One observes whether there is anxiety, apprehension, shame or irritability during the recital of the history. Does the patient perspire, tremble, weep, or seem agitated? On the other hand, is there too much of an air of calm or reserve or a denial of worry? The latter may be significant of a great deal of repression of emotion. It is important to note what comments are made in passing and also what the patient talks about during the physical examination. For instance, the patient with a very serious illness may insist upon talking about inconsequential things in order not to have the subject of the seriousness of his condition brought up. Contrariwise, the patient with a trifling symptom may be extremely overanxious and ask all kinds of questions pertaining to the ultimate outcome of his troubles.

Definitive Psychosomatic Diagnosis.   Just as in a consideration of somatic disease it is necessary to make a complete diagnosis before we can hope to apply scientific treatment, so in psychosomatic medicine it is equally necessary. Hence just as in general medical teaching we have always emphasized etiologic, anatomic and functional diagnosis, so in psychological medicine, as pointed out by Levine, it is necessary to make a clinical, dynamic and genetic diagnosis before one can stand on safe ground in regard to psychotherapy.

The clinical diagnosis in psychosomatic medicine refers to the structural and physiological deviations as well as to the underlying or associated psychological disturbance. For example, in the so-called organ neurosis, we would like to know whether we are dealing with a mild personality disorder such as hysteria or a severe personality disorder such as hypochondriasis. It is important, for example, in a functional gastrointestinal complaint to know whether the symptoms are on the basis of conversion hysteria or a part of the clinical picture of depression in which the mood disturbance is overshadowed by the somatic complaints. When one deals with depression there is often the threat of suicide.

Dynamic diagnosis refers to the meaning and purpose of the symptoms or behavior in terms of the particular personality and its structure. Coupled with the genetic diagnosis, which is derived from the longitudinal survey of the individual life history, it opens the way for comprehensive medical care.

In the development of the longitudinal study of the individual it will frequently be observed that psychosomatic disorders appear at epochal periods. Infancy, early childhood, later childhood, puberty and adolescence, early adult life, middle and late adult life, and old age periods have their own special problems as indicated in the accompanying table.

Correlation of Life Situation and Symptom Formation

LIFE SITUATION	SYMPTOM FORMATION
Oral Stage (first year of life)	
Food and love are being given to the child with no responsibilities exacted in return.	Refusal to nurse; fretfulness when nursing is over, or contentment? Protest to weaning (crying or vomiting)?
Anal Period (1–3 years)	
Responsibility of cleanliness and neatness has to be taken over in toilet habits and in other activities. This is not easy and the child needs much friendliness, understanding and patience to accomplish it without anxiety or detriment to personality development.	Is toilet training accepted or is child stubbornly resistive, wetting and soiling beyond usual age of established cleanliness? Is there constipation, temper tantrum, stubbornness, resentment, destructiveness?
Genital Period (3–6 years)	
Period of increasing general and sexual curiosity. Period of beginning tender attachment to parent of opposite sex.	Excessive masturbation, fretfulness, disobedience, aggression, cruelty, enuresis, poor adjustment to other children?

Correlation of Life Situation and Symptom Formation (Continued)

LIFE SITUATION	SYMPTOM FORMATION
Latent Period (6–12 years) Period of primary education, identification with ideals and authority.	How is social adjustment? Does he do well in studies? Does he mix well in classroom and playground? Is there sexual delinquency, truancy, aggressiveness, cruelty, poor sportsmanship, seclusiveness?
Puberty (12–15 years) Period of maturity and beginning activity of sex glands. Extra impetus given to entire emotional life, especially emotional patterns pertaining to love and sexuality.	Are there anxiety attacks; fears of disease, of death, of harming others; nightmares, irritability, social anxiety, seclusiveness, loss of appetite, vomiting, diarrhea, cardiac palpitation?
Adolescence (15–21 years) Period of secondary and college education. Often the need to leave the home and live among strangers. Beginning of love relationships. Planning for life work, career, home, marriage. The fields of competition widen. Conflicts over religion or ideals and current behavior.	Are there symptoms occurring on leaving home, on beginning or ending a love affair, because of inability to compete? Is there seclusiveness and anxiety? A period in which the incidence of somatic symptoms is high!
Early Adult Life (21–40 years) Decisions must be made about love, marriage, work, parenthood. Parental support drops away after 21, if not before. Responsibilities of adulthood are thrust upon one. They catch up with one whether he is prepared for them or not. May be stress of military service.	Symptoms may appear in relation to engagement, marriage, pregnancy, childbirth, loss of job, failure to adjust in marriage, or new environment. "War neuroses."
Middle Adult Life (40–60 years) Period when anticipated ambitions are lost or realized. Children begin to leave home. Women go through menopause. Both sexes have to adjust to changing values.	Women have to cope with the menopause and loss of companionship of the children. May not be resourceful enough, become depressed and anxious. For men it is the age of business success and failure. Of divorce. Reactions to physical disease. Cancerophobia, depression and suicide.
Late Adult Life and Old Age Period (60 years plus) Period of retirement for men, forced or voluntary. Dependency on children for support in both sexes. Problems of physical disease (geriatrics) and the need for care by others.	Symptoms of anxiety often appear after retirement, and many symptoms are due to the frictions incident to living with children and in-laws. Arteriosclerosis and senile dementia usually make social adjustment more difficult.

In approaching the patient from the standpoint of psychosomatic diagnosis one must realize that in dealing with the emotions one cannot separate treatment from diagnosis and that really as soon as one has made an initial contact with the patient the groundwork is being prepared for treatment. There is no sharp division between the period of diagnosis and the period of beginning treatment.

The System Review.   When the patient has concluded the story of the present illness it is best to review the various systems in order to round out the picture of the patient's illness, to make sure that important symptoms have not been overlooked, and thus to assist in establishing the diagnosis. Tension of emotional origin is usually reflected in more than one system of the body.

In some patients the system review may be deferred until the history nears completion. At times this part of the history can best be done while one is examining the patient. As the systematic physical examination proceeds one can inquire for symptoms regarding the parts examined. This may save some time and help the patient to relax. As one examines the genitals in men it is quite natural to inquire regarding sexual power. Women usually had better not be approached so directly on this question. Discussion of menstruation and perhaps contraceptive techniques will often more readily permit women to discuss sexual feelings.

HEAD.   *Headache,* one of the commonest complaints in psychosomatic affections, occurs either as the chief complaint or as an additional symptom. The subject will be discussed in greater detail in the chapter dealing with the central nervous system (Chapter XVI) but here it may be said that there are various kinds of headaches that may make one think of an emotional factor. Although the allergic approach has been emphasized in cases of migraine, it should always make one suspicious that an important personality disorder is present. Headaches which are described as a feeling of pressure on the head are often symbolic of problems that are weighing upon the patient. So, too, headaches beginning in the back of the head, referred from the neck region and sometimes extending down the back or into the shoulders, often represent tension expressed in the neuromuscular system. When one discusses with such a patient the fact that he is always tense, that he does not know how to relax, that his muscles are taut, and consequently that the tension is expressed especially in the muscles in the back of the neck, he will understand the origin of his headache and often produce material to confirm this suggestion. To refer again to the concept of body language one may think of "tossing the head" (disdain) and "stiffnecked" (obstinacy) as well as the common slang expression, "pain in the neck."

Patients often complain of being *dizzy* or light-headed. When organic cause has been ruled out, or evaluated, as for example in patients with hypertension and anxiety, we will find that this symptom is one of the commonest manifestations of emotional tension. It is one of the first expressions of insecurity, and if we think about it for a moment from a body language standpoint what better way is there to represent insecurity than for a patient to be unsure of his balance? It may become very pronounced, especially after the so-called *anxiety attack,* which is so often misunderstood and labeled a heart attack, hypoglycemia, hyperthyroidism or neurocirculatory asthenia. A patient may say that he has been perfectly well until the time of the attack and that since then he has not been himself. Not being himself often means that he is dizzy, heavy-headed, unable to concentrate and fatigued. What he does not tell you is that he has had a fear of death and that succeeding this he has thought "he was going to lose his mind." As we shall say later in discussing treatment it is very important to get these thoughts out on the surface where they can be dealt with adequately. The most superficial rationalizations of anxiety are fear of cancer, of heart disease, and of "losing one's mind."

In connection with this last idea there are often suicidal thoughts which are very disturbing to the patient. It is always important to get these most superficial ideas out before we attempt to deal with the deeper causes of anxiety.

The anxiety attack is discussed elsewhere (p. 38). All degrees occur from "weak feelings" in the abdomen and trembling of the legs, to actual panic states. As stated above it is essential for psychosomatic diagnosis that the attack be recognized for what it is—a symptom of psychological origin which must be handled by psychotherapy. *A great deal of confusion in the management of chronic illness results from the original misinterpretation of an anxiety attack.*

EYES. Problems regarding vision are by no means rare in psychosomatic affections. A history of many refractions; of frequent changing of lenses; of "heavy lids"; rubbing of the eyes; of pain, blurring, rings around the lights, or spots before the eyes that cannot be accounted for on an organic basis, frequently suggest that the eye is acting as a focal point for anxiety. Hysterical blindness and lesser impairments of vision of hysterical origin will usually be readily recognized. Then there are fears of becoming blind in connection with the scotoma of migraine.

NOSE. A very frequent problem indicating a probable psychosomatic disorder is vasomotor rhinitis. In association with real or alleged sinus disease it is a major problem in medicine and neither the allergic approach nor the attentions of the rhinologists are sufficient to deal with this disorder. Almost invariably it is a part of the picture of a psychosomatic affection.

EARS. Common complaints are tinnitus, buzzing and other peculiar noises. Although rarely the chief complaint they are often associated with other psychosomatic disorders. Patients themselves frequently volunteer that when they are tense the noises grow louder and that when they are relaxed the noises abate. Even when associated with Ménière's disorder there is still the need for psychosomatic exploration.

TEETH. Elsewhere we speak of the psychosomatic aspects of dental practice (p. 503). Here we need only remind ourselves that dentistry is the most mechanical branch of medicine, and yet the teeth can no more be divorced from the rest of the personality than can any other part of the body.

There are many implications from the standpoint of psychosomatic medicine. Grinding of the teeth (bruxism), especially at night; teeth as "foci of an infection"; peculiar sensations of the lips, cheeks, gums and tongue; bitter or metallic tastes; and atypical neuralgias of the face for which good teeth are often sacrificed, are some of the more common problems having to do with psychosomatic medicine. Nor must we forget that psychosomatic affections frequently follow dental extractions when the loss of teeth carries special psychological significance.

THROAT AND NECK.   The hysterical symptom of "a lump in the throat" is one of the most widely recognized indications of nervous illness. In addition to that, patients often speak of a tight sensation in the throat sometimes extending up into the ears and with this they frequently complain of "a sore throat," which is more or less continuous. This chronic type of sore throat for which no organic cause can be found is a frequent part of the psychosomatic picture. Incidentally it should be mentioned that patients who gag easily when the tongue blade is used or who volunteer the information that they gag easily, especially in the mornings, sometimes when using a tooth brush, are suspect from a psychosomatic standpoint.

Clearing of the throat is often an index of tension and frequently is associated with the so-called "post-nasal drip." This is a common symptom in neurotic patients, and while it may have some actual basis in vasomotor rhinitis and sinus disease it is frequently more troublesome to patients than the findings would lead one to expect.

The question of an enlarged thyroid gland frequently enters into psychosomatic problems. Aside from the presence of actual thyrotoxicosis there is the question of the coincidence of simple enlargement of the thyroid gland with neurotic illness. So often the latter is wrongly blamed upon the former.

RESPIRATORY SYSTEM.   The most frequent symptom referred to the respiratory tract is "sighing respiration" which is invariably indicative of an emotional component in the illness. Frequently spoken of by patients as shortness of breath, and sometimes mistakenly thought to be dyspnea of organic origin by physicians, the true nature of the complaint can always be elicited by discovering that it is just as apt to occur when the patient is at rest as when he is active and, moreover, the manner of the complaint—the patient placing his hand on the chest and saying that he has trouble taking a deep breath or cannot take a deep breath—indicates its emotional origin.

When actual asthmatic breathing is present there is still the necessity for looking into the personality for other indications of emotional disorder.

Neurotic cough is not a common symptom but it does occur, very often in association with "tuberculophobia." Usually it is blamed on cigarettes and, indeed, they may add to the problem. Invariably the patient tells you that he smokes only a few puffs and "throws the rest away."

CARDIAC SYSTEM.   The subject will be discussed in detail in the chapters dealing with the cardiovascular system but here it may be noted that the pain of cardiac neurosis is frequently at the apex, not necessarily related to effort, and practically always associated with sighing respirations, fatigue and heart consciousness.

In addition one must be alert to evaluate the symptoms when actual heart disease is present in order to decide whether they are not out of proportion to the disease and therefore to be accounted for on another basis. Again and again symptoms are blamed on hypertension which are really of emotional origin.

When hypertension and atherosclerosis both are present the differential diagnostic problems become very difficult and from the standpoint of the physician's peace of mind often the most disturbing in the whole realm of psychosomatic diagnosis. (See discussion of coronary artery disease, p. 209).

GASTROINTESTINAL SYSTEM. "The abdomen is the sounding board of the emotions" and more than any other system reflects disturbances in the emotional sphere. Hence it is that from mouth to anus occur a variety of symptoms included within the designation "functional disorders of the gastrointestinal tract." Just to list them would require much space. Peculiar or metallic tastes; burning of the gums and tongue; throat sensations already mentioned; swallowing difficulties; functional indigestion, especially to fatty and greasy foods; belching attacks; "nervous vomiting"; anorexia and chronic diarrhea; constipation and the irritable bowel syndrome with upper gastrointestinal symptoms; and pruritus of the anus are just some of the many "functional" disorders encountered. The problem of so-called chronic appendicitis has already been mentioned.

More serious psychosomatic problems are anorexia nervosa, cardiospasm, peptic ulcer, a host of disorders in connection with gall tract disease (with and without stones), and ulcerative colitis.

Not only in functional disorders of the gastrointestinal tract but in every variety of psychosomatic illness we find an extraordinary compulsion on the part of the patient to blame his illness on "something I *et.*" To this we usually reply, especially after we get to know the patient, "No, it's probably something you *met.*" So deeply ingrained is this idea that even patients who have apparently learned a good deal about the relations of life situation and symptoms will return again and again blaming new complaints on "something I et."

One of the great diagnostic problems in psychosomatic medicine is the evaluation of pain, and this is especially true in the abdomen. Even to the experienced observer it is often extraordinary how an intense pain will diminish or disappear when we understand and bring to the surface the emotional background. Sometimes this can be accomplished fairly readily as, for example, when the pain reflects the fear of cancer. When patients are told there is no organic disease and, emphatically, that there is no evidence of cancer, a stubborn pain which has resisted all previous therapeutic measures, often including surgery, will immediately diminish or disappear. This is usually discovered not by asking the patient "How is the pain?" but rather noting in the subsequent visit that the patient's emphasis is now directed toward another symptom or another part of the body and that concern over pain has receded into the background.

GENITOURINARY SYSTEM.   As would be expected symptoms referred to this region are very common in psychosomatic disorders.

Questions of menstruation and childbearing will often provide the way for a discussion of sexual adjustment. For example, how did the patient react to the first menstruation—surprised, frightened or disgusted—and whether the patient had any preparatory information from the mother. This will often lead naturally into the question of sexual preparation for marriage. The whole problem of frigidity and impotence, as we will later discuss, is of the greatest importance from the standpoint of human behavior and illness. Frigid women and impotent men have the kind of personalities that are subject to illness of emotional origin, and impairment of the sexual function stands as a revealing index to the personality make-up that may develop psychoneurotic or psychosomatic illness. Patients frequently mislead either deliberately or unconsciously in this regard. Because of our victorian background of repression in regard to sexuality, patients tend to regard sexual problems as of no importance in relation to their illness and evade questions or deny difficulties. The simple question, "What about sexual relations?" will often elicit the response that they are normal. Sometimes the patient knows differently; more often he, or especially she, does not. There is so much ignorance in this regard that even physicians frequently confuse the terms frigidity and sterility. But, as we have stated, these are matters that are usually best understood by allowing the patient to talk freely without asking too many direct questions and the way can often be paved by discussions of such matters as menstruation, contraception, and child-bearing.

Men frequently fail to confess impotence but will admit quick ejaculation, which is a lesser degree of impotence and just as significant as an indication of a predisposition to neurosis.

Frequency of urination, when it occurs during the day and not during the night, is one of the most frequent symptoms of nervous origin. However, even nocturia may be emotionally determined although it is usually an indication of organic disease and calls for extensive study of the genitourinary tract.

MENSES.   Dysmenorrhea is practically always an indication of difficulties in the emotional sphere. Generally speaking, the more severe the dysmenorrhea the more severe the neurotic disorder. Other disturbances of the menses also occur for emotional reasons and these will be discussed in a section devoted to the subject.

In general it may be stated that too much emphasis is placed on slight disturbances of menstruation both by patient and physician. So often the patient takes the attitude, "you can hardly expect me to be well when I have this menstrual difficulty." She thinks it is inevitable that she should be sick and often takes the same attitude with regard to having a child, dating all subsequent illness "from the time my child was born." She feels that the child has taken something out of her that she can never regain.

The physician often becomes a pathogenic agent when he approaches the menstrual problem purely from an organic standpoint, relying only on endocrine assays and endocrine products. It is true, of course, that the other symptoms of which the patient complains are often much worse in connection with the menstrual period and this is especially true of premenstrual tension but the problem is usually just as much psychological as it is endocrinological.

MUSCULOSKELETAL SYSTEM.   Aches and pains, in association with fatigue, frequently referred to as "fibrositis," are very common complaints of psychosomatic origin. If slight fever is also present the differential diagnosis will have to do chiefly with rheumatic fever, tuberculosis and brucellosis. The matter can and should be settled promptly—there is danger of invalidism in focusing too much attention on slight elevations of temperature (p. 522).

The explanation to a patient with fatigue and aches and pains that he is constantly in a state of tension, that he never relaxes, not even at night, and that his muscles are crying out in protest, will often be the first satisfactory explanation that he has had after having had innumerable physical studies. How often do we find the cause of fatigue to be emotional conflict that uses up energy which is then not available for other purposes! Such people can be compared to automobiles "running with the brakes on." Our job is "to take the brakes off."

People who cannot "stand a fight" and who therefore avoid situations that stir them up are usually very sensitive people, easily hurt, whose reaction to aggravation is to say, "well what's the use, it isn't worth fighting about." Nevertheless they pay in bodily symptoms, such as atypical neuralgias, for this inability to express anger.

When patients are tense, taut and uncommunicative, they will very often begin to talk when they are put at ease and muscular relaxation occurs, and of course the reverse is equally true, that when patients can be encouraged to talk their muscle tension often diminishes.

Patients who give the appearance of being calm and who deny being nervous will nevertheless admit that they have inner tension and that they "seethe or boil within." They are "burned-up" with indignation. Patients with hypertension and coronary artery disease, or other disorders involving smooth muscle, often give this impression whereas people who tend to have accidents are often impulsive people who are highly strung and tend to act out their conflicts (p. 529).

Pain in the lower back region is one of the diagnostic problems that present many difficulties. While today attention is focused on herniated disk we must not forget that the syndrome of low back pain and fatigue is often an expression of emotional conflict which frequently occurs in association with pelvic preoccupation on the part of both patient and doctor. Tired women with nagging or even "excruciating" pain in the back who are overconcerned about some slight pelvic abnormality and who are eager to have it corrected by surgery should be suspect from a psychosomatic standpoint and caution exercised before permitting such patients to be operated upon (see polysurgery, p. 496).

It is well known that the posture of the patient is often a gross index to his emotional attitude. He reflects, in the way he carries himself, the attitude that he has toward himself and the world. The dejected (depressed) patient shows his dejection in his posture and the confident, secure patient often reflects his attitude in the erect way that he carries himself. In this connection it may be said that the patient who is always willing to lie down has a passive attitude toward his illness, often aided and abetted by the physician who cautions rest and more rest; while the patient who insists on being up is often the individual with a lot of fight who makes a determined effort to recover from illness.

A subject which should be of great interest to orthopedic specialists is the question of supports and braces which are so often prescribed for individuals who really need inner (emotional) strength rather than a bolstering-up from the outside. They learn to depend upon these outside aids as crutches and see no need to look into their own dependent attitudes.

The social-psychiatric problems associated with rheumatoid arthritis are of great importance and will be treated in detail in the section devoted to that subject (p. 515).

SKIN AND APPENDAGES.   Vasomotor flushing of the head, neck and chest is probably the most frequent index of inner tension and is especially common in women. Often during the medical interview one can note the rise and fall of inner tension with the increase and decrease in the mottling of the neck and chest. We refer to this sign in regard to the psychosomatic postulates (p. 73) because not only may it be an indication of general tension but it may serve as an index to a specific problem that is disturbing the patient. We have noted with much interest the disappearance of such mottling after the use of rauwolfia.

Itching without an eruption is a frequent symptom of emotional origin and as already indicated is often localized in the anal and genital regions. Patients will sometimes volunteer that the itching is so intense that they scratch "until they bleed." Less readily volunteered and therefore all the more significant is the information that sometimes orgasm occurs in connection with such scratching. While allergic factors seem more important in acute attacks of urticaria, chronic urticaria must be approached as a psychosomatic disorder.

Loss of hair, as in alopecia areata, is a common symptom of psychosomatic disorders, and overgrowth of hair, especially on the face, arms and legs, also occurs in periods of psychoneurotic disturbances. Such disorders will need differentiation from endocrine disturbances.

Nail-biting, if persistent, is an important index to anxiety and should not be ignored. Often adults will say that the only times they were able to let their nails grow were during relaxed and happy periods in their lives.

Seborrheic eczema of the ear, scalp and nape of the neck often has an emotional component. Occurring as a chronic lesion in later life it is sometimes associated with acute flare-ups which involve other portions of the body. The so-called dysidroses, dermatitic or eczematoid eruptions of the hands, apparently occur in response to psychogenic factors. The emotional aspects of acne are important, but caution must be observed in subjecting young people to psychological study.

Again we must repeat that we do not think of the psychic factor as sole cause but only as one of the multiple factors in the development of these various skin disorders.

The Past Medical History.   INFANCY.   *Birth.*   Many questions regarding birth and the early infancy period cannot, of course, be answered by the patient. Sometimes the family can help to give a picture which is assuming more and more importance in personality development, that is, the first year of life. If an infant starts out as a fretful child with a feeding problem it is often so badly handicapped that the personality carries the traumatic experience as a focal conflict ready to be relighted when the experiences of adult life make their impacts.

A normal labor and a normal nursing experience in an atmosphere that provides emotional as well as physical security is probably the best insurance against psychosomatic problems later in life.

Nursing Experience.   More and more we hear of the importance of a normal nursing experience from child psychiatrists. It has not been fashionable in recent years to feed babies at the breast but there is no satisfactory substitute. The formula may not differ very much but the emotional content cannot be the same. A rigid feeding schedule and a hard weaning experience frequently establish the background for functional gastrointestinal disorders.

Feeding Problems.   Feeding problems are probably never entirely overcome. This statement will seem exaggerated when we think of the numerous individuals who had feeding problems in early life, changed over in adolescence and ate like gluttons to become fat and apparently very healthy people. But the difficulties of the feeding problem remain deeply ingrained in the personality and may reflect themselves in various subtle ways—if not directly in gastrointestinal symptoms later in life, then often in disturbances in character development which interfere with success and happiness.

Training Problems.   Just as bottle feeding has been popular in recent years, so has the effort to train children for bowel and bladder control at a very early age. As we have discussed elsewhere this often has its repercussions. A good rule to follow is for the child to receive information and training as its intellect is prepared for such information and discipline. Rarely does this happen before the second year. Frequently the story will be obtained of early training which breaks down when a new sibling appears. This regression often sets the pattern for other regressive behavior later in life.

Diseases.   The various diseases of early life should be enumerated and an effort be made to judge the behavior of the individual at the time. Frequently illnesses that required much medical attention and sometimes surgical intervention, such as ear infections and tonsillectomy, are traumatic experiences followed by neurotic behavior. Tonsillectomy in early life, which we have always regarded so lightly, has been found to have considerable importance from the standpoint of the psychological development (Levy).

CHILDHOOD.   It is always well to inquire whether the child was frail or strong because this will often give a clue as to the amount of care with which he was surrounded. A frail child will frequently be overprotected, surrounded with unusual care, making for dependency and passivity trends, while the robust child will be allowed to develop in a normal manner without pathological solicitude on the part of the parents.

People often wonder why children raised in the same family differ so much from a personality standpoint. Of course, many factors are involved but an important consideration is the position in the family. A first child will frequently be overprotected while the parents may be less solicitous about those that follow.

The various diseases, operations and injuries that occur in later childhood can be regarded from a psychological standpoint in the same way as those in early childhood although the individual is usually better prepared because of his intellectual and emotional maturity to deal with these traumatic experiences.

Frequently during this period behavior which is considered normal for the small child will be remarked upon, for example, thumb-sucking, nail-biting, bed-wetting, nightmares, fears, tantrums and masturbation. Parents and physicians often regard these matters as trivial—"the child will grow out of them"—but they may represent the prototype of serious psychosomatic disturbances later in life. It is true that to a limited extent any one of these "bad habits" can be regarded as a normal part of childhood. It is when the symptom is excessive, persists for a long time, or is associated with other habits that it becomes significant.

Questions regarding the kind of sexual education that the individual has had from its parents will frequently permit discussion of masturbation with the guilt and false ideas that are so commonly associated and that may be so distressing to the patient. We are so careful to rear our children in the proper intellectual atmosphere yet we make such serious errors in allowing their emotional education to proceed by chance. Sexual experiences of early life are very common and often serve as important screen memories for serious disturbances in personality development. In discussing sexual education or the lack of it we can often encourage the patient to talk further about his sexual development, thus providing helpful information about his behavior in adult life.

It is also during this period that questions regarding the social development may be informative. The shy child who keeps to himself and reads books instead of engaging in games is the kind of personality that often has difficulties in adult life. Even when he overcomes shyness in later years the emotional difficulty often remains within the personality to cause psychosomatic troubles. Socially poised and affable, such a person may nevertheless reflect his anxiety in the gastrointestinal tract.

It is also during this period—as the individual enters his school life—that questions regarding the social development will reveal the kind of person who adjusts well in later life or remains badly adjusted and susceptible to psychosomatic illness.

ADOLESCENCE.   Puberty and adolescence mark an important period of psychosexual development. Some of the difficulties of early life may disappear as the individual attains a better state of emotional adjustment but again many of the problems of early life are rekindled in this period

Again and again it will be found that the disorders of later life have their beginning in the adolescent period, although this may be established only after repeated interviews. It is not infrequent for an illness to appear just after an individual has overcome masturbation, which had been serving as an outlet for tension of emotional origin.

A history of "anemia," for which the patient received iron, or a period of a "near-breakdown," or a questionable diagnosis of chorea, is not unusual as early evidence of a neurotic or a psychosomatic complaint. Preoccupation with religious or philosophic concepts and bizarre behavior to which at first little attention is paid may mark the beginnings of serious mental disease.

Pain in the side in young girls is often the starting point of chronic invalidism, as we shall demonstrate by numerous case reports. Often the first conflicts that have to do with developing sexuality reflect themselves as a pain in the right side of the abdomen; then comes the diagnosis of chronic appendicitis, followed by operation. Unfortunately for the science of psychosomatic medicine the operation often does bring about relief as far as that particular pain is concerned. But the cause of the pain remains within the spirit of the individual and shows itself in another aspect of his behavior or in the production of other symptoms. Sometimes, of course, the pain is not relieved and then come operations for adhesions, followed by "polysurgical addiction" and chronic invalidism.

The beginnings of *menstruation* and the surrounding circumstances will often give important clues to the sexual development of later life. Dysmenorrhea may be first established in adolescence and may continue until the patient has had her first child. This early history, significant in regard to the emotional development, is sometimes neglected in dealing with women in their later years.

Religious conflicts, marked disturbances in parent-child relationships and school difficulties can occur in the adolescent period and indicate emotional maladjustment that may reassert itself later in life. Questions regarding social adjustment must, of course, take account of the normal social difficulties of this period.

The work life often begins during the adolescent period and conflicts surrounding this, such as rebellion against authority, usually having to do with the influence of the parents, or sibling rivalry, are often important as precipitating factors for psychosomatic illness.

The diseases of adolescence such as tuberculosis, venereal disease, chorea, rheumatic fever, and reactions to injuries of this period, are important in relation to the emotional health.

ADULTHOOD.   Diseases, operations and injuries assume great importance in adult life either as psychosomatic disorders or disorders with psychosomatic implications. Mention has already been made of the events leading up to operation or illness and here reference should also be made to accident-proneness, a subject to which Dunbar has made important contributions.

The *work history* will often give important clues to maladjustment because people, without realizing it, carry over in their relation to authoritative figures the attitudes which they had toward parents or siblings in early life. Thus it is that the beginnings of psychosomatic illness often will be found in conflicts surrounding work. Questions of prestige and financial reward, as well as jealousies toward other workers, are problems that frequently seem to precipitate illness.

So often we hear from patients who have illness of psychosomatic origin that they realize that "overwork is responsible." Our answer is that it is possible to work oneself into a state of illness but that the rule is "overwork plus emotional conflict." Moreover, the overwork in itself may represent the individual's effort to deal with his inner conflicts. Frequently the story is that he works hard but is in conflict with his superior or other people at work or at home, and this wear and tear plus the overwork brings about fatigue and other symptoms. Patients often will at first deny the conflict, as one of our patients with hypertension and headache who blamed his troubles on overwork and then in response to our suggestion regarding a personal problem admitted that his boss was the kind of person who said, "Now this is your department, run it" but then did not permit him to! "Burned up" inwardly, he had to "take it" with a smile.

When the family history is completed it is often expedient to inquire regarding the patient's *marital history.* Aside from the routine questions about when the patient married (year and age), number of children and their names, ages, health and emotional status, and the age and health of the *spouse,* inquiries regarding the family of the spouse, where they live, and hints as to their relation to the patient, may be obtained. Incidentally, it must not be forgotten that neurotics have a way of attracting one another and if their neuroses fit together the marriage may be successful.

Broken homes furnish the soil for psychosomatic illness. The age of the patient at the time the parents separated is important but it is well to remember that long years of incompatibility probably preceded the separation.

The question of marriage is one of the most important subjects to be investigated in relation to psychosomatic illness. Marriage is an emotional hurdle that brings about illness in a great many maladjusted people. Moreover, it is almost axiomatic that the emotional maladjustment of one individual is reflected in the personality of the marital partner. As said before, neurotics have a way of attracting one another and very often their conflicts fit together like lock and key. Therefore, while it is important to inquire and derive as much information as possible about the marriage relationship it is extremely unwise to try any superficial remedies for marital maladjustment. To listen and not to talk is the best piece of advice in regard to marital situations and the same applies to matters concerning extramarital relationships, separation and divorce. How often do physicians recommend marriage and parenthood to maladjusted people as a cure for their emotional problems! Not only does this "cure" fail but it often provides the background for additional neurotic and psychosomatic problems in the offspring. One should be extremely cautious about giving advice on the highly charged emotional problems of marriage.

Menopause has always been an important subject from an emotional standpoint and the climacteric is beginning to assume the same importance in men. One of the most frequent questions asked the physician by the woman with a psychosomatic disorder is, "Is this the beginning of the menopause?" and it doesn't make much difference what the age of the individual is, because the concern may start in the thirties and the same problem continues into late adult life. Now we are beginning to hear exactly the same question in regard to men, "Is this the change of life?" and so often in regard to both, physicians are in part responsible. When a symptom is not readily explained the physician often hints that it may be the menopause. This also provides an easy if not very satisfactory solution, that is, injections of estrogen for the woman and testosterone for the man. What is so often not realized is that the responsibilities and disappointments of middle adult life have much to do with the appearance of symptoms that are attributed to ovarian or testicular failure.

While this problem—how much is hormonal and how much psychological—can be worked out with considerable accuracy in the woman, easily performed tests are not yet available for the man and, as a consequence, the subject is much exploited in regard to men and their disorders of middle life. It is undoubtedly true that men do present a syndrome dependent upon testicular failure, which can be referred to as the male climacteric; still it can safely be said that most men who present such symptoms are really suffering from disorders that are primarily emotional in origin. They are in greater need of psychological understanding than of injections of testosterone.

Maladjusted people often seek their emotional satisfaction in the lives of their children. Just as the spouse frequently mirrors the emotional difficulties of the partner, so do the children of patients who present psychosomatic ailments frequently show a high degree of maladjustment and psychosomatic illness.

Feelings of inadequacy because of the failure to have children, or of guilt because of induced abortions, are often responsible for illness. Questions regarding the children, living and dead, including miscarriages and abortions, are of great importance to the psychosomatic history.

Childless couples who say that they were not very much interested in having a child or who made only slight effort to discover the cause of sterility are also very often emotionally immature people. The bachelor and, perhaps to a lesser extent, the spinster have been unable to make a satisfactory choice of mate, sometimes, to be sure, because of fate or circumstance but very often because of emotional difficulties. Next in order comes the childless couple who have achieved the hurdle of marriage but are unequal to the responsibility of having children. Then comes the couple with one child who felt the responsibility of the child so keenly that they were unwilling to have a larger family. It must be understood that in all of these examples there may be extenuating circumstances that nullify what has been said.

Interests, hobbies, recreations and habits may next be inquired into. The individual who is all work and no play is often preparing the way for emotional bankruptcy which may leave him with a psychosomatic illness. On the other hand, the very "successful" person who indulges in all kinds of community activities may nevertheless be a maladjusted person, neglectful in regard to the emotional development of his or her children, while seeking an unsatisfactory solution for his own emotional problem. So often patients refer with envy to the "successful" lives of these busy people, little realizing what problems this "busyness" may be trying to solve.

Patients often inquire regarding hobbies, wanting a suggestion from the physician. While a suggestion is sometimes helpful, for the most part people who have the capacity to do so will find their own hobbies and the individual who can readily lose himself in avocation or recreation is indeed fortunate. Again and again we see people in whom it is obvious that this is the saving grace that prevented emotional illness.

Patients with illness of psychosomatic origin will frequently retire from many of life's activities, circumscribing and impoverishing their lives. Physicians frequently add to this problem by recommending rest to regain health. "Go home and take it easy" is probably the most frequent piece of advice in the practice of medicine. For illness of emotional origin this kind of advice is rarely if ever helpful because people do not get well by resting nor can they run away from themselves on vacation. To rest is often "to stew in their own juices" and while vacation may provide temporary help by removing them from people to whom they are "allergic," just as often it fails to take them away from the problem because they carry the conflict within themselves. It is true that when people use up energy in emotional conflict they have less left for social and work purposes but they must be made to understand that it is not rest which provides the answer but rather an effort to solve their problems.

The question of *weight* is important in regard to the psychosomatic history. Marked weight loss always makes one think of organic disease but of course it may happen for emotional reasons. A striking example is anorexia nervosa in which the individual may be reduced to skin and bones. But it is also not uncommon for people to gain weight during illness of emotional origin. "Nervous hunger," which people frequently describe as a *void* in the pit of the stomach which they try to satisfy by eating, often results in weight gain even though the patient is complaining most during that period. The "void" is in the emotional life and cannot be satisfied by eating. Obesity in itself is frequently a psychosomatic problem or has important psychosomatic implications and a weight chart can often be correlated with a chart of the life situation.

Dietary habits are important in other respects. They sometimes reflect the atmosphere of the home in which the individual was raised and suggest the amount of emphasis placed on eating and bowel habits. Constipation often has its earliest origins in childhood when the overanxious mother creates anxiety in the child regarding the kind of food and regularity of the stool.

One must never neglect to inquire regarding *sleep* because insomnia or disturbances in the sleep pattern may sometimes be one of the few clues in regard to a psychosomatic disorder. It is also one of the commonest symptoms of psychosomatic disorder. Musser studied 300 patients suffering from relatively early psychosomatic illness to determine the common and important bodily symptoms which correlated closely with the development of the emotional disorder and found persistent insomnia in 57 per cent of the patients. This was often the earliest manifestation of emotional difficulty. The taking of sedatives has been widely commented upon in medical and lay publications and it does seem that the barbiturates and "tranquilizers" are almost as much abused as laxatives in the lives of our patients. Just as people addicted to the laxative and enema habit are apt to have illness of psychosomatic origin, so people who regularly take sedatives may be placed in the same category. Poor sleep is invariably (except in the presence of grave organic disease) an indication of emotional disturbance just as nail-biting is an invariable indication of anxiety of considerable degree within the personality.

The abuse of *tobacco* is also frequent in patients with psychosomatic disorders and, of course, addiction to *alcohol* and *drugs* is even more significant of psychological disturbance. The question where social drinking leaves off and drinking to combat pathological anxiety begins is sometimes hard to decide but the real dipsomaniac is not hard to recognize. In reference to the spouse as a clue to neurotic complaints the wife of an alcoholic is frequently as easily recognized as the patient himself. She complains bitterly, threatens divorce, makes repeated attempts to leave, only to return again and again, or on the other hand may assume an air of quiet martyrdom while she continues to suffer.

But it may also be significant when people completely avoid tobacco and alcohol. Their sensitiveness and overcautious attitude are indications that they may carry the seeds of neurotic disorder within their personalities.

Family History.   Probably the family history is the most important part of the psychosomatic history. Certainly it is the area in which the psychosomatic history differs most from the usual medical history. But again this is only in regard to emphasis and detail.

Simple questions, such as, "Who lives at home?" often provide the way for a great deal of information about the day-by-day activities of the patient and uncover many areas of tension that would ordinarily go unnoticed. One must often subject the family group to microscopic examination for sources of friction in the same way that the dentist systematically examines the teeth for defects. People frequently have sources of tension in their lives that they do not realize and cannot tell about in direct questioning but which come out as one surveys their life situation and gets to know the pattern of their day-by-day living. *Since it is usually the family group who harbor the emotional tensions out of which the patient's illness has developed it is very important to establish the relation of the patient to his family and to know the details about the family background.*

Parents.   Age and cause of death of parents are usually noted but rarely such important factors as the age of the patient at the time of the parent's death, the patient's reaction to the death, the circumstances surrounding the death of the parent, and the *anniversary* of the death which often unconsciously produces a reaction years later in the patient. We are paying more and more attention to the significance of the "anniversary reaction" in psychopathology and always note the exact time of the death of parents, siblings, and other key figures in the life of the patient. The question of any family conflicts following upon the death of a parent, for example, settling of the estate, and responsibilities developing upon the patient as a result of the death, are likewise important. As we learn to sharpen our observations of how the patient reacts to the medical interview one can get some idea, in the very way that the patient speaks about the parents, of conflicts that are important to him in his relationships to other people.

SIBLINGS.   Then one can discuss the siblings, noting them down in the order of their appearance, their names and ages, those who died as well as those who are alive, their health, marital status, emotional stability, where they live, getting hints about their relationship to the patient. Other people who came in contact with the patient early in life, such as grandparents who lived in the household, and other relatives and friends, may play an important part, and just as we are eager to know who constitutes the household in which the patient now resides, so do we want to know the members of the household in which he lived as a child.

Family history, remote as well as close, is important in regard to various diseases and especially the emotional stability and here one often encounters a good deal of resistance on the part of the patients. They are unwilling to confess to the "stigma" of mental and nervous illness. Frequently the use of the term "nervous breakdown" will serve better in an inquiry regarding the emotional health of the family. If one member of a family is unstable the others are apt to show some instability, so that a history of mental or nervous illness, psychosomatic symptoms, a number of divorces, alcoholism, vagabondism, or peculiar behavior in the siblings or other blood relatives may be helpful in establishing the diagnosis in regard to the patient.

The Physical Examination in Relation to the History-Taking.   In some instances the procedure may be varied and as the history nears completion one may stop for a moment and review the various systems, making certain that no important symptoms have been overlooked. Sometimes this part of the review can best be done while examining the patient because as the systematic physical examination proceeds one can inquire for symptoms regarding the parts examined.

As one reassures a patient while proceeding systematically with the physical examination muscle relaxation occurs and talking becomes easier. Frequently clues are obtained which can be pursued in the interviews which follow.

An important point should be mentioned here in regard to physical examination and laboratory investigation in the long-time care of patients with so-called functional ailments. To illustrate, let us refer to a middle-aged woman who had a long history of irritable colon. It was not difficult to relate certain emotionally disturbing situations, which tended to recur, to the rather frequent bowel upsets from which she suffered. On one occasion, however, pain and bowel disturbance continued and x-ray and sigmoidoscopic examination showed a cancer of the sigmoid colon.

This is one of the problems that troubles the physician—that he will overlook organic disease, especially cancer. And it can happen for the reason that so often we take our neurotic patients for granted—once we have established their pattern of behavior and the resultant psychophysiological reaction—and fail to make the periodic physical check-ups that are so essential in the long-time care of any patient. To the physician interested in psychosomatic medicine it is especially important to be on the alert for evidence of organic disease.

DIAGNOSTIC AIDS

Casual Remarks. One of the most important points in the taking of the psychosomatic history is to be aware of the importance of asides and apparent irrelevancies because so frequently important clues are obtained in this fashion. Much anxiety may be hidden behind laughter and jokes. The middle-aged man who with a laugh "guesses that he's cracking up" is often referring to his anxiety regarding his potency and future usefulness and the middle-aged woman with her half-expressed anxiety regarding the imminence of menopause is anticipating the end of her femininity. The fear of cancer is often expressed, not at the beginning, but at the end of the interview. When the patient is informed that she has no organic disease she allows us to know how deeply she feared cancer. Apparently casual remarks, made when the more formal part of the interview is over, often express the real motive for the consultation and indicate the problem that really concerns the patient. Women in conflict over the question of having a child, or another child, frequently do not express this concern directly but introduce it casually after talking about seemingly unrelated matters.

The Patient's Ideas of the Illness. In concluding a history or after one has had an opportunity to see a patient on several occasions and has pretty well concluded the study it is always wise to ask "What have you thought about the cause of your disorder?" One is often amazed at the ideas that people have about the cause and mechanism of their illness and, quite aside from getting out the important question of fear of cancer or fear of some other serious organic disease, one sometimes can deal effectively with distorted ideas that the patient has had, some of which he has arrived at on his own and others which have been furnished to him, often inadvertently, by the physicians whom he has seen. It is impossible to make progress toward an understanding of the patient's illness until some of these distorted ideas are dealt with. They are the first rationalizations of anxiety. It is not uncommon for a patient who has had an idea regarding ulcer, cancer, heart disease or "stroke" to accept reassurance but to hold in reserve the thought, "but if this condition continues I may develop such a disease." Consequently we often say, "You have no evidence of organic disease nor is there any indication that you will develop it."

At the same time in many patients it may be necessary to give reassurance as to the absence of any mental disease. Frequently the patient stammers out his gratitude because he has been greatly concerned about such things as cancer, heart disease or losing his mind but has not dared to say so. This reassurance will go a long way toward making him feel better and at the same it prepares the way for informing the patient that what he really suffers from is a disorder of his *feelings* rather than a disease of his body or mind. Then one can say that in order to confirm this opinion, certain tests should be made, arrange for them to be done, and make the next appointment, sometimes prescribing—with an explanation of what the medicine is for—sometimes postponing prescription until one knows more about the situation. It is important for the patient to realize that he is not a unique or peculiar person—that there are thousands of people who present exactly the same kind of a problem. Patients like this often imagine themselves peculiar or "different" and have a feeling of isolation. To realize that they are not unique is often very helpful to them.

Such patients are often told by well-meaning friends and physicians that they "must snap out of it" but that advice accomplishes nothing. People cannot "snap out of it" but with the help of an understanding physician they can work out of it.

Dreams as Diagnostic Aids.   One of the very great contributions made by Freud was the utilization of the dream as a means of helping the patient to understand the workings of the unconscious mind.

The dream represents the secretion of the mental apparatus and can be analyzed for diagnostic and prognostic as well as psychotherapeutic purposes, in the same way that the urine, the secretion of the kidneys, can be analyzed for diagnostic and prognostic purposes. To use another simile, dreams like x-rays give clues as to what is going on beneath the surface. One must have considerable training in psychodynamics, however, before much use can be made of dream material. Interpretation requires much experience on the part of the physician and cooperation in giving associations on the part of the patient. Certain indications may be very obvious. For example, the woman who finds no interest in sexual matters but who dreams repeatedly of sexual advances by men, like the old maid who looks under the bed, is readily recognized as being more preoccupied with sexual fantasies than she thinks. Repetitive dreams have special significance and often indicate a definite personality trend. The "peace-loving" person who constantly dreams of arguments and fights may be helped to recognize that there is a good deal of aggression in his make-up which he has not adequately expressed. And so it is with such dreams as those dealing with the death of relatives or friends, dreams of frustration, and dreams of semi-nudity—all may point the way toward definite conflicts in the unconscious mental life of the individual.

In experienced hands the dream can often be utilized to throw light upon the doctor-patient relationship and thus can render great assistance in helping the patient to understand his feelings. We must caution, however, that the dream is the royal road to the unconscious and that clumsy efforts to interpret may do more harm than good. A standard rule in psychotherapy is not to give information to the patient before he is prepared to take it and this is especially applicable to dream material.

Psychometric Testing.   Psychological tests formerly had to do only with intelligence, but in the last decade, and especially as a result of psychiatric experience in World War II, psychological testing has become an integral part of personality study. Just as the general physician relies on certain diagnostic procedures carried out in the medical laboratory, so he may also rely on certain diagnostic tests and procedures carried out by the clinical psychologist. While many tests have been devised, it is generally felt that no one test is adequate for total personality appraisal. An analogy might very well be made to the various tests that are used in laboratory medicine. Rarely does one test suffice for evaluating the total function of an organ. A great many tests, for example, have been devised for measuring kidney function; after long experience clinicians have pretty well agreed on a few, comprising a battery of tests, which in combination give a satisfactory pattern of measurements. The same thing is true of psychological testing for diagnostic and prognostic purposes. Question and answer techniques such as the Minnesota multiphasic personality inventory have been found useful for screening purposes, that is, for a simple test, quickly performed, which permits one to say whether an individual shows evidence of gross disturbance of personality so that further study may be made if indicated. Certain so-called projective tests, such as the Rorschach method, which tries to bring to expression the psychological structure of the subject without investigating historical antecedents, have been found of great value in the more detailed evaluation of the personality.

RORSCHACH TEST.   The name Rorschach is derived from the man who originated the test and pioneered in its development. Usually it requires about an hour to administer, and even a longer time to interpret. The test consists of ten bilaterally symmetrical, meaningless ink blots on cards which are presented one at a time to the patient who is asked to tell what they represent to him or what he sees in them. Half of the cards are black and white and half of them have color. The responses and comments when evaluated offer a remarkably accurate means of gaining information about the patient's reactions in terms of intellectual capacity, emotional control, quantity and quality of instinctual drive, special topics of conflict, and the manner of approach to various problems.

There are teaching centers in various parts of the country for instruction in the use and further development of the test. Both special training and considerable practice are necessary in order to use it skillfully. It has already proved of value in the differential diagnosis of psychotic and neurotic conditions since it shows the basic personality pattern, and its further usefulness is being constantly developed. The Rorschach test is also thought to be of value in helping to determine the lines along which the interest and activities of feebleminded and borderline cases should be directed.

In the field of psychosomatic medicine it should prove helpful in determining whether the personality pattern is closer to neurosis or psychosis, since very often a refractory case of psychosomatic illness is a masked psychosis. Moreover, since it measures the degree of affective control it should help us to be aware of energies which are not being utilized either socially or in work but are being dammed up or finding an outlet in a disturbance of the somatic functions. Furthermore, it may show more accurately than a history will reveal, the quality and quantity of instinctual drive which is being held in check. When one finds that a considerable amount of instinctual energy is being inhibited in the presence of psychosomatic disease we should suspect that this energy is playing a part in symptom formation. Hence, the Rorschach test may be useful not only to the psychologist and psychiatrist but also to the physician who is interested to know how misdirected emotional energies may disturb the workings of the body.

Psychosomatic Applications.   Harrower used the Rorschach method in a study of the personality changes accompanying cerebral lesions and later reported on certain "neurotic signs" which occurred frequently in a group of clinically diagnosed neurotics and infrequently in the records of control subjects. Although she found nothing pathognomonic of neurosis in any one of the signs taken alone, nevertheless taken together they were of value in differentiating those maladjusted patients whose physical conditions were mainly or entirely due to psychological factors; and they pointed to the basic psychological adjustment of other patients in whom organic lesions, responsible for the symptoms, were later found.

Kemple, working with patients in the general medical wards of the Presbyterian Hospital of New York, found that Rorschach study of hospital patients with rheumatic disease, hypertensive cardiovascular disease, coronary occlusion and fracture showed distinctive personalities associated with each illness syndrome. Recent psychiatric studies, however, do not substantiate these findings.

Limitations of the Test.   While the Rorschach test is the most valuable single test of personality, Rapaport and Schafer state that it does not yield in all cases a definitive diagnosis or a comprehensive description of adjustment or maladjustment, which is to be expected only from a battery of tests. They find that depressions or extreme inhibitions may occur in any clinical syndrome from schizophrenia to hysteria and, by obscuring all indicators, may invalidate the test. "A second limitation is that schizophrenics with 'well-preserved fronts'— usually the paranoids—are often able to go through the test giving a conventional and acceptable set of responses. A third major limitation is that neurotic conditions are frequently indistinguishable from normal adjustments. A hysteric and a very impulsive normal, a depressive and a stereotyped and inhibited normal, an obsessive-compulsive and a ruminative or well-endowed but rigid normal, each of these pairs may give similar test records. These difficulties cannot be met by 'refining' the Rorschach test but only by using it as one of a battery of tests, since they are partly inherent in the limitations of the test and partly in those maladjustment pictures which do not project themselves in Rorschach test responses."

THEMATIC APPERCEPTION TEST.   This is a story-telling projective technique which consists of twenty pictures. The patient is instructed to construct a story for each picture. The story reveals the personality problems which influence the patient's thoughts and actions. The assumption is that these stories have a relationship to analogous themes in the life of the patient. The test is frequently used as a supplement to the Rorschach test.

THE MINNESOTA MULTIPHASIC PERSONALITY INVENTORY.   This is a question and answer test which has the virtue of simplicity, ease of administration and economy of both time and expense. The actual scoring can be done by a secretary after a short period of instruction. The test is of assistance in indicating borderline conditions and mixtures of psychotic and psychoneurotic elements. It measures the patient's various personality disturbances as well as giving an indication of their severity.

THE CORNELL SELECTEE INDEX.   Mittelmann and his associates devised a simple method of personality evaluation primarily for group study which, however, can be used for the individual. Known as the Cornell Selectee Index it is a self-administered, pencil and paper procedure which can be given to any number of individuals simultaneously. It can be completed in ten minutes and scored within one minute with the use of a simple stencil. The simplicity of this instrument makes it valuable for use in large scale surveys while the information uncovered can be used in orienting the physician giving a psychiatric interview. One must recognize that it will show only gross abnormalities and hence is useful simply as a screen test to decide upon the necessity for further study.

Narcoanalysis and Narcosynthesis.   During World War II a psychotherapeutic method utilized by Grinker and Spiegel found great usefulness in the treatment of the emotional problems induced by combat experiences. It consisted of the administration of Pentothal sodium intravenously, permitting the patient to relive his battle experiences with a great catharsis of feeling, and this was followed by psychotherapeutic interviews which were often very helpful in relieving the individual and permitting his return to duty. Similar methods, using Sodium Amytal, had previously been tried in civil practice (Horsley) and have been used to some extent for diagnostic and treatment purposes since the war.

Ripley and Wolf from an experience with 500 patients with bodily disturbances, believed to be related to problems of personality adjustment, found the method useful in distinguishing between irreversible, structurally determined disorders and functional disorders of organ systems; in differentiating neurosis and malingering; and in the study of significant situational conflicts. Sodium Amytal (0.1–0.8 gm.) was used and no serious complications were encountered. The drug also proved useful in evaluating defects upon which were superimposed functional disabilities related to situational conflicts. In such conditions as migraine, asthma, hypertension and nasal disturbances, signs and symptoms often disappeared after injection, only to be exacerbated when discussion touched on points involving emotional conflict.

Patients with pains of undetermined mechanism, notably in back or abdomen, comprised the largest group successfully managed with aid of Sodium Amytal. Most suitable subjects for narcoanalysis were those with disorders of personality adjustment of relatively short duration. The drug was less effective in diagnosis and treatment of subjects with rigid personalities and long-standing patterns of disability. As a therapeutic agent, Sodium Amytal in no sense acts specifically or automatically. Temporary symptomatic improvement must be followed up with further psychotherapy.

For a variety of reasons this technique is not ideally adapted to office practice. There is some danger in the intravenous administration of a barbiturate without anesthetic equipment (oxygen) and there is always the question whether a person should be wholly or partly deprived of consciousness in a psychiatric interview unless a third person is present, and this violates a fundamental rule in psychological study. The method would not seem to hold the same promise in civil practice, which deals with problems usually related to the whole lifetime experience of the individual and in which multiple traumatic factors have occurred, unlike combat neurosis in which the impact of a single experience was the crucial factor in determining illness. For experimental purposes in hospital and clinic it is possible that information of diagnostic and therapeutic value may come from narcosynthesis but we caution against its indiscriminate use in private practice.

Hypnosis.   Much the same may be said about hypnosis, a technique which has been exploited on stage, screen and radio. However, much serious scientific work has been done from the standpoint of diagnosis and treatment of mental and emotional problems. Hypnosis provides a quick method of influencing the unconscious mental processes in some people and therefore it is conceivable that it might be of diagnostic help in certain psychosomatic problems. It is not recommended for any but the expert.

In general it may be said regarding all tests having to do with personality evaluation that no one of them is the equal of a skillful interview conducted by a well trained and experienced person. They may, however, furnish valuable corroborative information.

THE FORCES WHICH FAVOR PSYCHOTHERAPY

In some cases it is difficult for the patient to see the necessity of visiting a physician when he does not get a prescription, an injection, physiotherapy or an operation. To "just talk about himself" does not seem worth the effort, the time or the money. There are certain forces, however, which favor psychotherapy. The first is the distress which the patient has been suffering and which has been unrelieved by the application of the traditional medical or surgical therapies. The second is the standing and prestige of the physician who tells him that he needs psychotherapy. The third may be the family, who have a greater belief in the efficiency of psychotherapy than the patient, or who may be tired of putting up with the patient's long-drawn-out illness or distressing personality eccentricities. It must be admitted that resistance to psychotherapy causes many patients to make trials in every other direction and to suffer considerably before they will accept a treatment which calls for a scrutiny of their emotions and their relations to other human beings.

The Wish to Recover. The capacity for psychotherapy can often be judged on the basis of the material which we have discussed but it is especially the individual's wish to get well or the reverse, "the unconscious desire to remain sick," that we must try to evaluate. So often the patient repeats over and over again how eager he is to get well but we recognize that unconscious forces are working in just the opposite direction to perpetuate the illness. In fact, the more the patient complains, the more we may suspect that his "unconscious wish to remain sick" is the force which will exert itself.

Transference reactions which have to do with physician-patient relationships and which we will discuss again are important in evaluating chances for recovery. We have talked about "the good patient" who cooperates but is passively defiant and with whom it is difficult, if not impossible, to bring about recovery. We must also be suspicious of people who on the surface are affable and agreeable and apparently eager to cooperate but who beneath the surface are suspicious and skeptical and really refuse to cooperate.

A rough estimate which every physician is in a position to judge daily is the degree of obsession in regard to a fear such as cancer. Many patients present a fear of cancer as the first layer of their anxiety. If they are relatively well adjusted one can abolish this fear with ease. If they have a higher degree of maladjustment the fear will quickly return or be replaced by another fear.

AGE AS AN INDEX. One of the most important criteria for recovery is the age of the patient and the length of time that the illness has lasted. If an individual of middle age has been a semi-invalid, for emotional reasons, for many years, one is less hopeful about the chances of recovery than in a young person with an illness of relatively recent origin. Young people, of course, are more malleable than old. Another estimate of value is the strength of the precipitating force. If an illness appears for a relatively trivial reason and then maintains itself it is apt to be more serious from a prognostic standpoint than an illness which appears only under great stress and then lessens as the individual makes some spontaneous recovery. It is a question of the degree of predisposition and the impact of the environmental situation. If the individual was relatively well adjusted, as many of the men in military service were, and then met an extraordinary situation he broke down but recovered on return to civil life. On the contrary, a sensitive individual with a marked neurotic pattern to his personality may break down with psychosomatic illness for reasons that may seem to be trivial.

INTELLIGENCE. One often hears patients say "But Doctor, I ought to be intelligent enough to handle this problem." Unfortunately it is not so much a matter of intelligence as of feelings. *The will and the intellect are really weak instruments compared to the emotions.* When the emotions are involved, intelligence flies out of the window. In other words, the intellect has very little to do with these problems and therefore while it is a tool with which we must work in understanding and helping these patients it is not a matter of first consideration in judging their capacity to recover. One need not be gifted intellectually in order for psychotherapy to be done. If the intelligence is normal or near normal one may work with such people. Of course, a subnormal intelligence makes the approach difficult, if not impossible.

GAIN FROM ILLNESS.   The amount of emotional satisfaction permitted by the illness, in other words, what the patient gains from the illness, is a matter of great importance in assessing the capacity for recovery. Sometimes we must recognize that the illness is the best answer to the problem. Patients who have lived the better part of their lives, especially when they are so situated in relation to a marital or business problem that a realization of their shortcomings might prove disastrous, had better not be disturbed by efforts to show a relationship between symptoms and life situation. Under such circumstances reassurance and supportive therapy are indicated rather than efforts to make the patient aware of his emotional problems. In other words, we must judge not only the ability but the capacity of the patient to face himself.

IMPORTANCE OF PHYSICAL EXAMINATION

As indicated in the history-taking and examination outline, physical examinations in psychosomatic illness must be fully as painstaking and thorough as when physical disease only is suspected. It must never be forgotten that the neurotic personality may develop a physical disease. If anything, physical examination may need to be more inclusive for psychosomatic illness, owing to the fact that an important symptom in psychosomatic conditions is doubt and distrust. Consequently, as the treatment gets under way and the patient resists having the emotional pain underlying his symptoms uncovered, he may question whether the physical examination was adequate enough to rule out a physical cause for his symptoms. The physician must be in a position to show that the physical examination was complete and thorough. Laboratory studies are usually indicated, with x-ray studies if necessary, and if symptoms are referable to the nervous system neurological and supplementary examinations are necessary.

At the same time it must be remembered that the physical examination and laboratory studies have potentialities for harm as well as good if the patient misinterprets the significance of a test or reads something into the attitude of the physician that was not so intended. As Kaplan points out, speculations about tests are often distorted. For example, a basal metabolism test may seem to the patient to be a study of respiratory function rather than thyroid activity. Not infrequently patients consider tests part of the treatment, even though there is no intended therapeutic purpose. Just as people neglect their teeth for fear of being hurt by the dentist, so do they sometimes delay seeking medical care because of the fear of being physically hurt by diagnostic and therapeutic procedures.

EVALUATION OF THE FINDINGS

An intelligent and critical evaluation of the findings is one of the most important procedures in the management of psychosomatic illness. When there are evidences of personality disturbance and the diagnostic study rules out physical disease, or establishes how much of the problem is physical and how much is psychological and the relation between the two, then there should be no hesitancy in laying the problem before the patient. It is remarkable how many otherwise excellent physicians will postpone or delay such an evaluation of the illness or perhaps never come to a definite conclusion. Not only will the patient be benefited but the physician will add to his own satisfaction, to his reputation, and also enhance the prestige of medicine if he will cultivate the psychosomatic approach in his dealings with patients.

References

Alexander, F.: Psychosom. Med., *5:* 205, 1943.

Deutsch, F.: Psychoanalyt. Quart., *8:* 354, 1939.

Dunbar, H. F.: Psychosomatic Diagnosis, Paul B. Hoeber, Inc., New York, 1943.

Garrett, Annette: Interviewing: Its Principles and Methods, Family Welfare Association of America, New York, 1942.

Grinker, R. R., and Spiegel, J. P.: Psychosom. Med., *6:* 123, 1944.

Halliday, J. L.: Lancet, *245:* 692, 1943.

Harrower, M.: (a) Arch. Neurol. & Psychiat., *43:* 859, 1940. (b) Montreal Neurological Institute, Reprint No. 195.

Jelliffe, S. E.: J.A.M.A., *94:* 1393, 1930.

Kaplan, S. M.: J.A.M.A., *161:* 677, 1956.

Kemple, C.: Psychosom. Med., *7:* 85, 1945.

Kilgore, E. S.: J.A.M.A. *97:* 93, 1931.

Kubie, L. S.: Psychoanalyt. Quart., *13:* 503, 1944.

Levine, M.: Proceedings of The Brief Psychotherapy Council, The Institute for Psychoanalysis, Chicago, Illinois, Oct., 1942.

Levy, D. M.: Am. J. Dis. Child., *69:* 7, 1945.

Margolis, H. M., and Mendelsohn, H.: J.A.M.A., *161:* 309, 1956.

Mittelmann, B., Weider, A., Brodman, K., Wechsler, K., and Wolff, H. G.: Psychosom. Med., *7:* 220, 1945.

Musser, M.: J.A.M.A., *147:* 1030, 1951.

Rapaport, D. and Schafer, R.: Manual of Diagnostic Psychological Testing, Vol. 2. Josiah Macy, Jr. Foundation, New York, 1946, p. 27.

Ripley, H. S., and Wolf, S.: Psychosom. Med., *9:* 269, 1942.

Sherrington, C.: The Brain and Its Mechanism. Cambridge Press and The Macmillan Co., New York, 1933.

Stern, K., Boulanger, J. B., and Cleghorn, S.: Am. J. Psychiat., *106:* 851, 1950.

Chapter IV

Everyday Problems
of Psychotherapy

Retarded emotional development is fundamentally responsible for psychosomatic illness. In other words, if the intellectual age and the emotional age differ sharply, the background for illness of psychological origin exists. One might go further to say that man has four ages: first, his *chronologic age;* second, his *physical age;* third, his *intellectual age;* and fourth, his *emotional age.* For example, one can easily think of an adult who is chronologically forty, physically fifty, intellectually twelve, and emotionally only five. And it might be said that if these various ages are in harmony he is apt to be well and if they are in disharmony, he is apt to be ill. Such persons, and the world is full of them, furnish the soil for the development of psychosomatic illness. Psychotherapy, then, is a process which aims to bring about realignment of the emotions, and the psychosomatic approach takes cognizance of all factors—physical, intellectual and emotional—in preparation for comprehensive medical care.

Readjustment Is Difficult.   But now our first difficulty enters. Emotional maladjustments are regarded by the world at large as evidences of weakness. Hence, the patient who is told by his physician that "the illness is emotional in origin" often feels that he is accused of being a weakling. In spite of the great discoveries of Freud, now more than fifty years ago, the *will* is still looked upon as a supreme instrument which should control such weaknesses. By this time it ought to be common knowledge, certainly in medical circles, that strong forces of unconscious mental origin control our behavior, including the workings of our organs, and that these forces are beyond the influence of the will. Therefore, the patient who is to accept the advice that he needs psychotherapy must accept the fact that while his *will* is strong and his *mind* is normal, nevertheless he does need help as far as his *emotions* are concerned, and that he cannot be expected to do this for himself any more than he could be expected to deal with his own inflamed appendix. He must consult someone who is in a position to help him readjust his emotional life.

The Personality of the Physician.   This brings us to the question of the personality of the physician himself—not only his understanding of disease but his attitudes toward the behavior of sick people. The physician who is to be successful in the diagnosis and treatment of psychosomatic illness must have a real interest in human beings as well as in human disease. To a certain extent he must identify himself with the emotional pain from which his patient suffers. There are many physicians who cannot do this. Their personalities do not permit them to understand or sympathize with suffering of emotional origin. They must get quick results and if this is not possible they do not encourage the patient to remain under their care. Such physicians ought to know themselves well enough to see to it that the patient will get to someone who will undertake the care of these problems. What happens, however, is that the physician often errs in ways already indicated. Either he does not make a correct diagnosis or he does not tell his patient straightforwardly the diagnosis he has made. He treats him medically or surgically, or, sensing the patient's personality immaturities, he may criticize him for his inadequate adjustment to life in such a way that the patient is bound to leave him. Then drifting aimlessly the patient often ends in the hands of some charlatan or, at best, in the hands of some well-meaning but incompetent person on the fringe of scientific medical practice.

We repeat that the physician who is qualified to understand and treat psychosomatic illness not only must know disease but he must also be interested in people as human beings. To put it another way, he must have as much interest in psychopathology as he has in tissue pathology. He must be one to whom the patient feels that he can reveal himself. He must have great tolerance for human foibles. He must have an open mind for all the possibilities of the effect of an idea, and its charge of emotion, upon the body as a whole or any of its parts. He must be flexible in personality and he must be willing to believe that the safe ground of accepted knowledge, often called common sense, is sometimes made up of prejudices.

The Patient Wants To Be Important.   The physician should remember that the patient comes hoping to have his unique personality recognized as well as the individuality of his symptoms. In other words, it should be kept in mind that many patients wish to be the favorite or the most interesting patient to their physician. This comes from the simple wish everyone has at some time to be the favorite child. This should not be regarded as too much neurotic childishness. It is just a plain fact that when one is dealing with people from an authoritative position, one must respect their desire to be made to feel important.

The patient is deeply concerned as to whether he will be treated considerately—and with serious thoughtfulness. He has his own ideas about his illness which he may wish to present in the course of the history taking and examination. Generally, the physician will be wise to take them into account and give them respectful attention. He should not brush them aside as having no importance or as being insulting to his own omnipotent wisdom regarding the patient's state of health.

It should be kept in mind that if the physician is too disinterested or too casual, the patient may feel he has to exaggerate in order to get the attention he wants. If on the other hand he comes to a physician who he feels by conversation or demeanor is too pessimistic, then he may minimize the nature of his symptoms lest he hear "too much bad news."

In most instances, the patient hopes the physician will make a very personal plea for cooperation in the treatment program. Most patients want a clear-cut opinion, decision and formulation of treatment. It rarely helps the patient to be given an opportunity to choose between two possible courses. In certain cases, however, this may be helpful. For instance, a hernia operation, plastic surgery or certain diagnostic procedures may be done safely within a given period of time and this can be set at the patient's convenience. A pedantic or meticulous physician may make an unnecessary emergency out of procedures which can be approached with less urgency.

The patient will often appreciate some sign that the physician understands the cost of examinations and treatments and of time lost from work. Moreover, if a referral has to be made, some patients may prefer to make their own appointment, while others greatly prefer having the physician make such an appointment for them.

All these things take into account the individuality of people. The physician who knows his patients well will come to know their preferences. But when he is meeting them for the first time, a considerate discussion of these matters is helpful to both the physician and patient.

Preparation for Psychotherapy.   If a physician is interested in people and their feelings and ideas the patient will soon recognize and feel this. He will wish to impart his ideas and feelings to this physician. It is then up to the latter to know how to use the patient's verbal and active expressions of himself in order to show the patient the interrelation of his emotional life and the symptoms arising from them. After the physician has succeeded in showing him this relationship both patient and physician must come gradually to ignore the symptom and *treat the cause,* which is the personal emotional maladjustment. Before this process can begin, there must be some preparation for psychotherapy. This consists of a careful history, complete physical examination, including laboratory and x-ray studies if necessary, and finally a diagnostic summary and evaluation of the findings and presentation of the problem to the patient.

Situations That Precipitate Trouble.   In making a survey of the history one should pay particular attention to certain periods of life and phases of living which in certain people tend to be highly charged emotionally. At these periods the vulnerable personality tends to break down. These crises may appear at puberty, on beginning work, during a love affair, through disappointments in vocation or financial affairs, from a death in the family, by reason of the menopause, or through some incident of later life adjustment such as having a child marry and leave home. Many people believe that a neurosis or "nervous breakdown" results only from a major and obvious catastrophe in life. It is true that these major catastrophes can precipitate neuroses. Much more often, however, the onset of a neurosis is brought about by less obvious factors.

PERIOD OF LIFE.   Most neuroses have their onset between adolescence and middle age. This is the period of life in which increasing responsibilities have to be met. It is the period of greatest effort to establish a place in the economic and social world, as well as the period in which the individual is struggling for a satisfactory adjustment in his love life. Such a period, of course, is filled with many experiences of frustration and disappointment. If these frustrations and disappointments cannot be dealt with satisfactorily then an outbreak of symptoms will occur.

THE SINGLE WOMAN.   Many single girls develop symptoms in the period between twenty and thirty if they are not making a satisfactory adjustment in their love life. For many reasons they may be unable to compete with more fortunate girls. The resulting anxiety produces symptoms and the symptoms then serve the secondary purpose of producing a certain kind of attention and at the same time excusing them from the responsibility of marriage.

THE MARRIED WOMAN.   Often after marriage a woman becomes neurotically ill because her husband does not turn out to be the glamorous, attentive and demonstrative person she had expected. She may be unwilling to exert herself to effect compatibility but instead uses tears, sulking and inner resentment to express her dissatisfaction. Finally somatic symptoms appear.

Pregnancy may precipitate great anxiety or hostility in women who do not wish to become mothers. Emotional immaturity is usually responsible. Pregnancy to them means a distorted figure, seclusion from society, and sacrifice of time and effort when the child arrives. We have discussed this problem before. Women may not be fully aware of such feelings; consciously they may feel it their duty to have a child, but when they become pregnant vomiting may represent an unconscious effort to get rid of the fetus.

RELATIVES.   A domineering mother or mother-in-law can be the cause of anxiety, hostility and neurotic symptoms in either wife or husband. Well-meaning *relatives* may be a source of great conflict. They say, "I am not in the road one bit. I don't interfere with a thing that the young people want to do." And they mean it. However, they manage to make their disapproval felt in many disguises. A sigh, a raising of the eyebrow, fainting or a "heart attack" controls the environment for them.

CAREER.   Many women marry after having prepared themselves for a career or perhaps after having achieved success in work. If the marriage is unsatisfactory they toy with the idea of returning to work or to the career which they never had. Unable to adjust to marriage, too lazy or too fearful of criticism to return to work or to make a career for themselves, they suffer from a conflict which causes anxiety and symptom formation.

MENOPAUSE.   If a woman with a neurotic personality manages to get through life relatively symptom-free she may still break down at the menopause because of the many biological and emotional factors involved in the readjustments of this period. This is discussed in Chapter XII.

NEUROSIS IN MEN.   A man may show an outbreak of neurotic symptoms as a result of marrying, or of becoming a parent, because of anxiety over the increased responsibilities. He, too, may be disappointed in what he fails to obtain from marriage. The wife may not be so maternal as he would like or, on the other hand, she may be too maternal and too unromantic. Then, too, he may develop a neurotic illness if he does not progress as rapidly as he expected in his career. Finally, an operation or a prolonged illness may create an emotional need for being taken care of and having life made easy, and the strength necessary to resume former activity does not return. The wise physician will emphasize the excellent physical condition and the completeness of recovery and will point out some of these psychological trends in order to prevent this "failure of recovery." More will be said on this subject in a later chapter.

CUMULATIVE EFFECT OF LIFE'S PRESSURES.   As life goes on responsibilities become greater. If a man shows ability in his job increasing demands are put upon him; as a woman has more children her responsibilities increase. But nothing outstanding or dramatic occurs, and often the individual is not sufficiently aware of his increasing responsibilities, and certainly not aware of his inability to meet them. The strength of ego is related to the increasing pressure of reality, just as the boy who sets out to lift a growing calf daily for as long as he can—a stunt not infrequent in rural areas—finds one day that he is no longer able to do it. The growth of the calf is bound to outstrip the strength of the boy. The person who undergoes the personality breakdown which characterizes neurosis often feels only slightly different with his neurotic symptoms from the way he felt a month before. But the increasing weight of his responsibilities and consequent tensions and anxieties have been growing and he has not been able to grow correspondingly to meet them.

Terminology.   Having made a survey of the life history and symptoms in chronological order one should try to arrive at an exact diagnosis of the personality disorder. This is just as important and just as possible as in the case of physical disorders. The day has come to abolish the habit of labeling a "functional" case as simply neurotic. We must be able to understand the psychopathological basis of a specific personality disorder and then apply an exact diagnostic term. Treatment will thereby be facilitated, as we hope to show. The disorder usually will fall into one of the accepted classifications of psychoneuroses or psychoses or some combination of one or more of them. The term psychosomatic illness has not yet been exactly defined or generally accepted. Some physicians use the term psychosomatic illness synonymously with psychoneurosis and it is true that psychoneuroses and psychoses are often pychosomatic illnesses. Others restrict its use to disorders such as migraine, essential hypertension and asthma, in which the vegetative nervous system seems to be fundamentally involved. These conditions are now officially termed psychophysiologic disorders. We use the term psychosomatic illness in a wide sense to cover not only the physical manifestations of neurotic and psychotic disorders but also, and most importantly, the great variety of mixtures of psychological and structural disorders which make up the bulk of the practice of medicine.

The Meaning of Symptoms. In psychophysiological reactions there is value in pointing out the meaning of symptoms. What, for example, does a headache mean from the standpoint of behavior? Who or what is the cause of the headache and what does it symbolize? We have discussed this under the heading of "body language." But this must not be the sole aim of therapy. There are some symptoms which defy specific explanation but which disappear when the patient can participate in a well rounded life without anxiety. Vomiting may express disgust, aggression or guilt but to demonstrate what a symptom expresses should be a by-product of the therapeutic endeavor rather than an important therapeutic aim. The object is to free the patient from anxiety in his day-to-day living.

For example, a man of 24 complained of fatigue, headaches and spots before the eyes. The symptoms had begun two years before when he married and moved out of his mother's home. The mother was angry at him for marrying and for reducing the amount of money he had been giving her. He felt obligated to visit his mother two or three times a week and he always had to listen to the same reproaches—what an ungrateful son he was, what a scheming woman he had married, how hard it was for his mother to get along financially, how lonely she was. Fatigue and headache were pronounced and he had to give up work completely. The aim in this case was not to speculate on the meaning of the headaches and other symptoms but to help him with his fear of his mother's hostility. The physician became a substitute authority who *did* approve of his marriage and his attempts to emancipate himself from his family, and made him feel less guilty about ignoring his mother's reproaches in his struggle for a life of his own. Thus he was helped to lead a more mature existence, and relief from the headaches followed.

Transference as a Dynamic Factor in Psychotherapy. There are four dynamic events in psychotherapy:
1. Transference of emotion to the physician.
2. Recall of childhood memories.
3. Abreaction of emotion.
4. New orientation for future living.

As soon as the patient and physician decide to meet, transference begins. The term is freely used but poorly understood. It is not enough to assume that *confidence in the physician* is all that is meant by transference. We can best illustrate the phenomenon by returning to the situation which exists between child and parent.

REPETITION OF CHILD-PARENT RELATIONSHIP. The child has physical needs for food and protection and emotional needs for love and security. If these needs are fulfilled he will take for granted the goodwill of the world around him. Just as he receives kindness and goodwill so he is willing to return the same. Hence we can say his transference to human beings is positive. If he does not get enough love and consideration as a child then he will not feel so kindly toward others, and when he becomes an adult he may demand an excessive amount of love or he may express hostility directly. He may make his wants known in various indirect ways; for example, through gastro-intestinal symptoms, or through such habits as telling a long story of his symptoms to hold the physician's attention, exaggerating his complaints or demanding excessive service. He may be suspicious that he is not being treated well enough, thoroughly enough, honestly enough, skill-fully enough, and so on.

In brief, the dominant personality trends, which are in part the product of the early life environmental situations, will repeat them-selves in the relation between patient and physician. By carefully observ-ing and tactfully calling attention to these trends at appropriate times, and then showing how they are related to symptoms, we are able to make the patient understand the causes of his tensions and thus bring about improvement. For example, a man who has had a very dominating father may be acquiescent on the surface but hostile and defiant under-neath. He may show his resentment by failing to cooperate. A woman who, as a child, was made to feel that she could never succeed at any-thing may continue to belittle herself until she is shown how she is re-peating a childish and unnecessary pattern of behavior.

The difference between manifesting emotion with insight, or without it, is very great. A person may be morose, weep easily and frequently, and never change this behavior if he fails to understand the real reason for his depression. Abreaction presupposes that the emotion is acted out in the presence of the physician, who is trying to help the patient with a more constructive way of thinking and acting. *In this setting* the patient can see how immature and out of place his emotion is because he can relate it to some childhood situation. Gradually he attains a greater degree of emotional maturity which helps prevent his unreason-able childish emotions from appearing again. Or if they do appear, they have less force and finally they may disappear altogether.

Case 5.   Transference

A white man of 21 complained of occasional diarrhea, a bearing-down feeling in his lower abdomen, and fatigue. He said he had "colitis" and that a physician in another city had advised him to have his appendix removed. Nothing in the physical or labora-tory study confirmed the diagnosis of colitis or appendicitis.

We learned that he was the youngest of five children of an uninspired, impractical couple who lived without joy in life. Our patient had led a very seclusive, unsociable existence. He was advised against operation and psychotherapy was suggested. He refused to heed this advice; the appendix was removed and later, during which interval he had been working and was symptomatically unimproved, he returned to us. In this interview we inquired about his symptoms and tried to question him about himself and his reactions to life and the people around him but he remained apathetic and non-committal. We felt that we might be dealing with the early stages of schizophrenia and wrote to his parents stating that he was unresponsive to psychotherapeutic efforts.

Again the patient returned, this time a little less apathetic. He said, "I know I don't talk much, I only want to listen. I have always been that way." We explained the need for participation in life in order to find its values, saying, "One must *give* and *take* emotionally in order to enjoy life. If you allow your ideas and feelings to stagnate you will not be well and happy. Furthermore, you get out of practice in how to adjust to people and when you try again you are anxious and ill at ease and this affects the workings of your stomach and intestines."

The patient answered, "I'm surprised that it matters to you what I think, say or do. I guess it's because I just can't believe anyone is personally interested in me. I was the youngest of five children and I sometimes think I must have been an accident. All the older ones have done well and mother and father are proud of them. I never did especially well and no one ever seemed interested in me. Sometimes it seemed that my mother and father only spoke to me to tell me that there was no money to do the things that I wanted to do. So I got into the habit of keeping my thoughts and feelings to myself."

On the basis of our interest in him he soon demonstrated that he could reestablish friendships and also obtain a job. At first, he found it difficult to know what to say to his friends—"I don't know the expressions and slang used. In the three years that I have been sick and out of things I have come to feel like an old timer." He then discussed his fear of being laughed at and we assured him that "no one could be expected to know everything at 21," that "life was a matter of continuous learning." His emotional development continued and soon he reported that he "hardly noticed he had symptoms any more." Occasionally he fell into an attitude of indifference for a few hours and this was a warning to him "that he must get busy and do something," rather than stay in the rut of apathy that led nowhere.

SUMMARY

Here was an example of negative feelings being *transferred* to the physician. As a child the patient had been ignored by his parents, so, as a young man, he retaliated by keeping his thoughts to himself and further showed his resentment by apathy and indifference. We called his attention to what he was doing, at the same time showing our interest in him. He responded with friendliness or positive feelings, developed emotionally as well as intellectually, and became a healthier and more efficient person.

The Role of the Social Worker. Until recently, for reasons already discussed, there has been a suspiciousness between psychiatry and general medicine. For similar reasons social work is still looked upon with suspicion. Too often the social worker has been regarded by physicians as well as by people in general as a "snooper" or "do-gooder." People are generally reluctant to expose their weaknesses, betray their confidences, or "accept charity," and even resist militantly any attempt to get them to do these things. Nevertheless with growing prestige social work has developed as a profession with an established body of knowledge. There now exist some forty-odd schools of social work associated with universities, which furnish well established courses in graduate work. In addition to these courses the student is required to do field work in connection with recognized private and public agencies. The opportunities are great for social workers in many fields of endeavor and medicine is beginning to appreciate the role of social case work, and of medical and psychiatric social work, in their application to general medical problems.

Social case work deals with families or individuals in order to help them to lead more personally satisfying and socially useful lives. As Gayford points out, the object of the social worker is to help people help themselves and her work differs from that of the physician and psychiatrist in that she confines her efforts for the most part to current problems and environmental influences. While she may assist the physician or psychiatrist in helping the patient to release resources within himself, one of the social worker's chief functions is in changing the environment of the individual so as to reduce environmental pressures or to enrich the environment itself.

THE PSYCHOSOMATIC CONCEPT IN SOCIAL CASE WORK.   From the psychosomatic standpoint we speak of the medical and psychiatric social worker's concern with the social factors that help to make patients ill, the social problem which the illness creates, and the obstacles which may limit the patient's capacity to use what medicine has to offer. The psychosomatic approach to illness helps social workers to recognize that the tension and anxiety created by the demands of the social environment are the outgrowth of inner as well as outer pressures.

The request from a physician for the professional help of a social worker is frequently on the basis that the doctor "does not have time" to explore this aspect of a patient's problem. This is an unfortunate emphasis if it means that the physician delegates this task to someone else because he is too busy. The truth of the matter is that the physician needs the help of the social worker because he does not possess her special skills and he should use her in exactly the same way that he uses any other consultant: recognizing the need, that is, the indications, and respecting her professional judgment. Only in very recent years have physicians been presented with adequate information regarding the social component in illness (a condition which is yet true of only a few medical schools) and too many physicians still think of social workers as Lady Bountifuls, priers into other people's business, or clerks in the business office who evaluate the patient's ability to pay. It is the social worker's duty to bring to the patient and to the physician an appraisal of the social component which is different from that which the physician can obtain for himself. Nor is this just a psychiatric appraisal, although the basic knowledge which permits it is an orientation in dynamic psychiatry.

In other words, the help which the social worker can give and is called upon to give has changed considerably over the years. At one time she was regarded as we have mentioned above, then she became someone who visited the home and brought back a picture of the environment in which the patient lives, and now she has become respected as a consultant in the social component of illness.

COOPERATION OF PHYSICIAN AND SOCIAL WORKER.   In an effort to obtain integrated help for the patient the physician shares his professional thinking and planning with the worker, and depends upon her for an objective picture of the patient's social setting, the relationship with the family group, its socioeconomic as well as emotional resources. The social worker has her own special skills to help the patient in the interpretation of the medical problem, understanding the emotional conflicts that enter into the illness, and assisting in some of the many problems of the doctor-patient relationship. From the social worker must come the specialized knowledge of community resources for such problems as vocational guidance and other social needs related to the illness.

Hertzman indicates that when the physician is engrossed with the organic approach and neglects the patient as a person the social worker is forced to assume the responsibility for dealing with social and emotional factors. So long as the physician is not interested or is unprepared to use this material, however, it remains a separate part of the study; it is not incorporated into the total medical management. In such a situation physician and social worker operate in separate spheres. As the physician becomes more aware of the psychosomatic approach he will undoubtedly call more and more for the services of the skilled case worker.

The question is often raised, "Should not the physician himself do the work that is now considered the province of the social worker?" Our feeling is that he should have an awareness of this work and considerable understanding of it but that it remains a separate discipline to be pursued independently but constantly integrated in the teamwork of physician and social worker. We believe that not only will the social worker be utilized more and more in hospital and clinic practice but to an increasing extent in the private practice of physicians. Considerable experimentation has been done in making social work available for private patients on a fee basis and here and there one hears of a physician who utilizes the services of a social worker in his office. Soon medicine will employ psychological as well as physiological techniques in the consideration of the multiple factors that enter into the production of illness, in an effort to make a definitive diagnosis, and in preparation for comprehensive medical care. Then the services of the skilled case worker will be recognized as an integral part of the medical approach to all patients, those in private as well as public care.

Necessarily there will be some overlapping and duplication in the work of the doctor and the social worker but is this not always true of the various disciplines employed by the general physician? He must be aware of the many specialties and points of view that bear upon the medical problem and be prepared to utilize each to a certain extent, meaning that in a limited sense he can use the special skills (minor surgery, minor psychotherapy, and some of the skills of the social worker) but he must be able to recognize the point at which he will call for special help from each of these specialists.

From our own experience with social workers we are prepared to say that their understanding of the social and emotional factors can be of inestimable value to the physician. He cannot do the work of the social worker any more than the social worker can do his job, but both are essential in the psychosomatic approach.

PRACTICAL SUGGESTIONS.   A practical suggestion to the physician is in order. If he has been reared in the organic approach he may be unable to accept the help of the social worker. He may even look upon her as a meddler in personal affairs, one who is capable of interfering with the doctor-patient relationship. But this is far removed from modern social work, which is designed to help the patient to understand the social aspects of the life situation which has prepared the way for his illness, and to recognize the social problems it creates.

The social worker is very often sensitive to a condescending attitude on the part of the physician and leans over backward in her efforts not to antagonize him. This is not a healthy relationship. If the two are prepared to work together much can be accomplished.

Social case work has stated that one of the important considerations in dealing with the client is to find out what he wants for himself; this is the important issue, and not always easy to fathom because what he says he wants is often not what he actually wants. Medicine could well utilize this lesson in realizing that so often what the patient complains about is not in reality what is troubling him.

SOCIAL WORK AS A CAREER.   There is an intimate relation between medical illness and social breakdown. Surveys of the case load of private family agencies will show that an important medical problem exists in the background of social breakdown in a large number of cases and the reverse, of course, is equally true: Social problems help to create medical illness. Therefore there is a real need for physicians and social workers to understand each other's problems and to have considerable awareness of each other's training and qualifications. This means that more medical information must be introduced into schools of social work and more knowledge of the techniques of social work must be introduced in the schools of medicine. When this is done on a broad scale we will finally break down the misunderstandings between the two professions and find more mutual help. The social worker in any field requires a better body of medical knowledge than the average person and of course this is especially true of the medical social worker. Too often in the past the medical social worker has been a clerk juggling the finances of the patient in the business office of the hospital. This is a prostitution of the profession of social work.

Along with the many opportunities which now exist for a career for the social worker we believe that more and more they will be used in private offices and clinics. Indeed social work permits a very satisfactory career from a professional standpoint. We often recommend to both young women and young men who find it difficult to get into medical school, that they may be just as richly rewarded from the standpoint of a professional career in social work. The financial returns will not be large but the opportunity for helpful and interesting professional work should yield its own satisfactions.

EVERYDAY PROBLEMS OF EMOTIONAL SIGNIFICANCE

Work Adjustment.   As society grows older it seems to be paying more attention to the fact that human emotional growth is a continuous process. Possibly we are still thinking and talking about human development too much in terms of adjustment rather than growth. But undoubtedly if attention is paid to the necessity of creating conditions that will bring an individual into a healthy emotional equilibrium with his peers, growth is sure to follow. This concern for an emotionally healthy working climate has found increasing support in industry along with other fields such as education and religion. Whether pure altruism or an effort to reduce absenteeism and thereby promote greater efficiency is the motivating factor is not too important. The important thing is that regardless of motive the insights of psychiatry are being sought and utilized more and more by industry to sustain the worker in his job.

ATTITUDES TOWARD WORK.   There are a great many people who do not like their work. There are several reasons for this. Some never find work suited to their talents. Some are unable to obtain the necessary education or preparation for work they want. But many who do obtain work of their choice and the preparation for it still do not enjoy their opportunities. There are those who have unrealistic fantasies of what rewards a job should bring. Young men, for instance, find it uncongenial to begin at the bottom and believe their education and abilities should warrant large salaries and much prestige from the onset. Girls, too, in undertaking marriage have difficulty in beginning on a small scale and working on a small budget. They find homemaking and child rearing much more demanding of their time and energies than they had imagined, and they find that it requires specialized knowledge that they do not have.

Besides unrealistic concepts of the gains and rewards of a job some people are made anxious by the responsibilities of a job. They begin to fear rejection, criticism and ridicule or they fail to obtain the marks of approval and appreciation that they need. Consequently, they develop tension on the job. This tension may show itself in complaints, irritability and poor cooperation. And it may go even further and disturb body physiology to produce symptoms such as headache, fatigue, anorexia, nausea, diarrhea. The alert physician is always on the look-out for symptoms arising from tension at work.

We must realize that there are many people—perhaps an increasing number—who have never been taught the importance of cooperation— of doing something to help someone else and deriving pleasure from it. In our modern world with its many conveniences that make living so easy in the home, growing children have little to do in the way of work. There is less opportunity for them to learn cooperative living. Moreover, the philosophy of loving children has often been misunderstood to such an extent that great exertions are made for them and they are not asked to do anything in return. As a result they miss learning the joy of doing for others. They also seem to miss the important concept that work must be done by everyone if the individual and the nation are to prosper. Instead of feeling the need to produce, and learning early to enjoy concerted effort and service, they grow up with a great need to be served and taken care of by others. These "others" turn out to be husband, wife, employer, industry, community or government institution. It seems no exaggeration to say that as the standard of living goes up the wish to enjoy it with a minimum of effort goes up also and this produces many conflicts and many psychosomatic problems.

WORKING AND MAINTAINING PERSPECTIVE.   As a result of greater knowledge concerning the social and emotional factors in disease, in absenteeism and in the morale of workers generally, the physician finds it necessary to know more about the complex interrelations of the worker, his colleagues and his work. To use such knowledge can forestall serious emotional illnesses and physical disabilities. This is an important part of preventive medicine.

Few people have the ability to "look at themselves" as they progress in their work. We have already indicated that the young worker may bring eagerness, alertness and enthusiasm and expect great rewards for these qualities while underrating the value of experience. Patient counsel at this time can be the means of restoring perspective.

A little later a man—sometimes abetted by an ambitious wife—may be dissatisfied because advancement has not kept pace with his wishes. Single women between the ages of 25 and 35 may come to work hoping to facilitate marriage and will be dissatisfied with the job because it has not met their expectations in this regard.

A man may have anxieties about his children and if his wife is not a good manager he may bring these worries about family problems to work with him. This can impair both his morale and his efficiency on the job. Or he may displace a dissatisfaction onto his job which really belongs elsewhere. Women as they near the age of 40 may bring the emotional problems of the menopausal period into the job. Men and women both may find that this is one of the difficult periods of life in maintaining marital harmony. They may feel that they have given years of faithful service without having accomplished much. Often they have failed to keep pace with new developments. Instead of being able to look within, they blame the organization for not having had the proper consideration for them. Inflexible, they are vulnerable to unhappiness, irritability, depression of spirits, psychosomatic symptoms.

MORALE.   Good morale in a working organization is a valuable asset and one not easy to define. It is a constructive spirit of working together among all those in the organization. This working together must have certain goals. Cooperation, for example, has to be for the good of the organization and what it produces. There must be a goal of bringing something to the welfare of each individual in the organization. An organization may be well known for turning out a useful, well-made product or it may be known for taking a personal interest in its employees and their families. It may strive to have fair promotion plans, health insurance plans, good vacation plans, and so forth. The owner or the directors may choose their leaders and key men with great care. But unless there is the goal of caring for the individual, morale will never be too high. Important too is the attitude employees have toward the organization and this stems from the leadership of key employees. Management can do much to enhance good morale but the responsibility is not one-sided. The employee must bring his contribution to the morale of an industrial organization. This cannot be in the form of endless demands for more pay, fewer hours, and all other benefits. The worker, at all levels, has to have a positive attitude toward work and the opportunity for work. And no one group should determine how this shall come about. Certainly the home, the school, the church and the medical profession each in its own place helps to set the tone of the working morale of any nation or any community or organization.

The morale, of course, whether good or bad can always be made worse by emotionally sick persons in key positions. This should be borne in mind both by management and medical department and some policy made for the treatment or removal of such people.

The man who can promote good working relations should be highly prized. Such persons seem to be born and not made. But anyone in the position of supervisor can be helped by being given more knowledge about people in general and himself in particular. As it now stands, supervisors know more about the routines they follow and the equipment they handle than they know about the people under them.

The supervisor must be educated regarding social and emotional factors. In most instances the supervisor has been taught to handle the machine but not the man. The supervisor, in his limited sphere, is an executive charged with the handling of people. The extent of his production can be measured by his ability to correlate man and machine. Never in the history of industrial development, says Giberson, has there been greater need for complete understanding between medical advisors and personnel people.

"OVERWORK." A frequent explanation for mental and emotional illness is "overwork." Among the profession and even more among the laity "overwork" is ranked next to trauma of the head as a cause of mental illness. Smith studied the frequency with which "overwork" is blamed for illness in 91 patients who were seen for psychiatric consultation. Eighty-four of his patients (or 93%) had difficulties that were not directly related to the work itself but rather resulted from conflicts with other employees, an illness in another employee doing the same type of work, or a preexisting tension state. In only 7 patients could the emotional ills be directly attributed to the work itself. Overwork, therefore, is not so much a cause of illness as is *work plus conflict in personal relationships*.

THE ACCIDENT PROBLEM. It has been shown that emotional factors play a significant role in the occurrence of accidents. People differ in their susceptibility to accidents just as they differ in their susceptibility to mental and psychophysiological syndromes. Knowledge about accident-prone people and their identification is important not only for the desirability of transferring them to less hazardous areas but also to treat the emotional problems which underlie their behavior.

It has been noted that certain kinds of people are responsible for many accidents. A nagging or bullying foreman may have an adverse effect upon good morale. As a result, faulty attitudes are called forth. There is a blindness to potential hazards, faulty judgment and impulsiveness. Fear, inattention and a lessened sense of responsibility are found. In addition to the nagging, unfriendly foreman who calls these undesirable emotions into action, a wife, husband, fellow workman, or perhaps an encounter with a police officer or an unfriendly auto driver on the way to work, can also be the cause of trouble. There are factors such as fatigue, boredom and monotony. The psychological mechanisms usually are not especially profound. It is well known that an angry or dissatisfied man usually wants, consciously or unconsciously, to vent his feelings. He wants to vent them against the one who has caused him pain and this may be either the real person or some substitute for him. In the course, however, of venting this anger, he may feel so guilty that he includes himself in the damage or even damages himself exclusively. However, injury to others may also occur as well as injury to costly machinery or tools. It goes without saying that the same factors at work in industrial accidents hold in the accidents which happen at home and in automobile driving.

Marriage and Family Life

Courtship and Engagement.   Courtship and engagement often precipitate psychosomatic illness. Marriage is an emotional hurdle that some people cannot take at all, while others may stumble in the effort. Such persons, particularly women, are unhappy at the idea of leaving their own parents, dread sexual relations, and do not want the responsibilities of a home and children. To some women these ideas are partly conscious while to others they are completely unconscious. Whether partly conscious or wholly unconscious they can produce anxiety and this anxiety may be expressed in symptoms. Many women have postponed engagement or marriage time and again because of "poor health," not realizing that the "poor health" represented their anxiety about marriage. Hence the physician should be alert to these possibilities and when a young person has symptoms suggesting psychosomatic illness it is important to discuss the problem of marriage. The physician may then discover that the patient is planning marriage because it is "high time," "the thing to do," "a smart move," "an escape from home," "an easier way of living," "to please mother and father," or one of a number of reasons other than the mature one of making a home in the real sense of the word.

EMOTIONAL IMMATURITY.   A young woman who had been overprotected by her parents was courted by a devoted young man. As his intentions grew more serious and he talked of marriage our patient lost her appetite, slept poorly, complained of weakness and fatigue, became irritable and depressed, and cried a great deal. She spoke of her reluctance to move to another city and to leave her parents, even though the distance was not great. Her parents thought that she had a physical ailment and were surprised when it was pointed out to them how they had pampered and babied this girl until she was totally unprepared to face adult responsibility. When the meaning of her symptoms was made clear they promptly disappeared. However, this did not mean the cure was complete. Inquiry revealed that prior to this time she had had symptoms during periods of emotional stress and therefore it was important to continue her reeducation. To be satisfied with the mere removal of symptoms in such a case, particularly at this age period, is like giving rest and sedation to a patient with pulmonary hemorrhage and, when the bleeding stops, having no further concern as to where the bleeding originated.

Woman's most important responsibilities are bound up in the marriage relationship but she is often woefully ignorant of these responsibilities because her parents either would not or could not educate her properly. So many parents would rather have their daughters innocent and useless than informed and capable. This may be all right for a mother's peace of mind but it is difficult for the husbands and children of these "child-women." Emotional immaturity naturally cannot be changed in one session with the physician. This the patient and family must learn. But the physician too must learn to recognize the special importance of this phase of emotional immaturity. Too often he has prescribed sedatives and rest and allowed one more childish person to continue on the road of chronic fatigue and chronic illness when the everyday responsibilities have proved too burdening. Education for better adaptation will often have lasting good results and will make the difference between a fairly efficient person and a chronic invalid.

INCONSISTENT FAMILY ATTITUDES ABOUT CAREER.   Let us consider certain social and psychological phenomena that might create the conflict that would lead to invalidism. There are many things in our culture which frustrate both sexes in the fulfillment of their fundamental emotional needs. Women need to have appreciation and approval *as people;* they need also to have their childbearing and child-rearing potentialities valued. But no one does this—or let us say, few families or educational institutions do this. One very unhappy patient once said, "My mother and father never wanted me or my sisters and brothers to be men and women. They wanted us to be neuter spirits—the more neuter the better."

This expresses what a great many parents feel. They want their children to marry and have children. But they seem somehow to get sidetracked into encouraging the daughter toward a career or a job because they do not want to "have her on their hands." They push her in the direction of a job first and put marriage, wifehood and motherhood second. If young women were prepared instead, at home and in school, for wifehood, motherhood and homemaking they would be in a better position to cope with adult living. They might eventually find the man they marry to be important to them and they might be able to meet his emotional needs in a more satisfactory way.

Without this preparation, too many young women become insensitive to what it means to take care of their husbands or their children. They doubt that they are wanted by the community or by their husbands as sweetheart, wives, mothers or homemakers. They get caught up in the ambivalent game of debating whether it is better to seek a single goal of work with its implied simplicity or take on the more complicated and energetic, but less renowned role of parent, with its many demands from husband, in-laws, community, church, hospital, P.T.A. and so forth.

Too many parents are smug about all this and feel that their daughter is clever enough and pretty enough so that a young man will want to marry her no matter what her background. Fathers in particular think that it is important that a girl work and prove that she is capable of being self-supporting. This is of great concern and pride to them, but by the time a girl has spent enough energy and interest to please her father she is so far afield in some other libidinal investment than marriage and homemaking that the young man she marries is in grave danger of getting a confused, divided woman with only half of her energy available to please her husband and the healthy destiny of the human race.

In 1954 there were over nine million women at work—two million more than at the height of World War II. Some of these women must work, of course, but many of them have been driven to work by their parents whose upbringing has made them want to get away from home— to escape boredom or to raise their self-esteem—or escape from the necessity of settling down and helping some man to fulfill his destiny as a worker and family man. But once they are caught in the world of work they find that it is not fulfilling, it is not creative. It is sterile and lonely and it lacks participation in life, so that having children, changing diapers, wiping runny noses, going to P.T.A. meetings and coping with adolescent growing pains then becomes more desirable. This is but a part of the conflictual material that lies in the unconscious mind of every—or nearly every—working woman and should be taken into account by the physician when he is doing psychotherapy.

Marital Adjustments.   Marriage as a source of conflict has many implications for psychosomatic medicine. Physicians have always known that marriage and medicine had something in common; from ancient times to the present the advice to marry and have children has been a frequent prescription for certain ailments. But, paradoxical though it may seem, many illnesses arise from the marriage situation, and this fact has not been so clearly appreciated. Marriage is a social institution into which one should bring his best capacities. Human beings should be trained to make marriage an important part of their living, to share life harmoniously with someone else, and to provide a setting in which children may grow up happily and learn to be of use to themselves and others. Instead of this attitude one finds girls growing up looking for "a good catch," someone "to support them," to give them "a good home," "to take care of them." We find men fearing that they will be "caught," avoiding the "ball and chain," rebelling against losing their "freedom," and declaring that "no woman is going to make a sucker out of me." Even though these attitudes may be thought of as extreme and unusual, less pronounced but similar ideas are all too common since very few men and women have had any systematic or scientific preparation for marriage. A woman may drift along until advancing age frightens her into accepting an offer of marriage which is not especially attractive or a man may be drawn into marriage because in flight from loneliness he has sought the company of a woman and then marries because "she or her parents sort of expect it or take for granted."

INCOMPATIBILITY.   With as little thought as this given to the positive aspects of marriage it is little wonder that dissatisfaction and strife arise. Many small misunderstandings and annoyances come from the simple, lazy unwillingness of men and women to consider some of the fundamental differences in the habits and personality of each sex. For example, a man will be annoyed and scold because his wife takes longer to dress than he, yet he would be equally angry if she did not look well. A woman will be greatly annoyed because her husband plays golf with the boys on Saturday afternoon, yet she will not take the trouble to learn to play with him and she would be unhappy if he was not popular with his friends. If the wife does a good job of decorating a room, preparing a meal or arranging a party, she likes and needs appreciation. A man, too, after working hard to achieve a desired position, needs his wife's appreciation. But her only expression of satisfaction may be that "at last" they will be able to have a new coat, a trip, or a private school for Junior. Men and women in marriage should respect each other's goals and ambitions. The capacity to do this is an evidence of maturity and of the capacity for love.

If either party gets the idea of changing the other "for his own good" or is no longer able to feel that the marriage is a constructive partnership, then it is time to see the physician, a psychiatrist, or some person skilled in marriage counseling. The longer a man and wife continue to hurt each other or "get on each other's nerves" the harder it will be to make a fresh start with new ideas.

HOSTILITY IN THE MARRIAGE RELATIONSHIP.   People are thought of as marrying and living together because they are in love but, unfortunately, it is also true that people often live in hate rather than in love. Sometimes this hatred and hostility for the marital partner is outspoken; at other times, it is hardly conscious, and still more often it is deeply buried.

A middle-aged woman presented herself with a clinical picture that first was thought to be cardiovascular-renal disease. However, we were unable to discover any evidence of a cardiac disorder and the urine, blood pressure and kidney function were within normal limits. After vainly trying to understand the obscure illness, it finally became clear that the patient had a great deal of repressed hostility for an acoholic husband but could not bring herself to leave him. The husband suddenly died and we were amazed at the transformation that took place in this woman immediately afterward. Instead of grief, she had relief and her symptoms were immediately abolished.

A young woman, recently married, complained of generalized aches and pains and fatigue. While some of her symptoms had appeared soon after marriage, the fatigue dated from the birth of her child, two and one-half years previously, at which time, as she expressed it, "she gave all of her physical strength to her baby." She had been remarkably healthy during the period of pregnancy but had been sick since that time. Physical examination and laboratory studies failed to disclose any evidence of organic disease and the patient herself suspected an emotional cause. She stated that she was revolted by her husband and almost since the very beginning of her marriage had carried on an extramarital affair with a much older man. She was completely frigid with her husband and had fantasies of hostility and hatred during intercourse, but managed to have sexual satisfaction with her extramarital partner. Her reasons for dissatisfaction with her husband did not seem well founded, and it was clear that even before her marriage she had had great difficulties in her relationship to other people, especially the members of her immediate family.

While she recognized the psychological origin for her symptoms, she nevertheless was unwilling to do anything about it, i.e., anything decisive. She could not bring herself to leave her husband even though she despised him; she felt guilty over her extramarital affair, yet would not give it up; and she would not make any real effort to get at the source of her difficulties by psychotherapy. She contented herself with the partial solution of having another child, because "she was so well while she was carrying the first." This happens very often. *Certain neurotic patients enjoy a sense of well-being during the period that they are carrying a child, only to have symptoms recur after the baby is born.*

MARRIAGE FOR "THERAPEUTIC" REASONS.   In the kind of immature personality now being dealt with, marriage and children do not offer any help. On the contrary, they really only add to the problem. This last patient is a very good example of the kind of person that physicians ought not to counsel to get married in order to solve emotional problems. In fact, it may be added as a rule that it is unwise to give advice concerning marriage. If people are capable of accomplishing marriage for themselves, they will do so without urging, and if they are incapable of achieving marriage, to urge them to do so places a responsibility that the wise physician should be cautious about accepting. The same thing is true about the advice to have children. The fear of having a child is very common in neurotic women. It may be very slight or it may be very pronounced. The unwillingness of a newly married young woman to have a child during the first year of married life may be looked upon as almost normal for this day and age. It is one of the reasons why good *contraceptive* advice is a distinct aid to marital adjustment. But to women who have pronounced fears of having children, contraceptive advice is only a partial answer or no answer at all to their deeper psychological problems.

Often we see the problem of an immature person finding the hurdle of marriage too difficult and responding by the production of bodily symptoms. Too often such patients are told that if they will only marry their troubles will disappear. It is unwise to make such recommendations because, as we have said before, marriage should not be recommended for therapeutic reasons. *Marriage is an excellent institution and will no doubt persist but it is not intended as a short cut to the solution of emotional problems!* Neither are we justified in telling a patient not to marry but on the contrary we must allow the patient to make the choice herself, stating frankly that there is a cause and effect relationship between indecision over the marriage situation and the production of symptoms. It is perfectly possible that if such a person can bring herself to marry, sufficient emotional growth may occur so that the illness may be benefited, but quite the reverse usually occurs and the marriage situation adds to the emotional problem, causing more symptoms. This is especially true when one immature person selects another immature person as a mate and it is noteworthy that this unfortunate combination occurs with great frequency. The point is, of course, that we must be very cautious about recommendations in regard to such important problems as marriage, divorce and childbearing.

EDUCATION IN MARRIAGE.   When marriage is going badly and is producing resentment or illness let us counsel the partners, aid them in taking more mature attitudes, and thus try to make a more constructive institution out of marriage. We believe that often a marriage of two serious-minded persons need not end in divorce if they seek help early enough and each will take suggestions and try to do his part.

Case 6. *Adjustment through Education*

An intelligent couple who had been married for eight years and had had children sought help because of marriage difficulties. The husband complained that his wife was nagging, unsociable, frigid, neglected her appearance and was unappreciative of his efforts to advance himself and to become successful. He made an excellent impression and one got the feeling that marriage had given him a raw deal. No comment was made, however, and a desire was expressed to meet his wife and get her observations on the situation. She reported that this handsome, fine-appearing man had been dogmatic and dictatorial from the beginning of marriage. He took the attitude that since the man made the money he could make all the suggestions and give all the orders. On many occasions during the marriage he had walked out and stayed away a day or two in order to make her yield upon some small point. She was sensitive, came from a proud family, and had given up a good position to marry and she resented the "high-handed methods" of her husband. As for her lack of sociability and indifference to appearance she said, "He is obsessed with the idea of getting ahead. I want to get ahead too but I can't make a social life alone. He says 'make friends.' But I can't go to a country club dance by myself when he just has to see some man from out of town. I can't make dates for an evening and break them, at a moment's notice, just because he concludes at four o'clock that he has to work that night. We haven't had a vacation in four years. Sex has come to mean little to me. I don't think I was ever especially highly sexed but such feelings as I had have been pretty well cooled by his running out on me to discipline me, and by his faultfinding that I do not come up to his expectations as a wife."

After each had had the opportunity to express himself freely we felt that it was important to begin with suggestions to the husband. Fortunately he was the one who had come for advice and had expressed himself as ready "to do anything to improve conditions." We pointed out that he was overlooking his wife's personality make-up and, in fact, was overlooking certain things that are important in the make-up of any woman. We pointed out that he was expecting her to create a home and social life which could never become a reality without his cooperation.

We suggested that the only way to win back his wife's interest for greater emotional participation in the sexual relation was for him to act more like a lover than a faultfinding and harassed business man. It was a significant fact that the patient's father had been separated from his wife and while she had been willing to try to save the marriage the father always cruelly denied her any such opportunity. With this example of indifference to women's feelings before him it was understandable how our patient had been influenced in regard to his attitude toward women. We informed the wife of the necessity for being responsive to any new changes in her husband's attitude and in a short time we received an appreciative note about the improved state of affairs.

THE SEXUAL RELATIONSHIP IN MARRIAGE.   Elsewhere we discuss the emotional factors that have to do with varying degrees of impotence in the man and frigidity in the woman. A few more words will not be amiss on this important phase of marriage counseling which, by the way, is coming to be more and more a part of the physician's duty. It is a widely accepted fact that women are entitled to equality of sexual enjoyment with men. Man no longer uses his wife simply to gratify his own sexual desire without taking the time or trouble to gratify hers. By the same token it is now recognized that a wife is frigid who grudg-ingly or condescendingly acquiesces to the sex relationship without being able to participate emotionally. Such attitudes on the part of man and wife will do much to drive away possibilities for pleasure, and when mutual enjoyment fades from the sexual relationship a deterioration of other relationships is sure to follow.

Education in Sex Matters.   Investigation shows that the cause of marital disharmony and failure is, in most instances, failure in the achievement of a happy sexual adjustment in early married life. Studies on marriage also show that the failure to achieve this happy sexual adjustment has often been due to inadequate education in matters per-taining to sex. For instance, it is clearly stated by many authorities that women may not achieve orgasm with the first intercourse; in fact, that it may be some weeks or even months before it is achieved. If the man does not realize this and becomes impatient, reproachful or condemning, he may permanently prevent the achievement of this pleasure.

Most women are slower to become sexually aroused than the men, both in love-making before the sexual act begins and in the sex act itself. The man should control himself accordingly and will be rewarded by his wife's gratitude and his own sense of accomplishment. Both parties should educate themselves to be frank in expressing their individual desires. Each should come to know what acts or caresses give the keenest pleasure. Sexual intercourse with orgasm should bring about relaxation. If it does not, anxiety is present. The physician should help the patient to understand that shame and anxiety are acquired; they are not natural inheritances.

Pamphlets or books may not lead to a happy sexual adjustment but they do help to clarify thinking, to awaken certain emotions and to provide the way for further help. There are no rules in regard to fre-quency of intercourse but if the couple accomplish a satisfactory adjust-ment the question of frequency usually solves itself.

Contraceptive Advice.   In women fear of unwanted pregnancy may hinder the enjoyment of the sex act, but men, too, are affected by this problem. Both can be helped by trustworthy advice on contraception. Only in Massachusetts and Connecticut have laws been enforced pro-hibiting the dissemination of birth control information. Many larger communities have marriage counsel centers where engaged or young married couples may go for advice. Courses on marriage and family relationships are given in a few colleges. We believe that increasing demands will be made upon the general physician as a marriage coun-selor and therefore he should be prepared to give advice on all phases of the subject, including contraception and the fitting of contraceptive devices.

DIVORCE.   The physician's advice is frequently sought regarding the problem of divorce. The management of such problems requires the same scientific preparation and detachment as the management of a case of pneumonia or appendicitis. In other words, divorce is a *major opera-tion* in personal and social relations and one which the physician must

try to view scientifically rather than in the light of his personal prejudices. There seems to be an instinctive attitude in all human beings, and
physicians are no exception, that at the mention of divorce the first
reaction is to think of doing everything and saying everything which will
keep the couple together. Some people cannot believe that there is ever
anything salutary, helpful or constructive about divorce. However, it
would seem self-evident that the institution of marriage itself can be
improved only if people will take a more open-minded attitude toward
divorce and, by trying to ascertain its cause, learn how to prevent it.

Research on Divorce. An early divorce may mean strength in both
parties rather than weakness. Divorce is regarded as a social evil and is
disapproved of and those who take part in it are sometimes not supposed
to have the right feelings for society. But some of the people who stay
married out of fear, shame, laziness, or because they do not have the
courage to make an attempt to improve marital conditions are less
admirable than some who seek divorce. There has been research into
the causes of divorce just as there has been research into the causes of
crime and delinquency. What has been found is not unrelated to crime
and delinquency. It is that divorce grows out of emotional immaturity
in one or both parties. If divorce is a social evil then just disapproving
of it will not cure it any more than just locking up the delinquent will
cure him. Let us start by educating children in preparation for marriage, and let us counsel those in trouble.

MARRIAGE COUNSELING. When a physician is confronted with a
marital problem one safe rule is "never take sides"! Do not even make
suggestions until both parties have been seen and the story of each
heard at length. There may be an occasional exception to this but on
the whole it is a good rule.

It is generally fruitless for either married partner to attempt to conceal what he feels about the other. If there is anything short of love,
acceptance and cooperation in their attitude it will show itself in some
way. One couple, married ten years, who had grown apart agreed,
after some of their problems had been pointed out, "The trouble with us
is that we never told each other the truth in the beginning. We tried to
protect each other's feelings only to find out that this was useless as we
have hurt each other just the same." The man had a poor relationship
with his mother and had married his wife because she was ill and "he
felt sorry for her." She had married because he asked her to but she
had had no particular desire to marry; she had been overprotected by
her parents and would have been perfectly content to go on in the same
way indefinitely. The husband disapproved of her inadequacy from the
beginning. She was emotionally immature and sexually frigid. She
had little interest in his work and friends. She was always too fatigued
to be a companion to him in sports or recreation. "His energy made me
tired." Every time he asked her to do anything for him the thought ran
through her mind, "If I were home with mother I wouldn't have to do
this." She disapproved of his management of money and the friends he
brought to the house. Both thought it "the sporting thing to do" to
go on and say nothing. Although they could not keep their disapproval

of each other hidden they did not consider professional help until another woman entered the picture. In this case divorce was the solution for both parties, for each wanted it and agreed upon it, but it was regrettable that they came to this decision so late when it was not easy for either to make a new life and new attachments. There were no children so that phase of the problem did not have to be considered.

Constructive Elements.   We believe that strenuous efforts should be made to educate, counsel, strengthen, and hold a marriage together if there are constructive elements in it. But we also believe that neither the law, the church, nor the medical profession should blindly and arrogantly frown upon divorce. More possibilities for neurotic illness and social maladjustment arise in a family where marital discord exists than from any other source. Much as children need two parents for ideal personality formation they need peace, security and affection more. Better one parent and peace than two parents and an atmosphere of hostility, bitterness and reproach.

Advice to Have Children.   It is true that a certain number of immature people enter marriage thoughtlessly and get out of it in the same way. However, this is by no means the rule. On the contrary many intelligent, well-meaning people, after having made real efforts to make a success of marriage, and after serious consideration of all factors, may still want a divorce and their conclusions therefore may be entirely sound. A man and woman, who may have thought that they had something in common before marriage, but who, in a reasonable time afterward, find they do not and, furthermore, find that they are hurting each other every day in their relations together, may be proposing an entirely constructive social act when they contemplate divorce. If the couple have not been married long, friends and relatives are apt to say, "Oh, they are young yet. They have not settled down. They do not know what they want. They have to learn to make sacrifices." Lastly and worst of all—and unfortunately often by the advice of a physician—they are told, "What you need is a child—then you will have a common interest." We condemn this as stupid and dangerous advice. While it may succeed in holding a marriage together, who can say how many children are thus sacrificed on the altar of incompatibility?

In *marriage counseling* the physician should try to help people to think clearly on the following questions.

1. Did you have a common goal or goals when you married? What happened to them?

2. How have you been hurting each other? Has it been through neglect, indifference, nagging, argument, infidelity, disagreement over the matter of children, religious or educational differences, differences regarding friends, recreations, vacations, or lastly but not least, sexual incompatibility?

3. Why have you been hurting each other? Has the hurt one protested too much or not at all? Have you failed to be frank with each other?

4. Do you listen to each other and really try to understand what

the other is saying when discussions arise? Has an honest attempt been made to understand how the other person is being hurt?

5. How will children fare as the result of divorce? Has any plan been made for them which will give them reasonably healthy home conditions in which to grow up?

6. How will the other partner of the marriage manage if divorce is desired by only one member of the marriage? Usually this is more important in the case of the woman than in the case of the man, although not always. If young, the woman may wish to marry again and may have an opportunity to do so. Herein lies good argument for early divorce if it is going to take place. It gives both parties a better opportunity for rearranging their lives than if divorce is postponed ten or fifteen years.

7. Would either party be interested to try to change himself under the guidance of a physician or psychiatrist? If sexual incompatibility or other evidence of emotional immaturity is present would the person in question try a treatment period, to see what results might be obtained before going through with a divorce?

If these points are taken up with each of the marital partners and also discussed jointly and they still feel there is no hope for reconciliation or compatible living, then it is likely that the decision should be for divorce. If both parties agree, no suggestion should be made about having a child or having another child, or trying a separation for a while, or any of the wishful-thinking suggestions which are so often made under these circumstances.

Psychotherapy.   If there is some obvious personality maladjustment consultation with a psychiatrist should be urged. Sometimes skillful psychotherapy saves marriage. Again let us emphasize, however, that there should be no wholesale condemnation of divorce, since many times the people who carry it out are acting in better faith toward each other, toward their children, and toward the community at large than well-meaning friends and physicians who urge them to stay together at any and all costs. Few physicians realize how much mental pain and suffering may result from a marriage in which a disappointed, unhappy, frustrated individual is acting out his dissatisfaction upon the marital partner. It leads to neurosis, and even to psychosis, and aggravates existing somatic disease, not to mention the manner in which such an unhappy atmosphere warps the minds and careers of children. Those who would force two people to live together under such circumstances are more guilty of bad faith with society than the couple who would try to remedy their situation by divorce.

Value of the Kinsey Findings in Marriage Counseling.   The studies made by Dr. Kinsey and associates give information that is of tremendous value in the sexual aspect of marriage counseling. They point up the marked difference in both *attitude toward* and the *responses to* sexual relations. These differences are widespread and profound and must be taken into consideration by the physician-counselor and patient alike.

Briefly stated they are as follows: Most men are readily stimulated sexually by a variety of stimuli such as the sight of the woman as well as by particular parts of her body such as legs, hair, facial contour, make-up of face, type of clothing, gait, posture and gestures. Men are stimulated also by pictures of the female body, by perfumes, by stories of sexual adventure, not to mention contact with the woman herself.

Women, on the other hand, have relatively few avenues of stimulation. These have to do almost exclusively with tenderness, adoration or protective behavior of the man either in his active behavior toward her or behavior as portrayed in a movie, play or story, or by physical touch itself. When it comes to the latter, a woman takes longer to be brought to the point of sexual excitement than a man. This has been stressed again and again in books and articles on sexual technique but men forget it or ignore it too often and too easily.

There are other findings by Kinsey equally important for our problem of sexual incompatibility. These have to do with capacity for orgasm. The woman has been shown to have much less capacity for pleasure through orgasm in marital intercourse than the man in perhaps the following ratio. About one third of women never or rarely have orgasm. A third have orgasm about half of the time, and a third have orgasm more than half the time up to and including the 1 to 3 per cent who approximate the interest in and frequency of orgasm of the male.

From these statistics some of the following conclusions can be drawn: First, the husband cannot expect that the same things which excite him sexually are going to interest his wife, such as risque stories, pictures, verbal proposals of a sexual nature or sexual exhibitionism. Only the utmost consideration in daily living, tenderness, reassurance of her value and worth to him, the creation of a romantic atmosphere and physical petting of more than a perfunctory nature, are going to prepare the woman for an interest in sexual relations. Even with this effort on the part of the husband there will still be a great disparity in orgasm capacity to contend with. If the wife cannot remember that sex relations are productive of the pleasure of orgasm it is understandable that she will be less interested in initiating a sex relation and less enthusiastic about it once it has begun. The result is that husbands are prone to complain about refusal and rejection on the part of wives and wives are prone to complain that husbands are oversexed, inconsiderate and demanding. To keep mutual resentment from appearing over these differences or to reduce it once it has appeared, it is important for the physician to make these differences in capacity for arousal known to the marital partners and emphasize the fact that these differences are widespread. This helps to give the partners a healthier perspective. Second, with the differences in capacity for sexual pleasure through orgasm being what they are, it means that in most marriages compromises will have to be made with the husband demanding sex less often than he may want, and the wife participating more often than she may want. This should spare either party from bearing the whole burden of the differences while they work on personal problems tied up emotionally with sexuality.

There is such a thing, we believe, as being "oversexed," meaning that over and above the individual sexual drive there is a tendency to use the sex act neurotically for comfort, reassurance or relief of tension that should come from other sources. Moreover, it is to be borne in mind that in marriage it is not always the sexually active man who is paired with the sexually inactive woman. Occasionally it is the reverse.

Parenthood.   Parenthood is highly charged with emotion for both sexes but, of course, more so for the woman. How often the physician hears the comment, "I was perfectly well until my first child was born," or "I haven't had a well day since the birth of my youngest child." What does this mean? Certainly, in the great majority of instances it does not mean that pregnancy has produced or aggravated heart, lung or kidney disease. Usually it means that the woman in question was emotionally weak and unconsciously did not want the child in the first place. Then pregnancy and parturition probably stirred up false ideas which had been lying dormant within her. These ideas run something as follows. "Children spoil your figure." Children tie you down." "Children sap your strength." "Nursing a child weakens one." "Giving birth to a child tears you to pieces and you are never the same 'down there.'" Many women, after giving birth to a child, feel as though they have done their bit for the rest of their lives. From that point on this type of woman believes that others should take care of her. They "never get their strength back" because they never wanted to assume very much responsibility in the first place. By means of their invalidism they avoid further pregnancies, avoid marital responsibilities such as sexual intercourse, and are able to live a thoroughly self-centered life. In a word, they control their environment by illness.

EMOTIONAL BACKGROUND FOR INVALIDISM.   Because knowledge of body functioning preceded knowledge of psychic functioning it has been common practice for the medical profession to think only along the line of physical dysfunction. When a woman says, "Having a child sapped my strength," physicians are inclined to think in terms of anemia and glandular inadequacies, uterine displacement, lack of vitamins, etc., and ignore the fact that the woman is really referring to a lack of emotional strength and to a lack of enthusiasm about her job as a mother.

Children draw their energy for later life responsibilities from the love, attention, information, imagination and zest for living of their parents. How can a child become very enthusiastic about the joy of living when all she had heard was, "Don't bother mother, she's not well." "Don't make too much noise, dear, mother isn't strong." Or worse still, "Mother had such a hard time when you were born. She has never had her health since."

THE FATHER'S ROLE.   It is a refreshing sight to see a young woman enthusiastic about having a child, leading an active, healthy life during her pregnancy, and planning in an intelligent way to see that the child has what it needs both physically and emotionally. But the matter of caring for and being interested in children should not be left to the wife alone. Children need a father as well as a mother for the best results in personality development. In other words, the father is important not only as the provider but also as a contributor to the child's emotional growth. Modern life makes it rather difficult in some cases for fathers to spend a great deal of time with their children. This being so, it is all the more important that the quality of the relation between father and child should be exceptionally good. Modern machinery and appliances, both in urban and rural areas, have taken away the opportunity for father and son to work side by side. Men, to some extent, have ceased to be the head of the house in the sense that the mother makes decisions about clothing, school, hours of going to bed, and summer vacations. She does not have to work very hard to get this authority, as many men are quite willing to hand over all decisions while they concern themselves only with business and making money for the family support. Such a division of labor is of doubtful value. When the moral education of children is taken over by women the conscience tends to be formed by a female. Children growing up and constantly taking orders from women do not develop the kindly feeling toward the female sex which they should have. It leads to passivity in men and aggressiveness in women and this is not conducive to the best kind of relationship between the two sexes. *The father and mother should share the various decisions that come up regarding the child, whether the child is boy or girl.*

The father must learn to give more of himself in time and comradeship to children of both sexes. This is particularly true when the father's work is far removed from the family atmosphere. On the farm the children work with the parents and know the meaning of the work. In the shop this same state of affairs may also prevail. The children take an active part in the work and through this close association they come to know each other in a wholesome way. In other cases children grow up without having any real idea of what the father does to earn a living. He has never thought it important to explain his work and they have never thought to inquire about it. His particular knowledge of the world and the attitudes and values by which he lives should be made available to the child, since the children see the father in action less often than they do the mother.

One of the great problems with adolescents is what they are going to do with their lives. This problem is more frequent with children who have not been associated with their father's work. The father works hard to bring home the money to provide for the child's education but gives little consideration to the question of what this education is for.

No father can safely put off becoming acquainted with his child until some time when the child is half grown. A father who wishes to have the comradeship of his son or daughter at the age of fifteen must begin to cultivate the child's friendship when he is a baby. No grown child, for instance, can suddenly become friendly with a parent who has neglected him. The child will not feel that the parent's interest is genuine and he will probably be right in his supposition. The boy needs a friendly father as an example. A girl too, needs a father's interest, for through this interest she will develop a natural relationship with men. No girl who has been neglected by her father or who has been treated unkindly by him will be able to achieve the best kind of relationship with a husband. The same holds true for a boy and his mother. The mother must protect him as a baby and encourage increasing independence as he grows older. A husband and wife who have found happiness for themselves need only to share their lives generously with their children to fortify them for the problems of later life. *Slavish devotion to books on bringing up children is not a substitute for a wholesome family atmosphere in the preparation for living.* In general terms it may be said that when young people consult a physician about these problems his attitude should be that of a friendly parent rather than that of a detached scientist.

Convalescence after Illness or Operation

Physical factors alone cannot explain why convalescence after illness or operation is so long in some cases and so short in others. After an acute febrile illness some patients are soon up and back on the job. The same is true after operation. Others are very slow to "feel well" and convalescence is long drawn out. Some patients actually "never recover" from a certain illness or operation. The illness or operation is a crucial turning point in their lives. A state of semi-invalidism is maintained indefinitely; little or no work is done and former responsibilities are never taken up again.

UNCONSCIOUS WISH TO REMAIN ILL.   To understand this phenomenon we have only to remember that all human beings have an unconscious urge to return to the state of early childhood in which they had no responsibilities and were well cared for. In a severe illness or operation the emotional interest of the patient is withdrawn from the outside world and centered upon himself. An emotional regression to this infantile state is furthered by a general anesthetic or by unconsciousness which has been brought about by any other cause. The first few days after operation have been compared to the very early days of the child's life. The patient awakens from anesthesia usually to find a nurse who takes care of his every wish and need in the same way as the mother once did. The patient likes this and, in fact, may be as fussy as a child about having anyone but his nurse do things for him. He resents being left alone for any length of time and resents any interest on the nurse's part in anyone but himself. Instead of being understood and met and dealt with, this is sometimes resented by both nurse and physician.

THE AUTHORITY OF THE PHYSICIAN.   The surgeon or medical man often takes the place of the father, whose authority is accepted without question. The patient is in a very suggestible frame of mind and the physician or surgeon must be cautious in his comments regarding the patient or his illness. Many patients like to dramatize their illness or operation and a physician who intimates that the patient is lucky to have recovered, or who implies that a long convalescence will be necessary from such a serious illness or operation, may be suggesting something which the patient is all too ready to accept and to a much greater degree than the physician intended. It is natural for the physician, who is human, to want to appear as a benefactor in the eyes of his patient, but he should remember the patient may unconsciously want to be a chronic invalid, and in emphasizing the seriousness of the illness from which he has saved his patient, the latter may reach the conclusion that he is now a very delicate organism whose whole future existence is precarious. The patient may unconsciously use his illness or operation as a means of gratifying a need for dependence and inactivity, or if he does make an inadequate effort to carry on he will blame everything that happens to him on the results of that certain illness or operation. *Therefore, a very important consideration in the mind of every physician and nurse should be that it is part of their duty to combat the self-absorption which to some extent occurs in every patient.* This being the case physicians and nurses should encourage independence as soon as the physical circumstances permit in order to help the patient return to normal health. Often the nurse, in her eagerness to give "service" to the patient, brings about an abrupt change when she leaves, which is difficult for the patient to manage. It is better for the nurse to encourage the patient to be independent before she leaves rather than to cater to the desires of the patient up to the last moment.

It is so easy for the well-meaning physician, after an illness or operation, to show sympathy and goodwill by warnings of "be careful," "take it easy," "get back into things slowly," without differentiating between the patient who needs such warnings and the patient who *must not* have them. The physician who would be most kind must recognize this difference in people and act accordingly. Much chronic invalidism can thus be avoided. (See also Chapter XIX.)

Failure in Accomplishment

At some period in middle life it often happens that the anxiety underlying a psychosomatic disorder is due to a sense of personal or economic failure. A man may have failed to advance in his work or in his profession to the point that he had hoped or he may not have achieved financial security. A married woman may not have fulfilled her hopes to have a child or children, or her children have failed to fulfill her hopes for their accomplishments, or they may have "grown away" from her, or she may not have achieved her social aspirations or a career outside the home. Another woman has failed to acquire a husband, a home or children, or has failed to achieve her ambition in her career.

The physician should be aware that *spinsters* suffer the greatest emotional deprivation because they may not only be frustrated in their love life but also in their careers. They will often attempt to deny any sense of frustration or failure; they hasten to assure the physician that "everything is all right," "they are perfectly satisfied," "they wouldn't have had it any other way." However, such statements usually mean that the patient cannot bear to face her disappointment.

ACKNOWLEDGING FRUSTRATION.   If a sense of failure is suspected and this is pointed out to the patient he may ask, "Well, suppose I haven't accomplished all that I would have liked? If I dwell upon it won't it make me worse?" The answer to this is that it may cause more mental distress momentarily but that if the patient is seriously ill it is better for him to become conscious of frustration in order for him to realize that it may be the cause of his symptoms. In the second place it is only by acknowledging failure that he can analyze the causes and attempt to modify his attitudes and efforts for a more successful approach to the remainder of his life. The business man may thereby be helped to attack his problems more efficiently. A woman may be helped to become a more companionable and a more stimulating mother to her children. The spinster may be helped to deal more constructively with the problem of marriage and if marriage is not possible, perhaps she can be helped to plan a career or extend her circle of interests.

Problems of Aging

The nation is aging rapidly. In 1900 only 17 per cent of the total population of the United States were 45 years old or more. In 1940, 26.5 per cent were over 45, and conservative estimates are that in 1980 more than 40 per cent of our population will be over 45 years of age. Therefore, *gerontology,* the science of aging, has become an important study. This has been recognized in the development of a division on gerontology in the National Institute of Health.

The two terms, *gerontology* and *geriatrics,* must not be confused. Geriatrics is a special field of medical practice which deals with disease in aged individuals, and gerontology is the science of aging. *Senescence* is that part of the aging process which occurs after the peak of development. Although the changes of senescence are largely involutional, they do not solely represent decline. There are important compensations in certain functional capacities. Hence the unutilized potentialities of the aging are worthy of serious consideration.

Stiglitz states that the problems of aging with which gerontology is concerned are divisible into three major categories:

1. *The biology of senescence as a process.*

2. *The clinical problems of senescence in man.* Here questions are divisible into those relating to normal senescence and those relating to abnormality due to disorders associated with advancing years. Normal aging brings many changes, some obvious, others obscure, but all insidious and progressive. Chronological age is not identical with biological age. This we have already discussed. The common concept that senescence implies decline is erroneous for there is considerable compensation in certain functional capacities. Loss of physical strength and speed of reaction is often counterbalanced by increased skill and judgment. The popular phrase, "You can't teach an old dog new tricks," has done great harm. As a result many older people admit defeat before trying and opportunities for adult education are suppressed. Recent studies reveal that once this resistance to adult learning is overcome the capacity to learn is really very slightly diminished by aging. It would be better to say, "It is never too late to learn." This has a considerable bearing upon the psychosomatic problems of the aging. To distinguish certain phenomena of disease from those attributable to aging is most difficult. As we have tried to stress, the phenomena of disease are in many instances only exaggerations of normal reactions and do not imply new mecha-

nisms. The most significant of the geriatric disorders are cardiovascular-renal disease, arthritis, diabetes, cancer and certain syndromes of the climacteric. Of all these the cardiovascular-renal group, which includes hypertensive arterial disease and atherosclerosis, is the most significant. Arthritis also plays an immense role in disability, although its mortality is low. Not only are these disorders usually insidious in onset, but they are chronically progressive and bring about greater or lesser degrees of invalidism.

3. *Social-economic and psychological problems.*   The sociologic problems produced by increased longevity and greater life expectancy and the rising median age of the population are immense and complex. Industry is just awakening to the implications of the fact that the average age of employees is increasing at a surprising rate. Problems of placement and retirement, utilization and conservation of the health of older men in positions of great responsibility, the complexities of the workmen's compensation laws in relation to occupational exacerbation of preexistent disease, and many more questions are becoming increasingly important.

OLD AGE AND PRESTIGE.   In addition to the physical changes that occur with advancing years there are various sociological factors involving the adjustment of the individual to his environment which often result in emotional conflict. In our society old age is often regarded as an affliction and any skill and judgment acquired through years of experience is pushed aside for the energy and new ideas of youth. Old age receives little of the veneration so often accorded to the aged in such parts of the world as China or even in various parts of Europe. It is common practice in industry to view the man of 45 or 50 as being too old to learn or physically incapable of measuring up to certain standards of production. In an industrial world where speed and precision are so important the older person is usually thrust aside in favor of the greater speed, agility and endurance of youth. On careful thought it seems clear that the wisdom of experience, the mature judgment, the emotional stability and the capacity to teach the young would compensate for speed and endurance. Nevertheless, it is true that a marked preference by industry for younger men leads to insecurity on the part of the man who nears 50.

MENTAL CHANGES IN OLD AGE.   Of course, it is true that many human beings are unable to retain emotional and ideational flexibility as they grow older. They adjust badly to new ideas, they resist change, they are slow to make new friends, they have difficulties in memory, and what begins as a mild uneasiness often goes on to irritability, insomnia, and a general apprehensiveness and restlessness. To Overholser's excellent discussion of this topic we are indebted for many helpful suggestions.

What part cerebral arteriosclerosis, which interferes with nutrition of the brain, may play is difficult to determine. What begins as pessimism and mild mental depression often goes on to fears of death and delusions of persecution, and the afflicted individual becomes a menace to himself and a responsibility to others. He may wander aimlessly about the house or into the street. He may be careless with matches and fire, and, because of the breaking through of earlier repressed sexual impulses, he may make improper sexual advances to women or to young children.

Aging judgments may become so bad as to necessitate taking the man from his business. Sometimes such a person is permitted to harm a business because relatives and partners are afraid to hurt his feelings or are afraid to arouse his anger. It is often difficult to say when the memory defects, irritability and querulousness of old age have merged into actual psychosis. However, evidence of intellectual defect, the presence of marked insomnia, restlessness, delusions and hallucinations or other evidences of lack of control usually enable one to make a diagnosis of mental illness even though some parts of the personality are still intact. If cerebral arteriosclerosis is marked, or if an intracranial vascular accident occurs, the progression of mental symptoms may be greatly accelerated.

TREATMENT. *Prophylaxis.* Few people think concretely about how they will live after retirement or when they become older. They may vaguely assume that they will live with children without considering whether the children will want them or not. They may consider a small business without mapping out concretely what that business will be, whether they can afford it, whether they have enough health and money to start and run it and where it will be located.

Few people consider their chances of longevity. Actually it is computed that half of those in the United States who are now 50 will live twenty-five to fifty years more. Half of the women who reach 65 will live to be 80 and half of the men who reach 65 will live to be 88. The average American now has a life expectancy of 70—in contrast to one hundred years ago when the average life ended at 40. These figures tend to show what more people should prepare for.

As for the older people who are infirm, it needs to be kept in mind half of all working women are married. Hence an aged, infirm woman may not have her daughter or daughter-in-law around to care for her during the working day and this creates a problem. But what shall be done with her? Should she be institutionalized and if not who will take care of her? A whole problem has arisen over the aged who have no one to care for them and who cannot take care of themselves. Yet they are neither senile nor mentally incompetent. Social Security, Old Age Assistance and pension plans have made more older people financially independent. Yet little has been done to take care of their mental or emotional needs by recognizing their need to be useful and contributing citizens.

Many older people depend upon work as the means of maintaining their self-esteem. Hence their self-esteem declines when they are no longer employed and they become poor company for those with whom they live. It is not easy to get people to prepare for diversion when retired, but some industrial concerns help "about-to-be retired" individuals to retire *to* something rather than just retire *from* a regular schedule to idleness.

A case in point is that of a woman of 32 who married early at the age of 16. She had two children by this marriage but because of her husband's infidelity and alcoholism she obtained a divorce. She has married again but with two children of the first marriage in her new home *and* a mother who has cataracts and is "nearly blind," she is on the verge of a second divorce. Her husband wants to move into a housing project and *leave mother behind* because mother has injected contention into family life. The patient is in great conflict. To leave mother to shift for herself is gross neglect of filial duty. But mother at her best did not do too well as a mother and the patient does not want to leave her husband. What to do? Which way to decide? This is a case for psychiatrists and social workers to see the parties involved and offer their combined wisdom. Perhaps it would be better for the nearly blind mother to try to live alone and let the family work out their destiny. Or perhaps the family should be helped to take mother in. The solution of such cases involves the judgment of (*a*) each one's strength, and (*b*) each one's ability to change, and (*c*) the decision which will do the greatest good for the greatest number. No one should tyrannize.

A woman who loses vision and who has little social resourcefulness places a great problem upon her family which they may solve with their own goodwill and resourcefulness if they possess such. But if they do not, then community agencies must help them (*a*) to test the adaptability of each family member to the problem or (*b*) to care for the older person with the failing vision with whatever resources are available in the community and help the family to accept the decision without being handicapped by guilt and recrimination.

The man or woman who plans to be useful and valuable when retirement age is reached is the exception and not the rule. And he is so preoccupied in being useful that he never incurs sympathy. The other type of older person is so helpless, so demanding, so needy for the attention of others, so craving for deference that his care and living arrangements put everyone under a great strain. It would be desirable if older people could be indoctrinated in groups—either separate groups of men and women, or together. Churches are beginning to form groups for older people. So are organizations such as the Y.M.C.A., adult education groups and the like. Some communities have old age social groups; some areas such as Philadelphia have an organization called "Careers over Forty" where members help each other.

It should be a facet of our mental health program that each community have some program for older people, or more than one, sponsored by the local mental health association or by the local Health and Welfare Council. This should include discussion groups, recreations, education and hobbies. These activities preserve some mental health and give dignity to the aging process.

In the disorders of old age, no less than in any other psychosomatic problem, there should be some thought as to prevention. The child who is taught to be sociable and adaptable and resourceful will usually continue to be so in adult life and in old age. But education must not stop in childhood. *Adult education* is being looked upon with increasing interest. Community high schools are instituting classes in all kinds of subjects. Hobbies are discovered, as well as new forms of recreation, not to mention instruction in many subjects which contribute to intellectual improvement. People should be encouraged to attend these courses. They are of inestimable value as emotional investments against the impoverishments of later years.

A series of six pamphlets, "Notes for After Fifty," have been written by Edith M. Stern with Edward Linzer. They are available through the National Association for Mental Health, 1790 Broadway, New York 19, N. Y. Some of the statistics and insights of these pamphlets are recommended as a prescription for older people with problems who can benefit through some important reading. If the older person cannot read, the facts are in the pamphlets for the physician to give him.

Friction in the Home. Aging people are often problems in the homes of children. The differences in points of view cause frictions. The aging person may want to be a good sport and not get in the way but he or she cannot help giving unwanted advice. If there are children in the home the older people often try to supervise them—by an outmoded standard of values. The family physician often is reluctant to take part in family differences of this kind. However, if he wishes to relieve the emotional strains which are causing anxiety and producing symptoms, he may have to get acquainted with the two points of view, usually of daughter and mother-in-law, and suggest ways in which they can be reconciled. The aging parent or parent-in-law will often listen to advice from a physician when the same thing coming from a son or daughter would be rejected. The same is true when the son or daughter needs advice.

The Interests of the Children. When excessive irritability or attitudes of suspicion create too much friction in the home and cannot be corrected, it may be best to place the older person in a *nursing home* where he or she is associated with other people of the same age. If this can be afforded it usually makes life much more pleasant for everyone concerned. Often sons and daughters are reluctant to do this, fearing the older person may not like it, or may reproach them for having been pushed out, or that neighbors, friends or other relatives may accuse them of disloyalty. As a consequence an otherwise happy family life may be disrupted. In such cases the physician must try to think of the greatest good to the greatest number. A consideration of first importance must be the children in such a home. They must not serve as a buffer between the conflicting interests of different generations.

Mental Hospitals. Placing the psychotic aged person in a mental hospital is usually a last resort. When restlessness and insomnia can no longer be controlled by sedatives and hypnotics and when the aged person has lost control of himself in other ways, he must be given closer supervision and control than is possible in the average home. Sometimes depression of spirits is so marked in aged people that they contemplate and actually carry out *suicide*. It is not uncommon for the aged person to have such impairment in judgment and emotional control as to make sexual advances, and when this happens to small children it may have very unfortunate consequences. Certainly this demands the supervision which mental hospitals can give. When the mental state is one of slow progression, occurring in a person who has shown emotional and social limitations during most of his lifetime, it usually means a steady development toward greater dementia, unless early and active rehabilitation is begun.

References

Brown, M. L., Lucente, E. R., Alesbury, J. M., and Perloff, W. H.: Am. J. Obst. & Gynec., *61:* 200, 1951.

Deutsch, F.: Psychoanalyt. Quart., *8:* 354, 1939.

Gayford, M.: Personal Communication, May, 1947.

Giberson, L. G.: Clinics, *2:* 719, 1943.

Hertzman, J.: J. Social Case Work, *27:* 299, 1946.

Kinsey, A. C., Pomeroy, W. B., and Martin, C. E.: Sexual Behavior in the Human Male. W. B. Saunders Co., Philadelphia, 1948.

Kinsey, A. C., Pomeroy, W. B., Martin, C. E., and Gebhard, P. W.: Sexual Behavior in the Human Female. W. B. Saunders Co., Philadelphia, 1953.

Kroger, W. S., and DeLee, S. T.: Am. J. Obst. & Gynec., *51:* 544, 1946.

Overholser, W.: M. Ann. Dist. Columbia, *10:* 1, 1941.

Perloff, W. H.: Am. J. Obst. & Gynec., *59:* 223, 1950.

Perloff, W. H.: J. Clin. Endocrinol., *10:* 447, 1950.

Perloff, W. H.: Am. J. Obst. & Gynec., *61:*670, 1951.

Ross, W. D.: Psychosom. Med., *7:* 80, 1945.

Ross, W. D., and McNaughton, F. C.: Psychosom. Med., *7:* 73, 1945.

Smith, J. A.: J.A.M.A., *161:* 38, 1956.

Steinberg, A., Pastor, N., Winheld, E. B., Segal, H. I., Shechter, F. R., and Colton, N. H.: Psychosom. Med., *8:* 176, 1946.

Stern, Edith M., and Linzer, Ed.: Notes for After Fifty. National Association for Mental Health, New York, N. Y.

Stieglitz, E. J.: Technology Review, p. 358, June, 1941.

Chapter V

Treatment—Special
Psychotherapeutic Procedures

From what has been said in previous chapters regarding psychotherapy it is evident that one of the tasks of any psychotherapeutic technique is to reduce the amount of energy which enters channels unprofitable to the welfare of the patient. This energy then becomes available for useful purposes. Normal amounts of energy are an individual's birthright but the energy soon becomes attached to such emotions as the need for dependency, the desire for sensual gratification, the need for affection, prestige, love and security. If a man's need for security has been adequately met during his early years it is not likely that he will develop a hysterical paralysis of the legs when danger threatens on the battlefield. If a woman's craving for affection has been met satisfactorily during her childhood she is not likely to become overweight or to develop gastrointestinal symptoms when her turn comes to give affection to others or when she is deprived of it herself. If sexual curiosity has been satisfied and some normal outlet for sensual indulgence has been permitted in childhood a patient is not likely to suffer from hysterical blindness after witnessing a sexual scene. Emotions and ideas press hard for an outlet and if they are denied free expression through normal channels they are shunted into some organ or organ system, or find release in childish rather than adult behavior. "Every psychic tendency seeks adequate bodily expression." Hence, psychotherapeutic techniques hope to release energy being used in symptom formation so that it can be used in more constructive ways.

Resistance to Treatment. Since no human being likes to admit that he is childish or weak or that he differs too much from his fellows, he resists facing these facts. This *resistance* has always to be reckoned with in treatment. It grows out of the natural reluctance to discuss or relive unpleasant experiences. The more unacceptable the patient feels his emotions and ideas to be, the more he tries to avoid or circumvent any treatment which tries to bring them out. Treatment then can be approached from two directions. The therapist can help the patient to *suppress* his unacceptable ideas or he can help the patient to *bring*

Page 149

them into the open. With the latter technique he encounters resistance. This might be compared to treating a boil by sprinkling it with powder, thus hiding it, or opening it with a knife, which the patient resists. The dissimilarity here is that the boil will eventually open spontaneously, thus leading to recovery, whereas spontaneous recovery in most illnesses of psychic origin does not occur. Karl Menninger speaks of the principle of *suppression* and the principle of *expression.* The physician, in the suppressive method of psychotherapy, assumes an active attitude toward the patient's conflicts and endeavors to push them into the unconscious. In expressive psychotherapy the physician endeavors to bring the conflict into the open, where it can be viewed by physician and patient alike, so that an effort can be made to modify the faulty emotional trends. Under suppression Menninger lists terrorism, placebos, rest, hypnosis, suggestion, exhortation, persuasion, command and religious assurance. The methods using the principle of expression are mental catharsis, psychiatric counsel and psychoanalysis.

SUPPRESSIVE THERAPY

Terrorism.   Terrorism seems out of place as a psychotherapeutic technique and yet this method is used relatively frequently in an attempt to cure psychoneuroses, particularly of the hysterical type. An example follows. A physician was called to see a farm hand who had been discharged and who suddenly developed trembling and an inability to walk. The physician decided that the condition was hysterical. He ordered that the stove poker be heated red hot, stating that when this had been done he would apply it to the patient's back. When the red-hot poker was removed from the stove, and the physician advanced toward the patient, his trembling ceased and his paralysis disappeared.

While this "treatment" brought about normal functioning for the time being it did nothing to help the patient understand why he had to behave in such a manner and so, of course, it did nothing to prevent a future recurrence of the same symptom. Such therapy must be regarded as both unscientific and inhuman, and is only to be compared to the barbarous treatment accorded the insane a century ago.

Placebos.   The most frequent method of psychotherapy is the giving of placebos. These take the form of harmless drugs or hypodermic injections of sterile water combined with promises of improvement or cure. The physician implies that the medicine has great virtue and the patient, feeling that he has received some potent drug, is sometimes relieved of symptoms. The administration of the placebo is at least a recognition that the patient is suffering. This the patient appreciates and probably, in many instances, he gets well out of gratitude to the physician for the recognition. Certainly, the giving of placebos is far more satisfying to the patient than to be told that there is nothing wrong and that he need not worry about himself. Whether, in the long run, one method has more worth than the other is debatable. Strictly speaking, a placebo means an inactive or inert drug given to produce a satisfying effect upon the patient. But certain drugs of medicinal value are also given for their suggestive effect, without being specifically indicated. A timely example is *vitamin therapy*. This great advance in our understanding of health and disease has been prostituted by the placebo philosophy. Not only are vitamins administered in the relatively few conditions for which it has been proved that they are specifically indicated but in addition every obscure illness, physical or psychological, gets its complement of vitamins. The eagerness of the profession to find a physical answer to all medical problems, and the gullibility of the public, which also wants to swallow a magic pill to abolish any and all ills, find a common answer in vitamins. The *vita* part of the term is not without significance in this connection. Drug houses and department stores, candy stores and slot machines, peddle vitamins to the extent of millions of dollars annually—money which would go a long way toward real disease prevention. Apparently we must complete the swing of the pendulum as we have with "focal infection."

The physician who prescribes placebos, in whatever form, is not consciously dishonest. He wants to help his patient. He knows his patient expects drug treatment. He is aware of the resistance of the patient to the idea that his symptoms are the result of emotional conflict. He has seen the beneficial effects of suggestion by placebos in other cases and hopes that the same thing will happen again. When he runs out of placebos the patient runs out on him. The answer to this problem lies in an appreciation of the need for correct diagnosis of psychogenic illness and the adoption of an expressive type of psychotherapy rather than a suppressive one.

It is always a question as to who is being fooled by a placebo—the patient or the physician. Placebos have always been a resource of the harassed physician in dealing with neurotic patients but they have also been used in experimental work to determine the true effect of drugs apart from suggestion. Beecher and his associates at the Massachusetts General Hospital studied this problem by comparing the responses of postoperative patients to morphine and to a placebo. In a later study of the placebo reactor as well as the placebo response Lasagna et al. found that more than half of the patients experienced relief of pain from placebo injections. When two or more placebo injections were given, 69 per cent responded at least once with significant relief, while 14 per cent, the extreme reactors, responded unfailingly. The reactors also achieved more relief from morphine than the nonreactors, who made up 31 per cent of the group. Significant differences were found in attitudes, habits, educational background and personality structure between consistent reactors and nonreactors.

In general, the reactors were found to be less critical individuals. They were happier about their hospital experience and tended to minimize the postoperative discomfort they had suffered. Reaction and nonreaction were found to be independent of age and sex; women were not more likely to respond to a placebo than men.

Rorschach tests showed that the reactors differed from the nonreactors in being less hostile and more dependent on outside stimulation and support. Although they were more anxious, their outward orientation seemed to indicate that their anxieties could be more easily resolved.

Just as placebos have beneficial results, so may they produce toxic effects. Therefore a placebo effect may be positive or negative. Placebos can nullify or overbalance the pharmacologic action of drugs and produce side effects indistinguishable from those due to drugs. For these reasons Beecher states that "it should be apparent that 'clinical impression' is hardly a dependable source of information without the essential safeguards of the double unknowns technique, the use of placebos also as unknowns, randomization of administration, the use of correlated data (all agents are studied in the same patients), and mathematical validation of any supposed differences."

Fischer and Dlin conclude that the potency of the placebo is derived from and is a part of the emotionally invested doctor-patient relationship and that placebo therapy, if used, should always be an adjunct to psychotherapy.

Tranquilizing Drugs.   The tranquilizing drugs (or ataractics) have excited considerable interest. They produce an "emotional detachment," usually not a goal in psychiatric treatment, but one of immense importance when the detachment separates the patient from the acute excitement produced by his response to hallucinatory or delusional ideation.

The three main classes are: (1) The phenothiazine derivatives chlorpromazine and promazine, which presumably act on the cortex to produce a sedative effect, on the hypothalamus and thalamus to produce autonomic effects, and, with a depression of the alerting mechanism in the reticular formation, produce a quiescence which allows the patient to communicate his concerns without acute excitement. (2) The rauwolfia alkaloids, which have similar autonomic and sedative actions but require a longer period of dosage before effects are observed. (3) Meprobamate, a compound related to the internuncial neuron-blocking agent mephenesin, but with a longer duration of effect.

Side effects are a hazard. The main ones in the phenothiazine group, jaundice and parkinsonism, may have been lessened with the subtraction from the molecular structure of a chlorine radical. Agranulocytosis remains a constant hazard but is usually preceded by other toxic signs, such as a skin rash and fever. The rauwolfia alkaloids share the danger of parkinsonism but not that of jaundice. They tend to produce a depressive "turbulent" period. The least toxic is meprobamate which does not, however, appear to produce the same degree of "detachment" as the other drugs.

The search for new compounds is now directed toward lessening the possible toxic effects of present drugs; toward chemically or clinically related substances; toward chemicals which will antagonize such hallucinogenic substances as lysergic acid, mescoline, adrenochrome and serotonin; toward any preparation which will antagonize the action of drugs having recognized cerebral activity, such as anticholinergic substances.

These drugs do not appear to solve the problems of psychiatric treatment but rather add to them, because to effectively utilize these states of quiescence, active psychotherapeutic and sociologic measures to meet the return to "normalcy" which these drugs afford must be undertaken.

Another term which has been used to describe the action of these drugs, "chemical hibernation," suggests that while there is some organic fact of separation from internal or external stress during the period of drug administration, which may allow an internal reorganization of the personality structure, this cannot be relied upon. Very often these drugs may be unwisely used when more active psychotherapeutic measures should be undertaken to prevent progression or fixation of symptoms. Nonetheless, the improvement which these drugs offer patients suffering from the protean manifestations of psychosis should not be undervalued.

Meprobamate has been widely used in office practice for general tension and anxiety where it seems to reduce irritability and restlessness and promote generalized muscular relaxation and more restful sleep. Absence of toxicity and its non-habit-forming character have promoted its usefulness so that, as of this writing, its sale is threatening to exceed the sale of the barbiturates.

New preparations are being introduced almost as rapidly as antibiotics but we are conservative enough to believe that the total answer to mental and emotional illness will not come about in this fashion. They are undoubtedly useful but only as adjuncts to psychotherapy. We should not expect them to replace it.

Rest.   Rest and vacation are the first things that a physician thinks of in dealing with illness of emotional origin. He recognizes that the symptoms are due to external pressures of work or family life (which induce emotional conflicts) and he thinks first of reducing the pressures. It is felt, and rightly so, that in many instances rest will have a salutary effect. To be given permission by an authority like the physician to leave one's daily duties and go to bed does much to reduce anxiety and remove symptoms. In fact, about the turn of the present century, S. Weir Mitchell achieved fame for himself by prescribing the "rest cure." Believing that weakness and nervous exhaustion were responsible for illness of emotional origin he prescribed a definite regimen of rest and forced feeding. It worked very successfully because it catered to some of the most basic needs of the psychoneurotic individual. The patient was removed from the struggle of life; he was nursed and massaged, pampered and well fed. In short, he was treated as an infant and all of the infantile longings, called forth by the illness, were satisfied. Symptoms disappeared and in many cases the improvement continued for some time. In others, a frequent repetition of the rest cure was necessary. But a great many patients continued to be invalids for life and their characters were not improved by a treatment which provided so much secondary gain from illness. Rest has its value in relieving symptoms, but it does nothing to make the patient understand himself better. It does not show him what has made him ill nor does it cure emotional conflicts. The truth of the matter is that a "rest cure" or even a recommendation to "take it easy" does a positive disservice to many neurotic patients. A great many of these patients have to be told to "carry on in spite of symptoms," while the neurotic mechanisms underlying the symptoms are being worked out.

Suggestion and Persuasion.   Suggestion and persuasion are closely allied. Persuasion is added to suggestion in order to convince the patient that the suggestion is a good one and that in following it he will be benefited. In the same way command is combined with exhortation. If a patient suffers from paralysis of the legs it is suggested that there is no disease in his legs and that he can use them. This is repeated to him in various ways in order to persuade him of the truth of the suggestion. Then follows the command to use the legs. The aim of these methods is to make the patient cooperate by overcoming the forces which seek dependence and disability. Sometimes the method succeeds but very often the forces which seek dependence and relief from responsibility are too powerful to be overcome by any combination of suggestion, persuasion, command or exhortation.

Hypnosis.   A special and intense form of suggestion is utilized in hypnosis. The patient is asked to relax and is told that he is going to sleep. The hypnotist repeats his command in a low but firm voice. Sometimes he asks the patient to look at a bright object such as a ring, a coin, or some other small object. Or the hypnotist may stroke the forehead or the arms of the patient, repeating in a monotone some such formula as the following, "You are going to sleep. Your eyes are getting heavy. You feel very drowsy. Your eyes are getting heavier and heavier. The lids are closing. You are going to sleep." After a matter of seconds or minutes the patient enters a trance-like state of varying depth. In this sleeping state the patient may be given commands which he will carry out either during his trance, or after waking. This latter phenomenon is called *posthypnotic suggestion*.

Under hypnosis it can be suggested that pains will diminish, paralysis will disappear, that memory for certain events will be restored; in fact, almost any suggestion can be made, providing it does not conflict too much with the patient's training and fixed beliefs. It is said that patients who are hypnotized will not commit immoral or illegal acts, especially if their training has been highly moral.

EXPERIMENTAL VALUE.   Hypnosis has been known and used since the first part of the eighteenth century and has enjoyed popularity from time to time. It was used extensively by an Austrian named Mesmer and at time takes his name as "Mesmerism." It was also used by Charcot in Paris in the treatment of hysteria about 1870. Theoretically interesting, it has little practical value in treatment. It has had great value in psychological experimentation, especially from the standpoint of its contribution to psychopathology. The effects of hypnotism are not lasting. Through its use temporary dissociations of mental phenomena can occur and for the time being resistances can be overcome. For instance, dissociations can be brought about which will prevent the registry of pain impulses. A traumatic event which has induced paralysis can be dissociated so that function can once more take place. Painful affects which have produced defective memory can be dissociated so that memory returns. In other words, parts of the mind can be made to function without the knowledge of another part of the mind.

TEMPORARY CURE. Normal people under hypnosis can be made to laugh, to feel strange sensations in their bodies, to make ludicrous statements and to carry out ridiculous acts without remembering what took place. In emotionally ill people that part of the personality which disturbs normal function can be influenced by hypnosis. However, since this does nothing to bring about an understanding of the factors which produce the symptoms, the "cure" is only temporary, or the conflict takes some other form of expression.

Psychoanalysis has shown that it takes a conscious reliving of the unpleasant experiences to produce any permanent discharge of the unpleasant affect which is producing symptoms. This requires much time and effort. So hypnosis remains a therapy of suggestion, uncertain in its results and limited in its possibilities. At best it can cause a temporary shifting about of conflicts but it does not actually cure them. Furthermore it brings about a greater dependence upon some outer authority (the hypnotist).

A therapy which *reveals* rather than *conceals* the emotional pathology has greater value!

Religious Assurances. Undoubtedly many cures, more temporary than permanent, have taken place through religious assurances. These may take the form of affirmation, blessing, anointing, ingestion of consecrated bread, utilization of the sign of the cross, a visit to a shrine, or reassurance by a religious personage. When we attempt to explain this phenomenon scientifically we should bear in mind that love has a beneficial effect upon disturbances of emotional origin. The suffering child is helped by the security which he feels in the presence of his mother and father. Religion has much to do with mother and father figures. It is the childish parts of the personality which are in great need of love and reassurance in illness of emotional origin. Hence, when conflicts produced by guilt, hostility and sexuality produce pain and suffering, contact with a religious force may do much to bring relief. Physicians recognize the spiritual values of religion for themselves and their patients but they possess neither the religious training nor the desire to utilize religious assurances psychotherapeutically. A rare exception may be made; occasionally a patient is so inaccessible to psychotherapy that religion must be called upon to perform a function for which it is not intended. In the great majority of patients, however, as we have repeatedly emphasized, it is the direct working with the patient's emotional conflicts by the physician himself, based on his knowledge of the personality structure, which will have more controlled and more lasting results.

There is only one large religious order which specializes in healing the sick and its method of doing so does not deviate from the principles mentioned above. Christian Science has undoubtedly made many people feel better and function better, but it has also delayed scientific help to thousands of people until it was too late to be of any value. We feel that there is no power in Christian Science which is not possessed by a clergyman, priest or rabbi, none of whom attempts to heal the sick. They comfort and help the sick but the cure of disease is left in the hands of the medical profession.

EXPRESSIVE THERAPY

Psychoanalysis. Psychoanalysis is founded upon the psychobiological development of the individual. It is a medically orientated psychology; it is a psychology related to physiology. It teaches that physiological processes and psychological processes are indissolubly related in their development. It is a psychology of instincts. It shows how some of the most important emotional trends and ideas in the life of the human being are implanted in early childhood. It recognizes that these early life experiences and the resulting ideas and emotions are registered in the unconscious mind as forces which influence behavior. A psychology so intimately related to the functioning of the human body is obviously the best suited to the physician's use.

Psychoanalysis as a treatment aims at the redistribution of psychic energy. This means that when emotional trends are directed into wrong channels psychoanalysis attempts to make the reasons clear to the patient and thus help him in redistributing this energy into more constructive channels.

There still remains a misconception as to the nature of psychoanalysis. Some use the term to cover a single psychiatric interview which attempts to evaluate the existing personality disturbance. Others use the term to designate a few interviews in which the attempt is made to modify surface anxiety and correct a few faulty ideas. Psychoanalysis, however, is a major psychotherapeutic operation and it must take a long time. It follows a definite technique, as outlined by Freud, which consists of several sessions weekly over a period of a year or more, depending upon the severity of the illness.

Special qualifications are required for those who practice psychoanalysis. In fact, it was one of the first medical specialties to require certification of its members. They must have experience in psychiatric hospitals for a year or more. They must be trained in neurology. They have to undergo a *personal psychoanalysis* in order to be aware of their own personality difficulties. They must begin the practice of psychoanalysis under the control of those more experienced in the field and must have supervision in the treatment of at least two cases. They must attend lectures on the theory of psychoanalysis and on psychoanalytic technique, and they must attend seminars in which the clinical aspects of the neuroses and psychoses are presented. The discipline is arduous and the preparation may occupy five or six years. In this country most psychoanalysts are first physicians and psychiatrists, who then add to their psychiatric knowledge the training in psychoanalysis just outlined.

It is sometimes surprising how uninformed students of medicine and physicians regard the differences among neurologists, psychiatrists, psychoanalysts and psychologists. The *neurologist* is trained in the structure and function of the nervous system. He studies neuropathology, neurophysiology and the clinical phenomena of organic disease of the nervous system. The fields of neurology and psychiatry have become so extensive that it is practically impossible to be a first-class neurologist and at the same time a first-class psychiatrist. However, since there is a dearth of practitioners in these fields it is necessary, in many communities, for the specialties to be combined as neuropsychiatry. Nevertheless, the tendency toward separation should be encouraged.

The emphasis in the training of the *psychiatrist* has been on the psychoses. He has usually spent long years working in mental hospitals. Just as the neurologist has spent some time with psychotics in order to have some acquaintance with mental illness, so the psychiatrist has spent some time in neurology in order to be able to recognize some of the more common and more evident neurological disorders. However, the psychiatrist does not pretend to make a refined neurological diagnosis and usually refers such work to his neurological colleague.

The *psychoanalyst* is a psychiatrist who has received special training in the psychopathology of the unconscious mind, originated by Freud, and his work with patients is usually confined to the practice of this particular psychotherapeutic technique. *Psychoanalysis is related to psychiatry as microscopic anatomy is related to gross anatomy.*

The *psychologist* is not a physician and does not treat sick people. Psychologists can be divided roughly into three main groups composed of (1) the experimental psychologist who studies animal as well as human behavior; (2) the clinical psychologist who concerns himself with measurements of intelligence, tests of vocational aptitude, and is now attempting to develop some satisfactory measurement of personality values; (3) the consulting psychologist who uses his knowledge of mental life in personnel work and counseling with normal groups.

During World War II the psychologist became an important member of a team composed of psychiatrist, social worker and psychologist, and fortunately in many instances this teamwork has continued in civilian practice.

Harrower has said that the psychologist with his personality tests must do more than establish a diagnosis. He must assume the more positive role of assessing the dimensions and depths of the personality and exploring the individual's potentialities and resources. Thus his task would lie not simply in the diagnosis of a neurosis, but rather in a description of the type of personality in which neurotic symptoms were finding expression. In this way he can be of greater help to the psychotherapist who can then make use of this knowledge in planning for the patient's welfare.

Academic psychology, for the most part, has been very critical of psychoanalysis, but in embracing the Rorschach technique of personality evaluation, it has moved a little closer toward accepting the basic concepts of psychoanalysis. An appreciation of the workings of unconscious mental forces, as revealed by the Rorschach method, has made the depth psychology of Sigmund Freud a little more acceptable. Indeed, the Rorschach test has done for psychology what the psychosomatic concept has done for medicine, that is, provided a bridge of understanding between the organic tradition and a dynamic explanation of human behavior in sickness as well as in health.

INDICATIONS FOR PSYCHOANALYSIS.   Having tried to make clear what psychoanalysis is, we must say something about the indications for its use. For the most part, at present, patients come to psychoanalysis only when all other methods have been exhausted and all treatments have failed to help them. In brief, it is indicated in most severe neuroses. It is indicated in some cases of psychopathic personality such as alcoholism, sexual perversion, kleptomania, and other personality disturbances, providing that the patient has a strong desire to get well and there can be some co-operation and support from the family. Kubie summarizes the indications for psychoanalysis as (1) treatment for a fully developed neurosis, (2) to prevent neurosis from developing, (3) to prevent development or recurrence of a psychosis, (4) to find out the cause of some unhappy maladjustment in the personality. To these we would add: (5) to prevent a mild neurosis from becoming a severe and crippling illness as age advances and frustrations increase, and (6) to cure or alleviate the symptoms of psychosomatic disorder.

Treatment by psychoanalysis is preferably carried out early in life. Aside from the psychoanalysis of children, which is done for severe personality maladjustments, the next period of choice is early adult life. Clinical experience has shown that the adolescent period is not satisfactory. Since psychoanalysis means an inevitable change in certain fundamental attitudes toward life it is highly desirable that such a procedure be undertaken before too many irrevocable commitments have been made. A great many people make choices of career, marriage, parenthood, and other crucial decisions, in an effort to solve neurotic conflicts. In other words, these decisions are often symptomatic of their personality disorder. Therefore, if they are to be treated by psychoanalysis it had better be before, rather than after, these decisions have been made. Most analysts prefer patients under the age of forty, although the procedure may still have value after this age. It is especially important for a woman to solve her problems as early in life as possible, for if she wishes to marry and have children her time is limited, not to mention the limitation in opportunities.

THE TECHNIQUE OF PSYCHOANALYSIS.   Psychoanalysis is usually conducted with the patient lying on a couch while the physician sits behind him. In this position it is usually much easier for a patient to talk. As Alexander expressed it, "in the relaxed and matter of fact atmosphere of the psychoanalytic sessions the patient is encouraged to express himself in intelligible language instead of in the distorted language of his symptoms." The patient is instructed to say everything that comes to his mind, regardless of how inappropriate, irrelevant or personal it may seem to be. As the patient follows this rule certain trends of thought are manifested. Hostility, fear, feelings of dependency, sexual fantasies, ideas of suspicion, jealousy, and so forth, weave themselves into a pattern which expresses the patient's total personality. The material appears slowly—a little each day. As the material comes up its influence on the daily life of the patient is observed. Observed, too, is the reverse of this situation, that is, the influence of the daily life happenings on the material from the unconscious mental life. As Kubie puts it, "The patient's present life is a screen on which the past throws its shadows."

RELATION OF PATIENT TO ANALYST.   As these ideas and feelings are expressed a certain relation to the analyst is noted. Again to quote Kubie, "The analyst becomes a storm center of highly charged emotions." Hostility, fear, anger, and the like, which arose in other connections, are often expressed in relation to the analyst, whose own analysis permits him to tolerate their expression. After a variable time the patient begins to understand how unjustified these emotions are in relation to the analyst, who has tried to be entirely objective in his explanations, and he also sees that they have had their derivation from earlier life experience, usually the experiences of childhood. The reliving of the emotional experience, and the insight gained thereby, permit the mind to discharge the pathological material. This process is called *abreaction*. Psychic energy, which no longer has to be expended in repressing the pathological material, is now free to be turned into more constructive channels.

THE STUDY OF EMOTIONAL TRENDS.   In coming to the analyst several times a week, the patient has an opportunity to study his most basic emotional trends. Physician and patient focus their attention upon the feelings expressed toward the world in general and the analyst in particular, and the result is often most surprising to the patient. Having assumed that he was decisive he finds himself vacillating; having thought himself courageous he finds that he is timid; in his own eyes generous and magnanimous, he finds himself petty and parsimonious. Or, on the contrary, he may have considered himself stupid only to find that his ideas have merit. He has been handicapped by a feeling of inferiority and finds that his capacities are equal or superior to those of his associates. The opportunity offered by psychoanalysis to speak frankly and fearlessly about one's self reveals many things which the person has never before known about himself. Some people will fairly readily assimilate these facts and make some rearrangement of their lives. Others have so much hate, resentment, bitterness and distrust built up within them that they find it difficult to bring about any change in attitude.

TRANSFERENCE.   The relation of patient to physician is a phenomenon which has been given particular attention by Freud and his followers ever since psychoanalysis began. This tendency for emotion from another time and situation to occur in the psychotherapeutic session and to express itself in relation to the therapist is known as *transference*. The transference situation has many important implications for medicine in general and the management and utilization of this phenomenon is a most significant feature of psychoanalysis.

Alexander defines the transference as merely a projection of the past into the analytic situation, and the tranference situation, in reality, as nothing more than the relation between patient and physician. The transference manifestations occur under the continuous control of the ego and the patient is aware of their unmotivated nature. "The essential point is that in the transference, the adult with his stronger and more resistant ego faces in reduced quantity the same kind of conflict which as a child his weak ego could not solve. The solution of the reduced emotional conflict effects an increase in the resistance of the conscious ego, which becomes able to face mental conflicts and situations which were previously unbearable. This principle of analytic treatment can be compared with that of active immunization, by means of which the resistance of the body is partially increased by fighting small quantities of toxin."

In the setting of the psychiatric interview (when the attentions of the patient and the physician are not focused on the physical aspects of illness) there is time and opportunity for the patient to express his feelings, and that is when we are in the best position to see the basic emotional trends in action.

While the patient exhibits emotional attitudes which he has held toward a parent or someone else who has played an important role in his life, he is, of course, still able to react to the doctor as he really is. The doctor may be conscientious, kind and considerate, and this may be felt by the patient if he has some capacity for reality testing. In fact, some degree of being able to react emotionally to the present is essential to therapeutic progress. However, it is an important part of therapy to help the patient understand that some of his emotions are those of childhood and are now no longer necessary or useful. He must not only appreciate this intellectually, he must feel it emotionally. Indeed this should be stated in reverse, because what the patient feels and exhibits in his behavior is then explained intellectually.

When the patient's childhood attitudes are especially prominent he may see the physician and his role in a distorted way, but the physician must maintain his objectivity and allow full freedom of expression in order that the patient may get the necessary understanding of his problem. Many people in their day-to-day living have different moods, exhibit petty jealousies, become unreasonably angry over trifles, feel themselves exploited, blame others for lack of consideration, and they never change. In the controlled patient-physician relation, however, the setting is different: (1) The patient acknowledges that he is ill for emotional reasons; (2) he asks the physician to help him; (3) the physician remains objective and is neither critical nor punitive as (4) he explains how the mind functions and how to correct harmful attitudes.

Transference and the Physician.   Transference and countertransference are not solely the concern of the psychoanalyst. Fortunately (or unfortunately) the average patient-physician relationship engenders these same problems and they are even more difficult to understand because they are unconscious. For this reason the physician should be as free of mental conflict as possible in order not to confuse his patient's thinking any further. The less insight the physician has into his own emotions, the less likely he is to present the best attitude for the patient's recovery.

For instance, a physician may believe that women are by nature frigid; if he does, he will be of little help with the neuroses in which sexual difficulties enter strongly into the picture. He would, likewise, be a relatively useless counselor in most marital problems. Or the physician may be unable to stand anxiety in his patients without dosing them with sedatives. Or he cannot tolerate their displeasure and so will try to please them rather than do what is best for them. He may not like neurotic people and, being unaware of this, may mistakenly and sometimes cruelly subject them to painful, useless and expensive medical and surgical procedures. He may hold on to certain patients too long and fail to refer them for the expert help which they need. This may arise from his own insecurity represented by the necessity for a large income. Or, overconfident, he takes chances which are not scientifically justified.

Some pediatricians, feeling that children are "spoiled" by too much affection, teach the mothers to be frustrating rather than to give their affections freely. The obstetrician's inability to deal with the anxieties, questions and discomforts of the mother may result in so much anxiety and suffering during pregnancy and delivery that the number of children is limited. A surgeon with a great deal of unconscious hostility toward women cannot understand them, and when they come to his office unhappy and complaining, and very willing to attribute their distress to some bodily disorder, he, having the tools and knowing the techniques of cutting, thinks he may remove the discomfort (which often represents childishness, dependency and hostility) by surgery. He tries to remove a pain from the body which really resides in the spirit, or psyche.

Although these attitudes on the part of the physician are not ordinarily thought of as *transference* reactions the truth is that every physician gets into a transference situation with every patient the moment they meet, regardless of the problem. Each immediately brings many unconscious attitudes into the relationship, and these attitudes, of which both may be completely unaware, have great influence on the outcome of the illness.

The psychoanalyst has the kind of training which tends to reduce to a minimum these unfortunate attitudes. He does not claim to be completely objective. He merely claims to be relatively so, and he is always on the alert to keep his own immature attitudes and prejudices out of the picture, in order to give the patient the best opportunity for self-development. He also tries to pass on to his colleagues in the other areas of medicine some of the insight into interpersonal relations that will keep destructive countertransference reactions at a minimum.

Just as the patient transfers his emotions to the analyst so the analyst cannot avoid transferring certain feelings toward his patient. This phenomenon is called *countertransference*. But by his own analysis, made in preparation to practice psychoanalysis, the analyst is in a much better position to remain detached. The psychoanalyst, being human, does not relish being criticized, condemned and berated for months on end, but his insight and understanding make it possible for him to endure this without efforts to retaliate. So also the psychoanalyst is naturally pleased by his patient's gratitude and admiration but he does not allow this to deter him from pointing out his patient's shortcomings, when this is necessary. In short, the analyst has tried to obtain through his training as great an objectivity as possible concerning human emotions. Thus he can maintain an objective attitude toward the emotionally sick person in his attempt to help him to achieve emotional stability.

THE USE OF DREAMS.   Freud was the first to utilize the dream as a means of helping the patient to understand the workings of the unconscious mind. Some patients dream freely, one or more dreams every night, while others dream rarely. There is mental activity going on during sleep whether it is remembered as a dream or not. Some patients immediately accept the dream as meaningful while others have great resistance to "seeing any sense in dreams." Some dreams are very clear and understandable as *wish fulfillments.* A child dreams that he owns and rides a pony, or the business man, who must remain at work every day, may dream that he is attending a ball game. Other dreams, however, may be much more difficult to understand, as for instance a dream that a relative or friend is ill or dead or a dream in which one is in an embarrassing state of semi-nudity. Then there is the dream of being in a dangerous situation and great anxiety is felt. However, when the patient learns to associate freely to the various details of his dream it can be shown that they do make sense—that they attempt to reveal his forgotten experiences, his repressed desires, and his unconscious fears and dislikes.

To the psychoanalyst the dream represents the secretion of the mental apparatus, which can be analyzed for diagnostic and prognostic purposes, just as the urine, the secretion of the kidneys, can be analyzed by the general physician for diagnostic and prognostic purposes (p. 166).

Psychoanalysis, therefore, is a process of emotional reeducation. Emotions and ideas which have been unconscious are made conscious, with resulting better attitudes and more efficient living.

Hypnoanalysis.   Within recent years efforts have been made to combine hypnosis with psychoanalysis, for example: (1) in suggesting the recall of infantile experience or events surrounding the onset of illness or any other relevant associations, (2) in the recall of dreams and their interpretations, (3) to promote the analysis of the transference and (4) to make whatever interpretations seem necessary to insure the goal, a goal not only of symptom relief but of a better functioning ego.

This alliance between the hitherto dynamic but unwieldy hypnosis and the slower, tedious but better controlled psychoanalysis has been called hypnoanalysis (Wolberg). It is for a skilled psychiatrist to use and not for the average physician.

Mental Catharsis.   Mental catharsis is self-explanatory. It means talking to someone about your troubles. The one who talks usually feels better afterward even though the listener says nothing. He feels that someone has shared his trouble with him and hence he has less of a burden to carry. The listener, by withholding criticism, is usually regarded as having said, "I do not blame you. I understand why you feel as you do. You need not feel guilty. I might have done the same thing."

Such psychotherapy, of course, has distinct limitations. In the first place the patient talks about his conscious troubles, whereas neurotic symptoms have their roots in the unconscious mind. Hence the patient might talk endlessly without discussing real issues. Nevertheless, listening to another's troubles is a first principle in psychotherapy and such value as it has should not be lost sight of. A well trained and experienced psychotherapist can accomplish great good simply by directing a conversation, listening carefully and saying little, while a poorly trained and inexperienced psychotherapist can do real harm by talking instead of listening.

Psychiatric Counsel.   The most common form of psychotherapy is psychiatric counsel. Only a limited number of patients can be psychoanalyzed and, of course, all patients do not need such long and intensive treatment. In psychiatric counseling the physician attempts to learn as much as possible about the patient's ideas and trends of thought, in order to help him.

For this purpose the physician should have a background of psychoanalytic understanding. Every physician cannot be psychoanalyzed but information is readily available to acquaint him with the nature of unconscious mental processes. *Such knowledge is just as important for the practice of medicine as a basic training in anatomy and physiology.*

Psychosomatic history, thorough physical examination, laboratory and perhaps special studies prepare the way for psychiatric counsel in psychosomatic illness. With negative physical examination or symptoms out of proportion to the physical disease we are in a position to say to the patient, "I believe your illness is of emotional origin. Worry and anxiety can influence the function of the body and I think this is so in your case."

The patient may readily agree or may be skeptical. As a rule the patient says, "But there must be something the matter," meaning, of course, something physical. "This is not my imagination. I can't believe I'm neurotic. I hate neurotic people who do nothing but complain."

Illness Not Imaginary.   In the first place the physician must explain that he *did not say* the illness was imaginary. On the contrary, he has said it was just as real as though it were a physical disease. Patients must be taught to have as much respect for emotions as for bacteria. Pain in the abdomen from anxiety is no more imaginary than pain from appendicitis.

The physician can go on to say, "To have symptoms as a result of emotion is not a sign of weakness. Very capable people, doing the world's most important jobs, have emotional conflicts. Those who try to avoid conflict by assuming no responsibility are the weak ones. To be 'nervous,' to have anxiety, is only an evidence that energy is not being expressed in the proper channels."

Approximating Facts.   The patient then may say, "All right, if my symptoms are due to my emotions what can I do about it?" When we come to the point of helping the patient to "do something about it" we should think a moment of what the patient may be feeling. We must never be too eager to "tell," to "educate," to "advise." Learn to know what the resistances are to the patient's self-education. Much of what a patient "learns" in psychotherapy is self-evident truth except that the patient has not been quite aware of the situation. In fact, many times the physician has been surprised to hear his patient say, after being told about himself and what to do, "Why doctor, I knew that already." The point is that the patient has often known "that two and two were in his mind but he did not put them together to make four." The facts were there; the patient was aware of them; but they were isolated. The physician helps to approximate them.

UNDERSTANDING EMOTIONAL PROBLEMS.   But the physician must understand the emotional problems of his patient before help can be given. Sometimes the patient's greatest suffering is from immediate deprivations; sometimes from childhood deprivations. In still other instances it may be a combination of the two. An example of the first is a woman who developed insomnia, indigestion and mental depression. Her husband was cold and unromantic; there were financial worries; and they lived in an uncongenial neighborhood. The feeling of deprivation and the anxiety aroused by these immediate problems made the patient ill. Had the environment been more favorable she might have remained well.

Another woman, the oldest of eleven children, married happily at 23. She remained well until the age of 28 and then became ill with indigestion, fatigue and dizziness. Her husband was devoted to her and tried to get her the best medical care. For three years she was subjected to much medical and surgical treatment but continued to grow more depressed and disinterested in living. She had known many deprivations in childhood. For one thing she had been a feeding problem. Then when she was a year and a half old a sibling was born and when she was 3 years of age another came. Later the mother suffered a nervous breakdown and was very self-centered for a period of months. Our patient had to help with the other children and, being the oldest, had to assume much responsibility. Her own wants and desires were neglected. Falling ill at 28, with depression and lack of interest in her home and husband, meant that she was overcome once more with the same emotional emptiness as in her loveless childhood. In this case the childhood forces were more important in causing illness than any immediate deprivations.

In a third case a man wanted to enter a business project of which his father disapproved. He needed his father's financial as well as his moral support. When this was withheld the patient developed headaches, fatigue and constipation. There was obvious conflict over an immediate problem but his childhood fear of his father made the solution to the present problem doubly difficult and this had to be dealt with to give him relief.

NECESSITY FOR COOPERATION.   After we understand the patient's life situation we can make suggestions for help but the patient must cooperate as an active participant. Keeping in mind what has been said about passivity and the need for dependence in emotionally sick people, it is not difficult to understand that the patient does not relish the necessity for taking an active part in working out his cure. This dependent attitude of "letting the doctor do it" plus the physician's urge "to do something definite" accounts for the frequent submission, on the part of the patient, to operations, baths, electric treatments, diets, and so forth. The patient does not have to think or take much initiative. He submits and waits for results. In psychotherapy the patient must act.

He may talk and define his problem but there always comes a point when he must do something about it.

In the *first case* just cited, the woman suffered largely because her husband did not understand her need for affection. This brought up the question of whether the physician should see the husband. The patient was, of course, informed that this would be done tactfully, on the basis of a discussion of her health. Having received the wife's consent the physician informed the husband that her symptoms arose from unhappiness and anxiety rather than from tissue pathology and that it was to his advantage to understand the causes so that he could help her to recover. The husband was able to see the necessity for a more sympathetic interest in his wife's feelings.

We then explained to the patient that her neighborhood could not be completely unfriendly and that she could certainly find some people with common interests if she would only look for them. We said, "Make it your job to visit a neighbor this week and do not leave until you have found that you and she have at least two interests in common." She took up the challenge, found a neighbor who liked a certain radio program which they discussed, and also found that each had contemplated attending a night-school hobby class but had not wanted to go alone. And so they arranged to begin together. Considerable improvement in her symptoms followed.

The *second case* was more difficult to approach. Psychotherapy would have been easier if it had been done early. A long fixation on the physical aspects of her illness induced the patient to center a great deal of attention upon her body and she had grown distrustful that anything could be done for her. The first task was to have her accept the emotional basis for her illness. She had complained bitterly that no one understood her but when someone tried to understand her she turned once more to her somatic distress. We said, "You obviously have needed someone to interest himself in your feelings. Directing attention to your body has not helped. Now why do you try again to draw attention to your body when you have admitted that the trouble is in your feelings?" The patient replied, "I don't know. When I find what I want I don't seem to know how to use it."

She continued, "I love my husband so much. I'd give my soul to be well and be able to enjoy my life with him." We said, "You speak as though you cared but actually you seem compelled to give your thoughts and feelings to your own aches and pains. If you will turn your energy toward other interests and other people perhaps you will have less bodily discomfort." The patient would answer, "I don't see how you can take pain away without medicine." We said, "Perhaps you cannot see that far but let us proceed one step at a time. Use your goodwill and such effort as you have, to direct your attention outward instead of inward." She then complained of lack of appetite and we explained that just as she had no appetite for living so she had no appetite for food— that the symptoms represented behavior and not disease! On her next visit she reported a better appetite and began to show an interest in the emotional origin of her illness. In a short time she began to do her own housework again. In our interviews we continued to instruct her to dismiss the thoughts and feelings she had centered on her body and instead to direct them toward other people and other interests. Improvement was slow but, under the circumstances, satisfactory.

In the *third case* the patient could readily see that his symptoms arose in direct relation to his problem with his father. He felt thwarted by an insurmountable hurdle. When asked if he could not borrow the money elsewhere and go ahead with his venture he declared this was impossible. However, discussion showed that it seemed impossible only because he feared his father's disapproval of the venture. We asked him, "Does your father not want you to succeed? Does he not want you to use your own judgment and have the satisfaction of accomplishment?" He answered in the affirmative. We said, "Then why not go to your father and discuss your plans as man to man?" The patient still had anxiety about following this advice so we asked him to discuss his childhood relation to his father. He said, "I never asked favors of my father. I never dared press an issue. I couldn't bear to have him grow impatient or angry with me or refuse me anything. Yet I now know that he likes me and trusts me to a considerable extent. I've heard mother and his friends say so." We again pointed out that he was laboring under the same anxiety that he felt as a boy and that this prevented him from taking a convincing attitude with his father. He permitted his anxiety to convey the impression that he did not fully believe in the project, whereas the thing he was really afraid of was not the success of the project but the success of his appeal to his father. Finally after a third interview he saw his father, enlisted his interest and support, and his symptoms disappeared.

UNDERSTANDING THE BACKGROUND OF ANXIETY.   From these examples it may be seen that successful psychiatric counseling depends upon understanding the background of the patient's anxiety—whether the conflict is chiefly a product of the impact on the patient's specific emotional make-up of the present or the past external situation, or, as is usually true, a combination of the two. For this purpose we must have some understanding of personality structure and psychopathology. Then, to a large extent, we must ignore the symptoms and attack the basic sources of the conflict. When we say "ignore the symptoms" we mean "Teach the patient to carry on in spite of symptoms." Only in this way can improvement be brought about.

THE USE OF DREAMS.   Dreams can be utilized in psychiatric counseling although they cannot be as useful in this form of therapy as in psychoanalysis. In the latter treatment more time and attention can be given to associations to the dream and, with frequent repetition of ideas, there is a greater opportunity to see certain personality trends of thought or action. Thus understanding of the nature of his unconscious activity will more surely come to the patient.

Patients are often skeptical regarding the significance of dreams but some dreams are so clear that even the most skeptical person must admit that they have meaning. The woman who maintains that she has no sexual interest, but dreams repeatedly of sexual advances by men, should admit, when the opportunity is afforded of calling her attention to the idea, that a certain part of her mental life must have some interest in the subject. The man who insists that he has no resentment against his family, friends or employers, but who repeatedly dreams of arguments and fights with them, may be helped through his dreams to see an aggressive side of himself which he is repressing. One says to the patient something like this, "Mental activity goes on during sleep and some of the things you wish, some of the things you fear, and in fact anything that you feel strongly about may present itself in your dream pictures. The ideas may be disguised, they may appear in symbolic form, or they may be contained within what seems to be a lot of meaningless action. But, after all, dreams are a product of your mental activity and perhaps we can use them to help in understanding you."

The willingness or ability to understand dreams varies greatly among patients. Some patients are annoyed to have the physician try to see meaning in them. They require the actual feelings which they experience in daily living to convince them of the psychic forces existing within them. Other patients may volunteer dreams and ask to have them discussed. Often it is helpful to question as to whether there are dreams with a frequently recurring theme. *Repetitive dreams* have special significance. They indicate a definite personality trend (p. 162).

KEEPING MATERIAL SUPPRESSED. Sometimes a patient will ask, "If I do not like the people I am supposed to like isn't it better not to bring it out—won't it make our relations more strained?" Or a patient with greatly repressed erotic trend, especially if single, may ask, "If I have these tendencies won't it make a greater problem for me to become more aware of them?" The answer generally is "No," since we must not forget that we are treating the cause of symptoms and symptoms should be no more respectable than the emotion they represent. Secondly, when unconscious wishes are made conscious, with the exception of potential psychotics, there is still the healthy part of the personality to help solve the problem raised by hostility or sexual tension. The hate, jealousy and sexual tension in psychoneurotics are just additional facts of life which they must face and find a solution for, as other people try to do.

Their problems do not differ in kind from those of average "healthy" people—only the solution is more difficult and they need help. If a physician accepts such patients he should be aware of the sort of "trap" which these emotionally immature people set. They talk and act as if to say, "I'm just a little child. How can you expect me to struggle with those powerful forces?" With such an attitude the physician must be sympathetic but he must also try to avoid giving direct advice. He should give his patient the chance no one else has ever given him, that is, to think and express himself freely about what may be socially taboo. If undesirable thoughts or feelings are in the mind they are better managed when made conscious than when left unconscious. When the dream helps to make the unconscious more understandable it should be used as an adjunct in understanding and counseling the patient.

SOMETHING LESS THAN CURE. Now we must say something of the

other side of the picture. Physicians attempting psychotherapy sometimes must curb their zeal to accomplish too much. There are severe
neurotics and potential psychotics to whom some information, especially
if it is given carelessly, only serves to increase their anxiety. Unless they
can be seen frequently so as to gain friendly support and work over their
thoughts, they become worse. One should proceed carefully in the first
interview and see what the patient can tolerate. It is better not to probe
too much or attempt to enlighten too much at one time. This is particularly true in adolescents. A physician who is meticulous in administering
digitalis or insulin will tell a neurotic patient that he is lazy, cowardly,
doesn't love his family, hates his father, cannot face life, etc., and then
wonders why the patient is not better the next day.

REMOVING A SYMPTOM THAT THE PATIENT NEEDS.   Even the physician who proceeds more slowly and more carefully may try too hard to
remove a symptom which the patient needs. Remember that the symptom often represents the answer to a psychological conflict and in taking
the symptom away something must be given in its place or, stated better,
the patient must be helped to find something in its place. This takes
time, patience and resourcefulness. It can rarely be done by one or even
several "pep talks." The external situation may be impossible to solve,
or even when a solution exists the patient may not have available the
potential resources for the solution. Fortunately some modification of
the external situation or the patient's inner life, or both, can usually be
effected.

In an article entitled "What Price Healing," Jelliffe strikingly demonstrated that serious emotional illness may result when a symptom is
removed by medicine or surgery, without attention to the underlying
emotional make-up and the life situation. When psychosomatic illness
has become definitely "fixed," its pattern "set," it must be realized that
the emotional needs of the patient are being partially satisfied by the
illness itself and it may be necessary to allow him to keep his illness as
the best answer to his problem. For example, a woman of 55 suffered
from pains in the back and legs and occasionally in the joints. She was
carefully studied over a period of three years for evidence of physical
disease and none was found. She had had a barren childhood, a loveless
marriage, had raised two children, and both refused to live with her.
Her husband was dead and she was painfully lonely. But she had always
prided herself on her self-sufficiency. She could not be told that she was
lonely or that she needed friendship. To accept the idea that she was
lonely would be an admission of weakness which she could not tolerate.
To tell her that she needed friends was to make her realize that she had
never cultivated friends and was too rigid at this point to learn how. She
would keep a nurse for a while and either the nurse would leave because
of her constant complaining or she would find some excuse to discharge
her. Of course, she also changed physicians frequently. Since she had
money to spend for what she wanted, her son was advised to cease concerning himself about her and permit her to live the only pattern of
existence which was possible for her to live.

In other words, as physicians we sometimes have to admit that the illness must be allowed to continue—that, under certain circumstances, it is the best answer to a life problem.

GROUP PSYCHOTHERAPY

The time that must be devoted to each patient in individual psychotherapy has led various workers to attempt treatment in groups instead of singly. The procedure had been carried out with some success even before World War II. During the war, the larger numbers of patients made group psychotherapy a greater necessity than ever before, and it was used on an extensive scale. Although it will probably continue to be used since it can benefit a large number of persons at one time, it lacks many of the benefits of individual therapy and of course can never completely replace it. While the technique varies to some extent, the following plan is generally followed:

Technique. Instead of talking with one patient, the physician brings together a group with common problems and talks with them. From eight to twelve patients gather in a room of appropriate size; preferably the chairs are arranged in a circle, for this facilitates discussion. The physician acts as a leader and the relation of the emotions to bodily changes (the conversion of conflict into symptoms) may be simply stated. Tact and ingenuity are required to bring the patients into the discussion. The interest of the physician must not stray too far from the group to individuals or the therapeutic value becomes lost to the others. Yet he must be able to recognize and to call upon the more articulate members in the beginning to ask questions, express opinions, recount their symptoms, cite experiences which have produced symptoms or even those which have relieved symptoms. If a group shares fears of being alone, then the mechanism of helpless anxiety is discussed. Here are some of the consequences of the procedure:

1. There is expression of emotion (ventilation) which, plus the fact of recounting of experiences in the presence of others, reduces anxiety.

2. Personal problems seem less personal when it is learned that others have felt the same way, hence there is relief from guilt and feelings of inferiority.

3. The patient benefits from the experience of socalization in the group setting.

4. Inspired to offer a solution for another person's problem, a patient may find that he is offering the solution to his own.

While the physician is a member of the group he is at the same time its discussion leader. He may be consulted on a point of specific information or he may find it necessary to bring the subject back so that it may prove profitable to the majority. Frequently he presents a summary in concluding the discussion.

Some advocates of group therapy find it best to permit no additions to the group once it has started, carrying the same patients through the various sessions to a conclusion. Others feel that the introduction of new members does not impair the efficiency of the group and indeed has certain advantages to offer the new members.

No large-scale application has yet been made to specific psychosomatic problems but Ackerman reported some experience in psychosomatic disorders with such symptoms as headache, insomnia and fatigue. Heath, at the same meeting, described his experience in the treatment of merchant seamen, among whom was a group of alcoholics. Here the group meetings resembled the Alcoholics Anonymous meetings and after discharge the members of the group joined this organization.

Because there is little removal of infantile amnesia, and because the working out of transference phenomena is impossible, real depth understanding may not be reached in group therapy. Nevertheless the group method has much to offer and undoubtedly will find wide application, especially in a period when there are so few psychiatrists.

Group Psychotherapy as a Community Experiment.   An attempt has been made to examine how far a continuously changing population of patients and staff could develop its form of community within the framework of a military psychiatric hospital in England. Referring to the "Northfield Experiment" Lt. Col. T. F. Main speaks of the hospital as a therapeutic institution. He describes the demoralizing effect which the usual hospital may inadvertently have: "By tradition a hospital is a place wherein sick people may receive shelter from the stormy blasts of life, the care and attention of nursing and medical auxiliaries, and the individual attention of a skilled doctor. The concept of a hospital as a refuge too often means, however, that patients are robbed of their status of responsible human beings. Too often they are called 'good' or 'bad' only according to the degree of their passivity in the face of the hospital demand for their obedience, dependency and gratitude. The fine traditional mixture of charity and discipline which they receive is a practised technic for removing their initiative as adult beings, and making them 'patient.' They are less trouble thus to the staff. Hospitals which follow this orthodoxy are usually designed for the individual treatment of the individual patient by an individual doctor, not in a real social setting, but in a state of retirement from society. So, isolated and dominated, the patient tends to remain gripped by the hospital machine even in the games or prescribed occupations which fill in his time between treatments.

"Within such a setting, health and stability are too often bought at the excessive price of desocialisation. Sooner or later the patient, alone and unsupported, must face the difficult task of returning to the society in which he became unstable, and there regain social integration, and a daily sense of values and a purpose. This task is no light one for a desocialised man, however healthy he may have become . . . Treatment of the neurotic patient who suffers from a disturbance of social relationships cannot, therefore, be regarded as satisfactory unless it is undertaken within a framework of social reality which can provide him with opportunities for attaining fuller social insight and for expressing and modifying his emotional drives according to the demands of real life. In any case, the fact must be faced that radical individual psychotherapy is not a practicable proposition for the huge numbers of patients confronting the psychiatric world today. It is doubtful whether the hospital can usefully remain a building within which individual treatment is practised. Perhaps it must become a therapeutic institution. The North-field Experiment is an attempt to use a hospital not as an organization run by doctors in the interests of their own greater efficiency, but as a community with the immediate aim of full participation of all its daily members in its daily life and the eventual aim of the resocialisation of the neurotic individual for life in ordinary society."

In continuing the description of the Northfield Experiment, Major Bridger describes the program of admission, the natural way in which the patient meets the psychiatrist and the social worker; how the patient himself selects his activities; the opportunities for joining in recreation, which means more than just being shown a "good time"; and the intro-duction to the treatment ward where a democratic self-government obtains, and where "he can now embark on a secure but flexible pro-gram, involving not only the life in his ward and his selected activity, but also the social opportunities inside and outside the hospital." In these social relationships, individually and in groups, the psychiatrist has an opportunity to observe the behavior which will be of the greatest value in treatment. It is the integration of the patient into the hospital as a community which is important because, as Bridger concludes, "for all groups, whether founded spontaneously or not, whether large or small, it is true to say that the individual contribution has a value only in so far as it has a significance to the community; it is equally true to say that the individual can only experience full freedom and satisfaction in a society that recognizes his worth, and gives him the opportunity to develop in a spirit of warm human relationships."

The Northfield Experiment as described by Lt. Col. Main and his associates is social medicine in the finest sense and carries an important lesson for the future development of civil medicine.

THE GENERAL PHYSICIAN AND PSYCHOTHERAPEUTIC PROBLEMS

Treating the Discharged Mental Hospital Patient.   Every year a quarter of a million mental patients are discharged from hospitals into the community. It stands to reason that many of these discharged patients will require help of some kind and that they will be coming to the offices of general practitioners. Some will have a relapse of their psychotic symptoms, some will present complaints of psychosomatic origin. Some will fail to adjust to a job and may become truculent, unsatisfactory members of society. The discharged mental patient will usually need more understanding, patience and effort to help him adjust than is required for the average medical patient.

Some time will be required on the part of the physician to understand the make-up of these patients. He will need to learn what conditions have occurred since leaving the hospital which aggravated the patient's condition. He will need to ascertain what helps the patient as well as what upsets him. He may have to assess whether the patient is danger-ous either to himself or to others. Moreover, the physician will need to know about the patient's environment and how those in the environ-ment react to him. He will need to know how they feel about the patient as well as how the patient feels about them. Some families are able to tolerate very little unconventional behavior and would rather have the patient rehospitalized. Others may overprotect the patient so much that he is prevented from wholesome social and work contacts. Sometimes the community is unduly fearful of a patient who has been in a mental hospital and may be cool or indifferent to him which the patient may interpret as a hostile reaction.

Families are often unresourceful in planning a program for a discharged mental patient. They may not help him sufficiently to get a job if he is employable. If he is not employable or does not need to work he will still need opportunities, in the home or outside, for some limited usefulness or for some recreation. Suggestions may be made to those in the home environment as to how to provide these, or the patient and his family may be sent to local social agencies or recreational agencies in order to find constructive new directions.*

It may be necessary for the discharged patient to be returned to the hospital. A sympathetic and understanding family physician can do much to make this easier for both the patient and relatives. A kind but firm insistence on his part is usually necessary to overcome ambivalence on the part of both patient and family about going back to the hospital. It is well to keep in mind the importance of making it clear that a return to the hospital is a procedure undertaken for the welfare of many people and not as a punishment to the patient.

At times, when a discharged mental patient comes to see the family physician he will talk about his complaints, either physical or environmental. The fact that these complaints may be somewhat irrational can be baffling to the physician and he becomes disturbed because of their illogical character. However, he should bear in mind that just by listening and being reassuring he may be of much help to this particular patient and family. He should not be too quick to come to the conclusion that he "cannot do anything for this kind of patient," because the patient's conversation lacks logic or his complaints remain the same on a succession of visits. Contact with the family physician is often very beneficial. It will often keep down anxiety and tension in the patient and in his environment and will serve to keep him in the community rather than allowing him to return and take up a bed in the mental hospital. It has been said many times that what the mentally sick person needs is a friend—particularly a physician friend. A physician may have to look within himself and try to discover the reason for some of his own inner discomfort when a patient does not "talk sense."

LEARN HOW TO LISTEN.   Most general practitioners, in order to help with the large number of mentally sick people in the community, must be willing to deal with the patient who does not always talk sense completely. Most patients talk enough sense to be understood and worked with if the physician listens closely and tries to meet their needs. As the doctor learns to listen and finds that he is able even partially to understand these people, he will find that there are positive things in

---

* "Mental Illness—a Guide for the Family," National Association for Mental Health, 10 Columbus Circle, New York 19, offers practical advice to relatives of the mental patient through every phase of his illness.

them that need encouragement and that these words of encouragement will help to counteract feelings of despair and inferiority. These encouraging words are good medicine. If, for a few days, restlessness and tension become too great, one of the ataractic drugs may tide the patient over such an emergency and often make a return to the hospital unnecessary.

Sometimes explanation by the family physician to a potential employer may result in a job which has many beneficial effects. This is all part of a much needed community enlightenment in regard to mental illness.

Certainly patience and an interest in these discharged patients are in line with the movement to bring psychiatric practice out of the mental hospital. The physician must get over a feeling that when he deals with a patient with any degree of mental illness he is wasting time or is out of his element. Any patient well enough to be discharged from a mental hospital and able to live in a community has some if not all of his mental health. The general practitioner should be willing to work with and help strengthen that degree of mental health just as willingly and matter-of-factly as he accepts and works with the patient who has a partially healthy heart or lungs.

The Psychiatric Inpatient Service in a General Hospital. While the need for an "open" psychiatric section in a general hospital has been recognized for years, its actual utilization has gained ground slowly. One of the most convincing reasons for such a section is that it brings psychiatry into medicine instead of allowing it to lead an isolated existence. Such a section puts psychiatry where it not only helps the patient but is convenient and helpful to the referring physician, the specialist and the family as well. It permits ready consultation with other services. It permits an easy transfer of the patient from one service to another when care other than psychiatric is indicated. Additionally, it offers a unique opportunity to promote research in a more effective psychotherapy, for example, in the integration of the therapeutic group rather than a therapy based on locks, pills and suppressive measures of a physical nature. This opportunity is not similarly available in the private office or the closed mental hospital.

An "open" psychiatric section performs a useful educational function for the whole hospital since it enables everyone to see that with proper understanding, treatment and nursing care, people who are quite ill mentally and emotionally can be taken care of in a general hospital. It also tends to reduce the usual apprehension commonly felt by general physicians and medical personnel about emotionally ill people. The needs of the emotionally ill become better known throughout a hospital. The result is that patients obtain treatment earlier than they used to and hence there is a preventive effect on mental illness.

Finally, care of emotionally ill patients in a special section within a general hospital offers a unique opportunity for collaborative work on the part of many specialists in psychiatric and psychosomatic problems.

INDICATIONS FOR HOSPITAL CARE. There are many indications for hospitalization of emotionally disturbed patients who are not ordinarily thought of as being "ill enough" to enter the average mental hospital either public or private.

For instance, there are the psychoneurotic reactions that cause a patient great anxiety. Patients develop periods of panic lasting from minutes to hours during which they feel they are terribly ill or are going to die. Such patients are great burdens to family and physician. They call the physician day and night and they make great demands for reassurance, medicine and advice. Moreover, these patients even in ambulatory psychiatric treatment are often unable to derive enough insight and emotional support to progress. A period of hospitalization varying from two weeks to one month often gives them an opportunity to gain enough understanding of their neurotic problem so that ambulatory therapy can then be carried on much more satisfactorily.

Another type of patient who needs hospital care for a temporary period is one who lives in a family environment which has grown so uncongenial to him as to interfere with his progress in treatment. This environment may be either hostile, overprotective or sufficiently lacking in understanding so that a change is needed in order that psychotherapy can get under way. Of course, it should be added that a patient may have such a disturbing effect upon the family environment that they need a rest from him.

Another reason for a period of hospitalization is that certain demands can be made upon the patient which will enhance his emotional growth. It is well known that patients will cooperate with strangers when they will not with their own families. They will accept demands made upon them in a hospital environment which they will not accept at home.

The hospital relieves a patient of certain demands which are made upon him at home and gives him an opportunity to regress, to relax, and to be free from the necessity of living up to certain expectations until a desirable degree of ego strength has been achieved.

Hospitalization is often desirable for the purpose of studying at close range the patient's emotional reaction to new faces and new personalities in an around-the-clock fashion. When a patient has been complaining, for instance, that his regular environment has been inimical to him, it may come as a very important piece of insight to him to discover that he has the same feelings in the hospital.

Usually the patient is helped by seeing other people in various stages of recovery from emotional illness. It removes some of his feeling that he is "the only case of his kind" and lessens his sense of loneliness and isolation when he is in the company of other people who are working toward goals similar to his. Occasionally, it is true, a patient may suffer an adverse effect from association with other emotionally ill patients. But this is the exception and not the rule.

For the patient who is too involved in morbid thinking about himself, it is possible in the hospital environment to introduce certain diversionary as well as therapeutically valuable experiences such as occupational therapy, art therapy, bibliotherapy and sociotherapy.

It is often desirable to have a psychosomatic patient treated in the hospital environment so that a combined effort on the part of the internist and psychiatrist can be made. It is obvious that some patients need the security offered by twenty-four hour supervision of a trained therapeutic team.

Hospital care, by involving several psychiatrically trained people, may make it possible to meet more of the patient's emotional needs quantitatively as well as qualitatively and therefore enable him to make gains that are not possible in ambulatory psychotherapy.

Some of the public reaction and the reaction of the general hospital against admitting mental patients has been not so much because it is feared that patients will become violent and get out of hand (although this happens occasionally), but because doctors and nurses become upset by a patient whom they cannot understand and cannot treat. Some disturbed patients make the doctor, nurse and family so uncomfortable that in their bafflement they turn against the patient, thereby increasing tension, enhancing aggression and intensifying acting-out. (In short, the emotionally ill patient and the medical profession have been suffering from a lack of satisfactory communication.)

Psychiatric Referral.   Special problems are involved in referring a patient to a psychiatrist, even when the physician himself is convinced that it is necessary. It goes without saying that if he isn't convinced he doesn't make a good job of it. Often, psychiatric referral is employed as a last resort for a patient who is psychotic or for the neurotic patient who is so "fixed" in his neurotic obsession that nothing more can be done for him.

Referral of a psychotic patient is usually not too difficult. Hospitalization is presented to both the patient and the family in the same way as for any other medical problem and the family, frightened by the patient's behavior, is eager for a solution to the problem.

Referring a neurotic patient may be a more difficult matter because the patient sometimes objects with the question, "Do you think I'm crazy?" Even though the true function of psychiatry is much better recognized than it was before World War II there are still many people who believe that it deals only with the "insane." The physician should explain that the chief work of the psychiatrist is with people who have emotional or personality disorders and that he is an expert in the treatment of these disorders in the same way that another specialist is an expert in bodily illness.

Often the patient takes the attitude, "How is talking going to help me?" The suggestion can be made that perhaps he can recall some instance in which talking over a specific problem made him feel better or, on the other hand, someone else got relief discussing a problem with him. However, it should be made clear that more is involved than just talking—special skill is necessary and the psychiatrist provides unique help in understanding why and how the troubles have arisen as well as how to guide the patient into channels of healthier thinking and living.

Perhaps the money question will arise, and, of course, it is true that psychiatry is expensive but the fees are not out of line with the other specialties. Indeed, the psychiatrist's income ranks far from the top among medical specialists. People who object to psychiatric fees often spend fortunes seeking help along orthodox medical and surgical lines and often will spend a great deal on a "vacation" to escape from their troubles, usually without relief. The truth of the matter is that psychiatry is often economical rather than expensive when one considers these other expenses that so many patients have undergone, not to mention what is lost through impaired efficiency or actual loss of time from work.

Physicians are often prejudiced against psychiatry for a variety of reasons. They have sometimes had unsatisfactory experiences in sending a patient to a psychiatrist, or they find the psychiatrist uninterested in the physical aspects of the disorder, or they are unhappy about the fact that the psychiatrist does not give enough information about his contacts with the patient. These are understandable irritations and when they are added to the fact that the techniques of psychiatry seem "unscientific" and "interminable," it is little wonder that physicians often refuse to send patients to psychiatrists unless they are forced to do so. The psychiatrist does have a difficult job; patients often take a long time to grow up emotionally—which is the essence of psychotherapy—and the psychiatrist cannot divulge the confidences of his patient. The fact that psychiatrists are often very busy is another difficulty that the physician encounters. Often he has to call a great number before he can find one who has time for a patient. This too is understandable when one considers the difference in the case load of a psychiatrist and that of a general physician. However, if the referring physician is acquainted with the goals and accomplishments of psychiatry and the psychiatrist in turn has a healthy respect for physical medicine, they can often work well together and encounter less difficulty in making psychiatric referrals.

Perhaps the physician should ask himself whether he himself would see a psychiatrist for similar complaints or send a member of his family to a psychiatrist. If the answer is yes, then he can probably refer his patients when necessary and will be comfortable in meeting their objections. But if the answer is no or a hesitant yes, he may understand why he "can't get his patient to go to a psychiatrist." Unless he can deal successfully with the idea for himself or his family he will not be very successful in referring a member of his "patient family." But the effort he makes in reaching this understanding should bring him closer to success in referral.

SUMMARY

The following points summarize the psychosomatic approach to the everyday problems of the practice of medicine. Just as a history form cannot be followed without making some compromise to suit the individual patient, so may it be necessary at times to modify these suggestions.

General Principles of Management of Psychosomatic Disorders

1. Give the patient time to tell his story: Listen rather than talk.
2. Get to know the patient as a person rather than just as a medical case. Look for the person in the patient.
3. Make the physical examination (including laboratory studies) as complete as necessary: Exclude or evaluate physical disease.
4. Reassure: "No evidence of cancer, heart disease, mental disease, etc."
5. Explain: Disorder and not a disease (irritable colon—not "colitis," etc.); the symptoms are real (not imaginary) and although unpleasant will do no damage to the body.
6. If disease is present explain that symptoms are out of proportion to the disease (for example, headache, fatigue, etc., in hypertension).
7. Look for (and explain) the time relationship between onset of illness and emotionally disturbing events.
8. Encourage discussion of personal problems—family setting, marital situation, work, social life, etc.
9. Ask patient to give his own explanation of illness. Reeducate on the mechanism of symptom formation. Show patient how tension of emotional origin causes symptoms.
10. Instead of cautioning rest urge patient to engage in usual work and social endeavor. "Carry on in spite of symptoms." (This externalizes psychic energy—libido—and diverts attention from body sensation.)
11. If drugs are used explain their action: Avoid "mystery."
12. Try to desensitize (by repeated discussion) against noxious environmental influences (unfriendly relatives, critical employers, etc.). If desensitization is not successful and modification of environment is impossible then change of environment is indicated.

References

Ackerman, N. W.: Psychosom. Med., *8:* 118, 1946.
Alexander, F.: The Medical Value of Psychoanalysis. 2nd ed. W. W. Norton & Co., N. Y., 1937.
Appel, K. E., and Scheflen, A.: J.A.M.A., *159:* 1278, 1955.
Beecher, H. K.: J.A.M.A., *159:* 1602, 1955.
Beecher, H. K., Keats, A. S., Mosteller, F., and Lasagna, L.: J. Pharmacol. & Exper. Therap., *109:* 393, 1953.
Fischer, H. K., and Dlin, B.: Am. J. M. Sc., *232:*504, 1956.
Harrower, M.: Amer. Soc. for Research in Psychosom. Problems, Atlantic City, May 4, 1947.
Jelliffe, S. E.: J.A.M.A., *94:* 1393, 1930.
Kubie, L. S.: Practical Aspects of Psychoanalysis. W. W. Norton & Co., N. Y., 1936.
Lasagna, L., Mosteller, F., von Felsinger, J. M., and Beecher, H. K.: Am. J. Med., *16:* 770, 1954.
Lemkau, P. V.: J.A.M.A., *162:* 854, 1956.
Main, T. F.: Bull. Menninger Clinic, *10:* 66, 1946.
Menninger, K. A.: (*a*) The Human Mind. 3rd ed. Alfred A. Knopf, N. Y., 1947; (*b*) Man Against Himself. Harcourt, Brace & Co., N. Y., 1938.
Osborn, L. A.: J.A.M.A., *153:* 259–262, 1953.
Ozarin, L. D.: J.A.M.A., *161:* 940, 1956.
Wolberg, L. R.: Hypnoanalysis. Grune and Stratton, New York, 1945.

Part Two

Special Applications
to General Medicine
and the Specialties

Chapter VI

The Cardiovascular System

In spite of the enormous incidence of cardiovascular disease, _the_ _majority of patients who have symptoms referred to the heart region_ _do not have evidence of organic heart disease_. The reason is not hard to find. From time immemorial the heart has been the traditional seat of the emotions and hence acts as a focal point for anxiety. No other body organ is used so frequently in a symbolic way to refer to love and to hate, which, as W. C. Menninger pointed out, should lead us to think of the emotional significance of disturbances involving the heart. We are familiar with the universal use of the heart as a symbol of love, as in valentines, and the colloquial expressions "warmhearted," "loving with all my heart," "heart-felt." We speak of being "light-hearted" and of the heart "bounding with joy." But we also speak of being "broken-hearted," "heavy-hearted," and of "the heart growing weary." Then, too, we refer to the "faint-hearted" and the "chicken-hearted"; or think of the heart "racing with fear" or "fluttering or trembling." Hate and hostility are expressed in such terms as "hard-hearted," "heartless," and "cold-blooded" instead of "warm-hearted." The injured person is spoken of as suffering from "heartache," or of being "heartsick." All of these expressions have significance from the standpoint of *body language* as discussed in earlier chapters.

ANXIETY AND THE HEART

Do the expressions enclosed in quotation marks have any real meaning from the standpoint of psychopathology? Is there any actual relation of anxiety and the anxiety attack, also described in an earlier chapter, to disorders of the heart and the cardiovascular system? Anxiety neurosis stands in close relation to physiological changes and is therefore of utmost significance to all branches of medicine. This relation to physiological changes is especially close in the cardiovascular system. Moreover, anxiety neurosis, in its varying degrees, is probably the most frequent disorder of civilized life. The various forms of the anxiety attack were described by Freud more than fifty years ago. Not only did he call attention to such disturbances of cardiac function as palpitation, arrhythmia and tachycardia, but he also spoke of the disturbances of respiration and a host of physiological changes that are so often today regarded as evidences of vasomotor instability or autonomic imbalance. Furthermore, Freud emphasized the fact that these attacks are not always accompanied by recognizable anxiety. This, of course, is one special reason why they are so often regarded as indications of physical disease.

From the standpoint of psychosomatic medicine we can discuss the effect of the emotions upon the cardiovascular system from the following standpoints:

1. The effect of anxiety upon the normal heart, including the syndrome spoken of as neurocirculatory asthenia.

2. The effect of anxiety upon a diseased heart.

3. The relation of the emotions to the problem of hypertension.

ANXIETY AND THE NORMAL HEART (CARDIAC NEUROSIS)

Precipitating Factors.   Cardiac neurosis,* or so-called "functional heart disease," arises in predisposed persons who have been subjected to a precipitating factor. Such persons carry an unusual amount of anxiety in their make-ups. Then, under special circumstances, that anxiety is attached to the heart largely because the heart is regarded as the all-important bodily organ and is associated with the idea of sudden death.

This anxiety or even the personality predisposition may be anything but obvious and yet in reviewing the histories of patients with cardiac neuroses, it is interesting to note how frequently one obtains the story of some "nervous breakdown," either during the period of school life or in the course of some later period of stress. In an excellent paper on this subject Conner called attention to the following four groups of causes which may act as the precipitating events for the development of cardiac neurosis:

1) *The statement of some physician or life insurance examiner that the heart shows some abnormality such as a murmur or irregularity, of rhythm; or the rejection of the applicant for life insurance on the score of some heart disturbance or of "high blood pressure."* Sometimes it is the mere assumption on the part of the applicant himself that the heart must be diseased because two or three examiners were called in to listen to it. In a person predisposed, the slightest suggestion that the heart is not right may be enough to start the whole train of reactions that lead up to the development of cardiac neurosis. As will be stated in the discussion on neurocirculatory asthenia, this problem is of the greatest importance in the examination of young men for army service. Unusual attention to the cardiac examination or some casual remarks may be the starting point for later disability.

Hart questions iatrogenic factors as an important cause of cardiac neurosis. He correctly states that the cause is more fundamental than can be explained by a simple iatrogenic concept. He details the following: (1) There is usually lack of proof as to what the physician actually

* It is hardly necessary to say that we consider the designation "neurosis with cardiac manifestations" to be much more satisfactory, but because of tradition the term cardiac neurosis will probably continue to be used.

said. (2) Heart symptoms are often present long before the supposedly precipitating iatrogenic statement or suggestion. (3) There is rarely any evidence to show that patients with cardiac neurosis really fear heart disease; on the contrary, their over-all behavior indicates that they need and seek a tangible bodily defect, perhaps as a rationalistic lesser-evil defense against suspected mental illness. (4) Reassurance that the heart is sound, unless accompanied by other forms of positive follow-through treatment, not only may be ineffective but may indeed aggravate anxiety and other symptoms. Hart suggested that, on further study and reappraisal, cardiac neurosis which is iatrogenically caused may best be considered to represent errors not of commission but of omission, in failing to appreciate and treat the over-all medical needs of the patient.

We believe that people tolerate anxiety in respect to other organs and systems better than they do when it is attached to the heart but we agree with Hart that the most important error in dealing with cardiac neurosis is an act of omission rather than commission, that is, an attempt to reassure the patient without trying to understand the social and psychological problems that are responsible.

2. *The occurrence of some dramatic case of heart disease, perhaps with sudden death, among relatives or friends of the patient.* This is a frequent precipitating factor for cardiac neurosis particularly if the patient has been in close contact with the relative or friend or has actually nursed such a person. The continual emotional stress plus hard work and often lack of sleep prepare the way for the development of the first heart symptoms.

3. *The appearance of some symptom which calls the attention of the patient to his heart and leads to doubt as to its integrity.* This may be a sudden skip, a flutter or a twinge of pain, or it may be merely what is regarded as undue palpitation or dyspnea after some special exertion. Such disturbing symptoms are often first noticed during convalescence from an illness, such as an attack of grippe, or they may appear as a result of the excessive use of tobacco or coffee.

4. *Some profound and protracted emotional disturbance,* such as deep grief or prolonged anxiety, in which, however, there is at first no element of doubt concerning the state of the heart. This was strikingly illustrated by the innumerable instances of the condition known as "irritable heart of soldiers," "effort syndrome" or "neurocirculatory asthenia" which developed in military service. As a result of the profound and long-continued emotional disturbance incident to the process of volunteering or being drafted into the army, such cases were encountered in great numbers.

5. To these four groups we may add a fifth—*the occurrence of an anxiety attack* which causes rapid heart action and palpitation and frequently leads the physician to incriminate the heart.

Symptoms.   Under circumstances such as those that have just been discussed, pain in the heart region, fatigue, sighing respirations, insomnia, ringing or pounding in the ears, and faintness, dizziness, nervousness, irritability and flushes are apt to make their appearance. At first, there may be only discomfort in the heart region with the later development of other symptoms, particularly fatigue, which may be overwhelming and lead to complete invalidism.

The chief symptoms group themselves under the headings of (*a*) pain and distress in the heart region, (*b*) dyspnea and fatigue, (*c*) palpitation or heart consciousness, (*d*) tachycardia and other disturbances of rhythm, and (*e*) a group of symptoms which include all of the above in addition to evidences of vasomotor instability. This is often looked upon as a special form of cardiac neurosis, occurring especially in military life, and referred to as effort syndrome, neurocirculatory asthenia (N. C. A.) or "disordered action of the heart" (D. A. H.).

George Wolf and Harold Wolff made an important study of symptoms referable to the cardiovascular and respiratory systems occurring in patients with and without structural disease of the heart. A detailed, day-to-day physiological and psychological investigation was made of the way these persons responded to a standard exercise test as determined by cardiovascular and respiratory measurements.

The investigators took especial note of the reactions to persistent low-grade stresses and strains which are part of "everyday" living. Their results indicate that in a setting of adverse life circumstances and associated emotional reactions, performance in terms of respiration and work of the heart is costly. This high cost may manifest itself in cardiovascular symptoms which are not dependent alone upon gross structural heart disorder. This uneconomical performance may also manifest itself in impaired total efficiency of the individual. (See chart, p. 189.)

PAIN.   It has been estimated by Bishop that 25 per cent of all patients visiting the office of a cardiologist have cardiac pain as a primary complaint and more recently Master in a study of 1000 consecutive private patients seen in consultation found that 382 were suffering from "functional" disturbances of the heart and that pain or pressure in the chest was the most common symptom, affecting 64 per cent of this group.

Angina Pectoris and the Pain of "Functional" Heart Disease.   When characteristic effort pain with its peculiar distribution occurs in a hypertensive arteriosclerotic individual there is no problem of diagnosis— angina pectoris is present regardless of other findings. But under many other circumstances the problem may be a most difficult one. Intercostal neuralgia and spinal disease, hiatal hernia and cardiospasm, gallbladder and ulcer syndromes, as well as tobacco poisoning, are causes for pain in the cardiac region that must be borne in mind in regard to the problem of so-called pseudo-angina. The diagnostic problem is often difficult but if these various conditions are thought of the problem can usually be solved after careful study. Unfortunately the diagnosis of the anginal syndrome not infrequently must rest solely on subjective phenomena. Abnormal physical signs, x-ray and electrocardiographic evidence may be absent. It is important to recognize that the discomfort of the anginal syndrome appears, with few exceptions, when additional work is imposed on the heart. The abnormal sensation is usually of relatively short duration; it rarely lasts for more than a few minutes. It frequently disappears promptly when the patient rests and in the majority of instances after the administration of nitrites. Master found that any chest pain unrelieved by nitroglycerin was usually not caused by coronary artery disease, although there were exceptions to this rule.

In Harrison's study of 77 patients with angina pectoris the pain was in the substernal region in only about 50 per cent of the cases, and the discomfort was only mild or minimal in about the same number. He also found that aggravation by recumbent posture, improvement after eating, and nocturnal attacks occur more frequently than is commonly believed.

Harrison regards the most important features in the diagnosis of angina pectoris to be: (1) the history of relationship to effort, (2) the short duration of pain, and (3) the demonstration that the amount of muscular effort required to induce the pain is increased by glyceryl trinitrate. A very important aspect of this matter is that a large percentage of patients with angina pectoris also suffer from chest pain due to other disorders and that these disorders may be either related to the angina pectoris (as in myocardial infarction and reflex disturbances of the skeletal system) or unrelated to it (as in gallbladder disease, hiatal hernia, esophageal spasm, and the like). Owing to the frequent coexistence of two causes of chest pain, one of them may be overlooked unless unusual care is employed in obtaining the history, which Harrison finds is the one most important method of examination and in many patients more important than all the other procedures combined.

The same writer finds that when electrocardiograms are taken following muscular effort, changes of the S-T segments and of the T waves of such a nature as to be specifically suggestive of the presence of angina pectoris may be encountered in 50 to 60 per cent of patients. This was true not only of his study but of other studies that have been reported.

A word should be added regarding the relation of emotional factors to electrocardiographic changes. Wendkos has shown alterations in the T wave in the precordial lead in patients with neurocirculatory asthenia to be indistinguishable from those associated with structural heart disease. Anxiety may be accompanied by electrocardiographic changes in the absence of demonstrable heart disease as demonstrated by Crede et al. In the report of a case of a man of 27, subjected to various experiments, certain physiological disturbances due to anxiety were manifested by "abnormal" T waves, similar in contour to those seen in the pattern of left ventricular strain, but they appeared and disappeared rapidly. The changes were observed in limb leads as well as in precordial leads. Tachycardia and increased blood pressure usually accompanied the T wave inversion. Mainzer and Krause, in their study of the effects of fear on the electrocardiogram, showed that on the operating table immediately before induction of general anesthesia an abnormal electrocardiographic record was found to develop in roughly two fifths of 53 cases, when compared with the tracings of the previous day. Not only were these alterations observed in persons with cardiac disorders, where they merely accentuated the pathological character of the cardiogram already existing, but they occurred frequently in patients whose cardiograms had been normal. Although in a number of instances the changes disappeared when the patient was under anesthetic, or at least by the next day, in some cases they were still encountered twenty-four hours after the operation.

Therefore in cardiac neurosis careful analysis will usually show evident differences from true anginal pain. Rarely is the pain referred directly to the retrosternal region. Friedman found that patients suffering from functional cardiovascular disease experienced two separate and distinct types of precordial pain, which were not due to the same cause. The more common type was a sharp, piercing, transient pain at the left nipple which appeared to penetrate into the chest itself. The patients described it as a sensation of being "stabbed with a sharp needle," or being "torn" or "cut with a knife." Many patients became aware of irregular heart action in connection with this pain; others noted only the forceful heart action. Friedman believes that this particular pain originates from the nerve fibers in the heart muscle in association with arrhythmia or excessively forceful cardiac contraction.

The second type of precordial pain was a dull, aching, persistent discomfort, a combination of fatigue and pain, frequently described as "soreness." It was not so sharply localized as the other type of pain; it lasted for hours rather than minutes; and it was related to effort but did not come on immediately following exertion.

Some patients experienced both types of pain. Friedman confirms the observation of Wood, that patients with the dull type of precordial pain almost invariably used only the upper third of their chests in breathing. When such patients were asked to hyperventilate the majority complained of this dull precordial pain. When adhesive tape was applied to the chest in order to reduce the upper-chest breathing, forcing the patients to resort to abdominal breathing, the pain was abolished. Casts, too, were applied and kept on for a longer period but it is significant that when the casts were removed the patients reverted to upper-chest breathing and the pains returned. It is also interesting to record that when Friedman bound the chests of normal persons in the manner described (so that they had to breathe with the upper half of their chests) and then instructed them to exercise, the same kind of precordial pain appeared in these normal subjects. Friedman concludes, therefore, that the dull type of precordial pain is primarily due to the excessive use of the intercostal muscles in respiration.

But this pseudo-angina may have the characteristic features of true anginal pain and occasionally the recognition of its real nature must rest on the other factors present. For example, let us refer to the frequent problem of the obese woman of menopausal age with a labile blood pressure who complains of severe lancinating pain in the precordial region, breathlessness, and fatigue. Has she or has she not angina pectoris? If we remember that the pain of cardiac neurosis bears no definite relationship to effort, is frequently described as sticking, needle-like, or soreness; that it is often associated with inframammary tenderness and hyperalgesia, so that the pressure of the stethoscope sometimes elicits it; and that it may be accompanied by a sense of choking as well as sighing respirations, we shall have *no difficulty in the differential diagnosis particularly when we associate these symptoms with the whole picture and life situation of the individual with cardiac neurosis.*

Willius referred to a common error resulting from misinterpretation of the pain and soreness of inflammatory disease of the wall of the chest due to *fibromyositis* or *intercostal neuralgia.* Ordinarily, the painful sensations arising from this source are of rather long duration, often lasting for hours at a time; they occur when the patient is resting as well as when he is active and are likely to be exaggerated by deep breathing, coughing, and sudden movements of the upper extremities and body. At some time during the course of the trouble, regions of localized tenderness may be found on application of firm pressure over the ribs or sternum and in the intercostal spaces. Severe and fairly continuous pain occasionally is followed by the typical skin lesions of *herpes zoster.*

Another erroneous diagnosis of anginal syndrome to which Willius referred is due to *spondylitis* of the thoracic portion of the spine. Distribution of pain in the thorax and over its anterior surface is not uncommon as painful impulses are caused by impingement and irritation of spinal nerves by the hypertrophic arthritis. Under these circumstances, the pain is likely to occur on motion of the spine and when the patient is recumbent, particularly when considerable relaxation of the spine occurs and certain degrees of abnormal curvature result. Careful x-ray examination will permit the recognition of spondylitis.

Sometimes it is very difficult to exclude the *esophagus* and *upper digestive tract* as the source of pains which simulate angina. Special x-ray techniques and esophagoscopy studies have helped a great deal. It is a pretty safe rule to regard with suspicion any substernal pain that comes with effort regardless of whether the gastrointestinal tract seems to be responsible. *Tobacco* is a frequent offender in regard to pseudo-angina and had better be withheld whether or not the diagnosis of true angina is established.

The differential diagnosis of pain in the chest may be a most·difficult problem and is never to be regarded lightly. In any patient with pain in the chest, no matter how closely it may seem to be related to emotional factors, very careful physical studies must be made. In closing this discussion of cardiac pain, we cannot emphasize this point too strongly.

DYSPNEA.   Shortness of breath is the most common symptom of heart disease, but it also occurs for a variety of other reasons; for example, in lung diseases such as emphysema and bronchial asthma, in anemia and obesity, and in the air hunger of acidosis. But the dyspnea of actual heart disease occurs either directly as the result of exertion or in attacks of cardiac asthma. The dyspnea is determined by the vital capacity, which is reduced in patients with cardiac disease as a result of pulmonary congestion brought on by back pressure from the left side of the heart. Harrison referred to other factors, such as respiratory stimulation, the result of impulses arising in the moving muscles and in the distended great veins, as important in the production of dyspnea on exertion.

In the study by Wolf and Wolff, observations upon the respiratory function of patients and normal individuals showed that increase in the tidal volume and minute ventilation occurred in the setting of adverse life situations and associated emotional responses. They point out that increase in tidal volume may be brought about by such means as diminished oxygen capacity of the blood (anemia), impairment in alveolar oxygen transport in the lungs, increased oxygen demand in the tissues, acidosis, and obstruction in the air passage.

For our purpose we may conclude that cardiac dyspnea is in the main a reflex rather than a chemical disturbance and that its most important cause is congestion of the lungs. Therefore it seems strange that dyspnea of functional origin, which has nothing to do with congestion of the lungs, should be so frequently mistaken for the shortness of breath of organic heart disease. Here the dyspnea is due to anxiety even when the anxiety is not recognized. Indeed the shortness of breath often has a symbolic meaning. Although the patient describes "shortness of breath" careful questioning often will reveal that what he really has is a sensation of a weight on the chest—"a load on the chest"—which he can get rid of by talking about his troubles. It is an inability to obtain a deep breath plus a sensation that the air taken into the lungs is insufficient and does not enter deeply into the lungs. When an effort is made to overcome this sensation it leads to periodic sighing or "sighing respirations" and frequently the patient will demonstrate this in the course of an examination. For example, if he is asked to explain what he means by shortness of breath, he will place the hand on the lower sternum or epigastrium, take a deep sighing respiration and then often describe the feeling that the lungs seem insufficiently filled with air. Occasionally it is true that if the patients are suffering from severe emotional strain or anxiety, hyperpnea develops to the extent that hyperventilation tetany or syncope may result. Indeed, the test of hyperventilation in such subjects will frequently bring about such evidence of tetany as a positive Chvostek sign. It is of the greatest importance to differentiate this sighing respiration from dyspnea of cardiac origin.

A study of dyspnea and hyperventilation associated with sustained conflict, anxiety, humiliation, frustration and anger (in the paper by Wolf and Wolff already referred to) is illustrated in the accompanying figure.

The experiments indicate that the efficiency of the organism as evidenced in cardiovascular function was impaired (that is, the work of the heart was increased) under circumstances of conflict which resulted in reactions of anger, frustration, humiliation and anxiety. Respiratory inefficiency was apparent (that is, oxygen utilization was diminished) and was shown to be dependent upon impairment of the ventilatory rather than the respiratory mechanism of respiration.

PALPITATION.   "Heart consciousness," which comprises either tachycardia or arrhythmia or both, is a very frequent symptom in the cardiac neuroses and often leads to a mistaken diagnosis of organic heart disease. But it is also true that just as the heart may be speeded up by emotion so may it be retarded, and occasionally during anxiety attacks, especially in nightmares, great slowing of the heart occurs, apparently from vagal stimulation. More frequently, however, the heart is speeded up in its action and this together with premature contractions may lead to heart consciousness. Sometimes this is apparent only when the patient is lying on his left side or it occurs only in certain periods, but occasionally the patient is aware of the heart all of the time. When organic disease of the heart has been eliminated and when significant arrhythmias have not been demonstrated, one can feel quite certain that the awareness of the heart action is to be explained psychologically. Instances of actual

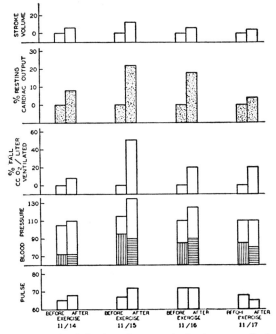

Figure 1.   Dyspnea and palpitation after exercise by hyperventilation and increased cardiac output in association with anxiety, frustration and anger. The per cent fall of cc. of oxygen per liter ventilated is equivalent to per cent increase in air ventilated per cc. of oxygen utilized. (Wolf, G. A., and Wolff, H. G.: Psychosom. Med., vol. 8, 1946.)

auricular fibrillation occurring during periods of emotional stress, which did not seem to have an organic basis, have been encountered.

Palpitation is sometimes the very first symptom of a cardiac neurosis. In the patient who has been prepared from the standpoint of his psychological make-up, certain life situations, such as prolonged emotional stress, plus such other factors as overindulgence in coffee and tobacco, will make a slight twinge or a skipped beat a sufficient stimulus to call attention to the heart and from that point on he may suffer from palpitation. Then, as Oille pointed out, if the physician gives medicine "to help prevent the irregularity" or makes the statement "the missed beats are not important if they don't get any worse," a cardiac neurosis has been established.

Wolf and Wolff suggest that changes in the intensity of frequency of stimuli caused by the beat of the heart may be associated with (*a*) increased stroke volume, (*b*) displacement of the heart or of tissues around it so that tissues ordinarily not stimulated by the beating heart are in a position to be stimulated, (*c*) occurrence of a beat out of phase with preceding and succeeding beats, and (*d*) rapid beating of the heart.

From their data they inferred that "significant change in stroke volume or in heart rate will cause mechanical disturbances such as traction and displacements within the chest, thus constituting adequate stimuli for the sensations interpreted as palpitation. It is, however, also apparent that the subjects' attitudes toward these sensations may become of major significance and be a factor in a chain of circumstances which accentuates or perpetuates the symptom. This may explain the frequent occurrence of palpitation in anxious patients with cardiac "neuroses," with or without structural cardiovascular disease. It may also indicate why patients who have apparently adequate stimuli such as occur in auricular fibrillation do not always experience palpitation. . . ."

In other words, certain attitudes as a result of conditioning in conjunction with minimal mechanical stimuli may pave the way for palpitation. Either alone may produce no symptoms. Having once suffered the experience of palpitation, should the patient develop anxiety or fear of heart disease, increased attention to this area of the body plus a stimulus in the form of exaggerated recoil of the heart or rapid pulse, associated with fear and anxiety, may potentiate the "vicious cycle" and the troublesome symptom of palpitation will prevail. It is generally known that palpitation associated with premature contractions will disappear upon reassurance that heart disease is not present, although the premature contractions may persist.

MURMUR. Probably no single objective finding leads to more false diagnoses of cardiac disease than a murmur. A systolic murmur can be found in a large number of healthy young adults if they are examined in various postures, in different phases of respiration, before and after exercise. These functional murmurs are also much more common during fevers. They are usually rather faint, but sometimes moderately loud, and are heard in the apical or pulmonic areas. Kilgore stated that if they are not very loud, not high pitched, if they are markedly changed by respiration and posture and not accompanied by other signs of heart disease (especially enlargement of the heart), by deficient heart function, or by a history of rheumatism or chorea, these systolic murmurs should not be regarded as pathologic. And in the case of borderline systolic murmurs—some of the louder ones, less clearly dependent on posture or respiration—the diagnosis of valvular disease, if suspected but not confirmed by other physical signs, should in general be held in abeyance until radiographic and electrocardiographic studies have been made.

The first point in the prophylaxis of cardiac neurosis enters in regard to this problem. If there is any question regarding the significance of the murmur the patient had better not be apprised of the fact or even made suspicious of heart disease until one can marshal his evidence in order completely to exonerate the heart. This is of special significance in regard to the recruiting of young men for military service. The beginnings of a cardiac neurosis can often be traced to the indiscreet remark of an examining physician who detects for the first time a systolic murmur at the apex of the heart unaccompanied by other evidence of organic disease.

Treatment. Separate chapters deal with treatment both of general and special problems in psychosomatic medicine but cardiac neurosis is so common and important an illness, with such individual characteristics, that some discussion of treatment will be considered here.

PROPHYLAXIS. The first thing to consider is prophylaxis. This means that in people predisposed because of their neurotic personality structure the physician must be particularly careful not to focus attention upon the heart in the course of a general physical examination, such as for insurance purposes, for military reasons, during recovery from infectious disease, or, more important still, during an anxiety attack. In the last instance, especially, our behavior must match our words, and when we tell such a patient that he does not have evidences of organic heart disease we must not say hesitatingly, "I do not *think* you have heart disease" but we must on the contrary say very definitely, "You do not have heart disease" and then instead of cautioning rest or giving "heart" medicine, which of course increases the patient's suspicion that we are not telling the truth or that we don't know, we must make the recommendation to "carry on in spite of symptoms."

Once cardiac neurosis has developed, the problem of eradicating the idea of heart disease from the patient's mind and reestablishing health becomes more difficult. In some instances it is relatively simple and a tactful explanation of the situation and reassurance may be all that is needed. But depending upon the severity of the underlying neurosis and the length of time that the cardiac symptoms have persisted, the problem may be very difficult. Under such circumstances the service of a trained psychiatrist may be necessary, but generally it is the attending physician who must assume the responsibility and care of such patients. We will discuss this question later.

IMPORTANCE OF HISTORY AND PHYSICAL EXAMINATION. It goes without saying that the first requisite is a careful history and physical examination. Often it is wise to carry out additional studies because a casual announcement after a hasty and superficial examination that "there is nothing the matter with the heart" will almost certainly fail to carry conviction. But there must be a point at which examinations stop and at that point one must say with confidence, "There is nothing the matter with your heart." Then if the patient can be persuaded to accept without resentment the idea that his symptoms are of emotional origin the battle is half won. From that point on, the liberal application of reassurance and encouragement will often accomplish a great deal. But the reassurance must be not simply that of the spoken word; the patient must be shown how to reassure himself by a demonstration that his symptoms can be made better rather than worse by the exercise and effort which he has been afraid to take.

Therefore we plan a program for the patient, of course using common sense in what we ask him to do. We do not ask a patient who has been incapacitated for months to go out and do a full day's work. On the contrary, we set an easy task at first. But we do say, "This much we know you can do and you must do it regardless of how you feel." That means that if you ask the patient to walk a block he must do so regardless of whether he feels faint or whether he feels that he will die before he gets back. It is kind of specious reasoning but we often say, "We will accept the responsibility for anything that happens to you" and this seems to be very persuasive to this type of patient.

Kilgore, in an excellent paper on the subject, emphasized the fact that once we have eliminated the idea of organic heart disease we must then tell the patient his slogan must be, "Carry on in spite of symptoms." This is a very successful way of handling such patients, and of course their confidence mounts in proportion to the degree of accomplishment.

DRUGS.   If medicines are used the patient must have a definite understanding that they are palliative rather than curative and that they have nothing to do with the heart itself. For example, if small doses of sedatives are used it is wise to explain to the patient that "they take the edge off his nervousness." The use of digitalis is, of course, a blunder. No intelligent patient could possibly be persuaded that his heart is sound if at the same time he is asked to take digitalis. If any rest in bed is to be recommended, and sometimes the patient will have to resort to some rest in the beginning, he must understand that this has nothing to do with his heart; that it is simply a question of having used up energy and that "his storage battery needs recharging." But for him to believe that the cultivation of a horizontal philosophy of life is going to cure him is erroneous because too much rest simply plays into the unconscious tendency to remain sick. In the final analysis it is the cultivation of an *erect philosophy of life* that is going to accomplish cure. The use of massage, hydrotherapy and gymnastic work must be looked upon from the standpoint not only of possible beneficial results but of the unhealthy suggestions that can come from such sources. Again and again it has been our experience that people who do not work directly with physicians, but rather in institutions that are developed solely from a commercial standpoint, are very prone to give the patient suggestions that are bad for him, not necessarily deliberately; by taking the pulse and commenting about it, taking the blood pressure and telling the blood pressure figures, referring to the muscle tone as bad or the circulation as poor, and so forth, they work harm rather than good. Subjects who develop cardiac neuroses usually do not tolerate coffee or tobacco well and we have found it useful to limit coffee and stop tobacco. This need not be an undeviating rule because some patients can tolerate both, but many tense people find momentary relaxation from the nervous cigarette habit but the end result is a bad one and the only way they can stop it is to quit rather than to cut down.

PSYCHOTHERAPY.   All of this, however, only leads to a consideration of psychotherapy, which is the fundamental method of treating the cardiac neuroses. Such management is very often rewarded by results that are just as satisfying as any in the field of internal medicine. We said before that this is usually a problem for the general physician. Certainly we cannot send all such patients to psychiatrists, not that there is anything reprehensible about sending patients to psychiatrists, but these problems are so numerous that general physicians must learn to deal with them. We have already pointed out that just as there is a minor and a major surgery so is there a minor and a major psychotherapy and many of the cardiac neuroses can be helped by minor psychotherapy. However, if a major disorder exists we must be able to recognize it and send such patients to psychiatrists. Furthermore, we must do our best to educate our patients and the medical profession to look upon psychic ailments in exactly the same way that they look upon organic ailments, that is, that there is no stigma to be attached to an illness simply because it is of emotional origin and hence there is no disgrace and certainly nothing to be ashamed of in consulting a psychiatrist.

Explaining the Illness to the Patient. Having determined then that we are dealing with cardiac neurosis (anxiety neurosis with cardiac manifestations), we first of all examine our patient as carefully as we can in order to rule out an organic disease but also, as mentioned in the beginning of the discussion, for the purpose of establishing a basis for psychotherapy. There is nothing so valuable as a thorough history and a complete physical examination in establishing a good relationship with the patient. It is then that you can say to the patient, and the statement carries conviction, "You do not have organic disease; this illness is of emotional origin." We use the latter term, emotional origin, advisedly because we find that it is the best way to explain to an intelligent patient that the illness is psychogenic. Patients often resent the term "just nerves" and they certainly resent the implication that the illness is "imaginary" or the impression that they sometimes gain from an unsympathetic physician that they are malingering. To say that the illness is functional does not offer sufficient explanation and patients frequently do not understand. To apply to the illness a term such as neurocirculatory asthenia, effort syndrome or hyperthyroidism is simply to delude yourself or to delude the patient. And yet this is frequently done just because the physician feels that he must give the illness a name and because he does not know how to approach the patient from an emotional standpoint. Hence the illness gets the name of a physical disease and often the unpropitious treatment that goes along with it.

One thing that we will have to discuss later is the unfortunate circumstance, as far as scientific psychological medicine is concerned, that no matter what you call the illness, if the patient has sufficient confidence in the physician, any kind of treatment may cause an alleviation of symptoms. Hence many physicians build up great reputations without really understanding the nature of such illnesses. What we are suggesting is that we call a spade a spade but attempt to do it in a way that the patient will understand. This, of course, is taking a chance with certain patients because, do what you will, they may resent the implication that the illness is emotional, largely owing to the belief that because we have "will power" and because we have intelligence, we ought to be able to handle "our nerves." But, of course, it is true that without help and without enlightenment a patient cannot handle anxiety of unconscious origin any more than he himself can handle an acutely inflamed appendix.

Organ Language.   To go on with our method of handling such patients, once we have told them that the illness is emotional we may use illustrations of how the emotions influence the functions of our body in order to show them that their emotions may be responsible for symptoms. Such examples as blushing, gooseflesh, vomiting, and diarrhea, as well as pallor, racing pulse and palpitation, occurring for various emotional reasons, are usually convincing. We say to them that if they have an emotional problem which they cannot express by word or deed, the tension arising from the emotional situation must express itself somehow and the organs of the body may take over the function of expression by a language of their own. ("Every psychic tendency seeks adequate bodily expression.")

Thus, if an individual finds it difficult to swallow it may not be that there is an obstruction in the gullet but it may be some situation in the environment that the individual cannot swallow. If the person "cannot tolerate something on his stomach" it may be something in his life situation that he cannot tolerate and the stomach is simply expressing it because he, for some reason, cannot; and if he has "a load on his chest" that is represented by sighing respirations or a "weight on the heart" that produces discomfort, the relation to his own illness is brought even nearer.

This kind of illustration will often permit a patient to talk freely about some problem that has been disturbing him perhaps more than he knew. Indeed, it is the very fact that such things are unconscious that makes it necessary for the body to express the emotions in such a primitive fashion as "organ language." Therefore we must strive to make the matter conscious and if we succeed it is likely that the particular symptoms will disappear. This discussion will usually have to do with the family group. For example, in a patient seen recently—a young married woman caring for a sick mother—the feelings of respect and devotion opposed to the inner resentment at the effort and cost and disruption of her own family life, led to anxiety which could not be dealt with as long as the approach was on the level of reassurance regarding the absence of organic disease, telling the patient that she must control herself, and giving phenobarbital. In other words, we must encourage our patients to talk about their "other troubles" in order to find out about the present trouble. To put it another way, *the more we can persuade our patients to talk about themselves as human beings rather than as medical cases the sooner we will come to understand their symptoms of emotional origin.*

This is usually best done by skillfully and tactfully *directing the conversation* rather than by asking direct questions. In regard to the latter point a word of caution is in order. It is often better to allow the patients to discuss matters of an intimate nature such as sexual problems without asking direct questions concerning sexual matters. If the patient has confidence in his physician he will frequently introduce these matters of his own accord but if it is necessary to ask questions it must be done in a way to indicate that such matters are perfectly natural, like any other natural function of the body, and that you are not asking as a matter of morbid curiosity; in other words, that you are scientifically and not morally interested.

Another point which may now be stated is that it is much better to listen than to talk. In other words, to give advice about important personal matters (such, for example, as marriage and divorce) is a distinctly dangerous matter for the physician to attempt. It is much better for him to listen, to direct, to allow the patient to see his problems, perhaps in a slightly different way, and then to come to his own conclusions about highly charged emotional matters.

Practical Suggestions.   We often say to patients who complain of palpitation that it is like the question of the horse and his rider. If the horse is whipped he will run but it is not the horse that is responsible —it is the rider. And so it is with the patient and his heart: It is not the heart that is at fault, it is the person himself, that is, his attitude and his feelings that are "making the heart run."

An important point is that the patient often seemingly agrees with the physician regarding the integrity of his heart but his skepticism prompts him to think (although he rarely tells the physician), "all right, the doctor says my heart is normal but if this keeps up, surely something will happen to it"; in other words, he hangs on to the notion that he is in for trouble, "that his heart will wear out"; "that he will develop angina or high blood pressure"; or that some other trouble confronts him which the physician cannot know about *even if he is telling the truth*. Therefore we often try to forestall this kind of thinking by telling the patient that his heart is normal and there is no reason why anything should happen to it.

The following case of typical cardiac neurosis occurred in an uneducated servant girl. It illustrates points which will be discussed in the treatment chapters, namely, that the poor develop neuroses as well as the rich and that the uneducated, if possessed of normal intelligence, can be treated by psychotherapy as well as the educated. Superior intellectual attainments are not necessary.

Case 7.   Cardiac Neurosis

A single, white girl, age 30 complained of *pain in the precordial region* and *fatigue*.

History and Symptoms.   Her trouble had begun six months ago. She felt tired and run down and then following a slight cold developed a sticking pain in the heart region. Her physician had found "a slight murmur, probably not important" and had recommended rest and a tonic to "strengthen her." Finally the pain and fatigue had become so pronounced that she could no longer work.

She had been a healthy child. Menses were established at 16, occurring every three weeks and usually attended by severe cramps. Because of the severe dysmenorrhea she had submitted to an operation at the age of 18 and one ovary was removed. On this occasion at the hospital the physicians "seemed very interested in her heart" and she then became suspicious that something was the matter.

The mother died at the age of 43 from "heart trouble." The patient was 15 at the time

She nursed her mother and helped look after the house during the period of her mother's illness. The father was living and well and one brother, younger than the patient, was well. There was no other evidence of heart disease in the family.

Physical Examination and Laboratory Studies.   The patient was fairly well-nourished. She seemed under considerable stress at the time of the examination. There was pronounced flush over the neck and upper chest; the blood pressure was 150/80; the heart was overactive but seemed normal in size. A slight systolic murmur was heard at the apex, but there was no shock or thrill. Palpitation over the apex area elicited tenderness. The remainder of the physical examination was negative.

Routine laboratory studies including the urine, blood count, blood Wassermann and sedimentation rate were within normal limits. Basal metabolism was normal. Fluoroscopic examination disclosed a normal sized heart and the electrocardiogram showed a normal tracing. Gynecological examination was negative.

LIFE SITUATION

Since her mother's death the patient had been employed in the house of a "well-to-do but stingy family." The patient was a passive person with a good deal of repressed hostility which was awakened when her mistress made what she considered unusual demands upon her. Discussion developed that the onset of the precordial pain had occurred just prior to housecleaning time. Then she remarked that each year she became ill right after housecleaning was over and this year she had become ill just before and, therefore, had been unable to do it because of the pain. Brief discussion brought out the fact that she considered that the housecleaning was too much for one person to do and that she resented the fact that her mistress, who could well afford extra help, insisted that she alone must do the work. Although she had never actually remonstrated before, she always became sick after the housecleaning was over (a belated and passive complaint) but this year her illness interfered with the job. Her manner indicated her deep resentment against her mistress and the simple expression of her unexpressed hostility, plus the suggestion of heart disease because of the mother's death from heart disease, was enough to indicate to her the cause for illness. When she was assured of the absence of heart disease and reassured as to her ability to carry on, and the explanation of the emotional background of the illness was made clear to her, she promptly recovered. A short time later she found another position and has remained well since.

Low Blood Pressure (Hypotension)

The problem of low blood pressure will be discussed again in relation to other conditions (pp. 241 and 447). At this point it is only necessary to say that, if anything, the concept of low blood pressure is even more open to criticism as an explanation for certain symptoms of unknown origin than is high blood pressure. When a patient speaks of weakness and fatigue it is so easy to say that "the blood pressure is low" or that "he is anemic," or both. It is much more difficult to examine the personality and study the life situation than it is to slap a cuff on the arm or have a technician do a blood count. A great many people go through life considering themselves victims of low blood pressure, with inadequate energy, easily fatigued, resting a lot and taking great care of themselves, often on the basis of a diagnosis of low blood pressure that really is unrelated to their symptoms. Their energy is low because it is consumed by emotional conflict and often it can be liberated by appropriate psychotherapy. Instead of cautioning these people to rest, and urging them to husband their energy, we ought to encourage them to do more instead of less. If for one reason or another we cannot undertake psychotherapy, at least we will not play into their unconscious fantasies regarding inadequacy and incapacity.

It is true, of course, that there is such a thing as essential hypotension but it is remarkably infrequent and has nothing to do with the thousands of inadequate people who limp through life leaning on the crutch of "low blood pressure" that has been furnished by some physician. We can say to these people, what has been proved by long observation, that low blood pressure is not a disease—it is more likely to be an indication of longevity.

Neurocirculatory Asthenia

Pain in the heart region, breathlessness and fatigue, to which may be added palpitation or heart consciousness, tachycardia and other disturbances of rhythm, faintness, dizziness, irritability and insomnia, as well as many other nervous symptoms, constitute a disorder frequently referred to as effort syndrome or neurocirculatory asthenia.

This disorder, designated by DaCosta as "irritable heart" in his description of this cardiac dysfunction noted in soldiers of the American Civil War, became known in World War I as "neurocirculatory asthenia." This latter name was suggested by a team of medical reserve officers (Oppenheimer and others) of the American Army sent to England to study the condition with Sir Thomas Lewis, whose term "effort syndrome" is the British equivalent.

From the very first description by DaCosta it has been recognized that emotional factors enter into the problem of neurocirculatory asthenia. However, the relative importance of the role played by the emotions has been the source of much dispute (Weiss).

Cohen and his associates (1951) have been studying this disorder for several years, and their many contributions are widely accepted as authoritative. Their studies are largely concerned with physiological measurements and long-term observations of the course of the disorder. Their experimental observations, which bear on the nature and severity of the symptoms and disability, demonstrate that abnormalities which are slight or absent at rest become pronounced with stress. Cohen's description of the disorder is the clinical picture of psychoneurosis, and since he holds the term "neurocirculatory asthenia" to be synonymous with "anxiety neurosis" and "neurasthenia," one would expect to find some consideration of psychodynamics and psychotherapy in his work. But this does not prove to be the case. A psychodynamic approach is excluded as unscientific, and simple reassurance with passage of time is held to be as effective as prolonged psychotherapy, psychoanalysis and other forms of treatment. Wheeler and his co-workers state that they are "unable to distinguish between patients with neurocirculatory asthenia as diagnosed by cardiologists and anxiety neurosis and neurasthenia as diagnosed by psychiatrists." Most observers would agree with this statement.

Margolin's remarks are to the point: "The syndrome which in 1917 was named neurocirculatory asthenia was originally observed in military combat situations. Anxiety neurosis, on the other hand, is a syndrome that was defined in a civilian environment. With the establishment of these two terms to cover a relatively unclassified group of somatic and psychic symptoms, anxiety neurosis and neurocirculatory asthenia began to appear as diagnoses in both civilian and military settings. It is important to realize that neurocirculatory asthenia as a term stresses the pathophysiological manifestations, whereas anxiety neurosis calls attention to the psychopathological phenomena. The significance of this distinction becomes apparent when the psychiatrist diagnoses anxiety neurosis in a patient who, according to the internist, exhibits neurocirculatory asthenia. In addition, this difference may be expressed by the patient's choice of his presenting symptom which may be psychological or physical. In fact, this unconscious selection may determine whether the patient will be referred to the psychiatrist or to the internist."

Cohen (1950) states that "cardiac neurosis is not a disease or diagnostic entity; most patients thus labeled probably have neurocirculatory asthenia." Most observers would turn this sentence around.

Miles and Cobb disagree with this disregard of the importance of psychogenic factors and look upon "neurocirculatory asthenia" and "anxiety neurosis" as opposite ends of a continuum, with the former diagnosis reserved for those patients who have evidence of a constitutional physiological deficit. They think of the differentiation in terms of a frequency distribution curve with a few relatively straight "somatic" cases at one end and a number of clearly "neurotic" cases at the other. The majority of cases they would regard as mixtures that fall somewhere in between, according to the proportions of the factors involved. They believe that this sort of division, rather than a clear-cut dichotomy, is of fundamental importance and still not sufficiently appreciated in medical thinking and teaching. They feel that the vagueness of the term "neurocirculatory asthenia," when defined merely by a list of symptoms, results in confusion and increases the difficulty of interpreting research data. It is not the label to which they object, but rather the concept of the disease that is implicit in a truly descriptive diagnosis.

Wittkower and his associates in a study of 50 unselected soldiers with "effort syndrome," delineated 5 personality types among them, and none was found to be emotionally well adjusted. The majority conformed to the obsessional type, but in an everyday view of their personalities important emotional problems might easily be overlooked.

Wheeler and his associates attempt to evaluate therapy by comparing a group of their patients with so-called neurocirculatory asthenia who were largely untreated, except by reassurance and the passage of time, with a heterogeneous group of subjects having psychologic disorders treated in other clinics by various medical and psychotherapeutic procedures, and conclude that their patients did just as well as the treated group. To make this type of comparison hardly seems adequate, and Walker feels that the deduction is supported by figures that could be used equally well to draw an opposite conclusion.

One would have no quarrel with a physiological study of neurocirculatory asthenia or any other condition so long as the author did not draw psychological conclusions from a nonpsychological study.

Cohen objects to the "anecdotal method" in the study of neurocirculatory asthenia, but it all depends on who is listening to the anecdote. It is like the interpretation of the microscopic image—it depends upon who is looking through the eyepiece. A person trained in psychodynamics listening to the story of a patient with neurocirculatory asthenia discovers (1) that the symptoms are those of psychoneurosis, (2) that the family history shows a high incidence of psychopathology, (3) that a long-term study of the life history indicates neurotic personality structure, (4) that a cross-sectional study of the life history at the time of onset of symptoms shows emotionally disturbing events that are specific for that particular personality, (5) that discussing this material brings out meaningful behavior on the part of the patient, and (6) that dealing with this material has psychotherapeutic value. Therefore, to neglect psychodynamic factors in patients with neurocirculatory asthenia means that one excludes from the field of observation the most important part of the clinical picture. This aspect is implicit in Cohen's treatment of the subject—in his use of the terms "anxiety neurosis" and "neurasthenia" as synonyms for neurocirculatory asthenia (even though he separates the terms from their psychological meaning); in his description of the disorder, which is identical with psychoneurosis; in his attempt to evaluate treatment by comparing the disorder with a heterogeneous group of psychologic disorders treated in other clinics; and even in his own treatment, which is largely concerned with reassurance and a study of "social" factors. We agree with Miles and Cobb that "unless one makes some attempt not only to measure the constitutional or physiologic factors but also to understand the psychodynamics of the illness and of the therapeutic processes as well, it seems unlikely that even the most objective and scientific investigations can prove fruitful." While we cannot measure human behavior with the same precision with which we measure the physiological disturbances which reflect that behavior, it is nevertheless true that neurosis has its own distinctive features to be discovered by personality study and that only in this way can diagnosis be correctly made and proper treatment instituted.

From the standpoint of the practical management of these disorders we think that the use of the term "neurocirculatory asthenia" does more harm than good. It calls attention to a part when the disorder is one of the whole. It implies that the circulation is somehow at fault. Our feeling is that medicine would be better off without the term "neurocirculatory asthenia," which only confuses the patient and often leads the physician to feel that he understands the disorder because he has given it an imposing name. There is less objection to the term "effort syndrome" (which leaves the way open for further investigation rather than closes the subject with a pretentious name), though the symptoms are not confined to exertion.

The term "neurocirculatory asthenia" has come to carry the connotation of constitutional inadequacy, which is so easy to incriminate, while the emotions are so difficult to study. But, as Walker states, the physician who believes that the patient has symptoms because he is made of "second-rate stuff" cannot hide this attitude from the patient. He also feels that it is more rational to focus attention on factors which can be modified rather than on those that only Providence can alter.

The designation "neurocirculatory asthenia" appeared on the horizon about the time when "shell-shock" was at the height of its popularity. The former seems to us just as bad a name as the latter because it is based on a misconception and perpetuates invalidism. If one refers to an illness of emotional origin in terms of organic disease, one fosters neuroticism. If it is called a disorder and explained in terms of behavior, the patient is immeasurably better off. To use an analogy pertaining to another part of the body: we have seen the rise and fall of the term "colitis" and the evil effects of giving this diagnosis to a neurotic patient with an "irritable bowel" syndrome. Neurocirculatory asthenia is just as bad a name as "colitis," and "irritable heart" is worse than "irritable colon," because people are more concerned about the heart than about the colon. It is the person that is at fault and not the colon, and the same is true in regard to the cardiovascular system in the patient with neurocirculatory asthenia.

Since neurocirculatory asthenia does not exist without neurosis or personality disturbance, we suggest that the condition be called neurosis, using the proper psychiatric designation, and adding qualifying terms if necessary.

The Syndrome in Military Life. "Neurocirculatory asthenia" seemed to be less of a problem in World War II than in World War I, probably because it became recognized for what it is, namely psychoneurosis with cardiac manifestations, and was classified as such rather than as heart disease. Then too, in the latter instance there was probably better selection at the time of induction into service. One of the reasons the British made so little headway with the disorder from a psychotherapeutic standpoint in the first war (returning only 20 per cent to front-line duty) is that in their management of the disorder valuable time was lost and the neurosis was permitted to consolidate; then of course it became more difficult to treat.

These deductions received confirmation in a large experience with so-called "effort syndrome" at the Mill Hill Emergency Hospital of London, England: 2323 cases treated at the Effort Syndrome Unit of this neurosis center, which permitted a number of studies on the functional responses of such persons. From this study the belief is stated that effort syndrome is largely a question of neurosis, and that the problem is one for the psychiatrist rather than the cardiologist. Three groups are proposed:

Group 1. Poor physical endowment is the primary factor in producing symptoms. Here one is dealing with a poor machine which shows excessive response to physical effort; the patient has effort intolerance which has been present since his earliest recollection.

Group 2. Similar to Group 1, but the patient responds in a neurotic manner to his constitutional inferiority. In this sense there is a psychological etiology but the constitutional factor is the basic one. The emotional reaction may take any form, depending upon the personality makeup. The patient feels that he has an effort intolerance but his disability may actually be less than he believes it to be. Such patients usually give a history of effort intolerance since childhood, whereas the mere disability of Group 1 frequently changes under stress to the neurotic attitude of Group 2.

Group 3. Primarily neurotic. Here the usual etiological factors determining a neurosis will apply. The form may be selected by the constitutional physical inferiority which, if present, colors the whole picture but is of only secondary importance; or it may be selected wholly on a psychogenetic basis. Such "illness" tends to be of comparatively recent origin and is particularly prone to result from the emotional and physical stresses of wartime.

A comparison of oxygen uptake, lactate rise and pulse area made after exercise in normal subjects, in patients suffering from anxiety states, and in effort syndrome patients, showed that the patients with anxiety states and those with effort syndromes had a significantly poorer exercise response when matched with normal controls.

If there is a postural circulatory defect the blood pressure drops and the pulse rate increases as the patient arises from recumbency to the upright position. Sometimes the blood pressure will not change so much as the pulse rate. Sometimes there are electrocardiographic changes to correlate with pulse and blood pressure changes. Voltage of T waves tends to be lowered in the erect position and P deflections in leads 2 and 3 show a higher voltage. This can be referred to as the electrocardiographic evidence of what has been called the postural syndrome.

It may be quite true that the vasomotor instability and the psychological disorder are parallel manifestations of the same basic fault. In one instance the poor physical endowment may be the chief problem, in another instance the personality disorder. It is largely a question of where the emphasis is placed. We believe that placing the emphasis on the "constitutional inadequacy" is a mistake. In the first place it is so often not true, and in the second place nothing can be done about it anyhow, whereas one can usually do something about a psychological disturbance.

In this connection Friedman found that most patients suffering from functional cardiovascular disease experienced transient giddiness. It usually occurred following rapid or abrupt change from the supine to the erect position. Experimental studies revealed that the symptom was most likely due to cerebral anemia arising from the retardation of the forward flow of blood. When giddy patients arose, it was observed fluoroscopically that a sudden, abrupt decrease in the width and pulsatile excursion of the pulmonary artery (conus) took place and the force of cardiac contraction was observed to dwindle although the rate increased remarkably. No such change was observed in normal individuals. A schematic representation of the probable mechanism underlying the giddiness of functional cardiovascular disease is shown in the accompanying diagram (Chart 1).

Differential Diagnosis. The great difficulty has been that, in keeping with our terminology referable to the cardiovascular system, our whole attitude and all observations have been limited to the cardiovascular system instead of including an approach to the subject from a psychosomatic standpoint. As to how these patients are classified, all depends upon the point of view. For example, some physicians think of them as endocrine problems, especially from the standpoint of the thyroid, and treat them as instances of hyperthyroidism; others think of them from a metabolic standpoint and speak of them as suffering from hypoglycemia or hyperinsulinism; others, impressed by the psychic dis-

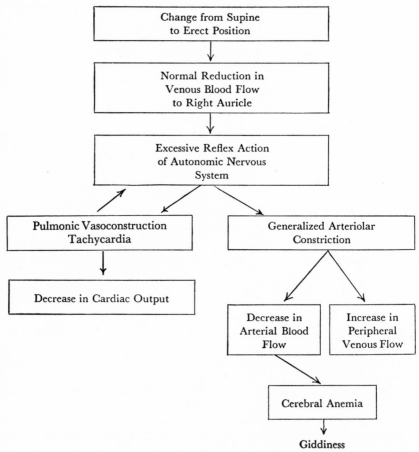

Chart 1.   The Probable Mechanism Underlying the Giddiness of Functional Cardiovascular Disease*

turbance, refer to them as instances of chronic nervous exhaustion, anxiety neurosis or neurasthenia, but the latter two terms are used devoid of psychic meaning and no psychic studies are made. Still others have been impressed by the slight fever that occurs in many of these cases and have studied them from that standpoint. A case will be cited in which this problem is encountered. Hamman, in two papers devoted to the "Diagnosis of Obscure Fever" and speaking of the *effort syndrome,* said, "The fever may persist for years and the most thorough investiga-

* Friedman, Meyer: Functional Cardiovascular Disease, Williams and Wilkins Co., Baltimore, 1947.

tion fail to discover any acceptable cause for it. The character of the symptoms and their long duration force us to look upon effort syndrome as a neurosis of obscure mechanism and origin. Unexplained, slight fever is so frequently present in this condition that we regard it as an important element of the clinical manifestations."

Friedman found low-grade fever, rarely exceeding 100.5°F., in more than 30 per cent of patients suffering from "functional" cardiovascular disease. He could detect no evidence that the fever was a manifestation of infection, either acute or chronic. He cautions reservation in the diagnosis of undulant fever in any patient who exhibits manifestations of functional cardiovascular disease, including fever, for over six months. Incidentally, Friedman holds that the presence of fever in this syndrome is a definite indication of hypothalamic involvement. Our own feeling is that unfortunately this brings us no closer to an understanding of this disorder.

Tobacco poisoning, tuberculosis, brucellosis and colitis are frequent terms used in connection with such patients. Altogether neurocirculatory asthenia seems to be a catch-basket into which are thrown a great variety of ill-defined conditions. Chart 2 summarizes some of the chief differentiating features.

RORSCHACH STUDY. Ross studied neurocirculatory asthenia by the Rorschach method (50 cases compared with 50 controls). He found that:

(a) Certain personality features are associated with neurocirculatory asthenia to a greater degree than would be accounted for by chance.

(b) These personality features include several which have been previously reported from clinical psychiatric study, namely, features characteristic of psychoneurosis, in particular a tendency to give up easily under stress ("hysterical quitters") and obsessive-compulsive traits.

(c) Sexually disturbing stimuli do not appear to cause as great difficulty for these patients as they do for miscellaneous civilian psychoneurotics, but other anxiety-producing stimuli are handled with even greater difficulty.

(d) When the neurocirculatory asthenia patients are divided into two groups, the more long-standing cases are found to possess the neurotic features to a more marked degree, while those of more recent onset show a stronger similarity to cases of migraine with persistence toward success and "ambitious perfectionism."

Many of the points mentioned in the discussion are illustrated by the following cases.

Case 8. "Neurocirculatory Asthenia" Induced by Military Service; Paranoid Personality

History and Symptoms. A white man, 36, was first seen in April, 1945. He complained of irregular heart action, weakness and fatigue, and said he felt unable to work. There was a sudden sensation in his chest that felt like "a balloon inflated." The condition had developed in the army and he had been discharged because of it with 60 per cent disability.

The illness began in October 1944, while he was in military training. He had to row upstream against a swift current until he felt exhausted, then the boat got stuck in the mud and everybody had to get out and push the boat to the river bank. Following this there was a "double quick" march for nine miles. When he reached camp the heart action

Chart 2. Differential Diagnosis in "Neurocirculatory Asthenia"

	Cardiac Neurosis	"Neurocirculatory Asthenia"	Hyperthyroidism	Chronic Infections (Tuberculosis—Brucellosis)
Family History	Unstable (epilepsy, neurosis, psychosis)	Unstable	Unstable	Stable
Past History	Poor adjustment (childhood neurosis, nervous breakdown)	Poor adjustment	Poor adjustment	Well adjusted
Precipitating Cause	Emotional stress, psychic trauma	Stress of military service	Emotional stress, psychic trauma	Sufficient exposure to specific organism
Clinical Picture	Precordial pain, fatigue, breathlessness, palpitation	Precordial pain, fatigue, breathlessness, palpitation	Goiter; exophthalmos; fine tremor; emotionalism	Febrile features conspicuous; anxiety features absent or inconspicuous
Physical Examination and Laboratory Studies	Normal cardiovascular system, rapid pulse while awake	Evidences of neurocirculatory instability—cold, sweaty and cyanotic extremities; flushing of face and neck; postural change in pulse, blood pressure, and electrocardiogram; slight elevation of temperature	Rapid pulse, awake and asleep; plus basal metabolism; response to iodine	*T. B.:* plus x-ray; plus sputum *Brucellosis:* plus skin, agglutination tests, and blood culture
Treatment	Psychotherapy	Psychotherapy and medical measures	Surgery plus psychotherapy	Medical measures
Prognosis	Depends on severity of underlying neurosis	Poor	Good	Good

was very rapid. Medical service was not immediately available, and when he did get to the dispensary "nothing was done for him." The rapid heart action and shortness of breath prevented him from sleeping. Finally an army physician told him that he had auricular fibrillation and kept him in bed for four days. Following this he was put through a thorough and "strenuous" physical check-up. Then he was discharged as physically unfit because of his heart. An electrocardiographic tracing was reported as auricular fibrillation with an occasional premature ventricular contraction.

The patient was bitter about his treatment in the service, referred to the army doctors in disrespectful terms, and felt that he had been given a "bad deal" because of the "excessive strain of the physical examination on top of 'what he already had.'"

After he had been discharged from the service his civilian physician reported that he had been well before he entered the service and that his work often required him to lift packages of 100 pounds in weight which he could do without ill effect. He told the patient that he suffered from "heart-muscle strain, that rest and relaxation would help him, and gave him medicine containing digitalis."

PAST HISTORY. In a more detailed investigation of his past history it was learned that he often showed fits of temper as a child and would get very angry at members of the family on the slightest provocation. He had suffered from headaches and fatigue beginning in high school and these had continued for about ten years. Then he became involved in a tempestuous love affair that "nearly drove him crazy." This broke up in 1940 at a time when "his nerves gave 'way." Gradually he recovered and was inducted into the army in January 1942. After his discharge he returned to his home and to his father's business. He reported much aggravation with his father, who conducted the business in a way of which the patient did not approve and would accept no suggestions from the patient. A younger brother and sister were unsympathetic to the patient's illness and only the mother, who was described as a hard-working, intelligent woman, "had any consideration for him."

Physical Examination and Laboratory Studies. Physical examination with special attention to the cardiovascular system disclosed no evidence of organic disease. The blood pressure was within normal limits; the heart was normal in size according to orthodiagram; and the electrocardiographic tracing was also within normal limits. Eyegrounds were physiologic. Routine laboratory studies were normal and glucose tolerance was normal.

LIFE SITUATION

Each time the patient returned he was encouraged to talk about his home situation and the burden of his complaint was always the same. He was disgusted with his father, whom he described as a stupid and obstinate man who refused to accept the patient's modern ideas about how to run the business. The son openly threatened the father with violence and on occasion was told "to get out if he didn't like it." But he felt unable to work and therefore was dependent upon his father for assistance. He was "humiliated" by the necessity of "borrowing" money from his father. This yielding to his dependency of course only infuriated him the more and while he recognized that the aggravation at home "exaggerated his condition," he continued to believe that his heart had been weakened by the overexertion and bad treatment which he had received in the army, that he was unable to undergo any real physical exertion, and that if he did so it would set him back for a matter of months. Thus, he was caught in the conflict of his impotent rage— acknowledging his dependence upon the father whom he hated. He would refuse to help in the store and would try to absent himself from home "to escape the aggravation." Finally he tried a succession of jobs as a salesman but they always involved more exertion than he felt he could undergo.

It was impossible to convince him that his heart was sound and that the whole problem was one of a disorder of his feelings rather than of his body. Although he expressed his feelings freely in the interviews this was so far from modifying the fury of his murderous impulses that he obtained very little relief. The family physician reported that both the mother and father were very much afraid of him because of his threats to the father. Moreover, the family physician also reported that any disturbance in the home was not the fault of the father and mother, but that they were kind and amenable people who would do anything for their children.

Finally the patient was called by the Veterans Administration for a resurvey and his disability was reduced from 60 to 10 per cent. He was more furious than ever with the injustice meted out to him, felt that we had conspired with the V. A. physicians, and broke off his treatment. During the time he remained under observation (April 1945 to November 1946) the only indications of improvement were his acknowledgement of somewhat lessened heart consciousness and his efforts to work, which he did for short periods of time.

SUMMARY

A young man developed the syndrome of neurocirculatory asthenia following an episode of physical exhaustion during military service. He had had previous neurotic difficulties and the illness was perpetuated by a home situation that gave rise to impotent rage. The paranoid personality of the patient indicated the poor prognosis and constituted a real threat to his family.

Case 9.   "Neurocirculatory Asthenia"; Long-continued, Low Fever of Obscure Origin; Questionable Endocarditis

History and Symptoms.   The patient was a rather attractive American-born Italian woman, 28 years old. She complained of fatigue, shortness of breath and pain in the precordium. She was well until September 1938, when she noticed a gradually increasing fatigue and was ordered to bed by her physician, where she remained for two weeks. Then she was somewhat improved until about Christmas time when she again became tired and "was in and out of bed for the remainder of the winter." In June 1939, her physician again ordered her to go to bed because she was so fatigued and because he thought that she had a "leak in her heart." At the same time she discovered that she had slight fever and from then on, following the physician's orders, she took her temperature four or five times a day. The temperature was never above 99.4° or 99.6°. In spite of a vacation at the seashore during the summer she failed to regain her strength, finally changed physicians, and was then referred to the hospital for further study.

The shortness of breath had been present for about four months. She described the shortness of breath as coming with slight exertion and demonstrated by placing her hand over her lower sternum and then stating that she felt as though she would like to take a deep breath but felt herself unable to do so. Thus she described the typical sighing respiration so common in functional problems. The pain was felt over the whole heart region and extended into the back to the angle of the left scapula.

PAST HISTORY.   The patient said she was a healthy child. Her father died when she was six, and the mother remarried two years later. The patient continued at school until the eighth grade, then worked in the store that her stepfather had established and also helped around the house. The menses began about eleven and had always been very painful. She married at 20 and became pregnant one year later. She had a hard delivery and a prolonged convalescence and was unable to nurse the child. During the hospital stay, following labor, she had slight fever. Shortly afterward she had to work very hard, taking care of the large household as well as the child.

Physical Examination and Laboratory Studies.   The patient was referred into the hospital as a case of "neurocirculatory asthenia" or possible endocarditis. The general physical examination showed a well nourished, young white woman, who did not appear ill. The temperature was slightly elevated, reaching about 99.6° in the afternoon. Aside from a slight systolic murmur at the apex of the heart, there were no physical findings to suggest organic disease. Moreover, the heart seemed normal in size and this was corroborated by the x-ray examination. The urinalysis was entirely normal; the blood count was within normal limits, both as to red and white blood cells, and differential count; and the Wassermann test was negative. Several blood cultures had been negative, and agglutination tests, especially for undulant fever, were negative.

LIFE SITUATION

This patient was born in America of Italian parents who enforced old world standards in bringing her up. She had few friends and was allowed no freedom during her adolescence. There was practically no social life, the family living very much within itself. She resented deeply the fact that she could not go on with her schooling and pictured herself as a person who would have derived much benefit from further education. She felt that she might have been able to go to college and "make something of herself." These were the thoughts which were disturbing her during her adolescence and during the period when she developed what she later looked upon as "nervous indigestion." It was also interesting that during this period she was very fatigued although this was brought out only by questioning—she did not remember it in connection with the story of the present illness.

Stepfather's Illness.   About three years ago her stepfather had an illness which was reported to be encephalitis, and then developed a change in personality. He began "to stare at the patient," especially at the table, and then made accusations to the mother that the patient was being untrue to her husband. He insisted that she was carrying on with men in the neighborhood and this caused her a great deal of concern. She insisted that there was no foundation in truth for these accusations, nor could she think of any possible reason why he should make these statements. Finally matters reached such a point that the stepfather threatened that she must either leave the house or he would. Without warning he carried out his threat one day in August, 1938; shortly, however, he had a change of heart, returned and suffered the patient to remain in the house, stating that he would change his attitude. It was true that he no longer made the accusations but the patient still felt that he stared at her and of course that he was thinking evil thoughts. *This period of emotional stress immediately preceded the beginning of her illness in September, 1938.*

Hostility Toward Parents.   She felt, and we thought with justification, that she had had a raw deal in life and so she carried a great deal of hostility within her toward fate in general and her parents in particular. Nevertheless, she did not dare to establish her own home which, of course, was what she wanted and could afford to do. She said "that it would be too hard on her mother and stepfather" who needed her financial help. Thus, she could not retaliate in any active way for the bad way in which they treated her. Nor could she tolerate any evidence of this hostility within herself.

TREATMENT

We sketched her problem for her as we saw it, that is, that the slight fever was inconsequential but that the fatigue was the important problem and that the cause of fatigue was emotional conflict; that she had had a very difficult childhood and adolescence, resenting the fact that she could not be educated and had to work, that she really had no chance for a good time like other young girls but immediately became interested in a young man whom she married. Then came the baby and lots of difficulties with it and then the episode with the stepfather. After we had sketched this outline of her history she said, "I did not tell you before but during the last year I have been afraid that he would come in during the night and kill me." When questioned as to why she had this thought she would give no answer and only after several months did she finally relate an episode of attempted seduction on the part of the stepfather which had been responsible for her great fear of him. She, of course, had always been too ashamed and too fearful of his vengeance to tell anyone about it.

Follow-up in Outpatient Department.   The patient was seen every two weeks in the outpatient department and at the end of a year she was much improved. It took considerable persuasion to get her to establish her own home but this she finally did and improvement was more rapid from that point on. Another source of tension with which we were able to help her was in regard to her son whose enuresis and soiling during the day was a great annoyance to her. We persuaded her to bring the boy to the children's outpatient psychiatric department and as a result of his treatment there he had been much improved. Gradually she was relieved of anxiety regarding the possibility of heart disease and no longer took her temperature.

The most important phase of the treatment, however, had to do with a personal contact which was established between a social worker, who was attached to the psychiatric department, and the patient. The worker was able to furnish an important link between the patient's visit to us and her behavior at home. By acting as an intelligent and sympathetic friend she was able to help the patient see the relationship between her illness and her life situation and, moreover, was able to provide her with sustained support and a feeling of security at times when her anxiety arose. She was an invaluable help to us in the management of this patient and we felt certain that recovery would not have advanced so far if it had not been for her help.

Follow-up.   The patient has been followed over the years and continues to be an effective person. There are occasional episodes of fatigue but no chronic invalidism which surely would have been her fate without psychosomatic help.

SUMMARY

A young white woman presented a clinical picture thought to be neurocirculatory asthenia. Slight fever also suggested endocarditis. The absence of a heart lesion was finally established. Too much attention was focused on the fever and not enough on the fatigue, which was emotional in origin. With the help of a social worker the emotional problem was handled and the patient restored to fairly satisfactory health which has been maintained for more than fifteen years.

EMOTIONAL FACTORS IN ORGANIC HEART DISEASE

As indicated in the previous discussion, many contributions have been made to the subject of the cardiac neuroses and it is quite generally appreciated that such disorders are psychogenic in origin and that psychotherapy is essential in treatment. But it has not been recognized that psychological factors are even more important in organic cardiovascular disease. In her comprehensive study of emotions and bodily changes Dunbar made particular mention of the work of Fahrenkamp and other foreign authors who have dealt with this problem, and both she and Wolfe in America have made notable contributions. The subject, however, needs repeated emphasis. For while a neurotic with a normal heart may suffer a great deal subjectively and may even have a disturbance of cardiac function marked by various forms of arrhythmia, the heart, certainly in the majority of such patients, remains structurally healthy. We are not considering the involved psychosomatic question of whether long-continued emotional stress can produce structural changes in the cardiovascular system. That is a problem for future determination. We are dealing here only with what are generally acknowledged to be unequivocal psychosomatic relationships.

Importance of Emotional Factors

The neurotic patient who has organic heart disease may add a real burden to the work of his heart, either through constant tension of psychic origin or, more especially, by means of acute episodes of emotional origin. This may hasten a cardiac breakdown which might be indefinitely postponed if there were no psychic stress. Thus the psychic factors may be even more important than the physical in producing incapacity. This is the problem which Dunbar and Wolfe have dealt with so effectively.

Wolfe called attention to the fallacy in medical thinking that if organic disease of the cardiovascular system is present, the physician is satisfied to let the matter rest without seeking to discover the psychic factor. The physician thinks "there is plenty of pathology present" to account for the trouble and looks no further for disabling factors. Hence, when such physicians examine a patient, no matter what his personality or complaints, if a physical defect is found the illness is apt to be attributed to that even if it is only a pathological curiosity. As far as the heart is concerned this is especially the case in instances of congenital lesions and well compensated mitral stenosis, and in many patients with essential hypertension. Repeatedly in nervous children with insignificant congenital lesions, in neurotic young women with mitral stenosis and normally functioning hearts, and in emotionally unstable women at the menopausal age with hypertension, the error is made of attributing the symptoms to the heart itself. We have already stated that this is one way for a physician to add to the neurotic problem. Both his organic training and his insecurity in dealing with cardiac disorders have been responsible for this attitude. But even better trained and more sophisticated clinicians make errors of a similar kind in many of the more complicated psychosomatic cardiac problems, especially those that occur in the hypertensive-arteriosclerotic group.

Chambers and Reiser studied 25 consecutive patients admitted to the Cincinnati General Hospital with heart lesions representative of those usually seen in a large city hospital (hypertensive, atherosclerotic, rheumatic, syphilitic, and so on). It was found that emotional factors had played a major precipitating role in the precipitation of congestive heart failure in 19 of the patients (76 per cent). While all of these 19 patients had been living under severe chronic emotional strain, in each of them the superimposition of an acute, emotionally stressful experience appeared to be the factor immediately responsible for the onset of cardiac decompensation. They were precisely the type of patients in whom the possibility of an emotional component in the illness is usually minimized or ignored by medical teachers and practitioners.

Emotional Problems of Coronary Occlusion

"Stress and strain" are regarded by the laity and the medical profession alike as an integral part of the problem of coronary occlusion but medical observations concerning these factors have been focused chiefly on physical exertion. Except for a few case reports, very little effort has been made to conduct systematic studies from a psychosomatic standpoint. Perhaps the organic tradition in medicine has encouraged us to think of coronary occlusion as a "purely physical disease," with emphasis on heredity, dietary factors and easily demonstrable coronary atherosclerosis; but the frequent onset of coronary occlusion during sleep or rest has also inclined observers to minimize emotional stress. Perhaps, too, the unwillingness to attempt psychiatric interviews with a very sick patient is another reason for the failure to study coronary occlusion from an emotional standpoint. Emotional factors have also been neglected in regard to treatment; physical rest and physical measures have been emphasized.

We do not wish to minimize the preexisting coronary artery disease that is the essential background for coronary occlusion. However, it has been demonstrated that emotional stress may be accompanied by measurable changes in pulse rate, stroke volume, cardiac output, peripheral resistance and arterial blood pressure (Stead et al., and Grollman). Clotting time and blood viscosity may also be influenced by emotional stress (Schneider and Zangari), so apparently physiological changes may be brought about that increase the work of the heart and impair its efficiency. Thus emotional factors might conceivably add to the burden of an impaired coronary circulation.

Previous Studies.   A few individual cases and only an occasional small series of patients with coronary artery occlusion have been studied from a psychological standpoint. Dunbar in a psychiatric study of 22 patients described a typical personality profile, and Arlow also found a clear-cut constellation of personality traits in patients with coronary artery disease. Both found evidence for compulsive competitive striving and concluded that the character structure of the patient predisposes him to coronary occlusion. Dunbar referred to the "coronary personality" as consisting of "compulsive striving, hard work, self-discipline, and great need to get to the top." Both emphasized the psychodynamic importance of the patient's childhood conflicts with authority. Arlow described an early competitive relationship with a much feared and envied parent (usually the father). He stated that the characteristic defense mechanisms used in dealing with this focal conflict were repression and identification, but that they served their purposes inadequately because the patient continued to reexperience his old conflict with authority over and over again as he unconsciously recreated in new forms the original situation of competition. He drove himself compulsively, through hard work and self-discipline, but success brought no sense of gratification or relief from tension.

Cathcart, a Canadian psychiatrist, was impressed with emotional factors in the precipitation of coronary occlusion in a series of patients whom he had seen in consultation, and in a study from a Finnish hospital Jarvinen concluded that some patients developed coronary occlusion while in the hospital from the emotional stress associated with ward rounds (see p. 220). Van Balen also studied a small series of patients and called attention to the fact that psychological factors may remain unrecognized unless a special inquiry is made with regard to this possibility.

Most of the large-scale studies on coronary occlusion by cardiologists minimize the importance of emotional factors in coronary occlusion. Master and Jaffe, studying the factors in the onset of coronary occlusion and coronary insufficiency, amassed a good deal of evidence to show that coronary occlusion is not brought about by events in the external environment. In their large series they found that about half of the attacks began during sleep and rest and since the majority of persons spend half the day in this way "these activities may be considered coincidental." Similarly, they conclude that the association of only 2 per cent of the coronary occlusion attacks with severe exertion is also coincidental. They argue that most persons perform some unusual effort at least several times a day so, if effort were a precipitating factor in coronary occlusion, the incidence of attacks during strain should be much greater. Even when coronary occlusion seems to have followed directly after effort they call attention to the fact that coronary thrombosis takes place over a variable period, occasionally several weeks prior to the attack, so that the occlusion had already completely formed. Therefore while "exertion may account for the appearance of symptoms and even death, it does not account for the coronary occlusion that had occurred spontaneously." Very little attention is paid to the question of emotional stress and this is generally true in papers dealing with the onset of coronary occlusion and in chapters on this subject in textbooks of medicine and cardiology. For example, Ancel Keys, long a protagonist of the nutritional approach to atherosclerosis, in speaking of coronary heart disease and the mode of life comments, "other factors beside the diet need more attention but it is fair to say that, except for physical exercise, no other clue is in sight. Even the concept that "stress and strain" is influential needs study because of the complete absence of evidence for its validity."

Nevertheless, there has been an important contribution to this subject. Miles, Waldfogel, Barrabee and Cobb studied 46 patients selected from the clinical material utilized by Gertler, Garn and White in their study of coronary heart disease in young adults. Miles et al. were interested in the relation of personality factors to the genesis of atherosclerosis of the coronary arteries. Their study was made on an average of 5.6 years after the attack of coronary occlusion so that it differs from ours in this respect as well as the fact that it was done on 46 young men with coronary artery disease (average age 41.7 years) and was controlled by a study of 49 healthy men (average age 39). A complete psychosocial survey was made, with special effort to see whether the coronary personality as described by Dunbar and Arlow could be confirmed. They could find no convincing evidence that the personality exhibited by the coronary patient, as compared to the control subject, could be implicated as a significant factor in the genesis of coronary artery atherosclerosis. "The coronary patients had tended to work harder, under more stress and strain, although this was not necessarily physically strenuous work. Only a few more of the coronary patients than controls showed a consistent tendency toward compulsive striving, ascetic self-discipline, and greater need to 'get to the top' in their chosen work. When the two groups were compared in terms of specific personality traits, the differences were very slight. The coronary group showed less tendency to introspection than did the controls and more difficulty in handling their aggressive tendencies. The similarities between the groups were more striking, however, than were the differences, and our findings, in the main, did not confirm previous observations."

Miles et al. assume that acute coronary occlusion with myocardial infarction can be precipitated by severe emotional stress but they did not concern themselves with this question and were only interested in the causal relationship that may exist between personality factors and coronary artery atherosclerosis.

Method of Study. In 43 patients suffering from myocardial infarction who were admitted to the Temple University Hospital, beginning in the fall of 1953, an effort was made to study the personality structure and life situation in an attempt to determine the role of emotional factors in the onset, course and recovery from coronary occlusion (Weiss, et al.).

In addition to the usual physical studies and medical management the patients were interviewed by psychiatrists. The interviews were begun as soon as the patient was comfortable enough to discuss himself freely—on the average the first one took place 9 days after admission to the hospital—and varied from three to twelve in number, averaging seven per patient of about an hour each. The interviews were conducted at the bedside. Whenever possible other members of the family were also interviewed, particularly the spouse, and a great deal of helpful information was obtained in this way.

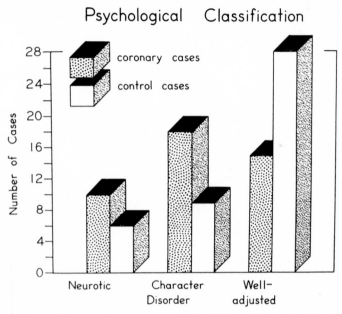

Figure 2.   Personality types in coronary occlusion. (From Weiss, E., Dlin, B., Rollin, H. R., Fischer, H. K., and Bepler, C. C.: A.M.A. Arch. Int. Med., vol. 99, 1957.)

An equal number of hospital patients matched for age, sex and race served as controls. Patients with coronary artery disease were excluded as well as those with obvious mental, nervous and psychosomatic disorders. The selection of control cases in psychosomatic investigation is always a difficult problem. For example, the high incidence of social and emotional problems in a hospital ward population is one such complicating factor. Miles et al. comment upon the problem of controls in the paper to which we have already referred, stating that "controls" are impossible to keep "controlled," and that the personality and theoretical convictions of the investigator inevitably influence the making of discriminating observations and the drawing of inferences.

We also felt that interviews were liable to be biased, especially when the diagnosis was known, so we tried to protect ourselves in this respect by weekly group conferences in which the material was reviewed and conclusions reached.

Results of Study. FAMILY HISTORY. A family history of heart disease occurred in 19 (44%) of the coronary group and 14 (32%) of the control group but psychopathology existed in the background of 20 members (46%) of the coronary group as opposed to 7 (16%) in the control group. Psychopathology refers to obvious mental or nervous illness or to evidence of pronounced emotional maladjustment.

PSYCHOLOGICAL CLASSIFICATION. The diagnosis of neurosis was established when the patient gave a history of symptoms of emotional origin that interfered with his relationship with other people or seriously impaired his capacity to work. This diagnosis was established in 10 (25%) of the coronary group as opposed to 6 (14%) in the control group (Fig. 2).

Character disorder was diagnosed when rigid and repetitive behavior interfered with the person's happiness and the security of his family.

Table 2. Psychological Stress Prior to Coronary Occlusion

	Coronary	Control
Gradually mounting tension	21	
Acute emotional stress	16	4
Anniversary reaction	4	
Anniversary reaction (suspected)	5	

From Weiss, E., Dlin, B., Rollin, H. R., Fischer, H. K., and Bepler, C. R.: A.M.A. Arch. Int. Med., *99*:628, 1957.

The neurotic character "acts out" his impulses; symptoms of emotional origin are few or absent. Eighteen (42%) of the coronary group fell into this classification and only 9 (21%) in the control group. This difference is statistically significant (P←.01).

Twenty-eight (65%) of the control group were considered well adjusted but only 15 (35%) of the coronary group.

PSYCHOLOGICAL STRESS. *Gradually Mounting Tension.* Study of the personality and life situation of patients with acute coronary occlusion compared with a control group (Table 2) showed that gradually mounting tension of emotional origin, months or years in duration, occurred prior to the onset of the occlusion in 21 (49%) of the cardiac group (Table 2). Analyzing the incidence of gradually mounting tension among the different age groups in men we find that it occurred in only 2 out of 8 (25%) over the age of 60 but in 18 out of 27 (66%) under the age of 60. The sample is too small for statistical analysis but the observation may be medically important. We found no evidence of gradually mounting tension prior to the onset of illness in the control group. In addition, 16 (37%) of the coronary group showed acute emotional stress which at least on four occasions (9%) was added to the gradually mounting tension just before the onset of the coronary occlusion. Acute emotional stress existed prior to illness in only 4 (9%) of the control group. This difference is statistically valid (P←.05).

Evidence for gradually mounting tension was not always obvious to the observer nor was it often apparent to the patient. Sometimes members of the family and especially the spouse helped us in obtaining such information. Increased smoking and drinking (which are sometimes blamed for the coronary occlusion) are often only the evidences of increasing tension of nervous origin. The same is true of irritability and suppressed anger, as well as insomnia, indecisiveness, withdrawal from social contacts, increased dependency on a spouse, obsessive thinking, preoccupation with bodily symptoms, inability to concentrate, disturbances in memory, impotence, depression and fear of insanity. An example follows:

Gradually Mounting Tension before Coronary Occlusion

A white machinist, age 43, was admitted to the hospital following an attack of coronary occlusion. He was a prematurely gray, passive and compulsive person. He had been dominated by his father, also a machinist, toward whom he had been totally submissive, and he had been betrayed by his first wife who was unfaithful to him. He took great pride in the quality of his work and, when he saw his work being destroyed as a result of the speed-up in the shop, he was filled with rage which he was unable to express. He felt himself heading for catastrophe. There were signs of mounting tension, such as increased concern about orderliness, neatness and bowel function, difficulty "getting himself going in the morning," obsessive thinking and decreased libido.

He described the events leading up to the attack as follows: "Everything had been O.K. at work until the last few weeks. Then they started a speed-up, smashing the equipment, and, because of the increased load on the machinery, as fast as we rebuilt it they smashed it again. Work used to be enjoyable but now I hated to get up in the morning. All the knocks I've had in life couldn't add up to this. The job got me down. I took my work home with me. Something had to happen. This [pointing to his heart] is the result. I couldn't talk to my family about it but I'm glad to get it off my chest."

No other precipitating factors could be demonstrated. There was no evidence of cardiovascular disease in the family history, no obesity, no hypertension or angina and no hypercholesteremia.

The patient appeared to profit from his interviews and made an uninterupted recovery from an acute anteroseptal infarction.

*Anniversary Reaction.** We have been impressed by the fact that the attack of coronary occlusion sometimes seems to occur on the anniversary of a significant event in the life of the patient. This is usually the death of some key figure with whom the patient had established a complex identification in which hostility is usually noted. The patient may be completely unaware of the circumstances and only when his attention is called to the fact does he recall the anniversary or the tension associated with it. In 4 (9%) of our cases of coronary occlusion this seemed to be true and in 5 others (12%) it seemed a likely possibility although we could not get enough confirmatory evidence to feel certain about it. There were no such cases among the controls (Table 2). We refer to this phenomenon as the anniversary reaction but we do not suggest that it is limited to coronary occlusion because it also occurs throughout the whole field of emotional disorders and psychophysiological reactions.

A story such as this is often obtained. A man approaching his 54th birthday, whose father died at 54 of heart disease, will show increasing

* Ferenczi credits Freud with the concept of the anniversary reaction. Hilgard used the term in relation to mental illness and Bressler in relation to ulcerative colitis.

evidence of tension, as previously described, and then in response to what seems to be an insignificant event or circumstance will suffer a coronary attack. When queried about any concern or worry prior to the attack he will deny it or refer only to the fact that he had been "overworked." He does not realize the significance of the anniversary of his father's death in regard to his own gradually mounting tension. The psychopathology is usually that of a hostile identification with the dead father. Perhaps the patient has had mixed feelings of respect and devotion but also fear and hostility toward a tyrannical father. He is bur-

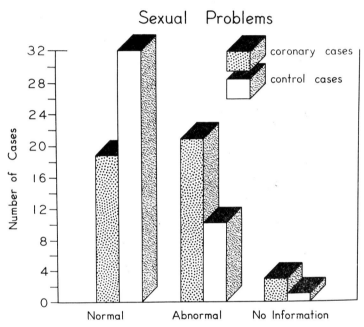

Figure 3.   Incidence of sexual problems in coronary occlusion. (From Weiss et al.: A.M.A. Arch. Int. Med., vol. 99, 1957.)

dened by guilt because of hostile feelings which may be wholly unconscious. He begins to believe that he too may die as the father did, and when he approaches the age at which his father died tension increases.

Sexual Problems.   The coronary age is also the age of diminishing potency. Sexual problems creating tension occur, especially among men. Since men are so much more likely to have coronary artery disease than women these tensions are of particular significance. In 21 (49%) of our cases there were important sexual problems and 18 (42%) of these occurred in men (Figs. 3 and 4). Loss of libido, premature ejaculation, a feeling of "growing old," or the "change of life," preoccupation with the idea of "loss of manhood," and compensatory efforts to prove oneself still a vigorous man (a frequent source of "stress and strain") are some of the problems that afflict men of this age. As previously mentioned in our discussion of evidences of gradually mounting tension, this is just another piece of evidence but one which is apt to be of greater concern and therefore in itself productive of more tension.

Sexual problems occurred more commonly in the coronary group than in the control group, 21 (49%) as opposed to 10 (23%). This is statistically significant (P←.05).

REACTION TO ILLNESS.   Because of the special significance of the heart the reactions to "heart attacks" are often unusual (Table 3). We

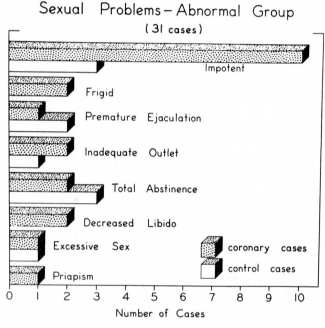

Figure 4.   Types of sexual problems in coronary occlusion. (From Weiss et al.: A.M.A. Arch. Int. Med., vol. 99, 1957.)

judged the reaction as normal when the well adjusted personality re-acted with concern and mood changes which, however, gradually disappeared as healing occurred. In 26 (65%) of the known reactions to illness* in our control cases it was regarded as normal or well adjusted but in only 11 (37%) of our coronary cases did we judge the reaction to be normal.

Denial of Illness.   Denial of illness of varying degree is apt to occur under many circumstances. It is extremely common in malignant disease, but it has special significance when it occurs in heart disease. Chambers and Reiser pointed out that it may have serious implications for the patient with heart disease. It may lead to self-destructive be-havior, such as the refusal to accept orders, "forgetting" to take medicine, and pronounced depression. Rigid enforcement of restriction in such

* Since the reaction to illness was not determined in 12 of the coronary cases and in 3 of the controls percentages will differ in this section.

patients may cause additional anxiety. They noted that the psychologic need to deny illness was often of such great intensity that it was actually less harmful to permit some activity than it was to impose the degree of inactivity which seemed indicated on the basis of physical considerations alone. In several of their cases it appeared clear that a permissive attitude toward the defense of denial was the best way to manage the patient. This has also been our experience in patients with coronary occlusion.

Incidentally, this points up an interesting observation regarding "clinically important" as opposed to "statistically significant." Eight (20%) of our control cases showed the phenomenon of denial whereas it occurred in only 6 (20%) of the known reactions in the coronary group and yet we felt that denial was more important in the cardiac group, for the reasons stated above, than in the control group where it was so often associated with the presence of malignant disease (6 out of 8 cases). Judging the matter only from a statistical standpoint might

Table 3.   Reaction to Illness Following Coronary Occlusion

	Coronary	Control
Normal	11	26
Denial	6	8
Depression	7	1
Regression	2	1
Mixed reaction	4	4
Died	1	0
No information	12	3

From Weiss et al.: A.M.A. Arch. Int. Med., *99*:628, 1957.

lead to a dismissal of the importance of denial in the cardiac group if clinical experience is not taken into consideration (Starr).

Depression.   Depression is a reactive mood disturbance often accompanied by hypochondriacal concern regarding the heart. It occurred in 7 (23%) of our cases as opposed to only 1 (2%) in the control group. It has special significance because it can easily be overlooked by the physician who is only concerned about the physical aspects of the heart disease. On the other hand it can be pronounced enough to mask heart symptoms and thus endanger the patient as well as pose a threat to the psychiatrist (Robertson).

Regression.   Regression is a phenomenon that may lead to psychological invalidism with hypochondriacal obsession concerning heart symptoms. Passive and dependent character traits are exaggerated and the patient may become an invalid, perhaps subsisting on insurance benefits. It occurred in 2 (7%) of the coronary group and in 1 (2%) of the controls.

The personality and training of the physician are important in regard to the above considerations because by encouraging denial or regression he may add to the patient's problem instead of helping him.

Tension During Rest.   Because coronary occlusion occurs so commonly at rest or during sleep it is assumed that "such patients could not be under strain." It may be quite true that hypodynamic factors are responsible but it must not be forgotten that tensions also occur during sleep. Grinding of teeth (bruxism) and nightmares are indications of the anxieties that give rise to tension during sleep. Bond called attention to this in recounting the dreams of patients who suffered coronary occlusion during the night. Physical rest is not synonymous with peace of mind; patients may be told to rest (or physical rest may be enforced) and yet they "stew in their own juices," creating tensions that can disturb the circulation.

THE "CORONARY PERSONALITY."   Miles et al. did not find an increased incidence of psychopathology in their coronary group as we did. However, they comment that since their study took place with an average interval of 5.6 years after the attack of myocardial infarction it was difficult to evaluate the kind of life situation associated with the acute attacks or to estimate the degree of anxiety and depression that had existed immediately after the attack. Nevertheless, they did feel that their coronary patients tended to utilize repression to a notably greater degree than the controls.

While our study was not designed to throw light on the question of the existence of a "coronary personality," an analysis of our material did not yield evidence pointing in this direction. Comparing their study with Dunbar's, Miles et al. raise the question as to the higher percentage of Jews in her study (59% compared with 35% in their group), suggesting that the features which she attributed to the "coronary personality" were really personality characteristics influenced by such cultural factors as family emphasis on education, ascent in the social scale and material success.

The percentage of Jews (35%) in our coronary group was the same as in the Miles study. Moreover, so far as the question of emotional factors preceding coronary occlusion is concerned, gradually mounting tension was just as common among Protestants and Catholics as among Jews. There were 9 Protestants with gradually mounting tension (60% of the Protestant group), 4 Catholics (66% of the Catholic group) and 8 Jews (57% of the Jewish group).

IATROGENIC FACTOR.   One of the most important and most difficult subjects in clinical medicine is the problem of anxiety and the heart. Many of the complicated problems that arise after coronary occlusion are of emotional origin and can only be understood when approached from that standpoint. Unfortunately the iatrogenic factor often adds to the problem through too much caution regarding physical exertion and inadequate attention to emotional factors. Many of the difficulties undoubtedly arise from the abuse of bed rest and precautions regarding activity and work. An anxious person with the symptoms of cardiac neurosis but with a normal heart can often be reassured and told to go about his business; an anxious person with a diseased heart cannot, but when he is told to rest and surrounded with other precautions he often becomes an invalid, more from the fear of heart disease than from the actual disease. Moreover, it seems to us that tensions of emotional origin can be as burdensome to the cardiovascular system as effort of physical origin, so that for both reasons one has to try to reduce anxiety in order to make such patients useful citizens again, within the capacity of their cardiovascular systems. Now and again such patients develop coronary occlusion or a cerebral vascular accident and the physician may be criticized for overlooking or giving insufficient attention to the organic disease.

Strangely enough, cardiac neurosis prior to coronary occlusion seems to be uncommon from our studies but when it does happen it can be very hard on a medical reputation. The physician attempts to reassure the patient by excluding organic heart disease and blaming the symptoms on emotional factors. Then if the patient develops coronary occlusion, no matter how long afterward, neither he nor his family easily forgives the physician who had said that "the heart was normal."

This poses a difficult question because the problems of psychosomatic relationships in cardiovascular disease may be very complicated, and depend as much upon an analysis of personality structure as upon an evaluation of the cardiovascular disease. Therefore, one has to try to determine the degree of psychological impairment as carefully as the degree of organic heart damage and judgment must be based on both. All of this means that the physician must understand the personality as well as the heart. Both have a structure that can be analyzed from a prognostic standpoint.

Surgery of the Heart

The newer developments in surgery of the heart have brought to light occasional serious psychological reactions such as depression and suicide. Fox and his associates at the Harvard Medical School made a psychiatric study of 32 patients undergoing heart surgery for mitral valvular disease. The prolonged adaptation to a disabling disease followed by the hope of surgical cure but also by the chance of sudden death produces reactions that often necessitate psychiatric observation.

Preoperative study gave some information concerning the nature of the patient's psychological defenses but it did not enable the observers to make accurate predictions concerning the patient's postoperative course. The development of unexpected postoperative complications sometimes brought out anxieties in patients who had shown no disturbance preoperatively or postoperatively up to that time. However, 6 of the patients had obvious emotional disturbances following the operation and since they had been seen preoperatively, emergency treatment was found to be more effective than in patients who had not been studied before operation. In some instances stress was so severe that the patients seemed virtually defenseless and were close to panic. In others the psychological defenses were inadequate and unsuccessful to such an extent that the patient bordered on psychosis. Psychological preparation for surgery remains an indispensable aspect of treatment.

In a review of the clinical records of 37 adult patients who had undergone mitral surgery, Bliss and associates found that 2 patients developed schizophrenic reactions after surgery and 2 others appeared to have experienced short-lived schizophrenic reactions. Six patients, although not psychotic, were anxious and depressed.

Kaplan studied 18 patients who had experienced mitral commissurotomy. He emphasized the fact that often the heart disorder became an important focal point in the personality of the individual and afforded gratification for dependency needs. Therefore, many of these patients felt threatened by any recovery from their illness, as this meant that they would be expected to adopt a more independent role in life. This was especially true of many women in the group who showed considerable anxiety over the necessity of accepting a mature feminine role. Sometimes patients developed new symptoms after the operation. One patient became psychotic and two others had mild psychotic symptoms.

In general it was found that the patient's reaction depended upon such factors as his premorbid personality structure, the degree of physical incapacity, the abruptness of onset, severity and duration of illness, and the relationship to the family and attending physician. "Poor reactions to the operation occurred so often that psychological evaluation seemed indicated in every instance where the operation is to be performed."

A fascinating personal account of thoughts and feelings while undergoing heart surgery has been described by a trained psychological observer in a book entitled "Straight to the Heart." George Lawton, a clinical psychologist who practices psychoanalysis, underwent a successful operation at the age of 54 and both he and his wife comment on the extraordinary changes that followed successful surgery.

Both urge that psychiatric consultation should accompany cardiac surgery.

Psychosis in Cardiac Disease

In order to complete our consideration of emotions and heart disease we ought to discuss the frank psychoses, of exhaustive or toxic nature, which occasionally accompany grave heart disease. This phase of the subject, however, is well treated in many textbooks of medicine and cardiology. Other than to say that the psychosis sometimes occurs very insidiously and that the form which it assumes depends upon the underlying personality of the individual we will deal no further with this subject. *One must be aware of the fact, however, that just as the emotions may influence the working of the heart so may advanced disease of the heart aggravate or precipitate emotional disorders.*

Case 10.   Coronary Occlusion Preceded by Psychic Trauma

History and Symptoms.   A middle-aged Italian woman developed coronary occlusion while a patient in the hospital. She had been a diabetic for many years. Her husband had had very little work for several months preceding her admission to the hospital and she could not afford the special food that she needed. She developed palpitation and finally asked the physician who had taken care of her for many years to send her into the hospital. He reported that "there was too much red tape and that she wouldn't like it— that she would come out and curse him for sending her." Finally she entered the hospital on her own initiative. She was told that it would take a few days to standardize her but this was not accomplished until the tenth day. She then prepared to go home.

A few days before, she had witnessed general ward rounds and had been very much upset by the demonstration of patients to a group of physicians and students. She told the nurse and interns that it must not happen to her. However, on the particular day in question she was resting in the sun parlor preparatory to going home when the nurse came for her and asked her to come into the ward. She said immediately, "What is it, class?" The nurse said "Yes," and the patient became very nervous and angry. She told the nurse it would be impossible, that "she would get sick—she knew what her heart could stand," but the nurse persuaded her to return to the ward. As she approached the ward she felt a pressing pain under the sternum, which she described as a "lump," and again she remonstrated with the intern as she entered the door. She was so upset that when the attending physician, who had known nothing about her feelings, asked her several questions, she found the strength of voice to answer only two and then could talk no more. She said, "I could not remember what happened after that." Then she added significantly, "I am like a child. If I am disappointed, it breaks my heart." When the class left she went into the bathroom thinking that she might be able to cry and that this would relieve her. She was unable to cry, came back to the ward, but finally "cried

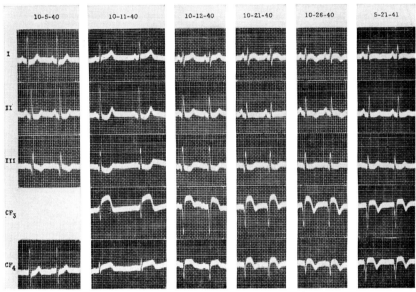

Figure 5. (Case 10).   Electrocardiographic tracings showing findings prior to coronary occlusion and serial studies following the occlusion.

her eyes out." As she did so the pain became sharper. She called for the nurse and insisted upon having the intern. Then she urged that her own physician be called and she reported that she was very sick "and was going to die." The intern later reported that she was having an "hysterical attack," saying that the patient had been one of the most difficult personalities that he had ever handled in any ward work. Nevertheless an electrocardiogram was ordered. It showed coronary occlusion! It is probably significant that everybody, from that point on, remarked how docile she had become. The patient made an excellent recovery. Serial electrocardiograms before and after the coronary occlusion are shown in Figure 5.

LIFE SITUATION

The patient was born and brought up in Italy in a peasant family with ten children. She had worked very hard but considered herself healthy. She married at 19 and very shortly afterward had a miscarriage. The following year she came to America. At 21 she had a pelvic operation and both ovaries were removed so that a surgical menopause ensued. She resigned herself to not having children and her husband "did not care." At times she spoke about bringing some children over from Italy but he said, "No, if we can't have our own, we won't have any." Her husband had been very good to her and they had led a quiet life in America. He had been employed as a laborer and always made a satisfactory living up until the few months prior to hospital admission, when work was scarce and their income was much reduced.

She was a meticulously clean housekeeper and could not tolerate dirt or disorder. She was very religious and had gone to church every day. During the last three or four years she had felt herself becoming quite nervous. She was always fearful that auto accidents might occur because they lived near a large boulevard where accidents were frequent. She could not stand to see people hurt. Two years before she had a bad fright when a burglar attempted to enter a house across the street during the night. She felt it "as a shock in the heart" and was paralyzed with fear. She went back to bed without waking her husband and "shook all night." Since then she had not felt right and her physician said that diabetes "was due to the shock."

SUMMARY

A middle-aged, neurotic and diabetic female felt humiliated and enraged by being presented to a class of students. Substernal pain developed which was thought to be part of an "hysterical attack" but the electrocardiogram showed coronary occlusion. Recovery occurred.

Case 11. Recurrent Congestive Heart Failure; Social and Psychological Problems

History and Symptoms. The patient, a woman of middle age, had been in Temple University Hospital on some twenty occasions over the past six or eight years.

She was a large, florid woman of Irish extraction who had mild diabetes and slight elevation of blood pressure and suffered from repeated attacks of heart failure. The attacks occurred in the following fashion. The patient became nauseated and vomited; then her body began to swell, and shortness of breath increased until hospitalization became necessary. In the hospital the time-honored remedies—morphine and oxygen, digitalis and mercury—proved effective, and in a short time the patient was much better. She got rid of about 20 or 30 pounds of fluid in a week or two, in the manner of a sponge that has been squeezed. She felt quite well again, went home, and the process was repeated. Within a few weeks or a month or two she was back in the hospital.

The reasons why this patient was so "refractory" to treatment were the subject of much discussion in our hospital. Why did she refuse to get well and stay well? In a medical conference her case was presented and discussed from the standpoint of determining the various factors that might be responsible for the frequent heart failure. The possibility of electrolyte imbalance, of hypermetabolism, of polycythemia or other complicating disease was discussed, but nothing was said about this patient as a person. Did her personal life have anything to do with the illness?

LIFE SITUATION

The patient lived with an only daughter in a tiny apartment near the Hospital. The daughter worked at one of the big plants in North Philadelphia. On the daughter's take-home pay of $41.00 per week the two had to live, and insulin, digitalis and special food had to be bought for the mother. The mother stated that since the money was insufficient to cover all the expenses, she ran out of medicine, became ill and was hospitalized. Although this appeared to be a fairly plausible explanation, like so many situations in life that seem so readily explained, if one probes a little bit deeper one will find that there is more to the story.

The patient confessed that often, just before she broke down, she had had a fight with her daughter. She became upset, "fed up" and started to "throw up" as though to say, "I can't tolerate this situation." Thus an attack was initiated. Now why did the patient fight with her daughter? Further inquiry revealed that it was the daughter who started the fights with the mother. The daughter, a single girl in her late twenties, was thinking, and sometimes said, "I have to sacrifice everything for you; you are a millstone around my neck. If I didn't have to spend my hard-earned money on you I could have clothes; I could have boy friends; I could go out and do the things that other girls do. But I promised Granny (the patient's mother) on her deathbed that I'd take care of you, and I intend to do it."

Thus we find that this patient lived in an atmosphere of considering herself a burden to her daughter, and felt that her life depended upon a deathbed promise. She was resentful but guilty, and, frequently, when she left the hospital feeling fairly well, she went home and kept herself busy doing things around the house to please her daughter. She prepared dishes that the daughter liked, cleaned the house, and performed other chores that she ought not to have done. Soon she was back in the hospital again.

There were many other aspects of this problem. For example, it was noted that these fights occurred just before the daughter's menstrual periods. The daughter had dysmenorrhea and suffered from premenstrual tension, becoming irritable and difficult just before her period. It was at this time that she was apt to fight with her mother and say the harsh things which she later regretted, but then it was too late—the mother was in the hospital. Therefore there was a somatopsychic as well as a psychosomatic problem. In other words, the endocrine balance of the daughter had to be taken into consideration in this involved medicosocial problem.

However, quite by chance we discovered an important psychological factor. The daughter was illegitimate and this was the source of much of her resentment and, of course, much of the mother's guilt.

FINAL ADMISSION

The final admission was in February, 1955, when death occurred. Autopsy demonstrated a large heart, weighing 600 grams, with hypertrophy of both the left and the right ventricles. This suggested pulmonary as well as systemic hypertension. There was pulmonary artery atherosclerosis. Nothing else of importance was found.

SUMMARY

An obese woman, with mild diabetes, had repeated admissions to the hospital because of congestive heart failure. Autopsy demonstrated evidence pointing to pulmonary as well as systemic hypertension but important social and psychological factors seemed to precipitate the repeated attacks of heart failure.

References

Arlow, J. A.: Psychosom. Med., 7: 195, 1945.
Bishop, L. F., and Bishop, L. F., Jr.: Am. J. M. Sc., 182: 19, 1931.
Bliss, E. L., Rumel, W. R., and Branch, C. H. H.: Arch. Neurol. & Psychiat., 74: 249, 1955.
Bond, D. D.: Postgrad. Med., 13: 487, 1953.
Bressler, B.: Psychoanal. Rev., 43:381, 1956.
Cathcart, J. P. S.: Personal Communication, 1953.
Chambers, W., and Reiser, M. F.: Psychosom. Med., 15: 38, 1953.
Cohen, M. E.: Proceedings, First National Conference on Cardiovascular Diseases. New York Heart Association, 1950.
Cohen, M. E., and White, P. D.: Psychosom. Med., 8: 335, 1951.
Conner, L. A.: J.A.M.A., 94: 447, 1930.
Crede, R. H., Chivers, N. C., and Shapiro, A. P.: Psychosom. Med., 13: 277, 1951.
DaCosta, J. M.: Am. J. M. Sc., 61: 17, 1871.
Dunbar, F.: (a) Emotions and Bodily Changes. 2nd ed., p. 210. Columbia University Press, N. Y., 1938; (b) New York State J. Med., 36: 1, 1936.
Dunbar, F.: Psychosomatic Diagnosis. Paul B. Hoeber, Inc., New York, 1943.
Ferenczi, S.: Further Contributions to the Theory and Technique of Psycho-analysis. Hogarth Press, London, 1950, p. 174.
Fox, H., Rizzo, N., and Gifford, S.: Psychosom. Med., 16: 186, 1954.
Freud, S.: Collected Papers. Vol. I, p. 76. Internat. Psychoan. Press, New York, 1924.
Friedman, M.: Functional Cardiovascular Disease. Williams and Wilkins Co., Baltimore, 1947, pp. 24, 51.
Gertler, M. M., Garn, S. M., and White, P. D.: Coronary Heart Disease in Young Adults. Harvard University Press for Commonwealth Fund, Cambridge, Mass., 1954.
Grollman, A.: Am. J. Physiol., 89: 584, 1929.
Hamman, L., and Wainwright, C. W.: Bull. Johns Hopkins Hosp., 58: 109 and 307, 1936.
Harrison, T. R.: Am. Assoc. Advancement Sc., Pub. 13, p. 231, 1940.
Harrison, T. R.: Am. J. M. Sc., 207: 561, 1944.

Hart, A. D.: J.A.M.A., *156:* 1133, 1954.
Hilgard, J. R.: Psychiatry, *16:* 73, 1953.
Jarvinen, K. A. J.: Brit. M. J., *1:* 318, 1955.
Kaplan, S. M.: Psychosom. Med., *18:* 221, 1956.
Keys, A.: Mod. Concepts Cardiovas. Dis., *25:* 317, 1956.
Kilgore, E. S.: (*a*) J.A.M.A., *117:* 258, 1941; (*b*) Am. Heart J., *5:* 9, 1929.
Lawton, G.: Straight to the Heart. International Universities Press, New York, 1956.
Mainzer, F., and Krause, M.: Brit. Heart., *2:* 221, 1940.
Margolin, S.: Presented before the Psychosomatic Forum, New York, 1950.
Master, A. M.: J.A.M.A., *150:* 195, 1952.
Master, A. M., and Jaffe, H. L.: J.A.M.A., *148:* 794, 1952.
Menninger, W. C.: Southwest. J. Med. and Surg., *21:* 281 and 324, 1937.
Miles, H. H. W., and Cobb, S.: New England J. Med., *245:* 711, 1951.
Miles, H. H. W., Waldfogel, S., Barrabee, E. L., and Cobb, S.: Psychosom. Med., *16:* 455, 1954.
Oille, J. A.: Canad. M.A.J., *45:* 1, 1941.
Oppenheimer, B. S., and others: Mil. Surgeon, *42:* 409, 1918.
Robertson, S. H.: Ann. Int. Med., *41:* 209, 1954.
Ross, W. Donald: Psychosom. Med., *7:* 80, 1945.
Schneider, R. A., and Zangari, V. M.: Psychosom. Med., *13:* 289, 1951.
Starr, I.: J.A.M.A., *160:* 672, 1956.
Stead, E. A., Jr., Warren, J. V., Merrill, A. J., and Brannon, E. S.: J. Clin. Invest., *24:* 326, 1945.
Van Balen, G. F.: Nederl. tijdschr. v. geneesk., *97:* 2074, 1954.
Walker, W. J.: Am. Heart J., *42:* 97, 1951.
Weiss, E.: Psychosom. Med., *14:* 150, 1952.
Weiss, E., Dlin, B., Rollin, H. R., Fischer, H. K., and Bepler, C. R.: A.M.A. Arch. Int. Med., *99:* 628, 1957.
Wendkos, M. H.: Am. Heart J., *28:* 549, 1944.
Wheeler, E. O., White, P. D., Reed, E. W., and Cohen, M. E.: J.A.M.A., *142:* 878, 1950.
Willius, F. A.: Proc. Staff Meet., Mayo Clinic, *13:* 11, 1938.
Wittkower, E., Rodger, T. F., and Wilson, A. T. M.: Lancet, *1:* 531, 1951.
Wolf, G. A., Jr., and Wolff, H. G.: Psychosom. Med., *8:* 293, 1946.
Wolfe, T. P.: Am. J. Psychiat., *93:* 681, 1936.

Chapter VII

The Cardiovascular System—
Essential Hypertension

There is little need to emphasize the importance of hypertension. According to the statistics of the Metropolitan Life Insurance Company every other individual in the United States past the age of 50 years dies of cardiovascular-renal disease. From other sources we have evidence that probably half of these deaths are due to essential hypertension; that is, almost one quarter of all people past the age of 50 years die of the effects of hypertension in one or another of the vital organs. Thus essential hypertension becomes the gravest problem of middle adult life, not even excepting cancer. The hypertension arises from arteriolar vasospasm (whatever its cause may be) and after it has continued for years a compensatory reaction in the arterial system results in a diffuse hyperplastic vascular sclerosis which, in conjunction with atherosclerosis, is eventually responsible for failure of such vital organs as heart, brain and kidney.

Our knowledge of the circulatory disorders has progressed in hundred-year cycles. It was about 1633 that William Harvey reported on the nature of the circulation and about 1733 that Stephen Hales, an English pastor, demonstrated the phenomenon of blood pressure in the horse. In 1833 Richard Bright correctly concluded that an increase in the peripheral resistance caused enlargement of the heart in patients with "chronic granulations of the kidneys," and about 1933 Goldblatt, by his brilliant researches, first produced in the experimental animal a form of hypertension which corresponds to essential hypertension in man.

According to Pickering hypertension is not a disease entity but a physical sign that may or may not indicate a pathological process. He describes it as merely one end of the distribution curve of observed blood pressure. It is based on an arbitrary dividing line between what is normal and what is alleged to be abnormal. He would define essential hypertension patients as that group of the population with arterial pressures exceeding a certain value arbitrarily selected and in whom no specific cause can be detected to account for the high pressure. He believes that the factors causing it are factors operating generally on the

Page 225

population. Of these factors, contributions of age, sex and inheritance can be defined approximately. The influence of environmental factors, which would seem by exclusion to be of great importance, remains to be explored.

Psyche and Hypertension.   It is generally admitted that psychic factors play an important part in essential hypertension. For example, it is always emphasized that we must allow for the emotional element in individual blood pressure readings. Also well known is the large part that rest and reassurance play in the medical management of hypertensive patients, both in relief of symptoms and in reduction of the blood pressure level. The early symptoms of hypertension are often exactly those of a *psychoneurosis,* and the relationship of emotional stress to the onset of hypertension and to the anxiety which is frequently responsible for the aggravation of existing hypertension is well known. Personality study of the hypertensive patient often reveals a deep-seated conflict which stands in close relationship to anxiety. This will be discussed in greater detail in the section on treatment of essential hypertension (p. 235). Therefore, it may be said that in spite of the organic nature of experimental hypertension, the psyche is not absolved as a factor in the etiology of hypertension in man. It is conceivable that a disturbance in the circulatory function of the kidneys could have its origin in impulses of central nervous origin.

The psychic factor thus becomes one of the multiple factors which enter into the pathogenesis of hypertension. An analogy might be drawn to the role of the kidney or the endocrine glands, either of which, in rare instances, may be chiefly responsible for the presence of hypertension but in most instances seems to play a secondary role, depending upon a constitutional or inherent tendency. "The psychologic factor is only one phase, although an important phase, in the composite of the degree and kind of renal, endocrine, and nervous participation" (Corcoran and Page).

In a study of 80 undergraduate college women, 40 of whom had blood pressure of 140/90 or over at the matriculation physical examination, and 40 of whom had normal blood pressures, Harris, Sokolow and their associates utilized psychiatric interviews and stress-provoking psychodramas in order to discover whether these techniques could differentiate the two groups. By personality study, it was possible to differentiate the prehypertensives from the controls in 69 per cent of the cases. In the stressful situation, the prehypertensives behaved less effectively, were less well controlled, less poised, and created a less favorable impression than the controls. The validity of these interpretations was reinforced by the agreement between observers' descriptions and the subjects' own self-appraisal.

These studies suggest to the authors that the prehypertensives are less able than normal persons to handle stressful or frustrating situations without becoming emotionally upset, and that they are therefore more likely to be subject to the autonomic accompaniments of emotion including repetitive rises in blood pressure. "It may be that such repetitive rises in blood pressure are part of the conditions leading to fixed hypertension."

In further studies of 14 hypertensive and 22 normotensive women Kalis, working with the same group, found that the responses of hypertensive women were more extreme—they were either more explosive or more submissive—than those of normotensive women. These authors agree that the personality characteristics present before the onset are relevant to the development of hypertension.

The Family History. Using medical students as subjects, Caroline Thomas has analyzed their family histories in regard to hypertension and related disorders and has also determined the incidence of certain circulatory, metabolic and psychological characteristics in the subjects themselves. In an analysis of 84 subjects with a history of hypertension in one or both parents compared with findings in 100 subjects whose parents were free from hypertension, she finds that circulatory lability is more prevalent in the offspring of hypertensive than of nonhypertensive parents. The heart as well as the blood pressure frequently participated in the pattern of lability. The percentage of subjects showing circulatory lability is higher than the incidence of hypertension in the parents' generation, suggesting that additional factors are necessary for the appearance of hypertension. Preliminary genetic analysis indicated that hypertension bears an etiological relationship to coronary artery disease, and that the same heritage is expressed more often as hypertension in females and as coronary artery disease in males. While in some respects hypertension behaves like a single recessive gene widely distributed in the population, it seems probable that a more complex genetic pattern is involved.

Experimental Observations of Renal Blood Flow During Stress. The blood flow in the kidney of the subject with essential hypertension is small in terms of functioning kidney tubular mass, that is to say, the hypertensive kidney is relatively ischemic as compared to the normal. Also, the degree of depression of renal blood flow parallels approximately the duration and severity of the hypertension. The order in which events proceed is indicated by the fact that the glomerular filtration rate in early hypertension is entirely within normal limits, but with advanced hypertension and reduction in the number of functioning glomeruli, the glomerular filtration rate is also gradually depressed. As the hypertension advances, the tubular mass decreases but always in such a manner that the renal blood flow is poor in terms of the existing tubular mass. These facts suggest that a defective renal blood flow precedes the onset of faulty excretory function. If kidney ischemia be at all relevant to the occurrence of arterial hypertension, renal blood flow studies in those with widespread vascular reaction to threats become of interest.

Pfeiffer and Wolff spoke of their investigation of the renal hemodynamics in subjects with essential hypertension, during a rise in blood pressure initiated by threats in the form of discussion of topics known to have a significant relationship to the personality structure. In 18 of

35 subjects with hypertension, without evidence of renal disease or abnormality of renal function as indicated by the usual clinical tests, renal
blood flow and glomerular filtration rate were ascertained.

Rises in diastolic and systolic blood pressure were induced by discussion of topics of personal significance, usually having to do with family
interpersonal relations, without, at the same time, inducing outward
evidence of strong emotional reaction. The rise in blood pressure under
such circumstances was accompanied by renal vasoconstriction which
was either proportional to that of the body as a whole or more intense
than necessary to compensate for the rise, reflected by decreases in renal
plasma flow of 17 to 25 per cent of control level. The increase of renal
vasoconstriction was located principally in efferent glomerular arterioles
although both efferent and afferent arteriolar constriction occurred. Fall
in blood pressure during induced feelings of security was accompanied
by vasodilation of the efferent and afferent arterioles.

"From these and other facts, it may be inferred that the kidney in
persons with arterial hypertension exhibits an abnormal vascular pattern,
characterized by increased arteriolar tone, and the latter may be further
increased by threats or assaults that evoke protective reactions of a
pressor nature."

A group of hypertensive patients were studied by Stevenson and
associates from the viewpoint of their personalities and responses to
stressful life situations in correlation with symptoms and measurements
of circulatory function.

The exercise tolerance test during relaxation in both hypertensive
and normal controls produced a slight elevation of mean blood pressure
and slight lowering of peripheral resistance. Following the discussion of
stressful life situations both groups showed an increase in cardiac output,
rise in blood pressure and fall in peripheral resistance. The hypertensive
patients manifested a greater rise in blood pressure, especially when the
reaction was characterized by restraint and resentment, indicating a
greater vasoconstrictor response in this group. The effect upon renal
hemodynamics was to lower renal blood flow and glomerular filtration
during the period of blood pressure elevation, presumably because of
constriction of the efferent glomerular arteriole. In sympathectomized
hypertensive patients, the response to stressful interviews was modified
but not profoundly affected. When the reaction to the interview was
one of defeat and resignation, a hypotensive response was sometimes
observed. However, in general, it may be stated that the hypertensive
displays a greater vasoconstrictor response to stress than does the normotensive.

Summary of Pathogenesis. A consideration of the material just
presented indicates that hypertension is a constitutional disorder in
which both hereditary and environmental (vasospastic) factors are important. Thus it would seem that normal vasomotor activity is superimposed upon intrinsic vascular hypertonus which is maintained
independently of the vasomotor nerves. In other words, we may assume
that there is an inherent vascular hypertonus fundamentally responsible
for increased peripheral resistance in essential hypertension to which

may be added vasoconstriction of nervous origin. Nevertheless, it must be acknowledged that the latter may constitute a considerable fraction of the peripheral resistance in persistent hypertension.

In an attempt to assign a proper relationship to the three systems of the body and to the various factors that play a part in the pathogenesis of hypertension a scheme has been constructed as shown in the accompanying diagram (Fig. 6). This makes an effort to indicate the relative importance of constitutional and hereditary factors (which make up the base of the pyramid) with regard to the interrelated systems of the body that have to do with hypertension—shown as the sides of the

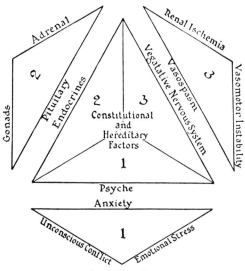

Figure 6.   Diagram to summarize discussion of pathogenesis. The base of the pyramid is made up of constitutional and hereditary factors; the sides consist of interrelated systems which are shown separately as triangles with their sides representing interrelated factors. (From E. Weiss: Psychosomatic Medicine, 1939, Vol. I, p. 183.)

pyramid. These systems are then shown as triangles with the sides of the triangles representing interrelated factors.

It is probable that the constitutional and hereditary factor in essential hypertension is responsible for the inherent vascular hypertonus previously discussed and that environmental influences produce the vasospastic factors which act as precipitating agents. Thus if one were born with a marked predisposition it would probably take little environmental stress to cause hypertension, whereas if the family history were relatively free and one were born with little predisposition then it would probably take a considerable degree of environmental stress to bring about hypertension. In this way we can assume two interacting processes with the environmental stress mediated by way of the vasomotor system.

CLINICAL PICTURE

It is well known that hypertension may exist for a long period without any symptoms whatever. When symptoms finally appear, they frequently arise from the organ or system that is bearing the brunt of the hypertensive-vascular disease process. Thus, the symptoms may be related entirely to the heart, or neurologic symptoms may predominate if the brain is chiefly affected. In terminal stages evidences of renal failure may dominate the clinical picture. However, as previously stated, many of the early symptoms are identical with those that are seen in psychoneurosis. Headache, dizziness, tinnitus, insomnia and fatigue are prominent symptoms and often are out of proportion to the amount of physical disease that is present.

The Problem in Medical Practice.   The problem often met in practice is as follows: An individual of middle age applies for life insurance and high blood pressure and perhaps albuminuria are discovered. Insurance is refused, and, frightened or angry, the applicant seeks the advice of his physician. General physical examination with special attention to the cardiovascular system, particularly in respect to the size of the heart, the condition of the peripheral vessels, including those of the retina, plus tests of kidney function,* will enable one to establish a diagnosis in the majority of instances. Tests to rule out pheochromocytoma should be done routinely. The problem resolves itself, with certain very unusual exceptions, into the differentiation of glomerulonephritis from hypertensive-vascular disease. Usually, it will be found that the patient is suffering from essential hypertension and the end result, perhaps five to ten years away, will be cardiac failure in about 50 per cent, intracranial accident (hemorrhage or thrombosis) in about 25 to 35 per cent and renal failure in probably less than 10 per cent. Other accidents and incidental infections account for the remainder of deaths.

If the end result is to be renal failure, the patient, usually over a period of years, will show gradual loss of concentrating power as determined by specific gravity tests of kidney function. The final event, renal failure ending in uremia, will be indicated by the onset of retinitis and progressive nitrogen retention. This change may come about with considerable rapidity; that is, patients who present the usual clinical picture of benign hypertension may quite suddenly complain of severe headaches, show a higher level of blood pressure, especially the diastolic element, increased eye signs (the result of actual retinitis), loss of renal concentrating power, nonprotein nitrogen retention and rapid progression to death. This acceleration of the hypertensive process has been called by Fishberg the malignant phase of essential hypertension.

Psychosomatic Symptoms

Ayman and Pratt showed that many of the symptoms of patients with essential hypertension closely resemble those seen in patients with psychoneurosis without hypertension. Closer study of their patients revealed that they really were suffering from psychoneurosis as well as hypertension. In a later paper Ayman divided the symptoms of essential hypertension into three groups:

* Concentration tests, urea clearance and intravenous urography are commonly performed. Unfortunately, there are no simple methods available for testing the circulatory function of the kidneys.

1. Psychoneurotic symptoms
2. Vasospastic symptoms
3. Organic symptoms

Headache and various forms of head discomforts, dizziness and constipation, as well as precordial pain, breathlessness of the sighing respiration variety, and fatigue often cannot be explained directly on the basis of the hypertension. They are out of proportion to the disease. When such patients are studied from a psychosomatic point of view it is often found that there is a great deal of conflict in their make-up and an inability to express their aggression directly, and thus it would seem that tensions which cannot be adequately expressed in words or action seek their way out in the circulatory system. We must repeat that psychological factors are not the only ones of importance in the clinical picture of hypertension, but they are important because their modification often results in benefit to the patient, regardless of whether the blood pressure figures are lowered or not.

Ayman suggests that generalized arterial constriction may be responsible for symptoms. It would seem to be largely a question of the intensity of the process and the rapidity with which it appears. Ayman points out, and we have frequently seen, patients with very high blood pressure, 250–300 mm. systolic, which may exist for years without symptoms. Yet in other individuals with lower pressures of more sudden onset, severe headaches, dizziness, spells of blushing and pallor, temporary pareses and even convulsions seem to appear on the basis of vascular spasm.

When the hypertensive vascular disease advances and vital organs are affected, it is of course true that many symptoms are caused by failure of these organs. Even here, however, it is important that we evaluate the part played by emotional as well as physical factors.

Headache.   Janeway observed that headache was the most frequent symptom of which his hypertensive patients complained. He described the typical hypertensive headache which appears on awakening as consisting of sensations ranging from a dull ache to severe pounding distress and as usually being located in the cervico-occipital region. But in addition, he noted that a surprisingly large number of patients had been subject to migraine throughout life. Gardner, Mountain and Hines found migraine five times as frequently in hypertensive patients as in a control group. Then there is a great variety of head pains, discomforts and peculiar sensations, such as dullness and fullness with or without vertigo, which occur in hypertensive subjects and are often referred to as headaches. The tendency is to attribute all these "headaches" to the hypertension. Certainly elevation of the blood pressure seems responsible for the so-called typical hypertensive headache. (Even here, however, the anxiety factor enters insofar as it is related to exacerbations of blood pressure.) However, the vast majority of peculiar head sensations and discomforts often designated as headache cannot be correlated with the blood pressure level itself. Here the emotional factor is directly related to the peculiar head sensations.

An example is a patient who had severe hypertension and constant headache. She had had a complete physical study. The blood pressure averaged 200/120. The heart seemed within normal limits as to size, as determined by the orthodiagram, and the electrocardiogram indicated only left-axis deviation, other features being within the limits of normal. There was no evidence of impairment of cardiac function. The eye-grounds showed arteriosclerosis of the hypertensive type, grade 1, but no evidence of retinitis. Urinalysis was negative and renal function, as measured by the urea clearance test, was within normal limits. An intra-venous urogram was normal. The conclusion was essential hypertension with symptoms out of proportion to disease.

After reviewing the studies, we said to her, "Sometimes tension is related to hypertension." She thought that over for a moment and said, "Well, I can improve on that formula. In my house, it is 'contention-tension-hypertension.'" Then she went on to tell of the role she played as a "buffer" between an irate husband and a lazy son who was in business with his father and of the constant quarrelling between them. The greater part of her sympathy was with the son. She was always trying to shield him. She was a martyr-like person and that kind always pays a penalty, absorbing punches which produce symptoms. This woman's headache was the "body language" means of representing her difficult life situation. It was just as if she would say, "My husband is a headache to me." Indeed he was. He was having an extramarital affair and boasted of it openly. He felt that it was indecent to smoke or drink, but the sexual appetites were normal and were to be indulged and no secret was to be made of the fact. By thus humiliating her in the presence of her friends he added to her problem. Perhaps as a result of the uncritical way this information was received she gained enough confidence to present her husband with an ultimatum and, contrary to her worst expectations, he agreed to end the extramarital affair. It made a great difference in her life. Thereafter, she was well as far as headache was concerned. It is true that this patient still has her hypertension. But the disappearance of the headache was an indication that the symptom was out of proportion to the disease and was related to the anxiety. The anxiety in turn was related to emotional conflict and the conflict could be understood by getting to know the patient as a human being and not just as a medical case.

Migraine presents a more complicated mechanism. It can hardly be assumed, as in the case of anxiety and hypertension, that migraine is so frequent in hypertension because the two are common disorders and therefore must frequently meet. Instead, there seems to be a common denominator, and psychological study gives a clue. Apparently there is an intimate relationship between the personality structure of the two disorders. Both present evidence of chronically repressed rage. Attacks of migraine occur when situations are met which intensify the rage without providing opportunity for adequate expression.

Constipation.   Most patients with hypertension see a connection between headache and bowel function. When they suffer from constipation they are ill, and when the bowel moves freely they are speedily relieved of symptoms. This, of course, is true for many patients who do not have hypertension, but in hypertensive individuals the relationship is especially obvious. Moreover, it is a relationship which is easily exploited and in which the physician becomes a pathogenic agent when he focuses attention on the bowel, as in the days, fortunately not now so common, when colonic irrigations were frequently prescribed for "autointoxication." It is very difficult to overcome a patient's prejudices —and even those of the medical profession—in this regard. But it does seem to be largely a psychological association, because relief comes too quickly after a bowel movement to be ascribed to physical causes, and, in addition, deeper psychologic study often shows the relationship between ideas of obstruction, "poisoning" and pain in the head.

Vertigo. Patients frequently refer to the symptom of vertigo, which occurs in a great many instances with the head discomforts just described, as dizziness and giddiness. Differentiating syncope, which does not imply a disturbance of equilibrium, and true Ménière's syndrome, one often finds that the symptom of vertigo bears a definite relation to an anxiety state. Frequently in association with ringing in the ears and sometimes with numbness and tingling of the extremities, it is the result of psychic stress.

The early symptoms of anxiety are usually expressed through the cardiovascular, respiratory, gastrointestinal and genitourinary systems. It is after the anxiety state has persisted for some time that the symptom of vertigo makes its appearance. When it occurs in association with hypertension the vascular disease often is held to be responsible. However, it is well to bear in mind that, like organ language elsewhere, vertigo (unsteadiness) frequently is the symbolic representation of insecurity, and this is just as true when it occurs in association with hypertension.

Case 12.   Hypertension and Vertigo

A woman of 55 with a moderate elevation of blood pressure and pronounced symptoms of cardiac neurosis recently suffered an attack of severe vertigo. She was thoroughly studied at the hospital and no evidence of organic disease other than moderate elevation of blood pressure was found. The study included a complete neurological survey.

As one of us was leaving her room after the last interview, a casual comment seemed to have more bearing on the vertigo than all of the examinations just completed. In the course of the conversation, she said, "You have much to live for (meaning the profession of medicine) while I have nothing."

She had always aspired to a career in medicine, encouraged by a dominating mother who directed her own ambitions to the daughter. Instead she married a man whom she idealized as a perfect person "not primarily interested in woman as a sexual object," only to find that he made constant sexual demands. She never attained sexual gratification but had five children in rapid order. She devoted herself to her children, now grown, and following the death of her mother from heart disease she developed a mild depressive reaction from which she had not recovered. The discovery of the hypertension permitted her to focus her anxiety upon her heart and the fear of death from a "stroke."

With psychotherapy she was able to recognize and express the hostility against her husband but she had more difficulty with her guilt-laden death wishes against her mother. It was with great difficulty that she was able to see her mother's domination and her own need for her mother's love, which had determined her pattern of submission, the development of unconscious wishes for her mother's death to relieve herself of this burden, and the ensuing guilt, which increased her own need to act the dutiful daughter. Then from this identification she punished herself with her mother's symptoms of heart disease, especially after anything that she considered self-indulgence or ostentation. After the heart "pain" there was a secondary depression associated with her feelings of helplessness and inadequacy.

During the course of treatment her depression diminished and she was able to engage in more activities, such as joining a class in music appreciation from which she derived great pleasure. The atmosphere at home improved. Then on her own accord she suggested diminishing the frequency of her visits to the psychiatrist and immediately after this had the attack of severe vertigo that resulted in the hospital study. We thought of the symptom as representing symbolically her fear that she might not be able to maintain her balance without supportive therapy but perhaps on a deeper level it had to do with fear of "falling" in a sexual sense. Certainly unconscious depreciation of femininity colored her whole life as a disappointment that could not be fulfilled. The substitution was to have children and be a perfect mother, but with her children grown and no longer needing her care the illness was precipitated by the death of the mother with whom she was strongly identified. When she no longer had the gratification of motherhood the pains in the chest acted as a constant reminder of her inadequacy. They meant, "I can never hope to attain the goal that mother wanted for me," and a life of leisure and self-indulgence only added to her woes.

Cardiac Neurosis.   Pain in the precordium, palpitation, dyspnea and fatigue are a group of symptoms frequently associated with cardiac neurosis. Fatigue may be a prominent part of the clinical picture, in fact, the most prominent symptom, although again and again the patient speaks of pain in the heart region and only after considerable discussion is it brought out that really the most important symptom is fatigue, that it occurred first, and that only later was the pain added. One of the commonest causes of fatigue is emotional conflict, which steals energy that is not then available for useful purposes.

When these symptoms are present with a normal cardiovascular system and the general medical examination otherwise is negative, it is not as a rule difficult to assign them to their proper sphere—the emotions. When hypertension is present, however, it is almost invariably held to be the responsible factor. It is under such circumstances that psychosomatic study will frequently reveal that symptoms are out of proportion to disease, that there is much conflict in the personality make-up, and that it depends on repressed hostility. Moreover, a specific as well as a temporal relationship will be found between the onset of the symptoms and a psychic event.

When pain in the chest is associated with hypertension in a middle-aged individual, and especially in the presence of physical evidence of cardiovascular disease, the problem becomes a very difficult one from the standpoint of management. It is all very well to advise a young person invalided by cardiac neurosis but with only moderate elevation of blood pressure and no evidence of cardiovascular disease "to carry on in spite of symptoms," and to encourage him to do the things that other people do. But in the presence of electrocardiographic evidence or other indications of coronary disease, one assumes a heavy responsibility in encouraging such patients to carry on; yet to caution rest on the one hand and try to give reassurance on the other is so often worse than useless. To the young physician treating such a patient, and to psychiatrists as well, it poses a very difficult problem; the sudden death that may occur in patients who have been encouraged to carry on, or who are undergoing psychotherapy, may bring the criticisms of the community down upon the head of the unfortunate practitioner. And yet to play into the unconscious fears of the patient by cautioning rest and more rest leads to greater and greater degrees of invalidism. Moreover, as the patient waits for his arteries to harden the questionable benefit of the physical rest is more than offset by the physiological burden provoked by psychic stress. The only advice that we can offer in this regard is that the patient must be evaluated as carefully as possible, both physically and psychologically, and then an effort made to advise him correctly regarding his activities.

TREATMENT

Let us take again the example of a middle-aged man refused by a life insurance company because of high blood pressure. His physician rules out glomerulonephritis and decides that the patient is suffering from essential hypertension. Then, all too frequently, attention is concentrated on the effort to "bring the blood pressure down." The patient demands to know the blood pressure figure; on each visit to the physician he waits with anxious concern to hear the latest reading and frequently he has ideas of "stroke," "heart failure" or "Bright's disease" in the back of his mind.

Just what has been done to this poor patient in the effort to "bring his blood pressure down"? Because of an ill-founded idea that protein was responsible for hypertension and kidney disease he was for years denied meat and eggs, especially red meat, which for some reason was looked upon with particular dread. Then his diet was rendered even more unpalatable by the withdrawal of salt. One would sympathize with this half-starved victim of good intentions except that he probably was not able to eat anyway, his teeth having been removed on the theory that focal infection had something to do with hypertension. Even before this period he had sacrificed his tonsils and had had his sinuses punctured because of the same theory. In case he actually had been able to eat some solid food, in spite of these previous therapeutic measures, the slight colonic residue was promptly washed out by numerous "colonic irrigations," especially during the period when the theory of autointoxication was enjoying a wave of popularity. To add to his unhappiness he was often told to stop work and exercise, and of course was denied alcohol and tobacco as well as coffee and tea. Then to cap the climax of his difficulties, the unfortunate person with hypertension was referred to the neurosurgeon, who was prepared to separate him from his sympathetic nervous system.

Now he is rendered hypotensive with potent ganglionic blocking agents and dulled with "tranquilizers." Hardly a voice is raised in protest. Shapiro, however, in a courageous paper, questions the widespread use of hypotensive drugs. In his studies the drugs were administered to a series of patients with hypertensive disease of all degrees of severity. Special efforts were made not only to standardize the conditions under which blood pressures were read but also to determine the spontaneous course of the disease in each individual and to carefully evaluate the nonpharmacological forces impinging upon the patient and the physician during the experimental or therapeutic situation. By the observations of a third party he and his associates found it possible to correlate changes in the enthusiasm of the investigator for the drug, the patient and the study, with significant changes in the patient's blood pressure. These variations in blood pressure were statistically evaluated and found at least equal to those produced by the specific drugs and capable of potentiating or partially masking its effects.

In one study to determine the variations in blood pressure during salt restriction, an actual rise in blood pressure, often following an initial decline, was noted in several patients in conjunction with an increasing resentment of hospitalization or with the occurrence of events outside the hospital that created anxiety in the patient.

In another study Shapiro found that (1) mere inclusion of a patient in a special study, even when no specific treatment is prescribed, may exert a hypotensive effect; (2) the giving of medicaments exerts an additional effect that must be controlled by placebo-drug alternation; (3) in some instances, placebo alternation may reveal that the hypotensive effect of the drug has been masked; (4) the changes induced by the nonpharmacological stimuli in the experimental situation can be of at least equal magnitude to those resulting from the drug per se.

Shapiro concluded, as Ayman many years ago had shown, that the symptoms of hypertensive vascular disease are largely nonspecific, except for those that arise from complications such as heart failure, encephalopathy and renal failure. Both Reiser et al. and Weiss et al. had also made this observation. The relief of headaches, malaise and easy fatigability that many patients exhibit is notoriously unreliable as an index of improvement. That is why the statement, seen in so many reports on the treatment of hypertension by various medical and surgical methods, "the level of blood pressure was not influenced, but the symptoms were relieved" means nothing because it fails to take into consideration the important psychological factors that enter into the problem. Symptoms regularly disappear with almost any therapy.

In designing an experiment for the assay of hypotensive agents Shapiro suggests: (1) the necessity for control periods during therapy and after therapy, as well as prior to treatment; (2) the establishment of maximal conditions for randomizing suggestion from the physician, as well as in the patient, by employing a double blind technique of drug-placebo administration, alternated in a random fashion; and (3) the elucidation of the underlying psychodynamic patterns in the patient under study and observation of the interplay of psychological forces in the experimental situation, so that systematic errors produced by these factors may be identified and their influence determined.

Psychosomatic Aspects of Treatment

The knowledge that "every psychic tendency seeks adequate bodily expression" gives a practical hint in dealing with hypertensive patients. An explanation to the effect that inner tension which cannot be released through ordinary channels (action or words) may manifest itself in the circulatory system by adding to the problem of hypertension represents a rational approach insofar as the patient is concerned. This often leads to a discussion of problems which are of considerable interest and importance from the standpoint of illness.

A case, reported in detail elsewhere (p. 246), is interesting from this standpoint. The patient, a young man working for a trucking company in Philadelphia, had rather severe hypertension. His father, who had worked for the same firm, was killed in an accident, and the family was denied compensation. Our patient was "burned up" about it. He wanted to get into union activities where he would have an opportunity to avenge his father. He had been denied this opportunity because it meant "too much work and excitement." We gave him permission. In addition to working eight hours on the job, he had to work six hours for the union. He was an organizer and worked hard, yet he actually improved during the two years he was engaged in union activities. He improved as far as symptoms were concerned and even his blood pressure was lower. Then the union broke up and again he was "burned up." He was "choked with rage," and his blood pressure went up again. As soon as he was denied an outlet for aggression along the lines of avenging his father, up went his blood pressure and symptoms returned. So we think there is something in the personality of a hypertensive patient that suggests a relationship between hostile impulses that cannot find an outlet and elevation of blood pressure. It is not the whole answer—not by any means. We do not maintain that it is the basic cause of hypertension. A patient can be "burned up" all his life and unless he has a predisposition to hypertension, he probably will not get it. Given the predisposition and an aggressive personality with no outlets for aggression, then in all probability hypertension will develop.

Personality Studies.   Studies of the emotional lives of patients with hypertension have been published by Alexander, Saul, Dunbar, and Binger.

Dunbar calls attention to the increased tension and sometimes spasm of voluntary or smooth muscles or both that may be alleviated as unconscious conflicts became conscious. She feels that this tension is part of the whole defense mechanism, psychologically and physiologically a general attitude of being on guard. Often its significance is elaborated in terms of accompanying disturbance of tonus in other systems, especially in the gastrointestinal and the genitourinary tract. Dunbar finds that hostile impulses against which the patient is on guard are as a rule relatively near the surface and accessible to treatment. As these impulses emerge to consciousness there is usually a rise in the blood pressure curve followed by a drop to a lower level as the material is worked through. There are also transitory psychoneurotic manifestations of a phobic or compulsive nature in the course of such treatment. Dunbar has dealt with the subject in detail in her comprehensive book entitled *Emotions and Bodily Changes* in which, among the many studies reported, considerable attention is given to the opinions of Fahrenkamp, whose psychophysiological studies on hypertension are noteworthy. He also feels that psychic factors play a decisive role in regard to the blood pressure level in all stages of the disorder and therefore that in all hypertensive patients the major emphasis should be on the treatment of the psychic element. However, it is impressive that this psychologically minded physician does not accept the existence of a functional hypertension of purely psychogenic origin, since he has never seen a patient who completely lost his hypertension. In other words, in his experience the tendency of the circulatory system to pathological reaction remains demonstrable.

HOSTILITY AND AGGRESSION.   Other investigators, notably Alexander and Saul, find that hypertensive patients show external friendliness and self-control, beneath which there are strong aggressions and anxiety. The anxiety grows out of the danger which these repressed aggressions would create for the security of the individual if they were allowed expression. It is as if the inner psychological tension (force) of the aggression found expression through heightened arterial pressure. We are all familiar with the every-day comment to the person who is about to explode with anger and resentment, "Now, think of your blood pressure!" Of course by discouraging or threatening the person who would relieve his anger by words or action one might be doing just the thing to cause a further rise in the blood pressure.

Latent hostility and repressed aggression are found in every neurosis, but the difference, as noted in hypertension, is explained by Saul who finds the hostility in hypertensive persons to be intense, chronic, inhibited, near to consciousness and perhaps to motility, but not adequately repressed or bound as in an organized neurosis. He finds these people are neither able to satisfy passive, dependent wishes nor to gratify the hostile ones and hence they remain blocked in both directions. Such a psychological structure may develop as follows: With the continuance of the problem of achieving social position, prestige and a high standard of living, the individual has difficulty in controlling his hostile aggressive feelings. Competitive urges stem from aggression but aggression is often punished and hence fears accompany the aggression. These fears lead to inhibitions which in turn limit an adequate expression of aggressive feelings. This hostile impulse accumulates and increases in intensity, requiring further inhibition in order to keep such impulses from the patient's view or the view of others. The vicious circle goes on and the result is that in some people the emotional energy so generated finds release only through the blood-pressure-controlling physiological mechanisms.

Psychosomatic Observations.   In an effort to throw further light on this subject Binger and his associates made detailed psychological and physiological studies of 24 patients with hypertension. No effort was made to prove "psychogenesis"; on the contrary, the authors refrained from drawing conclusions regarding the role of psychic factors in the etiology of essential hypertension.

While all of their patients presented evidence of a disorder of the personality which could be classified as "neurotic," the appearance of an organized neurosis with specific symptoms was the exception rather than the rule. A particular configuration of tendencies was consistently found and an approximate composite picture of the personality and its development described. Regarding this personality these workers say that "the failure of the integrative functions of personality, the inadequacy of the characteristic defenses against anxiety, the inefficiency of the repressive mechanisms and the inability to develop an organized neurosis, rather than the nature of the underlying 'instinctive' drives, are what appear to differentiate this disorder from other seemingly similar ones."

EARLY INSECURITY. The outstanding feature of personality study was found to be an early sense of insecurity. In the majority of cases it was possible to discern a critical shock-like reaction wherein the patients felt overwhelmed by danger against which their usual defenses were ineffective. In general the situation which seemed to epitomize the major threat was separation from a parent. The discovery of hypertension or the first appearance of its prodromal symptoms usually occurred in such emotional settings and followed acute emotional disturbances. Study of the childhood of these patients showed that death of the parent or separation occurred in 12 out of 24 cases. In 23 of the same number of cases the existence of high blood pressure was first observed after the occurrence of an emotional disturbance such as illness or death of a relative; injury, illness, or other trauma to the patient; changes in the patient's life such as separation from parents, marriage, illness of a child, loss of a job, or loss of savings. In 13 of these 24 cases the emotional disturbance seemed to be mainly a reaction to a serious illness or death of a relative. The common factors were loss of security or exposure to the aggressions of the persons on whom the patient was dependent.

PERSONALITY DISORDER. Binger et al. point out that unlike such disorders as asthma and migraine, in which the psychological setting of an attack can easily be studied, it is difficult to show a correlation between psychological situation and physiological response in a disorder like elevated blood pressure, which is not episodic and in which there is not even always a parallel between the level of blood pressure and the existence and severity of symptoms. They review previous observations such as those of Alexander and Saul and agree with the description of the conflict situation in which aggressive impulses are inhibited but not deeply repressed, yet, "the assumption that psychic factors causative of the somatic disturbance are of a specific nature, is by no means clear." The authors regard their investigation as a clinical study contributing to the nosology and development of hypertension but not to its etiology. They do not consider the disorder of the personality as the cause of hypertension; rather they prefer to regard the disorder of the personality and the "constitutional vasomotor instability" as different aspects of the same fundamental pathological process.

EVIDENCE AGAINST SPECIFICITY. The frequency with which emotional factors may play a significant role in influencing the course of hypertension has not been adequately clarified. Reiser, Brust and Ferris have rendered a service by summarizing their general observations concerning the relationship of emotionally stressful life situations to the course of hypertensive disease in 230 unselected patients. Special attention was paid to the natural course of the disease, the role of emotional factors, physiological mechanisms involved, and the response of the patients to various pharmacological agents and therapeutic procedures. The studies represented a multidisciplinary integrative approach, including the disciplines of psychiatry, internal medicine, surgery, pathology and physiology.

The frequency with which the patients responded in a favorable manner to a sustained therapeutic relationship was quite striking and supported other evidence indicating the important role of emotional factors influencing the course of hypertension. A majority of patients experienced marked symptomatic relief and functioned more effectively in their environment, and, in a period of observation which averaged 21 months, there was usually an absence of objective evidence of progression of the disease. In a small but significant percentage of patients an actual regression of structural changes and blood pressure levels was observed.

As part of a comprehensive study of hypertension, Reiser et al. investigated 12 patients who were in various stages of the transition from benign to malignant hypertension. In each of these patients, examination of the relationship between the life history and the medical course of the disease revealed that the precipitation of the malignant phase could be chronologically correlated with emotionally significant life situations or events. While psychomatic correlations were specific within the individual patient, the data did not reveal any specificity of personality structure or conflict situations for the group as a whole and thus did not explain the selection of this organ system. "The findings are consistent with the view that the specific choice of the hypertensive vascular mechanism may be related to an additional factor, or factors, such as the presence of a predisposing renal lesion in patients with coexistent renal disease, but as yet unknown in the patients with essential hypertension."

Weiss et al., in a long term study of 150 patients with hypertension, conclude that the symptoms of hypertension usually rise in a social setting of emotional stress. They feel that one must always question their relation to the high blood pressure itself, and make an effort to understand them from the viewpoint of behavior. With the discovery of the hypertension the "blood pressure phobia" begins and often dominates the clinical picture; the new symptoms are only an exaggeration of the premorbid personality trends. These symptoms respond readily to psychotherapy, but there is no evidence that the course of the hypertensive vascular disease can be influenced by psychotherapy. Therefore, while hypertension in itself is not an indication for psychotherapy, the emotional problems which occur in association with hypertension are, and because they are so common, psychotherapy is indicated in the great majority of patients with hypertension. There is no reason why psychotherapy cannot be combined with medical and surgical treatment.

Hypertension occurs in all types of personalities, from normal to psychotic, but there is a great preponderance of neurotic personalities with strong compulsive trends. Weiss et al. were unable to discover any specific personality conflicts or specific personality structure that seems related to the hypertension. Repressed hostility is not peculiar to hypertension, as opposed to other psychosomatic disorders.

From these observations, it would appear that the hypertensive predisposition and the personality fault are parallel disturbances, the one inherited and exhibited in the somatic sphere, the other manifesting itself in the emotional life through thoughts and feelings. When the life situation becomes sufficiently disturbing for the particular personality, the hypertension may appear as one aspect of the personality decompensation. Having appeared, it usually pursues an irrevocable course.

The failure to deal adequately with hypertension stems in large part from the concern about "bringing the blood pressure down," and from the failure to recognize the emotional origin of most of the symptoms that are attributed to the high blood pressure.

On "Bringing the Blood Pressure Down."   It is freely admitted that the height of the blood pressure is one index to the condition and prognosis of the patient with essential hypertension but to put all of our attention on the matter of bringing this blood pressure down is to do the patient an injustice. We say this whether or not psychic factors are fundamental in hypertension.

Perhaps at this point something should be said regarding home blood pressure readings as used in programs of treatment based on adjusting the dosage of ganglion-blocking drugs. Freis points out that home recordings encourage the patient's cooperation, teach him to recognize side effects of hypotension, and aid him in managing situations which disturb and raise his blood pressure. We, as well as others, have been reluctant to adopt this technique, believing that the patient's attention should be directed away from, rather than focused on, blood pressure figures, but Corcoran, Dustan and Page also recommend home blood pressure readings and believe that home readings do not tend to fix a neurotic obsession with blood pressure. In two groups of patients, one recording home pressures and the other not, they found the incidence of psychiatric disability in the two groups the same, one in ten, over a three year period. While they do not recommend home readings for the majority of patients with hypertension they do feel that they are necessary adjuncts to the use of ganglion-blockers.

Redefining Objectives.   We must redefine our objectives in the treatment of hypertension. The consideration of pathogenesis must impress us with the necessity for the total evaluation of the patient with hypertension. This will represent a combined physical and psychological study. When we do such a study we will realize that many symptoms occurring in hypertension are of emotional rather than physical origin and that *the incapacity is often out of proportion to the disease*. Hence the importance in a great many patients of reeducation along the lines of "carrying on" rather than urging rest and more rest. Menninger champions this idea on the basis that self-directed aggression may be turned outward by the authority of the physician and that extroversion of the aggression, if not too strenuous, may be of advantage to the patient. We have repeatedly proved this to our own satisfaction in patients who have been invalided by the *knowledge* of blood pressure rather than by the physical effects of the hypertension itself.

Some Practical Points. An explanation that tension of emotional origin which cannot be released through words or action may seek a way out in the circulatory system, thus adding to the problem of hypertension, often provides a stepping stone to permit patients to talk about themselves as persons rather than as cases of high blood pressure. It makes sense to the patient to say, "in medical language high blood pressure is known as hypertension, and tension makes hypertension. Therefore, let us talk about the causes of your tension."

To advise the individual involved in mental conflict "not to worry" is valueless, especially when, as is so often the case, no concerted effort is made to find out what is disturbing him. Too often the physician is satisfied that there are no problems disturbing the patient after he has inquired, "Are you worried about anything?" and has received a negative reply. Most of the time the patient really does not know just how much he is disturbed nor does he relate the factors actually responsible for his discontent. He is much more apt to project his worries into questions about his blood pressure, heart, brain and kidneys. Careful inquiry will bring out that his fears are exaggerated and that the reasons he assigns for them are illogical.

There is only one approach that has any merit, that is, to *encourage the patient to talk about himself as a person rather than as a medical case.* This will permit some insight into conflict situations and lead often to some relief of anxiety, which is closely related to the high blood pressure. Although this approach does not offer a complete solution of the hypertensive problem and does not even apply to all patients, it is a practical method of dealing with a set of important factors that may be modified, whereas the constitution of the individual cannot be touched. It is an approach heretofore not sufficiently practiced. We are too much concerned with physical measurements in hypertension—the blood pressure figures, the percentage of renal function, the size of the heart, the electrocardiographic tracing, the amount of retinal sclerosis—all of which are essential in the study of the hypertensive mechanism but give incomplete information from the standpoint of the total evaluation of the patient. They should represent the beginning and not the end of the study. We are too little concerned with the emotional life, which may hold the key to the satisfactory management of the hypertensive patient.

There is no objection to the effort to lower blood pressure as long as this does not constitute the sole approach to the problem of high blood pressure. This applies to the most recent methods of dealing with hypertension by medical and surgical means. In some patients sympathectomy will produce a prolonged drop of the blood pressure. One may say to patients who have hypertension and anxiety (due to the meeting of inner conflicts and external pressures) that our objective in their management is to "take off some of the load." If we can do this by helping them to achieve some insight into their emotional problems, with consequent lowering of tension, well and good; if we can do it by environmental manipulation, fine; but if we have to resort in addition to drug therapy or to surgery (sympathectomy) by all means let us use a combination of efforts to help our patients with hypertension. While we believe that essential hypertension cannot be eradicated by any psychotherapeutic process, no matter how intensive or prolonged, we feel also that almost every patient with essential hypertension can be benefited by psychotherapy.

PSYCHOANALYSIS.   Binger and his associates had the following to say: "The problem is that of treating a severe character neurosis in which anxiety, depression, and suppressed aggression are the cardinal psychopathological features. The method of choice will vary from cheerful neglect to deep psychological exploration. The latter . . . is a matter for the expert. What is to be hoped from it we cannot say. There is as yet no evidence that psychoanalysis or any other psychotherapeutic procedure can reverse the physiological process or change the destiny of this disease—be it benign or malignant. The problem is an open one. It needs further investigation. The ground has now been cleared for such an undertaking."

Because of the involved emotional problems frequently presented by patients with hypertension, however, psychoanalysis is sometimes advised.

A young man with essential hypertension and angina pectoris was referred for analysis because of serious personality problems. It was a long and difficult analysis, but the patient made great social improvement and became a more effective personality. Nevertheless, the cardiovascular disease was uninfluenced and, indeed, showed evidence of progression.

One should approach a problem like this from the standpoint of the psychologic difficulty. It is not that the hypertension needs analysis but that the patient needs analysis (p. 251). At the same time one must bear in mind the physical threat imposed by the cardiovascular disease. Will the stress of the work of analysis threaten such a patient? Has he a chance to live out enough years to make the investment in time, energy and money worth while? Should one ask the analyst to assume such a responsibility in the face of coronary disease and the threat of sudden death? When coronary artery disease exists in a patient with a seriously disturbed personality, we have to question whether to advise analysis or to be satisfied with superficial psychotherapy and reassurance.

Conclusions

The organic tradition in medicine has been responsible for a narrow view of the etiology and treatment of essential hypertension. The psychosomatic approach does not neglect the physical problems involved but includes a consideration of the role of the emotions. It does not mean to study the soma less; it only means to study the psyche more. It emphasizes the multiple factors in etiology and pathogenesis and attempts to evaluate the resulting composite clinical picture. Such studies indicate that emotional factors apparently are intimately related to the development of hypertension in some patients, to the production of symptoms in

Know

many others, and enter into the question of treatment in nearly all patients with essential hypertension.

A common problem seems to be the presence of emotional tension due to chronic repressed hostility. If this inhibited aggression can be relieved by psychotherapy anxiety is diminished and blood pressure may be lowered. Even if the blood pressure is unaffected, the treatment often benefits the patient by making him a healthier and more effective personality. Our objectives in treatment should be readjusted. We must not limit our efforts to "bringing the blood pressure down." There is no reason why we cannot combine physical (medical and surgical) methods with psychotherapy but we must go beyond the physical aspects of hypertension to the personality of the hypertensive individual in order to be successful in the management of such patients.

The following cases have been selected to illustrate various psychosomatic problems in hypertension and their management.

Case 13.   Essential Hypertension, Unrelated Symptoms, Obsessive Personality, Improvement with Reassurance

History and Symptoms.   A 42 year old white woman was seen in the out-patient department with a history of headaches, palpitation and pain in the heart region which had begun fifteen years before. At that time she was told that she had high blood pressure. She consulted a number of physicians, then went to the clinic of a woman's hospital, but "felt no confidence in women physicians." After trying osteopathy she came to our clinic. She felt as though her head would "explode" and as though something were "probing" to get out—"something was running or flowing down inside the head on the left side."

The past history otherwise was negative.

The mother had been hypertensive for a few years but was now 77 and only recently had had "a light heart attack." The father had died of cirrhosis in April, 1940; he had been an alcoholic.

A sister suffered from migraine, and one brother had been turned down by the Army because he was nervous.

General physical examination showed moderate elevation of blood pressure, varying between 170/100 and 180/114 mm. of Hg, but in spite of the long history of hypertension there was remarkably little change in the cardiovascular-renal system. The heart was normal in size, urinalysis negative and the kidney function good, and there was only slight attenuation of retinal arterioles, with a mild degree of sclerosis of the peripheral branches.

The patient was reassured about her physical condition and was asked to describe in more detail the onset of her difficulties. She told us that at the time she had felt confused, and had suffered from headache and a sense of rushing or being pushed all the time, and that she had thought of a "mental condition" because a cousin of her husband's had had some kind of a "mental condition" for many years. However, a physician told her that it was high blood pressure, and from then on she accepted that explanation of her illness.

LIFE SITUATION

She had gone to public school to the eighth grade and then had had various jobs until she married at 19. There was one child, a son, now 22.

Her father had been a brewer, born in Germany, an alcoholic; the mother was a good-hearted, kind woman, much upset by her husband's drinking. The patient had been afraid of her father, who was very strict. She had had to give up school at 14, just before finishing the eighth grade, because the father was sick and out of work; afterwards, the father worked now and then but "drank most of the wages."

She had known her husband for several years before marriage. For the first five years they lived with her parents. He worked as a bank clerk, and was still with the same bank.

Fifteen years ago (at the time her illness began), she was very proud of the new home they had recently built, and when they were about to leave on a vacation she cleaned the house thoroughly, her usual practice. On her return she was amazed to find some cockroaches in the kitchen. She put roach powder about the house and then became upset on finding all the dead roaches. This continued all through the summer; she kept putting roach powder around, finding dead roaches and became "obsessed and frantic," so that she couldn't sleep or eat, and lost weight. She called in an exterminator, who "laughed at her"—he regarded the problem as so insignificant. But she would get up in the middle of the night and crawl around on the floor to look for roaches. She was so ashamed of her obsession that she would sometimes send her husband to the movies so she could look for roaches without his knowledge. She dreamed of them. The trouble continued for five years, the patient says, but she admitted that when summer came around she was still uneasy and looked for roaches.

It was at this time that she went to her physician because of a "confusion in her head" and a fear that something was going wrong with her mind. It was then her doctor told her that high blood pressure was the cause of her trouble.

She had always been an excessively clean, meticulous person about herself and the house. Now she said that this had lessened somewhat, that she was silly, and that she would never be that way again.

The patient was a very neat, attractive, gray haired woman in her early forties, gentle and soft voiced; she spoke in terms of high praise of her mother and husband. She had had a great disappointment in her son, who refused an education. She had wanted him to be a physician "from the day that he was born."

The patient said that nothing else in her life ever upset her as much as the roaches. She had never discussed it before because she was afraid of being thought silly. She said that she was always a perfectionist, and that the roaches represented an imperfection. She felt that having them "was close to being a sin," which gave us some insight into her obsession with dirt.

She was presented in psychosomatic conference and later was disturbed by such thoughts as "Did I do right—did I answer correctly?" She felt guilty when she was questioned about her religion; she was ashamed to admit that she did not go to church.

She was still fearful that something would happen to her mind and that, if it did, it would also affect her boy's mind. When she was given a Rorschach test it increased her doubts about her sanity, and for a week afterwards, until she was once more reassured, she had considerable headache and "confusion" in her head. The Rorschach test showed her compulsive trends, indications of sexual difficulties and some paranoid tendencies.

Although she improved remarkably after her interviews, the blood pressure was still elevated.

Follow-up. One year later the patient continued free of symptoms. Her son had married and had entered military service, and she had resigned herself to the situation as "other mothers have to do." She confessed that she still got a little uneasy when spring approached and she thought about roaches. The blood pressure continued to be moderately elevated.

SUMMARY

An instance of hypertension arising in the setting of an emotional illness, compulsive in nature. Apparently the blood pressure elevation had not been constant, because so few changes had occurred in the cardiovascular system. Certainly the blood pressure elevation has nothing to do with her symptoms now, and probably did not have in the beginning of her illness. It is also likely that, with so little impairment of the cardio-vascular-renal system, the blood pressure is not even a threat to a normal span of years.

Case 14. *Hypertension and Unrelated Symptoms. Anniversary Reaction. Mental Depression with Recovery*

History and Symptoms. A white man of 49 was seen in December, 1954, complaining of tension, with a feeling of being numb all over, tightening in the head, weakness, inability to concentrate, blurred vision and a feeling that his arms and legs were "like lead." The symptoms had begun in August, 1954, with headache and a "tightening inside of the head."

He had had similar trouble seven years before at which time hypertension was discovered. He was treated for high blood pressure, and within a few months felt better and had paid no further attention to his blood pressure until the present illness.

A physician referred him to a diagnostic clinic where he was given a thorough survey and told that his blood pressure was over 200, and that "he was in the first stages of cardiovascular disease," that the heart was enlarged and the aorta dilated. He was placed on reserpine and hexamethonium and although there was some lowering of blood pressure his symptoms continued.

On physical examination the blood pressure was 220/130 and there was slight enlargement of the left ventricle. Urinalysis was negative; kidney function good; and the eye grounds showed attenuation and sclerosis grade 1 of the retinal arterioles but no evidence of retinitis.

The patient had insomnia, felt worse in the morning, improved slightly toward evening, was unable to do his work, remained passively at home, overconcerned that he was disturbing his wife and family; in short, the picture of depression.

Attention was taken away from his blood pressure, he was reassured about his heart, and was told that he suffered from an illness of emotional origin.

It became clear that the illness of seven years before had also been a mild depression which had been blamed upon high blood pressure.

LIFE SITUATION

The present illness really began when he was "forced out of a large business" with great loss of self-esteem. He had difficulty adjusting to a new business, was much concerned about financial security (although there was no real threat), angry at his wife "for her casual attitude toward his financial problem," and felt as though he were "in a treadmill."

During the summer of 1954 he became more and more tense and in August headache was pronounced. Then came the diagnostic study and the diagnosis of hypertension.

When queried about his life situation in July, 1954, he said that "July is always an eventful month for us." That meant that in July he had married, had a birthday, his daughter was born, and several family deaths had occurred, including that of his father. Each summer he congratulated himself when he got through July without an unpleasant incident.

The father had died of coronary occlusion and it seemed clear that the patient was identifying with his father in this respect. The diagnosis of hypertension and preoccupation with the idea of heart disease had been the trigger to precipitate depression in this compulsive personality.

As we rehearsed this "anniversary reaction" and then discussed the background factors relating to his job and family situation, the depression lifted and symptoms disappeared. The blood pressure remained the same. In other words, the symptoms were unrelated to the hypertension and therefore could not be influenced by blood pressure-reducing drugs. They could only be dealt with by understanding their psychological origin and treating the patient along emotional lines.

Case 15.   *Early Essential Hypertension. Recurrent Attacks of Acute Hypertension with Hypertensive Encephalopathy*

History and Symptoms.   A young white man, 29 years old, was first referred to Temple University Hospital on the service of Dr. W. Wayne Babcock, December 12, 1935.

The diagnosis was acute gangrenous appendicitis which was proved at operation. The blood pressure during spinal anesthesia gradually dropped from 140/78 to 86/48. The patient later reported that he had been "scared to death of the operation," that he knew it was a "pus appendix" and that he was fearful that peritonitis would develop. Ten days postoperatively a note on his record stated that he "seemed somewhat hysterical." The blood pressure had been normal and the general physical condition seemed satisfactory so that he was discharged on December 24, 1935.

The same evening he felt dizzy, became delirious and had to be restrained. The following morning he reported that he was "blind in both eyes." He was sent to the psychopathic ward of the Philadelphia General Hospital, where he remained for three weeks. There, according to his later statement, he was treated for "high blood pressure and uremia." From their records it was noted that when he came home from the Temple

University Hospital he developed "terrible pain in the suprapubic region which extended into the testicles . . . it made me almost hysterical." He woke up unable to see and became very agitated. At the hospital he had auditory and visual hallucinations in which he saw funny faces and men teasing him. He cried a great deal and was restless and noisy at times. On discharge from the Philadelphia General Hospital, at the end of three weeks, he reported that he was so weak that he was unable to walk. Because of this weakness and nervousness he was readmitted to Temple University Hospital on February 11, 1936.

Physical Examination and Laboratory Studies.   Emaciation was pronounced. The skin was warm and moist. The blood pressure during this stay in the hospital varied between 160 and 180 systolic, and 110 and 120 diastolic. There was no evidence of thyroid enlargement. The heart seemed normal in size; the aortic second sound was accentuated. The eyeground examination showed evidence of an acute vasospastic retinitis without organic sclerosis (Dr. Gibson). The nasal retinal arteries were especially constricted. The temporals showed moderate attenuation. There were a few hemorrhages and exudates in the right retina and many in the left. The spinal fluid was clear and no abnormalities were detected.

A psychiatric examination found the patient well oriented and suggested that he had previously suffered from an organic delirium.

The urine examination showed no albumin although there were occasional hyaline casts. Renal function was normal. The blood count showed a moderate degree of secondary anemia. All blood chemical studies, including glucose tolerance, were within normal limits and the basal metabolism was plus 6 per cent.

Additional History.   During this stay in the hospital opportunity was afforded for a more satisfactory history. We were told that he had been a healthy child, nursed until one year and then was very difficult to wean; he would not eat and lost much weight. He had diphtheria and scarlet fever in childhood from which he made a good recovery but otherwise had no serious diseases until the present illness. Since about the age of 16 he would get a "bilious" headache about once a month unless he "warded it off" with a laxative and he reported that his father had suffered from the same kind of headaches.

He completed the eighth grade of school. He married at the age of 20. His wife had two children, one of whom died in infancy and the other was living and well.

His father suffered from valvular heart disease and his paternal grandfather died of a stroke after the age of 60. The mother had gallbladder disease and the maternal grandfather died of uremia. The patient was the oldest of a family of six and there was nothing remarkable in the medical history of his brothers and sisters. None of them had hypertension.

After his discharge from the hospital he was carefully followed by his physician who recorded that the blood pressure gradually diminished from 150/110 to 130/88. This last reading was obtained on May 22, 1936, after the patient had returned to his job as truck-driver in a large concern, and had been working for about a month. Meanwhile, his weight had increased from 114 to 127½ pounds and he felt very well.

Hypertensive Encephalopathy.   On May 28, 1936, at 4 P.M., he witnessed an automobile accident and although no one was injured the patient became terribly excited over "what might have happened to some children who were playing in the path of the truck." He "knew that he would get sick again," and after a few hours of restless sleep he awakened with abdominal pains, nausea, vomiting and diarrhea. (Later his physician reported that the first illness, that is, the appendicitis, had begun similarly—"like gastroenteritis with diarrhea.") Nausea and vomiting continued and also the diarrhea. Sleep was restless and fitful and on June 2nd the patient reported blindness on awakening but there was no evidence of this when he was examined by his physician later in the day.

Abdominal examination was negative but the blood pressure was now 160/100. That night he developed *convulsive seizures*. By midnight he was mentally clear but the blood pressure was 190/110. He was readmitted to the Temple University Hospital on the service of Dr. Charles L. Brown on June 3, 1936. On this admission the blood pressure, taken four times daily for a week, remained constantly at 200 to 210 systolic and 140 to 160 diastolic. There were almost no fluctuations. Even during sleep the blood pressure on several occasions was found to be 175/125. Weakness, however, was not so pronounced as before. The temperature on occasions was slightly elevated to 99.4°; the pulse varied from 90 to 120 and the leukocytes ranged from 15,800 to 22,450. Sedimentation time was 10 mm. in one hour and the other laboratory findings were within normal limits. Now the eyeground picture was stated to be acute vasospastic retinitis with arteriosclerosis, grade 1; but the functional (spastic) element was still the predominant feature. There were some retinal scars where previous exudates had been.

Psychologically it was found that the patient had been sleepless and restless ever since witnessing the accident, whereas previously he had always been an excellent sleeper. He kept recalling the accident and thought how "terrible" the consequences might have been. It was obvious that in this patient there was a great deal of unconscious anxiety which, following operation, had resulted in a psychosis, but had then subsided, during which time the patient improved and remained well for more than a month. Then after the accident anxiety broke out again, not quite to the former extent but with pronounced insomnia and a constant feeling of tension.

Following discharge from the hospital in June, 1936, the patient constantly improved. The weight increased and the blood pressure gradually diminished. During the latter part of June it was reported on several occasions at 140 to 150 systolic over 115 to 120 diastolic. By the latter part of July the blood pressure had dropped to 120/90. The weight had increased to 121½ pounds, and the patient felt perfectly well, eating and sleeping normally, and once more returned to work.

During this period more detailed information bearing on his life situation was obtained.

LIFE SITUATION

According to the mother he was a normal boy, the oldest of six children. Other than difficulty in weaning there were no behavior problems although there were occasional nightmares. He completed the eighth grade at school and began working at the age of 17. For some time he was employed as a clerk with a refining company and there he "first developed a fear of operations; a friend had the wrong kidney removed." There he also saw many accidents and deaths and it was largely for that reason that he gave up the position. He was always afraid of hospitals ("a fear of being cut").

He only vaguely recalled any masturbation. He began his heterosexual career at 14 with an older girl but often suffered from premature ejaculation. After marriage, although his wife was frigid, he indulged in excessive intercourse and asked whether perhaps that might be responsible for his present difficulties. Occasionally again he would suffer from premature ejaculation. With his illness he lost desire for intercourse. Then when desire returned he could not maintain an erection. Since the illness he developed nocturia. He would awaken with a "water" erection and complained of a pain in the testes.

Marriage.   He married at the age of 20. He became interested in his future wife through a challenge. A friend was attentive to her and expressed himself to the effect that she could not be taken away from him. The patient finally succeeded in winning her away and after a nine months' courtship they were married. During this period he did not have intercourse "because he had too much respect for the girl." His attitude toward his wife was one of extreme jealousy; the following incident is an example: She had been visiting her physician for gynecologic treatments. The patient would go along and wanted to stay in the room while the doctor treated her. "I didn't trust the doctor." His wife did not approve but suffered him to remain. The treatments affected him "in the stomach."

A child was born a year after marriage but lived only three months. The patient was nervously upset for a time afterwards.

Employment History.   For the past eight years he had been employed as a truckdriver for a large concern. On occasions he worked many extra hours; once he worked a hundred hours in one week. Nevertheless, he was always in debt. This was especially so just before his illness. In addition he felt the strain of trying to prevent accidents and stated that although he had a reputation for handling the truck well he, nevertheless, had many accidents and "the more I tried to avoid them the more accidents I had."

Beginning in the fall of 1937, he began to interest himself in *union work*. He stated that his father, who had worked for the same company, had always resented the company's "restrictions" but did nothing, but "my mother is a fighter and I must have inherited it from her." Furthermore, his father was killed by a truck in July, 1937, and the company was fighting compensation. This "makes me more determined than ever to fight the company union." He missed his father very much, because he used to talk to him about union activities. He threw himself into the work with great intensity and after working seven and one-half hours a day on the truck he would then engage in union activities for another five or six hours and in spite of this fact, at the end of six months of such constant pressure of activity, he had gained weight and his blood pressure still averaged 135/90! He stated that when he was under a nervous strain his muscles grew taut and that he perspired freely but that he was able to relax when he left the tense atmosphere. Now and then he felt cramps in the muscles especially of the arms and legs. He became an official of the union and in addition to the long hours of work managed to do a great deal of study. He often worked eighteen out of twenty-four hours and rarely got more than six or six and one-half hours in bed. His activity in the union dated from April, 1937, and in January, 1939, his blood pressure was still 135/90 and he was enjoying excellent health.

Retinal Studies.   In October, 1936, Dr. Gibson had found the eyegrounds almost normal. There was very slight attenuation of the nasal arterioles with arteriosclerosis, grade 1, of the hypertensive type, in the periphery of all four arterioles, and residual scars of previous retinitis. All vasospastic features had subsided and a remarkable increase in the caliber of all vessels was noted. In July, 1939, Dr. Gibson found "retinal arteriolar sclerosis, grade 1, of the hypertensive type. There is a very mild attenuation of the arterioles without exaggeration of the reflex stripe. The retinitis has completely subsided. This is a most unusual remission in the retinal picture of hypertension."

Elevation of Blood Pressure.   In September, 1939, for the first time since his recovery the blood pressure was definitely elevated (160/105). Union activities "folded up" in the early part of June; he was bitterly disappointed, anxious to do something about it but could not stir up any enthusiasm among his associates. When talking to them he became so "hot under the collar" that he lost the power of speech. He felt very keenly that something should be done but "just couldn't push things through." The injustice was "burning him up" and he felt himself "boiling inside." He had a constant feeling of tension and could not relax.

Coincidentally there had been a recurrence of *premature ejaculation* and a feeling that he could not be satisfied sexually. It seemed very obvious that his throttled aggression manifested itself in the sexual sphere and in his general feeling of not being able to relax, of being irritable and easily angered. We explained that the tension which he used to get rid of in union activities was bottled up and had to find an outlet in bodily symptoms.

Final Hospital Admission.   The blood pressure continued to be elevated until the final admission to the hospital in June, 1944, when he developed evidences of malignant hypertension and died of renal failure.

SUMMARY

A young white man of 29 with pronounced "mutilation anxiety," first seen in December, 1935, developed high blood pressure and an acute psychosis following an appendectomy, when he became fearful that peritonitis would develop. An acute vasospastic retinitis developed but the heart and kidneys seemed unaffected. The hypertension gradually subsided but in the spring of 1936, following an anxiety-producing episode, hypertension, vasospastic retinitis and hypertensive encephalopathy again occurred. Once more the blood pressure and eyeground changes subsided as anxiety was reduced and for the next three years the patient remained well, having maintained a normal blood pressure (135/90) since July, 1936.

For almost two years during this period he felt well and the blood pressure remained normal in spite of excessive work. The long hours and intense activity were employed, however, in union activities where he was able to give direct expression to his aggressive impulses. Union activities ceased in the spring of 1939 and in September he was once more suffering from tense feelings, experiencing sexual difficulties, and the blood pressure was once more elevated. It seemed clear that this coincided with the period of "throttled aggression." The blood pressure remained elevated until his death in June, 1944, of malignant hypertension.

Case 16.   Hypertension and Anxiety. Marked Improvement from Superficial Psychotherapy

A white man 55 years old first consulted us in May, 1937, complaining of "high blood pressure."

History and Symptoms.   At the age of 20 he had rheumatic fever, rested for a year and according to his statement "did not think of his heart again." The tonsils were removed the following year. Although he stated that he was not concerned about his heart he began to have an annual physical examination a few years later. Always he was told that he was normal. Eight years ago he took out a large insurance policy and was told that his blood pressure at that time was 140/90. The following year in his annual physical examination his blood pressure was found to be 150/100 and his physician recommended weight reduction. He dieted, lost weight, and in two weeks' time his blood pressure was 140/90 and remained at about that level for the following several months.

The next record that he knew about was 1932 when the blood pressure again was 150/100, and about August, 1935, he took another insurance examination and was turned down; he was told that the blood pressure was 180/100. This, he said, was the beginning of his concern about his blood pressure. He was then examined by many physicians and finally was told by a heart specialist, in regard to his hypertension, that he should go home and "take it easy," which he interpreted to mean that he was on his last legs. Then real anxiety attacks began and on his way to another physician he stopped to see a lawyer and have a will made, urging that it be completed immediately because he felt that he had only a few days to live.

Physical Examination and Laboratory Studies.   Physical examination showed an obese white man whose blood pressure varied between 190 and 200 systolic, and 110 and 120 diastolic. The heart seemed slightly enlarged to the left and x-ray showed the heart size at the upper limits of normal. The aorta was slightly elongated but not dilated. The electrocardiogram showed slight changes in the T waves in leads 1 and 4 and suggested myocardial degeneration. The urine was normal and renal function, measured by concentration and urea clearance tests, was within normal limits.

The eyeground studies showed arteriosclerosis grade 2 plus, of the hypertensive type. There were innumerable localized areas of narrowing of the retinal arterioles with attenuation of the reflex stripe and generalized narrowing of the arteriolar tree. The impression was of a rather advanced, fairly progressive vascular lesion.

During his study the patient discussed his occasional headaches which extended down into the neck and shoulders and also described a painful penile erection which occurred three or four times at night. The first attack had occurred eight or ten years before. He had been informed that this had some relationship to the prostate gland. It was some time later that he recalled that these attacks had occurred a short time after hearing a discussion of cancer of the rectum.

LIFE SITUATION

The patient was of humble origin. He first had limited schooling and then worked at manual labor in an effort to save money to put himself through school. This he accomplished, and finally achieved a position of success in the business world. After jilting a girl whom he had known intimately for many years, he married another who "seemed very kind and considerate" but immediately after their marriage "she changed" and according to his statement "from then on made life miserable for him." They had two healthy children.

Most of his visits now had to do with his marital difficulties. On one occasion his wife suddenly left home but in spite of the fact that he exhibited a great deal of hostility for her he nevertheless urged her to return, which she finally did.

So much of his anxiety seemed to surround the fact that he accused his wife of being psychotic—and it seemed to us without real justification—that we urged that he bring her to the psychiatrist. This he did, with her consent of course, and she remained for several months under the care of the psychiatrist, who reported that she was a maladjusted but not a psychotic person.

Fear of Psychosis.   Consequent interviews with our patient persuaded us that these accusations of psychosis regarding his wife were really projections of his own fears for his own condition. It was as though he said, "No, I am not psychotic; you are." In fact, on one occasion he said, "Perhaps I am losing my mind and I ought to see the psychiatrist." He was reassured that no hint of mental disease was present; that it was simply a question of an emotional disturbance.

Improvement.   Within a period of a few months he began to improve and by the following year reported that he felt as well as he had ever been. At the same time he stated that his wife was very much better since seeing the psychiatrist. For the first time he began to make some physical efforts such as polishing his car and at our suggestion doing a little gardening, which he very much enjoyed. In fact, he had alway enjoyed gardening but during the last few years had been so fearful of straining himself that he had given it up.

His blood pressure was not very different; it varied between 170 and 200 systolic, and 110 and 120 diastolic. All during these months he had troubled dreams but as he improved they diminished and finally disappeared. The night-time penile erections with the pain in the rectum also disappeared. He occasionally had a slight headache which seemed to occur every time he was reminded of high blood pressure, a stroke or heart disease. His visits to us were spaced out. Each time he reported himself well and working to advantage. He had great fun in his gardening and to his great satisfaction his son was also interested and worked along with him.

He was still gun-shy of the blood pressure apparatus but said he was not so afraid of death and was more like his former self.

The eyeground report in 1939 follows: "Retinal arterial sclerosis grade 2, hypertensive type. The right superior nasal retinal artery is spasmed out. There are numerous small retinal scars and areas of pigment proliferation in the retina.

"Impression: There has been no increase in the sclerosis since the examination in 1937. There is less attenuation and less spasm. Apparently he has had an acute retinitis which has become absorbed."

Reeducation. Here is another example of great improvement in a hypertensive individual without a real alteration of the blood pressure figures. Nevertheless, by a process of reeducation, removing anxiety over the blood pressure figures themselves, trying to understand the whole personality and the family situation, assisting the patient in achieving the sublimation of which he was capable by gardening and other outdoor activities, we succeeded in obtaining good results. This is an example of the kind of patient in whom a short period of *hospital study* at the beginning was very helpful. *It facilitates a thorough physical study in order to evaluate the cardiovascular-renal situation properly and at the same time furnishes an opportunity to get to know the patient as a human being as well as a medical case.* Also it takes the patient away from his environment in order that reeducation can be promptly instituted. In other words, it is often possible by this abrupt change to bring about some alteration in the patient's attitude toward himself and life. As a great English physician once remarked, "It enables you to make a philosopher of the man before the disease does it for you."

Follow-up. The patient continued to lead a busy professional life until 1944 when he had a mild stroke from which, however, he made a good recovery. In the following year he retired and moved to Florida. Reports a year later stated that he was in good condition and enjoying life.

SUMMARY

No far-reaching changes occurred in this man's personality or hypertensive state, yet he became a very different person from what he was in 1937. He carried on his occupation very successfully, was an efficient individual enjoying an ordinary degree of happiness, and his marital situation had been vastly improved. All of this came about with a relatively simple and superficial psychotherapy which consisted in: (1) reeducation regarding his blood pressure disturbance; (2) trying to understand his anxiety which he had focused on his heart and blood pressure; (3) improvement of his domestic situation by getting help for his wife; and (4) encouraging him to obtain satisfaction from a hobby which served as an outlet for some of his aggressive impulses.

Case 17. Early Essential Hypertension; Psychoanalysis; Social Recovery but Hypertension Persists

History and Symptoms. A white man of 31 was first seen in March, 1944. He had been called before the Induction Board in October, 1940; two doctors had examined him, and he thought he heard the term "aneurysm" used in connection with his case and "hasn't been right since." He had many symptoms referred to the circulatory system, and dull headaches and depression.

Later he was rejected by the Board, he says because of hemorrhoids, and still later

252 Applications to General Medicine and the Specialties

received occupational deferment until June, 1944. The previous summer he had contracted gonorrhea, "had been knocked out by sulfa," and then his old symptoms, which had been in abeyance, returned.

He had never had a serious illness, but gave a history of repeated fainting, usually in connection with hospital experiences, such as visiting a sick friend, so that he "hates hospitals."

The physical examination showed that the blood pressure was somewhat elevated, varying between 160 and 180 systolic and 95 to 120 diastolic, but was otherwise negative for evidence of organic disease. In particular, the cardiovascular-renal system seemed to be normal, so that the hypertension was thought to be of the essential variety.

The patient said that his parents had separated when he was 4 or 5 and had finally been divorced five years ago, when the patient was 26. There were six siblings, but there was nothing remarkable about the medical history other than that the mother was subject to migraine headaches.

The patient was seen about once a month (he lived in another city) and the blood pressure remained about the same but symptoms diminished. However, from time to time he continued to have various anxiety symptoms and mild depressions, and in 1947 it was possible to refer him for analysis. The analysis continued for about two years, and the following notes were sent to us by the analyst at the end of this period.

PSYCHOANALYTIC DATA

"He is the youngest child who has known all of his life that his mother regards him as her favorite, but wanted him—both before his birth and ever since—to be a girl. He has been very much attached to her and has been desirous of, and very rebellious against, giving in to her wishes. Thus, he wore long hair and "sissified" clothes until a very late age, when he finally insisted upon becoming more boylike. His three older brothers did not include him in their play or work endeavors, which led him to feel inferior, hostile and depressed. His overly religious severe father seemed forbidding to the patient, who nonetheless felt ashamed and inferior 'not to have a father like other children' when for several of his childhood years the father abandoned the family. He was relieved when at 14 his father returned. But then, as always, it was the mother who was careful, energetic, and who saved money, and it was she who seemed to the patient to be a good example.

"He had a great deal of castration anxiety which had to do with his many syncopal attacks. Thus visiting a cousin in the hospital who had been circumcised, the patient fainted, and from then on he feared and hated hospitals. As he reached his late teens, there developed a severe conflict between his fears of approaching girls sexually and his overaccentuated urges to conquest. The latter won out, and he has since had continuous Don Juan activities in which numbers of conquests were very important to him. Among them all, only four were 'special.' They were all tremendously appealing to him sexually. Each was dark haired and about five feet tall. His mother was dark haired and five feet tall.

"As the analysis proceeded he has grown steadily better able to separate the infantile hangovers from present day reality situations. After he had learned about his wish to be feminine, to give up his penis to please his mother, he began to stack this wish up against his masculine competitive longings and to assign them their correct roles. When he had worked over the Oedipus attachments to his mother, he became less interested in promiscuity. His fears of marriage as a 'cutting down upon' his freedom gradually diminished to the point where he could accept being a father. He then legally married the girl he had been living with—a dark haired girl, five feet tall. When pregnancy occurred, he was pleased and proud; since a baby girl has been born, he is quite able to accept the father's role. He is a fairly considerate husband. He is able to show sympathy, affection, self-sacrifice. He can be critical for cause, both at home and more realistically in business relations with men. When his mother died several months ago, he accepted it in average fashion.

"Recently we have cut down to two sessions per week, and he is polishing up various details and synthesizing matters. His episodes of anxiety are not yet totally absent, but he is able to minimize them and can always find for himself what had re-animated a bit of the old castration dread. His breadth of vision has markedly widened."

He was not seen between the time he started analysis (October, 1947) and March,

1950. His physical condition was unchanged except that he had gained about 30 pounds in weight (he was very tall and had been quite thin, so that it was possible for him to carry this increased weight); but the blood pressure figures were the same, and eyeground examination showed the generalized narrowing of the arterioles that is indicative of a preorganic hypertensive change. Otherwise the cardiovascular-renal system was normal.

The patient was seen a year later and again two years later, and although he reported himself free of symptoms, making good in business, successful in marriage and the father of a fine child, his blood pressure has continued to be elevated at the same figures as had been previously obtained.

References

Alexander, F.: Psychosom. Med., *1:* 173, 1939.

Alexander, F., and Saul, L. J.: Psychosom. Med., *1:* 139–153, 1939.

Ayman, D.: J.A.M.A., *95:* 246, 1930.

Ayman, D.: (*a*) J.A.M.A., *95:* 246, 1930; (*b*) J.A.M.A., *96:* 2091, 1931.

Ayman, D.: M. Clin. North America, *28:* 1151, 1944.

Ayman, D., and Pratt, J. H.: Arch. Int. Med., *47:* 675, 1931.

Binger, C. A. L.: Bull. New York Acad. Med., *21:* 610, 1945.

Binger, C. A. L., Ackerman, N. W., Cohn, A. E., Schroeder, H. A., and Steele, J. M.: Personality in Arterial Hypertension, The American Society for Research in Psychosomatic Problems, N. Y., 1945.

Bright, R.: Guy's Hosp. Rep., *1:* 338, 1836.

Corcoran, A. C., and Page, I. H.: J.A.M.A., *116:* 690 (Feb. 22), 1941.

Corcoran, A. C., Dustan, H. P., and Page, I. H.: Ann. Int. Med., *43:* 1161, 1955.

Dunbar, F.: (*a*) N. Y. State J. Med., *36:* 423, 1935; (*b*) Am. J. Psychiat., *92:* 1095, 1936; (*c*) Am. J. Psychiat., *91:* 541, 1934; (*d*) Emotions and Bodily Changes. Columbia University Press, N. Y., 1938; (*e*) Psychoanalyt. Quart., *8:* 18, 1939.

Fahrenkamp—cited by Dunbar (*d*), p. 228.

Fishberg: Hypertension and Nephritis. 4th ed. Lea and Febiger, Philadelphia, 1939.

Freis, E. D.: M. Ann. District of Columbia, *23:* 1, 1954.

Gardner, J. W., Mountain, G. E., and Hines, E. A., Jr.: Am. J. M. Sc., *200:* 50, 1940.

Gull, W. W., and Sutton, H. G.: Tr. Med. Chir., *55:* 273, 1872.

Harris, R. E., Sokolow, W., Carpenter, L. G., Jr., Friedman, M., and Hunt, S. P.: Circulation, *7:* 874, 1953.

Huchard: Traité Clinique des Maladies du Coeur et de l'Aorte. 3rd ed. Paris, 1899.

Kalis, B. L., Harris, R. E., Carpenter, L. G., and Sokolow, M.: Presented to the Western Society for Clinical Research, Feb. 1956.

Menninger, K. A.: (*a*) Bull. N. Y. Acad. Med., *14:* 198, 1938; (*b*) Man against Himself, p. 378. Harcourt, Brace and Co., New York, 1938; (*c*) Bull. New York Acad. Med., *14:* 198, 1938.

Pfeiffer, J. B., Jr., and Wolff, H. G.: *in* Life Stress and Bodily Disease. Research publication, Association for Research in Nervous and Mental Disease. Williams and Wilkins Co., Baltimore, 1950, p. 929.

Pickering, G. W.: Ann. Int. Med., *43:* 919, 1955.

Reiser, M. F., Brust, A. A., and Ferris, E. B.: Psychosom. Med., *13:* 133, 1951.

Reiser, M. F., Rosenbaum, M., and Ferris, E. B.: Psychosom. Med., *13:* 147, 1951.

Saul, L. J.: Psychosom. Med., *1:* 153, 1939.

Shapiro, A. P.: J.A.M.A., *160:* 30, 1956.

Shapiro, A. P., Myers, T., Reiser, M. F., and Ferris, E. B., Jr.: Psychosom. Med., *16:* 478, 1954.

Smith, H. W., Goldring, W., and Chasis, H.: J. Clin. Investigation, *17:* 263, 1938.

Stewart, H. J.: Bull. New York Acad. Med., *14:* 681, 1938.

Stevenson, I. P., Duncan, C. H., Flyn, J. T., and Wolf, S.: Am. J. M. Sc., *224:* 286, 1952.

Thomas, C.: Am. J. M. Sc., *224:* 367, 1952.

Von Basch, S.: Ueber latente Arteriosclerose. Vienna, 1893.

Weiss, E.: J.A.M.A., *120:* 1081, 1942.

Weiss, E.: Emotional Factors in Cardiovascular Disease, Charles C Thomas, Springfield, Ill., 1951.

Weiss, E., English, O. S., Fischer, H. K., Kleinbart, M., and Zatuchni, J.: Ann. Int. Med., *37:* 677, 1952.

Chapter VIII

The Gastrointestinal System

FUNCTIONAL DIGESTIVE DISTURBANCES

The abdomen has aptly been called "the sounding board of the emotions." It is well known that the student before examination may develop anorexia, nausea or diarrhea. The business man may get indigestion, heartburn and actual abdominal pain at the time of important conferences or in connection with financial reverses. The worrisome housewife develops indigestion and constipation when there is trouble with the children or housecleaning to be done. Even the child who is not making a happy adjustment with his playmates in the school yard may have an attack of vomiting some morning about school time.

In spite of the fact that this relation between psyche and soma is well known, it is surprising how little attention has been given to this matter in the actual management of gastrointestinal disorders. Psychotherapy in gastrointestinal illness has been handled rather superficially in medical articles and textbooks. Advice to avoid worry and strain and to get plenty of rest, and investigation of the work conditions or marital relationship for sources of tension, have been the extent of psychotherapeutic investigation. It is hoped that we can carry our readers further into an understanding of the connection between emotional problems and gastrointestinal illness and, by the discussion of cases illustrating various disorders, show the relationship of personality trends to symptoms.

Organ Language. It is understandable that the abdomen should be the sounding board of the emotions since (1) it is so well supplied with autonomic nerve fibers, both of the sympathetic and parasympathetic systems—the lines of communication between brain centers and the viscera—and (2) the behavior patterns of the gastrointestinal tract which have been utilized in infancy are carried to the brain and lodged there in that reservoir of memory, the unconscious mind. Given the proper stimulus, and without awareness on the part of the individual, impulses may be sent out by way of the autonomic nervous system from the unconscious mind recreating that same infantile behavior pattern. The tense business man may bluster about and struggle consciously to be effective while unconsciously there is a strong desire to be a little

Page 254

boy, once again under the protection of his mother and father and depending upon them for his sustenance, rather than trusting, as a mature person would, that a big order from some uncertain source may come his way. Security and sustenance are indissolubly related in the unconscious mind through the very nature of a human being's infantile existence and hence, *if security is threatened* later in life, the organ which regulates sustenance may be disturbed in its normal functioning. The gastrointestinal tract is phylogenetically the oldest system in the body and hence most likely to be used to express an emotion which cannot be dealt with through the regular channels. When urges such as loving or being loved, giving protection or being protected, are not successfully carried out with the mind (emotions), this oldest system of the body will be called into service in a vain attempt to solve the problem in a primitive way. This is what we have referred to as "organ language." Since it is not intended for service of this kind, the gastrointestinal tract is doomed to failure and its misguided effort to be of service for such psychological purposes causes dysfunction and discomfort which results in illness.

A notable deficiency in psychosomatic theory has been the inability to point to a mechanism of emotion that would account for the variety of ways the effective qualities of experience may act on autonomic centers. MacLean in his studies on the "visceral brain" (p. 62) has shown that this area, the limbic system, is largely concerned with visceral emotional functions and appears to be so strategically situated as to be able to correlate every form of internal and external perception. In other words, the possibility exists in this region for bringing into association not only oral (smell, taste, mouth) and visceral sensations, but also impressions of the sex organs, body wall, eye and ear. MacLean states that these relationships of the rhinencephalon have far-reaching implications in regard to psychosomatic medicine. While intellectual functions are carried on in the newest and most highly developed part of the brain (the neocortex), our effective behavior is dominated by a relatively crude and primitive system (visceral brain). This situation, says MacLean, provides a clue to understanding the difference between what we "feel" and what we "know."

Emotional Trends.   The first important studies of gastrointestinal illnesses were made by Franz Alexander and his co-workers of Chicago. They studied the psychological structure and life situations of patients suffering from functional disorders of the gastrointestinal tract as well as of those who have suffered from peptic ulcer and colitis. Their studies led to the conclusion that the gastrointestinal tract, because of its three major functions of taking in, retaining and eliminating, was especially suitable for the expression of these three elementary emotional tendencies, particularly if their normal expression through the voluntary motor system was inhibited. They found some correlation between certain personality trends and different disturbances of the gastrointestinal tract and also a relationship to the part of the tract involved. Thus, the upper end of the tract, according to its normal function, was well suited to express the receptive or taking-in tendencies, whereas the lower end of the tract was more suitable for the expression of the retentive and giving trends.

GASTRIC PROBLEMS.   The important personality trends in the gastric neuroses and peptic ulcer cases were intense unconscious receptive and acquisitive wishes which the patient could not admit to himself. It was thought that the stomach symptoms were conditioned by the repressed receptive and aggressive taking-in tendencies which served as chronic psychic stimuli to the stomach function. In other words, many patients who have a strong, unconscious need for affection, a strong desire to be appreciated and taken care of, psychologically translate these trends as a need to be fed. At the same time they cannot admit these impulses to themselves and as a consequence *overcompensate* with a demonstration of great energy and great endeavor. They are afraid to be dependent or ineffectual. Nevertheless, their strong unconscious tendencies to be dependent cause reactions in the gastrointestinal tract so that the stomach tries to serve a double function. It tries to serve the function of emotional reception of love as well as acting as the organ of digestion. This is too difficult for the stomach to accomplish because the need to be taken care of (fed emotionally) is acting as an unusual or foreign and constant stimulus. This stimulus is responsible for overactivity and excessive secretion beyond the digestive needs. Moreover, this "need to be fed and loved" trend is being opposed by a stronger need to reject the unacceptable idea of dependency and ineffectuality and this conflict may result in stomach symptoms. More will be said on this subject in connection with the discussion of peptic ulcer.

BOWEL PROBLEMS.   The trend of the colitis cases was quite different in that such patients unconsciously felt that they had the right to take and demand for "they always gave sufficiently." They did not feel guilty or inferior because of a desire to receive or take because they were already giving something in return for what they received. This something they gave was the childish substitute of feces for real values— sometimes "given" to express aggression. It was pointed out in the chapter on psychopathology that during the period of training in sphincter control the child's first "stock in trade" was his excretions. Up to the time of the beginning of toilet training much has been given to the child and little asked for in return. Then during the bowel training period he learns to attach unusual value to his feces because he is praised so highly for producing them. With his willingness to understand the rules of cleanliness he can give "gifts" of the contents of the bowel or bladder to those who care for him. The emotional value attached to feces may never be sufficiently relinquished to other life values such as work, cooperation, money or artistic talent. Later in life such people may fail to produce anything worthwhile in these fields and feeling anxiety, guilt or shame about this, which they cannot admit, they fall back upon the childish pattern of "giving feces." This may sound fantastic to one who has given little thought to such matters or to one who has failed to live closely with the thinking and behavior of children or neurotics.

So often we hear it said that the application of more common sense is the answer to these problems, but it takes more than common sense to understand the seemingly irrational behavior of children or the closely related unconscious trends of the neurotic. What it really takes is "uncommon sense" plus a knowledge of psychopathology. It is not to be forgotten that it is during the period of toilet training that a personality trait called *ambivalence* becomes predominant. In other words, the child often develops conflict because of his own desires which are at odds with the wishes or demands of his parent. One part of him loves his parent and wants to *control* the bowel movement as the parent wishes. Another part of his personality defies such wishes and says, "No, I hate you and do not care about control. I care more for my comfort and pleasure than for your love and I'll spite you by moving my bowels any time I wish." *Underneath a surface attitude of love may rest strong hostile feelings.* Hence a poorly built up control easily breaks down later in life to show an emotion such as hostility by means of a disturbance in bowel function.

Constipation. In patients with constipation the dynamic emotional trends express the idea that since the individual took or received nothing he was under no obligation to give. Alexander and his colleagues assumed that the constipation was a reaction against the obligation to give. Here again we must think of the relationship between mother and child during toilet training and remember that constipation or incontinence may express lack of cooperation on the part of the child. He holds back either to spite the parent or out of a fear that his bowel movements may prove harmful or offensive. He not only believes that his bowel movements offend when deposited in the wrong place but he stretches this belief to cover bowel movements at any time or place. Nearly everyone is familiar with the person who cannot urinate or defecate in the presence of others, for example, in a public toilet. It is a short step from this inhibition to the development of constipation even in privacy. Constipation may be a kind of "anal impotence," in some cases growing out of anxiety over offending. In other cases it may mean indifference or stubbornness about producing something for others.

Incidence of Functional Disturbances of the Gastrointestinal Tract. Psychosomatic disturbances of gastrointestinal function occur in healthy people subjected to unusual emotional stress; they are among the commonest manifestations of emotional stress in neurotic people. Of 269 neurotic patients encountered in a medical outpatient department Friess and Nelson found that 41.5 per cent mentioned gastrointestinal symptoms as their chief complaint. The abdomen is, indeed, the sounding board of the emotions.

Among the patients with "functional gastrointestinal disorder" are many who complain of *heartburn.* Contrary to the general opinion this is not due to excessive gastric acidity. Investigation shows that a change in the tonus of the esophagus probably produces the symptom. Tumen and Cohn studied 120 consecutive patients referred because of a variety of gastrointestinal disturbances and found 30 per cent who complained of heartburn. Acid regurgitation, belching, nausea, constipation and diarrhea were other symptoms complained of by this group. Nervous tension appeared to be the outstanding cause of heartburn. An explanation of the functional nature of the problem, education in proper eating habits and, occasionally, more intensive psychotherapy made the major contribution to relief of the patient.

In a study of 3000 cases from a clinical and roentgenological viewpoint Dwyer and Blackford found that gross lesions in the stomach and duodenum accounted for gastric symptoms in only 15 per cent of the cases. In a consecutive series of 15,000 patients with chronic dyspepsia examined in the Mayo Clinic, 15.5 per cent had deformities which were interpreted as being the result of peptic ulcer. A little more than 2.6 per cent had gastric carcinoma. This made a total of 18 per cent of patients whose digestive disturbances were the result of gross organic diseases of the stomach and duodenum. In commenting upon this material Eusterman stated that these, and a few other rare lesions, would account for about 20 per cent of the cases of chronic gastric disturbances. But he added that in private general practice the percentage might not exceed 10. He concluded that gastric disturbances arising reflexly from abdominal viscera other than the stomach are responsible for from 30 to 40 per cent of all cases and that in his opinion the neuroses constitute about 25 per cent of the total. Then from 15 to 20 per cent of gastric disturbances are attributable to disease of organs remote from the stomach, but only on infrequent occasions are such gastric disturbances the sole expression of an extragastric disorder.

CHRONIC DYSPEPSIA.   Rivers and Ferreira, also from the Mayo Clinic, studied 4223 cases of chronic dyspepsia and divided them into four types: *organic, reflex, systemic* and *functional.* Under organic causes of dyspepsia they included diseases or anomalies involving the tissues of the stomach or duodenum. Among the reflex causes of dyspepsia they included diseases of the appendix, gallbladder, biliary ducts, pancreas or intestines and renal stone or other conditions which reflexly disturb the chemistry or mechanics of the stomach or duodenum. Among the dyspepsias of systemic origin they included those due to disturbances of metabolism, toxemia, deficiency diseases, or dysfunction of the organs of internal secretion. Functional dyspepsias were assumed to include the disturbances in normal gastroduodenal activity not resulting from demonstrable disease elsewhere in the body. Of this type they mentioned the various gastric neuroses, constitutional inadequacies and habit dyspepsias and the various dyspeptic manifestations of chronic nervous exhaustion. Their functional cases totaled 25 per cent as shown in the accompanying chart (Chart 3).

TESTING ACCURACY OF DIAGNOSIS.   In an effort to test the accuracy of the diagnosis of nervous indigestion, Wilbur and Mills studied the records of 354 patients who after examination at the Mayo Clinic received the diagnosis of functional or nervous indigestion or its equivalent and who were reexamined at the clinic more than seven years later. In 303 cases no evidence of organic disease was found in the follow-up examination. The results suggest a diagnostic accuracy of at least 85.6 per cent for functional dyspepsia in that series. There were 39 cases in which organic disease of the gastrointestinal tract was found at subsequent examination, but in 19 of the 39 a final diagnosis of duodenal ulcer was made and this represented the most common diagnostic error in the series. We will comment later on whether this represents a serious error in the etiological approach to peptic ulcer.

DIAGNOSIS BY EXCLUSION.   Thus when chronic dyspepsia is approached even from a purely organic standpoint the incidence of functional disorders is at least 25 per cent. We have commented previously on the inadequacy of this type of investigation which for the most part represents diagnosis by exclusion. The point that we particularly wish to make is that the diagnosis of functional illness must be established not simply by exclusion of organic disease but on its own characteristics as well. *In other words, neurosis has its own distinctive features to be dis-*

Functional	24.7%
Peptic ulcer	9.0%
Cholecystic disease	8.6%
Cardiovascular disease	5.6%
Migraine	4.5%
Constipation	3.9%
Arthritis and fibrositis	3.8%
Organic nervous disease	3.7%
Pelvic disease	3.6%
Cancer stomach	3.0%
Chronic appendicitis	2.2%
Genito-urinary disease	2.0%

Types of dyspepsia (total cases)

Systemic	37%
Functional	25%
Reflex	22%
Organic	14%
Undetermined	2%

Chart 3.   The twelve most common causes of dyspepsia in order of frequency. (Rivers and Ferreira: J.A.M.A., *110*:2132, 1938.)

covered by personality study. Only in this way can serious errors in diagnosis and treatment be avoided. If this is true then it must naturally follow that personality studies are just as important in the problems of chronic dyspepsia as laboratory investigations. This applies not only to problems in which evidence of structural disease has been excluded but also to patients who present evidence of physical disease and emotional factors such as ulcer and cholecystic disease. Just as we cannot limit ourselves simply to the exclusion of organic disease in the so-called purely functional group, so even more importantly is there the necessity for study of the emotional life in patients who present evidence of an organic lesion.

PSYCHOSOMATIC STUDY.   Physicians with greater interest in psychological medicine find a much higher percentage of patients with symptoms referable to the gastrointestinal tract in whom emotional factors are chiefly responsible for the illness. Stevenson, in a study of 150 patients presenting themselves to a gastrointestinal clinic, found that there was an important emotional problem in two thirds of the cases and Robinson, in a thoughtful analysis of 50 patients with digestive complaints, found that in two thirds of them no organic lesion or unhygienic habits could be discovered to account for the symptoms. Moreover, the latter author felt that many patients have digestive symptoms as a manifestation of personality disorder before they develop organic disease of the digestive tract and that the latter might be prevented if they were successfully treated. This seemed to be especially true with respect to peptic ulcer. He went on to say that functional nervousness, including fatigue and anxiety, was by far the greatest detectable cause of recurrences of peptic ulcer symptoms, and in many instances it seemed likely that the same etiological factors were initially responsible for the ulcer. He thought, therefore, that the question could legitimately be raised as to how many of these patients might have escaped peptic ulcer if their functional nervousness had been recognized and treated in the first place.

In an analysis of the records of 5000 consecutive patients studied at a diagnostic clinic Gregg and Snowden found that 47.7 per cent of all patients with even comparatively severe symptoms referable to the digestive tract had no evidence of organic involvement. Another analysis by Emery of 2839 patients of whom 19 per cent had applied for relief of gastrointestinal symptoms found that only 50 per cent presented evidence of organic disease. Of these 2839 patients 1000 were from the wards of the Peter Bent Brigham Hospital, 1000 were consecutive out-patients, 839 were from general practice and in addition there were reports from 500 consecutive autopsies.

We made a study of 100 consecutive patients encountered in the practice of internal medicine who were considered to have psychosomatic gastrointestinal problems. Forty-four cases were classified under neurosis with gastrointestinal symptom formation; 30 as somatic disease plus symptoms in part of emotional origin; 14 as vegetative neuroses.* Seven cases fell in the group of psychoses with gastrointestinal symptoms and 5 were labeled as hypochondriasis. Among the neurotic cases with gastrointestinal symptoms 21 were listed as anxiety state, 16 as conversion neurosis, 5 as compulsive neurosis, and there were 2 phobias.

Thus, as is well known, every variety of personality from the well adjusted to the psychotic may have psychosomatic disturbances of the gastrointestinal tract. As in other surveys the percentage of somatic disease represented about one third of all cases seen. This leaves, so far as the gastrointestinal field is concerned, about two thirds of the cases in which the gastrointestinal symptoms appear to be wholly or in part of psychogenic origin.

We are persuaded from our own studies that emotional factors are the *chief* cause of gastrointestinal complaints and many other authors besides those cited could be quoted in support of this viewpoint. Nevertheless, if we took only the organic studies above referred to, in which diagnosis is established by exclusion, we would still have the very con-

---

* A distinction is made between somatic disease with emotional factors, such as structural alterations of the gall tract with stone formation, and the vegetative neuroses. In the latter are included cardiospasm, peptic ulcer and ulcerative colitis.

siderable number of 25 per cent of all patients with chronic dyspepsia labeled as functional, and to be approached, therefore, from a psychological standpoint.

The cases which follow will illustrate some of these syndromes and call attention to the relationship between personality trends and symptom formation.

Case 18. Constipation Related to Social Anxiety; Good Response to Brief Psychotherapy

History and Symptoms. M. F., a white girl, aged 19, complained of constipation of several years' duration, headaches, ulcers in the mouth and fatigue. She had never been seriously ill and there were no other symptoms of importance except that she had had enuresis until she was 16. Her father and mother had never been compatible and the patient had always been aware of tension in the household. Finally the parents separated and the four children, of which our patient was the youngest, remained with the mother. At this time the enuresis ceased.

The general physical examination showed no evidence of disease and it quickly became apparent that more important than the symptoms complained of was a high degree of social anxiety in a hysterical person which had interfered with her social development. From a genetic standpoint, insecurity in personal relationships was of course related to the insecurity of childhood and the constipation apparently was a reflection of the tension growing out of social situations. One such situation which seemed to cause the most trouble was an attempt to compete with a pretty cousin. Anticipation of such competition would bring about headache and constipation which were aggravated by erroneous ideas regarding bowel obstruction and toxic poisoning.

Improvement. The origin of the symptoms was made clear and when she was reassured about the insignificance of the constipation and encouraged by the physician, who assumed the role of a friendly parent in trying to give her a little more self-confidence and urging her to cultivate new interests and friends, she improved remarkably and blossomed out into a friendly creature who in turn "found everybody more friendly." Incidentally constipation no longer was a problem.

Recurrence. During a period of a year and a half her progress continued and then suddenly new symptoms appeared. She suffered from vertigo and had pain in the epigastrium. It was not difficult to ascertain that she was forced again to compete with a very attractive young woman in a new circle of boys and girls in which she felt insecure. Once more a single interview succeeded in pointing out the source of anxiety and permitted once again the opportunity for more reassurance and the acquisition of more confidence.

Role of Psychotherapy. Here, without mentioning psychotherapy, the physician assumed the parental role, taking the attention of the patient away from the symptom and attaching it to life circumstance. It would be fine for this young woman to have the advantages of psychoanalysis but since that is clearly out of the question we must get along with less. There is no doubt that transference played the important role and was deliberately utilized. Re-education regarding the emotional development was the basis of the brief and, in this case, superficial psychotherapy, although of course psychotherapy is not necessarily superficial just because it is brief. Nor is there any denying that the patient remains dependent on the physician and will have to return from time to time as she encounters new situations. Is it not better, however, to treat a patient with constipation in this manner than to make this young woman dependent upon laxatives or enemas and perhaps start her on a career of gastrointestinal invalidism? So often we find the criticism leveled at the psychotherapist that he does not cure people—they remain dependent upon him. No one expects the diabetic specialist to cure his patient; when he regulates the diet and adjusts a dosage of insulin and carries his patient along successfully everyone is satisfied. Why cannot the psychotherapist be permitted the same privilege of administering reassurance and enlightenment in regulated dosages, knowing full well that in the greatest number of instances he cannot hope to achieve cure but only strive to make the patient a healthier, happier and more efficient individual?

Case 19.   "Nervous Indigestion"; Traumatic Precipitating Event

History and Symptoms.   A white man, age 27, stated his complaint as "nervous indigestion." Since the fall of 1934 he had suffered from attacks of "nervous indigestion," and he had been under the care of many physicians. Complete studies had been made which failed to reveal any organic cause. His principal digestive complaint was nausea which came in attacks when there was any variation from his established routine. Further inquiry revealed that the nausea was preceded by loss of appetite, considerable belching, a feeling of tension in the throat, and the fear that he might vomit or have an involuntary bowel movement. Because of these fears he tried to plan his days in such a way that he was never far from a lavatory and it was only after some time that we learned how far his business and social life had been restricted by this necessity. With an attack he had considerable anxiety, the hands and feet became cold, and he perspired freely. The attacks had become more frequent and he had lost a few pounds in weight.

He had been a sickly child, had had considerable ear trouble and many operations. He felt that he had been much handicapped by his frequent hospital experiences and long illness and that it was only about the time of puberty that he began to develop as a healthy person should. During his teens he considered himself in excellent health.

The mother had died suddenly of heart disease at the age of 52 in 1931. The father died from a gunshot accident at the age of 57 in 1934. More will be said of this shortly. An older sister was in good health. The grandparents had been long lived and there was nothing else of medical importance in the family history.

Physical Examination and Laboratory Studies.   The patient was tall and thin and seemed somewhat pale. Temperature, pulse and respirations were within normal limits and the blood pressure was normal. The general physical examination disclosed no evidence of organic disease. Ordinary laboratory studies were within normal limits and a gastrointestinal x-ray series, including a barium enema, showed no evidence of abnormality. Gastric analysis showed a fairly high acid curve but no other indications of abnormality.

LIFE SITUATION

The patient's family had always been in comfortable circumstances and he had been a pampered child, chiefly because of the many illnesses during his childhood. He had grown up to be a healthy young man, however, and considered himself well adjusted. He took an active interest in his father's business and during the summer months when he was not at school he frequently acted as his father's chauffeur.

In the fall of 1934 he was hunting with his father when a gun was accidentally discharged and his father suffered serious head injuries which shortly proved fatal. In spite of the fact that he was in no way responsible for the accident he continued to blame himself for his father's death and it was at this time that his "nervous indigestion" began. As time wore on and more and more people in whom he had confidence assured him that he was blameless, his digestive disturbance improved somewhat but he was never completely free of discomfort.

Meanwhile he had married and apparently had adjusted well to marriage and had also begun a business career in which he was getting along satisfactorily. His illness, however, had circumscribed his activities severely so that he felt that his opportunities for advancement were limited so long as his illness continued. On close questioning it was revealed that it was not so much nausea which disturbed him as the idea that he might embarrass himself and the people around him by the necessity for vomiting or having an involuntary bowel movement and hence he could never allow himself to be far away from a toilet. His days were planned so that he would always know that he was going to be near a toilet and his appointments were planned with special regard to meal time so that he would be unlikely to vomit. This in spite of the fact that he never once had vomited. The constant thought in his mind whenever he made any social plans or business appointments was "suppose I take sick—what shall I do?"

TREATMENT

On reviewing his early life history it became clear that he had always suffered from an overstrict conscience and that as a young man he could never forgive himself for any mishaps, actual or fancied. For example, he had done less experimenting with sex than the average young man and yet he could not get rid of his guilt over what were relatively minor transgressions.

The next point of importance which developed was that although he had stated at first that all guilt over his father's death had vanished, it became quite clear with detailed conversation that he still held himself responsible and when anything happened which reactivated his guilt an attack of indigestion, which was in reality an anxiety attack, would occur.

Overconscientious Personality. We pointed out that he was the kind of personality that was overconscientious and overscrupulous and hence burdened with excessive guilty feelings and that he therefore was bound to react as he had to his father's death. He confessed that he always labored under the feeling that he did not deserve to be happy. After this conversation, in which he had an opportunity to air his feelings thoroughly, he felt considerably elated and engaged in some frivolity with his associates at his place of business. He later stated that in the middle of this sudden happiness a thought had flashed through his mind, "something terrible is going to happen." It thus became clear that he did not have the capacity for enjoyment unless at the same time he envisaged the possibility of suffering.

Toilet Training. Conversation with an old family retainer who had acted as his childhood nurse revealed that he had been subjected to very strict toilet training and that during his first year or year and a half he cried a great deal when he was placed on the toilet, and finally a physician had said that there was something the matter with the rectum and a minor operation was performed. After that he became very docile but developed some fears, such as fear of the dark, and during the period of his ear infections he frequently became "hysterical when attended by the physician."

On subsequent occasions it was pointed out to him that his fears of vomiting or of having a bowel movement and thus embarrassing himself and other people were probably related to his overstrict training in childhood when he became docile on the surface but probably resentful and spiteful underneath. And now it would seem that his fears of "making a mess" were probably related to unconscious wishes to do just that in order to gain attention. In other words, fears, in reality, are often disguised wishes, and so we can readily understand that as a pampered and spoiled youngster whose attention had been focused unduly on toilet training he may have turned to this means of attracting attention from his caretakers even though it involved censure or punishment. Now as an adult his conscious wish was just the reverse, that is, to be neat, clean, orderly and over-conscientious, but still existing within him were certain infantile patterns of behavior which translated themselves into bodily symptoms.

Results of Treatment. For the first month or six weeks he was seen once a week and was given an opportunity to relate the intimate details of the hunting accident which preceded the onset of his illness. It was revealed to him how his overconscientious personality was bound to react to his father's death by his self-accusation of being responsible. By airing this matter on several occasions, combined with the reassurance that we were able to give him, and the conviction that he had taken more responsibility than he should have, his anxiety gradually diminished and his digestive attacks became less intense and occurred at longer intervals. Combined with this was the explanation concerning his early life toilet training and bowel habits and how they in turn were now related to his present difficulty. He became a much happier and more efficient person and was finally able to plan his days so that he no longer thought of the question of being near a toilet. No longer did his "life surround his bowel movements."

Follow-up. Although relieved of his digestive troubles he continued to be disturbed by social problems for which he was referred for psychoanalysis. After completion of a successful analysis he has remained well, effective and happy.

SUMMARY

A young man developed "nervous indigestion" following his father's death from an accident for which he felt responsible. Guilt reactivated infantile patterns of behavior of the gastrointestinal tract. After much medical investigation and treatment, satisfactory recovery followed psychotherapy.

Nervous Vomiting

In a review of 140 cases of functional vomiting Wilbur and Washburn found that in most cases there were characteristic clinical and diagnostic features. Continued vomiting which is usually without effort, nausea, or significant abdominal symptoms and which occurs within an hour after meals is typically functional. Most patients were women between the ages of 20 and 40 years, who, while they were relatively healthy in appearance, presented evidence of instability of the nervous system. In 60, or 43 per cent of the cases in the series, operation, and particularly appendectomy, had been performed for the vomiting without benefit to the patients.

Many types of treatment had been tried but the keystone of treatment was psychotherapy.

The following case is illustrative:

Case 20. Nervous Vomiting; Repressed Sexuality

History and Symptoms.   A young married woman was first seen in February, 1940, complaining of attacks of vomiting, which were usually most pronounced in the morning.

The trouble began about three years before and on two occasions during that period she had hospital observation but no organic cause had been found. The diagnosis on both occasions had been spastic colitis.

Menstruation had been established normally and was always regular but she was often troubled with vomiting at the time of her menstrual period. The patient had been married for a little more than two years but had not been pregnant.

Physical Examination and Laboratory Studies.   The patient had lost a few pounds in a recent severe attack of vomiting but still was a well-nourished person without signs of obvious illness. The general examination disclosed no evidence of organic disease. Gynecological examination was negative.

Routine laboratory studies and basal metabolism were within normal limits. Gastric analysis and gastrointestinal x-ray series disclosed no abnormalities. Biliary drainage and cholecystogram were normal.

LIFE SITUATION

The patient reported that her fear of eating in the presence of others led her to shun people and thus her life was more or less secluded. She became a burden to her husband and parents by restricting their social lives and making increasing demands on their attention.

Her illness began at the age of 11, shortly after the birth of her youngest sister. At that time, she developed fears for her father's safety whenever he failed to return home promptly. These fears continued for several years. At 17 she suffered from attacks of nausea whenever she had a date with a young man. On one occasion, when kissed by a man, she suddenly became sick and began to vomit. The vomiting persisted for several days, during which time she was conscious of what she described as a "sexual" odor which had emanated from the man. Shortly thereafter she was courted by another man whom her mother urged her to marry. She resented her mother's interference, but submitted to her wishes, and, as will be seen, characteristically reserved the right to punish her later. On the day of her marriage she felt nauseated and the wedding trip had to be shortened on account of her persistent vomiting. On her return home, she spent a week with her mother until her symptoms subsided. Sexual relations during this period were impossible because of vaginismus. When they did take place later she was, for the most part, frigid.

Dependence on Mother.   During the few years of her married life, there had been a number of recurrences of vomiting. The attacks usually occurred when she was angry with her husband or parents. On one occasion, she began to vomit after being advised by a physician to have a child. This, by the way, was his therapeutic advice as a cure for her vomiting. During a period of vomiting, she was troubled by disturbing thoughts concerning the death of relatives. She stated that there seemed to be a "devil" inside her which the vomiting served to get rid of. When well, the patient was a comparatively adequate housewife, but during attacks she became helplessly dependent and spent most of her time with her mother. She had even crept into bed with her mother and cuddled up like a baby and at times had insisted that her mother literally feed her with a spoon. In addition, her vomiting became particularly violent in the presence of her mother, although when alone she could usually control it. She said that she could not give her mother the satisfaction of seeing her comfortable. Once, when her mother remonstrated with her, the patient replied that the mother had no reason for complaining since she, at least, was well; furthermore, she must suffer because the patient was her child. One could readily see the personality of a self-centered individual who had very little consideration for others and tried to dominate them in a passive and dependent way.

Vomiting an Expression of Hostility.   Her resentment against her mother at the time of her marriage was based on her belief that her mother was rushing her into marriage in order to get rid of her. This led to a half-conscious desire to punish **the** mother by her illness, which was actually expressed when she said that her **mother** deserved to suffer for making her get married when she wasn't ready for it. In her anxiety to obtain affection, however, she had to convince herself that she was in love with her husband lest he leave her. On the other hand, however, she felt that he did not really love her, but had married her because of her money. She suspected that he preferred his own mother to her. This unspoken accusation always came up whenever she quarreled with him; at which times she would feel a surge of intense hatred against him, associated with death wishes. This was tied up with the suspicion that her father did not really love her but preferred her mother, which caused her to be resentful against him. The attacks of vomiting at such times were the result of her unexpressed hostility because her passive nature would not permit her to express her hostility directly.

TREATMENT

As she was permitted little by little to understand some of the forces that were responsible for her vomiting attacks they diminished in number and intensity and for a period of about one year she enjoyed freedom from vomiting. Then came a recurrence however, in connection with conflict over having a child. Psychoanalysis was recommended, which she carried out successfully and, in the following five years, she has had two children and has remained quite well.

SUMMARY

A young white woman, with markedly repressed sexuality, developed frequent vomiting attacks after a marriage to which she had assented because of her mother's urging. Her passive and dependent nature did not allow her to express hostility openly but instead her unconscious mental forces caused her to vomit as though to say, "I cannot stomach this situation." Gradually she was made aware of some of her hostile feelings and, following successful psychoanalysis, no longer had to resort to vomiting attacks to express herself. This led to considerable improvement not only in her gastrointestinal function but also in her ability to taste more fully of life in general.

Mental Depression with Digestive Symptoms

Elsewhere we will discuss the clinical importance of recognition of depression as a definite clinical syndrome. One of the characteristic features of this symptom picture is a digestive disorder. The following case is illustrative.

Case 21.   Two Attacks of Mild Depression with Digestive Symptoms, Precipitated by Financial Losses

A man of 40 complained of loss of appetite, sleeplessness, depression of mood, "all-gone" feelings and shakiness.

History and Symptoms.   He had always considered himself a healthy person and had never suffered from a serious illness.

Father and mother were living and well, as were three brothers and two sisters. There was no mental or nervous disease in the family.

He had always been successful in the real estate business until the depression began and then he had lost a great deal of money. He had tried to keep the knowledge from his wife because he didn't want to disturb her but gradually he found himself sleepless and then came loss of appetite and symptoms related above.

Physical Examination and Laboratory Studies.   The patient was a well-nourished, robust, white man with normal blood pressure and normal cardiovascular system. The remainder of the physical examination was negative except for the presence of a few hemorrhoids which he attributed to recent constipation. Routine laboratory studies were negative.

LIFE SITUATION

A review of his life situation indicated how dependent he had been upon his real estate holdings for a feeling of security, and it was pointed out that now that he had lost considerable of his estate his "all-gone" feelings and his feelings of shakiness indicated his insecurity. It was obvious that he was in no critical situation from the viewpoint of his financial standing and a discussion of this fact seemed to revive his spirits somewhat. He was placed on ¼ grain phenobarbital three times a day and in a week reported that he was sleeping slightly better but still felt depressed in mood, especially in the morning. His treatment was continued and it was recommended that he once more interest himself in golf, in which he had been active previously but had given up when things were going bad at the office. One month later he reported that he was feeling quite well again. After this the patient was not seen for a period of seven years.

Recurrence of Depression.   Once more he complained of "all-gone" feelings in the lower abdomen, loss of strength, no ambition, awakening early in the morning with a feeling of depression, loss of appetite, and a loss of weight.

He himself observed that the same financial circumstances were at work now as had been true on the previous occasion. Not only was business bad but he felt himself under great financial strain. He felt that he had gotten over his previous depression quickly and that he had been well since and he hoped that the same thing might happen once more.

Again physical examination failed to disclose any evidence of organic disease and once more he was reassured when he had an opportunity to discuss his actual financial situation which was in no sense critical. Again it was pointed out to him that he had always been the kind of person who had to accumulate funds and real estate holdings in order to feel secure and that on two occasions in question his losses had been great enough to threaten his security. Hence, he became depressed, symbolized his weakness with his "all-gone" feeling in the lower abdomen, and at the same time lost his appetite as he had lost his zest for living. Once more he was placed on mild sedation and once again he responded although some depression of mood continued for several months.

SUMMARY

A middle-aged white man who presented the clinical picture of mental depression complained chiefly of digestive symptoms. Recovery followed superficial psychotherapy. Recurrence at the end of seven years followed the same precipitating cause. The importance of recognizing the mental depression rests not only upon the psychological approach to the digestive symptoms but on the greater necessity of recognizing a serious disorder of the personality often leading to suicide. This point is discussed more fully elsewhere (p. 47).

GALLBLADDER DISEASE

As previously stated one of the most frequent causes of chronic dyspepsia is gallbladder disease. When a patient has suffered from attacks of gallstone colic and studies demonstrate the presence of gallstones it is universally recognized that operation is essential for cure. Nevertheless, the role of the emotions in the possible development of gall tract disease; in the precipitation of attacks of colic; and in the preparation of the patient for surgery and then recovery from operation, is a matter with which general medicine has not sufficiently concerned itself. We are beginning to realize the importance of emotional factors in the so-called "noncalculous cases" which, in reality, are often simply upper digestive tract reactions to an irritable colon rather than actual gallbladder disease (Tumen). To remove such a gallbladder is very similar to the problem of the removal of the appendix in so-called chronic appendicitis. All of the evil consequences of *polysurgery,* plus the additional complications furnished by the difficult anatomy of the gall tract, are apt to follow.

The following cases illustrate some of these points.

Case 22.   Mental Depression; Repeated Hospital Admissions; Cholecystectomy

History and Symptoms.   A 43-year-old white woman complained of crampy pains in the right upper quadrant of the abdomen, referred to the right shoulder region, right pubic region and, in fact, over almost the entire abdomen; frequency of urination during the day, and some burning sensation; loss of appetite; loss of weight; occasional vomiting; irritability. The patient had consulted many physicians and had had many hospital admissions.

PAST HISTORY.   The first hospital experience was in December, 1934, when salpingo-oophorectomy and appendectomy were done. The hospital reported a pathological diagnosis of bilateral pyosalpinx. In March, 1935, the patient was admitted to the same hospital suffering with an abscess of the hand. A good recovery was made. In December, 1935, she was first admitted to the Temple University Hospital for abdominal complaints but did not remain more than twenty-four hours. She refused x-ray studies and signed a release in order "to go home for the holidays." About one year later she was again admitted to the Temple University Hospital, following an attempt at suicide by taking bichloride. She remained in the hospital three weeks. In January, 1937, she was admitted to another hospital where a diagnosis of possible gallbladder disease was made, because of the same complaint, *i. e.,* abdominal pain. In November, 1937, she was again admitted to the same hospital for four weeks with the same diagnosis. In December, 1937, again she was admitted to the same hospital, diagnosis undetermined. January, 1938, she was admitted to still another hospital where she remained for five days. No diagnosis was made. She returned to the previous hospital, was operated upon for gallbladder trouble and the gallbladder was removed. Following cholecystectomy deep jaundice developed. Five days later an end-to-end suture of the cystic duct was performed. The patient remained at home and felt fairly well for about two months but then the same symptoms returned and increased in severity. She continued to come to the surgical outpatient department and finally was admitted to the hospital once more.

FAMILY HISTORY.   The father was a drunkard and the mother was a highly nervous person. Three brothers were living; one had tuberculosis, one was highly nervous, a third was apparently healthy.

MARITAL HISTORY.   The patient was married at the age of 17, had two children, and then separated from her husband because "he ran around with other women and contracted a venereal disease." She believed, probably correctly, that this was responsible for her first operation.

She had been married to her second husband for eighteen years and had one child by him. She stated that she loved this husband but was sorry that her ill health had made her a burden to him. He was a textile worker but for the past five years had been irregularly employed.

There were symptoms in many parts of the body: blurry vision, headaches, and occasional tinnitus; "a lump in the neck causes nausea"; dyspnea and constipation; frequency of urination; shooting pains and aches in the right leg and weakness of both legs.

Physical Examination.   Temperature, pulse, respirations and blood pressure were normal. Fingernails were badly bitten. There was a vasomotor flush over chest and abdomen. The patient was fairly well nourished and appeared quite comfortable. There was a small nodule in the right lobe of the thyroid gland. It was fairly soft and possibly cystic. The remainder of the physical examination revealed nothing unusual. The heart was normal, the lungs were clear. The abdomen was soft and easily palpable without indication of tenderness or rigidity. We were unable to make out any organs or masses. The extremities were normal.

Laboratory Studies.   December, 1935, first admission; urine negative, blood count good, serological tests normal. October, 1936, admitted with a diagnosis of mercurial gastritis following attempt at suicide.

After recovery a gastrointestinal x-ray study, including cholecystogram, was negative.

Operation, January, 1938: histological report on gallbladder, "cholesterosis," gross description indicated a normal gallbladder. No stones were found.

Here then, was a woman approaching middle age, who had had ten hospital admissions in the past four years. She insisted that she had had constant abdominal pain for more than that length of time. She had been constantly disturbed by the idea that she might have a cancer. Many doctors had told her that she was "nervous rather than sick" and one even intimated that she was "crazy."

Our complete studies failed to show any evidence of organic disease other than the small nodule in the thyroid gland. There was no question that the first operation was a justifiable one; it is doubtful if the same could be said of the second. It was probably done for the reason that a great many gallbladder operations have been done, that is, because of the patient's complaint of excruciating and intractable pain, and insistence upon "something being done" in spite of negative x-ray study. Unquestionably surgeons are becoming more reluctant to operate for supposed gallbladder disease when pain of the type described by this patient is the chief symptom and the findings are negative.

LIFE SITUATION

The patient maintained that she was well until 1934 when she had her operation for pelvic infection. Upon closer questioning, however, we discovered that there was a period of anxiety and depression in 1926, at the time of her mother's death. At that time she also had the same pains and discomfort as on her hospital admission.

Childhood.   This patient's childhood was a most unhappy one. Her father drank and mistreated the entire family, and on more than one occasion seduced her sexually. She was always afraid of her father and never felt comfortable in his presence. Her mother seems to have been a passive person who contributed very little to offset the cruelty and lack of affection shown by the father. The patient described herself as always a worrisome person, never happy and never having enjoyed any social life. Her only pleasures were cooking, sewing, ironing. She had never made any close friends or taken an active interest in anything outside of her home. She was extremely irritable and depressed, and cried a great deal. She was very discouraged about herself and very pessimistic about the future.

Mental Depression.   We seemed to be dealing with a woman who had been a chronically depressed person all her life, and at times the depression had reached the degree of psychosis. In 1936 there seems to have been a genuine suicidal attempt.

As in all other severe emotional disturbances there was some conversion of anxiety into somatic symptoms. However, in most cases of psychotic depression somatic symptoms are not in the foreground; instead there is a great deal of guilt and self-condemnation usually over real or imagined sexual advances and over digressions, real or fancied. With what we knew of this patient's childhood there was no doubt that she had a great deal of hostility and guilt over sexual feelings aroused in her at an early age. Many patients, instead of emphasizing self-condemnation, find a solution through punishment by somatic suffering, *i. e.,* somatic symptom formation. We were sure that in this case the sexual seduction by the father had weighed heavily upon the patient's conscience.

As we observe depressed people we often wonder how it is that they can condemn themselves for so long and suffer so much. We wonder why no one can reassure them. The answer seems to be that the quantity of guilt is so great that a long period of expiation is necessary in order to balance the imaginary sins committed. This patient complained of a terrible feeling of loneliness and sadness which at times was almost unbearable. *From her long list of hospital admissions it would seem that she could endure her feelings only for a certain period of time and then she had to enter the hospital and offer herself up for study and operation in order to relieve her guilt feelings.*

The Unconscious Wish To Be Sick.   This was the most important question, that is, "the unconscious will to remain sick." *We could not escape the notion that she achieved a certain satisfaction out of her suffering.* This is a very important consideration in medicine and in this kind of patient is of paramount importance. Because such a patient is really eager to be operated upon and because of her very insistence upon the continuous and excruciating nature of the pain from which she suffers, one can easily understand how she may prevail on a very sympathetic surgeon to operate. This is particularly true when such patients meet a surgeon who is not loath to operate. Thus, we can say that a willing and even eager patient who derives a certain satisfaction from being hospitalized and operated upon and a surgeon who is ever ready to wield a knife is a very unfortunate combination. A great many patients with numerous scars on the abdomen serve as testimony to this combination.

We felt that following operation this patient should have entered a sanatorium and remained there for a period of at least six weeks where she could have had rest, relaxation and diversion, and a beginning could have been made in reeducating her emotional life. She needed to become acquainted with her feelings of guilt and hostility, and to realize how much energy she had been using up all these years keeping them repressed. She needed to learn how to enjoy something else besides cooking, sewing and ironing, and remaining isolated within her own home.

Unfortunately no such sanatorium exists for a patient with a small income. A suitable private institution would cost at least $50 weekly. We felt that unless this patient understood more of her psychic problem, and how it was producing symptoms, then it was highly probable that she would remain just as sick or grow worse.

Furthermore, the danger of another suicidal attempt was always present in a patient as emotionally ill as this one. Any patient who attempts suicide is very sick emotionally, whether neurotic or psychotic. Such persons in one stroke seek to destroy a body they despise and a mind which feels detached from the world.

It was emotional misery which had to be treated in this patient. The husband and two daughters seemed to be of the kind who could give some cooperation. Any relief which could be produced in her emotional state would give a corresponding improvement in symptoms relating to her body. Once the patient had begun to see these connections a beginning would have been made toward a return to health. To be realistic, an entirely symptom-free individual was not to be expected in this woman who had suffered so much over so many years. Probably the best we could hope for was improvement with greater efficiency and less suffering. It is difficult to help a patient who has so few memories of a happy adjustment to everyday life. But even though the therapeutic task was formidable the eventual results would probably be better than symptomatic drugs or surgical treatment could produce.

SUMMARY

A middle-aged woman had repeated hospital admissions because of abdominal pain. On one occasion she attempted suicide. Finally the gallbladder was removed but symptoms returned. Personality study indicated that symptoms of mental depression antedated the hospital admissions and, in reality, constituted the main feature of this clinical problem. Unfortunately we were unable to follow her after she left the hospital.

The following case also shows a recurrence of "gallbladder symptoms" after removal of the gallbladder. A good result followed superficial psychotherapy.

Case 23.   Chronic Dyspepsia; Cholecystectomy

History and Symptoms.   A white woman, 47 years old, complained of pain in the epigastrium and in the gallbladder region, nausea and heart burn, headache and fatigue. A peculiar feeling in the back "like cold water" extended down to the buttocks. The first attack had occurred twenty-two years ago after the birth of a son. She had been told that the trouble was due to gallbladder disease and the gallbladder was removed. A few years later, however, the same trouble recurred and she had been having attacks which lasted for several weeks at a time ever since. In the summer preceding her present illness an attack had lasted for two weeks and during that time there had been some looseness of bowel as well. There had been no other serious illnesses in the past medical history.

The father had died of a stomach ulcer twenty-two years before, that is, just before the onset of her illness. The mother had only recently died of heart disease. Three sisters and a brother were living and well.

The patient had been married for twenty-five years and had two children, one 22 and the other 20, both of whom were well. The husband was living and well.

Menses had always been irregular and painful and the menopause had been established at the age of 42 without untoward incident.

The patient had always been heavy but there had been a gradual increase in weight since her marriage until she weighed 185 pounds. She had always chosen her diet carefully and especially in the last two years because of the digestive disturbance. She felt that cream and milk made her "bilious" and she had cut her diet down in many other respects, eating very little meat, fish or eggs, so that her protein intake was less than average.

Physical Examination and Laboratory Studies.   The patient was an obese woman with normal blood pressure and normal cardiovascular system. There was slight tenderness in the epigastrium but no organs or masses could be made out. Aside from a few varicose veins the examination of the extremities was normal.

Routine laboratory studies, including sedimentation rate and basal metabolism, were within normal limits. Gastric analysis showed normal motility and low acid values. A gastrointestinal x-ray series, including barium enema, was normal. Biliary drainage showed an absence of cholesterin and calcium bilirubin pigment in the centrifuged specimen so that on that basis we felt reasonably sure that gallstones were not present.

LIFE SITUATION

The patient described her life as a happy one. She had been brought up in a comfortably fixed and what she considered a cultured family and had never known serious hardships. At 26 she had married a man who had always been very kind to her, and her children had brought them great pleasure.

In discussing her married life she kept referring to the fact that her husband was very generous and very kind, that he had been successful in business and enjoyed a fine reputation among his business associates and in their social group. The emphasis that she placed on his fine qualities sounded as though she had more to say on the subject, so that while no particular reference was made to the matter upon the first two or three occasions when we saw her, a note was made to reintroduce the subject on a subsequent occasion.

Meanwhile with reassurance that there was no evidence of organic disease and the recommendation that she enlarge her diet to include proteins such as meat, fish, and fowl, she reported considerable improvement.

Marriage Problems.   On the fourth occasion that she was seen, which was about six weeks after her first visit, she reported that she had been very uncomfortable on that day in spite of the fact that she had eaten very little. She stated that her mouth was dry and that she had an ice-cold sensation in the back which was the same "as her mother complained of just before she died." Conversation was directed along the lines of her day-by-day activities for the two or three days preceding the onset of this difficulty and it became clear that she was disturbed about her son who was about to get married and she, like so many mothers, felt that the girl was selfish and not quite suited for him. Although the engagement had been known for some time the marriage date had just been decided upon, which brought the acute realization to her that she was about to lose this fine son to what she considered a scheming and designing, selfish girl. When this matter was discussed her behavior revealed that she had a great deal of feeling on the subject. The opportunity was provided to discuss the young lady's qualifications dispassionately and it was pointed out somewhat jokingly "that all mothers felt that way about their sons."

This afforded an opening for discussing her own marriage. With a great deal of reluctance, and with constant apologetic statements that her husband was a very good man, she brought out the fact that her chief problem had been that she considered her husband beneath her from a cultural or class standpoint, that he was a coarse and uncultured fellow while she considered herself a refined and sensitive person. She had never really been happy and had never been free of the thought that she was married to a clod or peasant. The feeling with which she discussed the matter revealed how intensely she felt. It was obvious that beneath these feelings were the physical problems concerning her inability to be demonstrative with him, or for that matter to receive his affections. Consequently she lived a life of fantasy and romance so far as her secret feelings were concerned but felt like a caged animal in regard to her actual life. She had always been frigid with her husband and on many occasions had considered leaving him but had been held back by the thought of her children. But even at this late date she harbored the fantasy that once her children were married she would establish a home of her own. She had a great deal of self-pity and at the same time some apprehension and guilt about discussing for the first time in her life her real feelings about her husband. Still, the matter was received in an uncritical fashion and she seemed to derive a great deal of relief over having unburdened herself at last.

SUMMARY

A middle-aged woman had had her gallbladder removed for epigastric pain but trouble recurred. The remainder of the symptom picture was that of anxiety. Long-standing marital maladjustment, which had been "suffered in silence," stood in the background of the physical complaints. Uncritical listening and reassurance brought relief.

PANCREATIC DISEASE

Interesting clinical observations of patients with pancreatic disease by Savage, Butcher and Noble emphasize the complicating influence of psychological factors. In patients with carcinoma of the pancreas, depression and anxiety appeared to be related to: (1) the fact that the diagnosis is often missed and the patient left in a state of chronic uncertainty; and (2) some peculiar characteristic of the pancreas, possibly related to its parasympathetic connections, which makes the patient more aware of the seriousness of the onslaught upon his organism. The nature of this manifestation deserves study since it may touch upon the basic problem of anxiety.

The study of patients with pancreatic necrosis revealed a long history of somatic and psychological maladjustment often associated with the use of alcohol and the establishment of a vicious self-destructive cycle. There was a high incidence of mental disturbance during the acute attacks of pancreatic necrosis.

In chronic pancreatitis, persistent anxiety, depression and narcotic addiction were prominent psychiatric problems. This has been confirmed by Dlin in a study of seven cases.

In another report Savage and Noble state that at least 26 cases of verified carcinoma of the pancreas have been reported in which the symptoms of depression, anxiety and insomnia dominated the clinical picture. They estimate that 10 per cent of all cases of carcinoma of the pancreas are complicated by psychiatric problems. They report two additional cases of carcinoma of the pancreas, in both of which psychiatric conditions were diagnosed. Both patients received psychotherapy and carcinoma of the pancreas was not suspected. Both patients showed frank psychiatric symptoms and were typical of the cases of carcinoma of the pancreas that had come to the attention of the psychiatrist. They were in the involutional age group and had minimal organic findings and localizing signs. The authors emphasize that the alleviation of symptoms by suggestion and psychotherapy is not incompatible with malignant disease, and if the patient improves the diagnostic error is perpetuated.

THE IRRITABLE COLON SYNDROME ("MUCOUS COLITIS")

The irritable colon syndrome is a disorder rather than a disease. Therefore the term is preferable to "mucous colitis." When patients are told that they have "colitis" they think in terms of organic disease (and are often treated as though they had an organic disease) whereas if they are told that they suffer from irritable colon, due to tension of emotional origin, they are apt to regard the disorder less seriously. Then, instead of continuing to search for the cause of "colitis," they can be taught to look upon the irritability of the colon as a manifestation of behavior. Instead of being so concerned about their extra bowel movements and so preoccupied with bowel function, they learn to adjust themselves to their few movements and instead of regarding themselves as invalids or semi-invalids they think of the bowel disturbance as a minor handicap and go about their business.

One difficulty enters into this concept on the part of the physician and patient and this applies to a great variety of psychophysiological reactions. The physician and patient, after a time, may take the reaction for granted, look for an emotional disturbance in connection with each exacerbation of the disorder and neglect routine physical studies. This was brought home to us quite forcibly in a woman of advanced years who had had an irritable colon syndrome for the greater part of her life but complained of more persistent pain; sigmoidoscopic examination disclosed cancer of the sigmoid colon.

White, Cobb and Jones regard the manifestations of "mucous colitis" as manifold and inconstant and often overshadowed by other symptoms. They consider that mucous colitis is probably responsible for the removal of more undiseased appendices than any other cause and Tumen believes that more than half of the patients initially labelled as having chronic gallbladder disease are eventually identified as having unstable colons. A total of 60 patients were carefully studied by White, Cobb, and Jones over a period of two years. Of these, 57 were studied psychologically with sufficient thoroughness to afford considerable insight into the role of precipitating emotional factors as well as the types of personality encountered in persons with this syndrome.

Clinical Syndrome.   In general, patients with irritable colon syndrome suffer from constipation or diarrhea with some form of abdominal pain. In most cases the stools are small and are either mushy or composed of hard pellets. As a rule the symptoms are seen in patients who have a labile autonomic nervous system with associated cardiovascular instability. The lower abdominal pain is generally accompanied by upper abdominal symptoms such as nausea, heart burn, belching and sour eructations. Cardiovascular symptoms such as palpitation, sweating, faintness and "neurocirculatory asthenia" are often encountered. On physical examination the sigmoid colon is often palpable as a firm "rubber hose." In general the diagnosis is based on the presence of either constipation or diarrhea as a major complaint, the presence of distress in the lower part of the abdomen related to bowel function, absence of organic disease of the colon and x-ray demonstration of disturbed colonic motility and tonus.

Emotional Factors. Diarrhea as a symptom of nervousness has been recognized for centuries. Moreover, from the very first it has been known that the emotions had something to do with mucous colitis. J. M. DaCosta described the syndrome with accuracy, noted the condition of the rectal mucosa through a speculum and recognized the tense, emotionally unstable nature of the patients. Thus he was responsible for delineating the syndrome to which he gave the name "membranous enteritis." Although infection has been held responsible no one has succeeded in isolating a specific organism. Allergy, of course, has been suspected but repeatedly throughout the literature one meets with the belief that mucous colitis is a secretory and motor neurosis of the intestines.

Severity of Neurosis. Of the 60 cases of mucous colitis studied by White et al., 57 were divided into two groups, a more neurotic group, handicapped by neurotic symptoms or personality problems, and a less neurotic group, composed of persons whose personality problems were not incapacitating. With 4 exceptions all of the 28 less neurotic patients showed a close relation between emotion and aggravation of symptoms. In the more neurotic group there were 29 patients and of these only 17 showed a close relation between emotion and colonic symptoms. No specific personality type was found and the authors could only conclude that mucous colitis appeared to be a somatic response to a type of nervous tension. Mental states conducive to this response appeared to be anxiety, resentment and guilt. Associated depressive, neurasthenic and hypochondriacal features were often present and in about half the cases a rigid type of thinking, similar to that seen in the obsessive-compulsive state, was present. Diminution in energy output was also characteristic of the group as a whole. Most of the persons required more than the average amount of sleep. Asthenia was present in the great majority and in some cases was incapacitating. There was a high incidence of sexual difficulties; two-thirds of the women were frigid and libido was diminished in the men.

The Organic Approach. P. W. Brown of the Mayo Clinic in a discussion of "Doctoring the Bowels" presented the matter dramatically. We quote his graphic description.

"The following hypothetical history portrays a composite picture of this group which is under consideration: A patient of either sex, but usually a woman between the ages of twenty-five and forty-five years, comes in with the chief complaint of stomach and bowel trouble. During the narrative her memory is frequently refreshed by reference to her notes.

"Her abdominal troubles date back five to twenty or more years, and consist chiefly of distress from gas, bloating, soreness in the right lower abdominal quadrant, and constipation, with occasional attacks of diarrhea which follow catharsis. The stools often contain considerable mucus, and if they are hard, bloody streaks are noticed. The distress has been present more or less all these years, and bears no regular relationship to meals or types of food. The woman never has been strong, although able to attend to usual duties and social demands. Moderate exertion, such as that accompanying a morning of shopping, or having a few guests for dinner is followed by much abdominal distress and fatigue. Dull headaches and a nagging backache are added burdens.

"Further the woman gives the history that because of the distress referable to the abdomen and back, she submitted to an operation, in the hope that appendectomy and straightening of the uterus might help. Prior to operation, a roentgenologic examination had suggested the presence of chronic appendicitis. Relief was obtained for about three months, when the same or even more marked symptoms recurred. Opinions were expressed that perhaps the gallbladder or adhesions might explain the symptoms. In view of the occasional bloody streaks in the stool and anal discomfort, treatment of hemorrhoids was carried out with relief of these local symptoms. Some time later the question of possible focal infection was raised and tonsillectomy was performed. As symptoms persisted, further investigation resulted in a diagnosis of 'chronic colitis.' In consequence, a succession of diets was recommended: no fried or greasy foods, no starches, no meats except fish and breast of chicken, proteins and carbohydrates not to be taken at the same meal, commercial vitamin substances to be included in the diet, only raw fruits and vegetables, only cooked fruits and vegetables, and so on. These diets have resulted in a distaste for food, fear of everything to eat, loss of weight, and actually more or less a state of deficiency. As a logical accompaniment of diet the arch demon, colonic irrigation, was invoked, and the irrigations soon made the mucus and distress worse, in spite of thorough flushing. Other roentgenologic studies resulted in a report of falling of the colon and stomach, for which an abdominal support was prescribed. Almost incidentally, reference is made to peculiar or difficult environmental, social and economic problems, but these are the basis of much, if not all, of the physiologic disturbances. At present the patient eagerly asks, and all in one breath, 'Is the gallbladder diseased and will its removal cure colitis? Will continual abdominal irritation make a cancer? What can be done to restore the normal position of the fallen organs? Just what should my diet be? Are my adhesions causing my trouble?'

"Physical examination reveals an apprehensive, undernourished woman. The abdominal wall is relaxed and all muscles are flabby. A large tonsillar tag is present on the left side. Tenderness is present on palpation of the cecal region. Bimanual examination of the pelvis discloses only retroversion of the uterus.

"The laboratory data are as follows: Roentgenologic examination of the stomach gives evidence of an apparently normal organ. A cholecystogram indicates that the gallbladder is functioning normally. The mucosa of the rectum is normal. No roentgenologic evidence of organic disease of the colon is elicited. The roentgenograms depict the expected influence of the abdominal support on the position of the colon.

"The present condition in this hypothetical case is obvious; it is the end result of *doctoring the bowels*. Interpreted as a group, the diagnosis in such cases is that of functional intestinal disturbance associated with a state of physical and nervous exhaustion. Usually there is a greater or less degree of biologic inferiority, for which the patient is hardly to blame. It is this, with the characteristic emotional, nervous instability, that makes for so much difficulty. We are so constantly harassed by the fear of missing something that we may fail to appreciate how profound are the physiologic disturbances produced by nervous and emotional strain. Although we may need special guidance in some cases, this is not a problem for the psychologist or psychiatrist. It has been suggested that undergraduate training unwittingly stresses organic disease at the expense of a broader and more sympathetic appreciation of emotional and nervous problems. There need be neither thought of curtailing the instruction in organic disease, nor of deprecating correction of organic conditions of nervous patients, but by a fuller understanding of the emotions we may be of greater service."

The following cases illustrate some of the points that have been discussed.

Case 24.   Irritable Colon ("Mucous Colitis")
The Conflict of Marriage and Career

History and Symptoms.   A young white woman complained of "colitis," pain in the abdomen, worse after eating, and excessive gas. She also complained of "feeling nervous."

The past history was negative. Menses began at the age of 11, had always been regular and were not painful although for a few days before the period there was some feeling of tension.

The present trouble began while she was at college during a hectic period when she was cramming for examinations. She had an attack of "intestinal grippe" and then the colitis began. Prior to that time she had been constipated on occasions but at the time of which we speak she had five or six bowel movements daily accompanied by considerable amounts of mucus but no blood. She was given bismuth and after about two months the condition subsided. After that she had trouble "only when nervous" but for a few weeks she had been so distressed by the necessity for frequent movements that it was interfering with her work and pleasure. Following graduation from college she obtained a position in a social agency and in addition took courses in a school of social work.

When her bowels were disturbed she also suffered from poor digestion and had some abdominal pains and bloating. She stated that her appetite was poor and that she "filled up easily after eating." There had been no loss of weight.

In addition to the above complaints she had found herself more nervous and irritable during the month prior to this study.

The mother and father were living and well except that both were subject to indigestion. There were two brothers and two sisters; one sister had been operated upon for exophthalmic goiter and the remainder of the siblings were well.

Physical Examination and Laboratory Studies. The general physical examination disclosed that she was somewhat overweight and that the blood pressure was slightly elevated (150/100). The hands and feet were cold and moist. Examination of head and neck was negative. The heart rate was rapid but the heart was within normal limits and the sounds were normal. The lungs were clear and resonant throughout. The abdominal examination showed slight tenderness over the descending colon. Urine examination was normal; blood count was good; the examination of the stool showed the presence of mucus but no other abnormalities were detected. The blood sedimentation rate was within normal limits. Basal metabolic rate was plus 5 and the gastrointestinal x-ray series, including a barium enema, showed a normal gastrointestinal tract. Incidentally a small dermoid cyst of the right ovary was apparent in the x-ray film but it was obvious that this had no significance from the standpoint of her illness.

LIFE SITUATION

This young woman immediately revealed herself as a tense, highstrung and unstable person who talked the language of modern psychology and casually considered the idea of intensive psychotherapy for herself. She explained that while she was a junior in college, her mother became nervous and depressed and had to be examined by a psychiatrist, who stated that the mother's condition was due to the menopause. At the same time the patient suffered from sleeplessness and the college physician recommended that she too should consult a psychiatrist. This period corresponded with the former attack of "colitis." She stated that as the mother's condition improved, she, herself, became better.

Already she had determined to major in psychology and to embark upon a career of social service. However, her work in the social agency had not satisfied her and she had become increasingly aware of her limitations so far as advancement in her work was concerned; but at the same time she had been unable to decide between a desire to perfect herself for further progress in her career and an offer of marriage. For about a year a man many years her senior, whom she described as cultured, traveled and intelligent, had been attentive to her and recently had made a proposal of marriage. She could not choose between marriage and a career but admitted that the thought of marriage and its responsibilities were very disturbing to her.

The patient was informed that the conflict between marriage and a career probably had some relation to her illness and that it would be helpful to her if she were able definitely to make up her mind. She was seen again a month later and was much improved and announced that she had given up the idea of marriage and had determined upon a period of intensive study to perfect herself for her career.

Principles of Management. The problem of the psychotherapeutic management of such a case as this one is to realize that we are dealing with an emotionally immature and hence weak individual who cannot meet certain life situations in an adequate manner. In the process of treatment he is given an opportunity to release certain tensions and expose psychic weaknesses. The physician who understands and is sympathetic to the idea that it is not reprehensible for patients to have such psychic weakness has the opportunity to strengthen them psychologically by discussing better ways of adaptation to their specific life situation.

The physician should try to find out by careful history-taking what the bowel function is trying to express, then introduce the formulation to the patient and try to get him thinking of the bowel as misbehaving or as trying to express some attitude he does not recognize or accept consciously. For instance, it can be pointed out that those lacking courage move their bowels under the influence of fear rather than attacking the enemy in the usual fashion. Instead of using the voluntary muscles there is regression to a childish symbolic expression of aggression through the bowel. This reeducational effort helps the patient to meet his situation with the mind rather than by means of "organ language," *i. e.,* diarrhea; and as the individual becomes stronger and able to express his emotions on a more mature level, his bowel, too, should become stronger and better able to "control" its action.

Case 25.   Irritable Colon Syndrome; Anniversary Reaction

A white man, 36, first seen in February, 1953, complained of "trouble with his insides; something isn't working right." He had suffered from loose stools for years. He also complained of poor sleep, dizziness and poor appetite. There was a questionable history of duodenal ulcer four or five years before and also questionable hypothyroidism—neither had been confirmed.

A friend had been told that "his stomach trouble was nervous but had to have a stomach resection."

The patient had bilious attacks as a youngster. The father had always had stomach trouble which "was not properly diagnosed." He died following an operation for appendicitis. The patient was then 17.

LIFE SITUATION

The patient is an only child and has helped support his mother since his father's death. The mother objected to his marriage in 1943 and he had not seen a great deal of her since, although he continued to support her and keep in touch with her.

The mother became ill in 1953, was operated upon in June, and died from metastatic cancer.

The patient was bothered by thoughts that now that he had a happy family his mother was not able to join them and that he had not seen enough of his mother or done enough for her. He had a flare-up of difficulties. He was convinced that "there was something organic" so that he had to have a very thorough survey, including a gastrointestinal series, to reassure him.

Thereafter, he remained well until June, 1954, when he had another attack lasting a few weeks which he attributed to hard work, long hours and irregular meals. But it also happened to correspond to the *anniversary* of his mother's death and it was quite obvious that this had stimulated the former guilty feelings in regard to her. Rehearsing this material led to improvement and he has remained well since.

Case 26.   Irritable Colon Syndrome

A white man, a physician, 36, first seen in July, 1951, complained of diarrhea which began in 1937 while in professional school. At that time it was so disturbing that he remained out of school for a year, improved, but had had flare-ups since, lasting a week or two. The previous year he had a thorough study including a complete gastrointestinal x-ray series and sigmoidoscopic examination; the findings were negative.

He knew "there is some kind of a tie-up between the nervous system and diarrhea but which causes which?"

LIFE SITUATION

He was always a serious minded, conscientious and perfectionistic person who worried about examinations at school and was much concerned about the fact that his father, a machinist, had to make sacrifices to see him through professional school. The patient himself worked in order to help pay board and tuition.

There was no evidence of disease in the general physical examination and we confirmed the diagnosis of irritable colon syndrome but urged the patient to regard it as a disorder, "not a disease." We also talked about his conscientiousness and perfectionism. He spoke of the pressures under which he lives, how he can't stand getting behind in his work— he would rather lose patients. He doesn't like to be under obligations to people; especially he cannot be in debt.

We saw him again about six weeks later and once more we talked about his difficulties in getting through school. His father had wanted him to be an engineer but the patient insisted on studying medicine and hence felt very guilty toward the father, especially because the father had to borrow money to help him go to school and purchase equipment when he finished. It was a great sacrifice for the father who had to reduce his standard of living. Since then the patient had tried to pay him back but his father refused to accept the money, which only increased the patient's guilt.

He has had frequent dreams of practicing without a license and much anxiety that "they would catch up with him." Thus he indicated his guilt about doing something illegitimate. He could not tolerate the mantle of authority—couldn't do something better than his father. In other words, he dared not take his father's place.

After rehearsing this problem in some detail the patient was able to state on a subsequent visit that he was fine, and one year later he reported that he was still well. He knew this indicated real improvement because for the previous several years he always had flare-ups at this time of the year. Now he occasionally has a little looseness of the bowel for a day or two but he adopts the attitude "so what," and goes on about his business. He has been a little less demanding on himself, does not push so hard in his professional work, and both his wife and office assistant had noted that he was more relaxed.

Case 27.   *Irritable Bowel Syndrome and Impotence*

A white man, 31, complained of belching and burning in the epigastrium. The trouble had begun two months before with belching, constipation and some looseness of the bowel. He had taken drugstore remedies, limited his diet and "was afraid that he had an ulcer."

He had always been healthy, "had been a big eater, and able to digest anything."

Physical examination showed a robust, well nourished, white man with no evidence of organic disease. It was noted that the patient gagged easily and when we tried to do gastric studies he was unable to swallow the tube. Routine laboratory studies were negative and the gastrointestinal x-ray series was normal except for hypermotility of the intestinal tract.

We reassured the patient about the absence of ulcer, and other organic disease, and explained his illness on the basis of irritable bowel syndrome. We told him that emotional factors were important in this kind of problem.

LIFE SITUATION

He talked about the strain of hard work but it was only on a subsequent visit that he discussed impotence, which had begun about three months before, that is, just before his gastrointestinal disturbance. He had not mentioned it because "he didn't think it was relevant." He had always been potent except for an occasional premature ejaculation but on one occasion after his wife had returned from a vacation he had felt a pain on orgasm and had thought of injury. Then he became impotent for about a month but recovered spontaneously.

Following reassurance and some insight on this question he became practically free of symptoms "except for slight belching" and six months later reported himself well with the exception of occasional belching and slight looseness of the bowel on infrequent occasions. But he "paid no attention" to this and carried on in spite of it.

SUMMARY

A young white man suffered from indigestion on the basis of irritable bowel syndrome. A temporary period of impotence had immediately preceded the onset of the irritable bowel syndrome. Reassurance was responsible for considerable improvement.

ULCERATIVE COLITIS

The problem of ulcerative colitis focuses attention on the question of the interrelationship of psychic and organic disease. The general outline of this topic was discussed in the introduction. Here we need only say that we are not interested in trying to prove that psychological factors are directly or solely responsible for ulcerative colitis. Indeed, we do not believe it. In line with our thesis that all illness should be regarded from the standpoint of the whole organism, we are interested in psychological factors in ulcerative colitis only as one part of a complicated psychosomatic problem.

Emotional Factors.   When we come to a consideration of ulcerative colitis, we find general medicine less impressed by psychic factors in the etiology than in mucous colitis. The opinion is frequently expressed, "Yes, it is easy enough to understand that mucous colitis is a functional disorder but you can't tell me that psychic factors can produce actual ulcers of the bowel." We would be the last to see a direct relationship between psychic factors and ulcer formation. As in many other disorders involving the vegetative nervous system we consider the psychological panel only one phase of this disorder. Some such scheme as that erected for the discussion of the pathogenesis of essential hypertension might apply equally well to ulcerative colitis so far as the part that the psyche plays is concerned (p. 229). However, it is an important phase upon which not a great deal of work has been done. Murray presented some impressive psychological case studies and Sullivan, from the medical standpoint, stressed the importance of psychogenic factors in etiology and considered psychotherapy of the utmost importance in treatment. He felt that when the emotional conflict is solved, the intestinal motility returns to normal, the chief irritative factor is removed from the colon, which can then take care of its bacterial invaders, and the disease may promptly disappear.

PERSONALITY STUDY.   Daniels made an intensive psychological study of a case of ulcerative colitis associated with hysterical depression. The patient was a woman of 32 with a history of three previous attacks of ulcerative colitis. Daniels observed her during most of the five years of her fourth attack. Between the third and fourth attacks the patient had two pregnancies. The first pregnancy was terminated by giving birth to the fetus in the toilet, which acted as a great psychic shock, and the second pregnancy was followed by a prolonged attack of tachycardia and a period of partial amnesia.

Psychiatric investigtaion revealed deep unconscious hostile trends and suicidal drives. The patient was treated by intensive psychotherapy and by this means was able to emancipate herself from her family. Then the social service department assisted her in reestablishing her own home. This was an essential step in treatment. Hay fever and asthma appeared for the first time during this transition and there was an acute flare-up of palpitation and diarrhea when she made the actual step of moving to a new home. Although some frequency of stool persisted and there was an occasional diarrhea brought about by the emotional factors, there was no further clinical evidence of ulcerative colitis. The colon showed chronic changes which suggested that complete recovery was unlikely and the persistence of depressive personality trends further modified the prognosis. The greater severity and duration of the last attack seemed to have been due to an altered life situation with conflict related to a neurotically conditioned marriage reinforced by the child-birth for which she was ill-prepared. Various medical procedures had relatively little effect on the disease process and it seemed fair to assume that psychotherapy had been an important factor in the arrest of the disease and in her social recovery.

DEPENDENCY. In another contribution to the subject Daniels states that such persons are apt to be self-centered and dependent. This dependency is shown particularly toward the mother or a mother substitute, frequently an older sister, and is often maintained by an enforced docility on the part of the patient, who says, "My mother would rather have me sick at home than well and away." Dominating in-laws frequently take over this family role.

Furthermore, the ulcerative colitis patients are sexually immature and do not carry responsibility well. They are apt to break in a crisis and have been called the "giver-uppers." In this way they are the opposite of the peptic ulcer patients who as a rule are aggressive and seek responsibility. The males with ulcerative colitis are inclined to be passive, pathologically attached to their mothers, frequently unmarried; the women, who are more frequently married, are apt to be the "fussy" type of housewife.

RELATION TO PSYCHOSIS. Daniels further noted mental depression in association with this disease. He pointed out the importance of recognizing this to be a primary emotional disturbance rather than a secondary reaction to an uncomfortable and disagreeable disease. The depression is usually reactive in nature following some loss or frustration. The psychic structures of ulcerative colitis and manic-depressive psychosis suggest a possible relationship that deserves further study. In regard to precipitating factors it seems that acute upper respiratory infections, emotional upheavals, and possibly pregnancy are the most frequent elements entering into the onset of the disease. The rigid and immature personalities of the majority of these persons make them unable to tolerate reverses or crises well or to undertake the necessary steps in emotional sexual maturity of engagement, marriage and child-bearing. While many such women get safely through pregnancy, an attack often follows after childbirth. In the men a frequent conflict is that between attachment to the mother and a desire to get married.

Sickness or death of a near relative, particularly the mother, seems especially traumatic in these cases. Losses of money or financial worries also act as precipitating factors.

BEREAVEMENT AS PRECIPITATING FACTOR.   Lindemann, in a study of 45 patients with ulcerative colitis, noted that various forms of bereavement are the most important precipitating factors. In 26 of 45 patients a close relationship existed between the loss of an important person and the onset of the illness. Dependency became a threat to the patient after bereavement because of a tendency to primitive behavior patterns, colored by fantasies of extreme violence, and asocial behavior marked by aggressiveness and overcritical, demanding, and "spoiled-child" attitudes.

Lindemann cautions against early attempts at exploration with the usual psychiatric techniques. He suggests that the contact must be brief, not permitting the development of regressive tendencies, hostile feelings or affectionate attachment. "The relationship must, rather, be an identifying one, in which the patient copies the behavior patterns of the psychiatrist, and makes use of them in the same manner as he previously did with the patterns of the person who is lost." After such a relationship is established, it is often possible to review the bereavement with the proper emotion of depression and sorrow. The patient may go through a period of "nervousness" and worry, which might, superficially, appear detrimental to visceral functions, but is necessary for readjustment.

Psychosomatic Observations.   In a brilliant and comprehensive review Engel comments upon many of these points. His review, based upon the published reports of psychological data in more than 700 patients with ulcerative colitis, included observations in 39 patients of his own. He found obsessive-compulsive personality traits to be common even though none of the patients had a well developed obsessive-compulsive neurosis. In brief, these patients tend to fall into a population group having preponderantly pregenital personality traits, especially compulsive and dependent features. They show a defect in their capacity to relate to people, with a tendency to retain features of their early mother-child symbiotic relation; there is a failure to resolve this symbiotic relationship, which genetically and dynamically also appears to be related to the distinctive characteristics of one parent, usually the mother, who also cannot relinquish this relationship with her child. Sexual maturity is not achieved and the patients tend to make marriages which assure continuation of the same kind of relationship; ulcerative colitis develops in settings in which the important relationship in fact or in fantasy is threatened or actually disrupted, when at the same time the patient feels helpless to cope with the new situation. Remissions occur when effective relationship is again achieved; in similar situations, when more effective adjustive mechanisms are operative and when the affect is other than that designated by such terms as helpless, hopeless, despairing, etc., other symptoms, notably headache, rather than colitis develop. There is a vulnerability to psychotic reactions greater than in the general population.

With impressive consistency Engel found defects in personality structure long antedating the onset of colitis, a characteristic type of dependent and restricted relationship with people, consistent psychopathology in the mothers, and failure to achieve full heterosexual development.

Engel speculates upon a psychosomatic formulation which stresses the significance of the mother-child symbiosis in determining the particular personality development and vulnerability to separation, relates the tissue reaction of ulcerative colitis to biologic changes occurring consequent to traumatic separations, and attempts to account for the choice of organ (colon) on the basis of constitutional and experiential factors in the mother-child transaction.

STUDIES IN CHILDREN.   In a study of ulcerative colitis in children, Sperling found extremely ambivalent mothers who subjected their children to early and deep frustration. All the mothers showed an unconscious wish to be rid of their children. The children reacted to the treatment with hostility and an intense need to hold their position and developed "strong oral and anal sadistic tendencies." The author found that these children were unable to tolerate any psychic tension. They were in a permanent state of frustration, which caused rage and an irresistible urge for immediate discharge. The slightest additional frustrations provoked exaggerated reactions. Although essentially it is the degree of regression that differentiates ulcerative colitis from conversion reaction and mucous colitis, the author believes that it is the quantity of sadism that perhaps determines the depths of the regression itself. The severe form of ulcerative colitis shows great resemblance to melancholia in behavior, personality structure and dynamics, and seems to represent the somatic dramatization of the same conflict that is expressed psychologically in depression. Psychoanalysis is difficult in these cases and, according to Sperling, should include the mother.

Combined Therapy.   In discussing therapy Daniels pointed out that the severity of the condition made medical and sometimes surgical treatment necessary. However, in selected cases he regarded psychotherapy as definitely the treatment of choice and actually necessary to get results. Since the patients are usually severely ill physically, frequent contact with the physician over long periods of time is desirable for general medical supervision and to give opportunity for observation, collecting of necessary history and prolonged psychotherapy, either superficial or deep. Some of the cases encountered were largely situational while others had a deep neurotic structure which no one but a psychiatrist experienced in psychosomatic medicine should attempt to treat. Daniels emphasized that it may take weeks or months of observation before relationships between the precipitating elements and the disease become clear. While the problem of a domineering mother or her substitute is one of the most frequent relationships to overcome, the relief of repressed hostility as well as gradual help in bringing the patient to greater emotional maturity is in general the chief aim of the treatment.

Psychotherapy can be carried on while the patient is receiving other therapy. The privacy of a room for interviews is important. Daniels also stressed the importance of having other members of the house staff and nursing personnel acquainted with the nature of psychotherapy, and of realizing that following psychotherapeutic interviews the patient might be upset. They should not regard this as a sign that the patient is worse but as a necessary part of recovery through relief of tension. The help of the social service staff is frequently required in making plans for environmental changes and relief from difficult social and family situations.

PSYCHOSIS AND ULCERATIVE COLITIS.   Clinical experience has shown that many psychosomatic disorders, such as ulcerative colitis, often seem to be substitutes for psychosis and occasionally, when one is successful in removing the disorder, a pychotic state appears instead. Hence the necessity for caution in regard to therapy. The experienced therapist will often deal superficially with these disorders rather than subject them to deep psychotherapy. Although Engel is not impressed by this alternation of ulcerative colitis and psychosis we have recently studied a striking instance in which the patient, with a long history of diarrhea due to ulcerative colitis, became depressed and constipated, and when the depression was cured by electroshock therapy, the diarrhea began again.

Physical and Emotional Immaturity.   Our own observations support the suggestions that ulcerative colitis is frequently precipitated by emotional factors and that psychotherapy is invaluable in treatment. We have been impressed by the physical and emotional immaturity of patients with this disease. We are not impressed by the argument that this immaturity is dependent upon the disease. As in many other psychosomatic problems we believe that it is the other way around, that is, the immaturity is an index to the kind of personality that is apt to develop a disorder of the vegetative nervous system in which psychic factors play an important part.

In a discussion of Sullivan's paper Jones stated that in easily two-thirds of 100 cases which he and Urmy had followed at the Massachusetts General Hospital psychogenic disturbances seemed responsible for bringing on exacerbations, and that in the whole group acute upper respiratory infections, emotional or nervous upheavals, and possibly pregnancy, were the most obvious elements entering into the onset of the disease. "That there is an infection of the colon is obvious, but that it represents a specific disease due to a single organism is still, I believe, far from obvious." This statement was made in 1935 but we believe that it still holds.

The following case is typical of the kind of personality and psychological background of many cases of ulcerative colitis.

Case 28.   Ulcerative Colitis

A white woman of 25 complained of frequent, bloody bowel movements.

History and Symptoms.   Except for an occasional attack of tonsillitis she had always been in good health. The menses had been established at 15, and had been regular and normal. She married at 22 and had a child one year later. Frequent bowel movements with blood-streaked stools began shortly after the birth of the child.

The father, aged 57, and the mother, aged 53, were living and well. Three brothers and four sisters were all living and well. There was no history of serious bowel trouble among any blood relatives.

Physical Examination and Laboratory Studies.   The patient was a pale, poorly nourished, young white woman with the physical appearance of immaturity and a timid, whining manner. Examination was negative except for slight tenderness on deep pressure over the lower left quadrant of the abdomen. The sigmoidoscopic examination showed a markedly inflamed and ulcerated lower bowel. Barium enema findings were in conformity with the diagnosis of ulcerative colitis affecting principally the descending colon.

Shortly after admission to the hospital the temperature rose to 105° F., then dropped to normal with peaks of lesser magnitude on alternating successive days during the first ten days. Then there was slight irregular fever until discharge from the hospital one month later. She improved during her hospital stay, apparently from topical treatment.

LIFE SITUATION

The patient had an insecure girlhood. The parents were incompatible and there was a great deal of contention in the household which the patient seemed to feel more than her brothers or sisters did. They were a hardy lot who openly entered into the family quarrels while the patient, who gave the impression of a refined and lady-like person, suffered the quarreling in silence. She married at the age of 22 and a short time before the marriage her fiancé, who had been working in Philadelphia, decided to settle in a small town. This was very distasteful to the patient but she did not attempt to express her unwillingness to leave Philadelphia. Then immediately after marriage she became pregnant, although she did not want to, and suffered from severe nausea all through the pregnancy. About six weeks after the baby was born she first noted blood in the bowel movement. Her local physician apparently did not regard it as a serious symptom. However, the bowel movements increased in frequency and the blood increased in amount. She harbored a great deal of ill-feeling for this physician who had made light of the first symptom. She also showed a great deal of resentment in many other aspects of her life. Although she stated that there were no special problems disturbing her, she confessed that she did not get along well with her in-laws who lived in a nearby town and whom her husband insisted upon visiting frequently. She had a child-like *resentment* against them, saying that they held her in little esteem because she did not have a dowry to give their son. Her sexual life during marriage had been unsatisfactory so that she had been resentful of the necessity for permitting intercourse. Her conscious attitude in the hospital ward was one of constant complaining and constant discussion of how long she must remain, insisting that she must get back to her child, and yet it was apparent that she was really satisfied to remain in the hospital as long as we wished her to.

She maintained her improvement after leaving the hospital for a period of about two weeks while she remained in Philadelphia. Then she went home, financial difficulties arose, and the bowel trouble returned. With a second pregnancy the colitis was aggravated and following this incident she never fully recovered. There was constant family dissension, and the patient died of a perforation of the bowel nine years after the onset of the disease.

SUMMARY

A young white woman, presenting the emotional and physical aspects of immaturity, developed ulcerative colitis following marriage and the birth of an unwanted child. Her manner was childlike, complaining, and resentful, and it was felt that her personality plus the problems of her life situation had much to do with her illness.

Case 29.   *Ulcerative Colitis Alternating with Depression*

The patient is a 39-year-old white male who has suffered from ulcerative colitis for the past six years. His colitis cleared for a brief period of time three years ago, when he suffered from a depression accompanied by a suicidal attempt, but recurred when he recovered from his depression.

He is a meek, mild, frightened, somewhat effeminate man, afraid of expressing his anger, but who feels overwhelming hostility. His hostility is always accompanied by a sadistic feeling of guilt. He is above average intellectually, but is so bowed down by his physical and emotional symptoms that he is completely crippled and unable to fend for himself.

LIFE SITUATION

The patient has never been able to establish an adequate relationship with his harsh, cruel, vicious father, or his psychotic mother. Early in his life he was forced to assume a feminine role in his home and to replace his mother, by taking on her duties such as cooking, caring for the children and caring for his father.

At the same time he had a frank homosexual experience, at the age of 11, which was not entirely unpleasant to him. To appease his father and to avoid castration he partially accepted the feminine role in which he was placed and gained pleasure from this masochistic submission to his father. This, too, however, was intolerable to him—homosexuality and submission to the father meant being a woman which also involved being a castrated person. So the patient sought further protection from these anxieties by regressing to an anal-sadistic level.

His guilt over his sadism, however, was intense and cruel and also involved castration or punishment by authority, so he sought a further escape in a regression to a narcissistic level, as if he were saying, "If I love myself no one can punish me." His entire libido is directed upon his own body and here he found his satisfaction. He was able to soil himself as he did when he was a child; he was able to force his wife to care for him; and he was able to cause guilt feelings in the men toward whom his anger was directed.

It is interesting to note that when the patient became depressed he was no longer preoccupied with his own body and his diarrhea cleared up. This patient demonstrated a severe narcissistic neurosis with obsessive-compulsive and depressive features, which manifested themselves primarily through his ulcerative colitis. The borderline between psychosis and psychoneurosis is so slim that it is only through the reality of his psychosomatic illness that he is prevented from escaping into psychosis.

References

Alexander, F.: Psychoanalyt. Quart., *3:* 501, 1934.

Brown, P. W.: Proc. Staff Meet., Mayo Clinic, 7: 651, 1932.

DaCosta, J. M.: Am. J. M. Sc., *89:* 321, 1871.

Daniels, G. E.: Psychosom. Med., *2:* 276, 1940.

Dlin, B.: Personal Communication, 1956.

Dwyer, M. F., and Blackford, J. M.: Radiology, *14:* 38, 1930.

Emery, E. S., Jr.: Gastroenterology, *6:* 477, 1946.

Engel, G. L.: Am. J. Med., *19:* 231, 1955.

Eusterman, G. B.: J.A.M.A., *107:* 1232, 1936.

Friess, E. C., and Nelson, M. J.: Am. J. Med. Sci., *203:* 539, 1942.

Gregg, F. J., and Snowden, R. R.: Rev. Gastroenterol., *8:* 432, 1941.

Lindemann, E.: *in* Life Stress and Bodily Disease. Research publication, Association for Research in Nervous and Mental Disease. Williams & Wilkins Co., Baltimore, 1950, p. 706.

MacLean, P. D.: Psychosom. Med., *11:* 338, 1949.

Murray, C. D.: Am. J. Med. Sci., *180:* 239, 1930.

Rivers, A. B., and Ferreira, A. E. M.: J.A.M.A., *110:* 2132, 1938.

Savage, C., Butcher, W., and Noble, D.: J. Clin. Exper. Psychopath., *13:* 9, 1952.

Savage, L., and Noble, D.: J. Nerv. & Ment. Dis., *120:* 62, 1954.

Sperling, M.: Psychoanal. Quart., *15:* 302, 1954.

Sullivan, A. J.: Am. J. Digest. Dis. & Nutrition, *2:* 651, 1935.

Tumen, H. J.: Northwestern Med., *41:* 42, 1942.

Tumen, H. J., and Cohn, E. M.: J.A.M.A., *139:* 292, 1949.

White, B. V., Cobb, S., and Jones, C. M.: Mucous Colitis. Psychosom. Med. Monograph I. 1939.

Wilbur, D. L., and Mills, J. H.: Ann. Int. Med., *12:* 821, 1938.

Wilbur, D. L., and Washburn, R. N.: J.A.M.A., *110:* 477, 1938.

Chapter IX

The Gastrointestinal
System (Concluded)

CARDIOSPASM

Cardiospasm is a disorder of the swallowing function in which contraction of the lower end of the esophagus is followed by dilatation of the proximal portion, often to enormous size. A variety of terms other than cardiospasm, often based upon the etiological concepts of the author, occur in the literature. These include idiopathic dilatation of the esophagus, phrenospasm, megalo-esophagus and preventriculosis.

Probably the first recorded instance of cardiospasm was by Thomas Willis in which he described the vomiting of an otherwise healthy man and attributed it to closure of the mouth of the stomach, either by "Tumour or Palsie." He prepared a rodlike instrument of a whale bone with a little button of sponge fixed to the top which the patient used as a ramrod. By this means the patient fed himself daily for a period of fifteen years and was alive and well when the report was made in 1672.

Etiology. The term cardiospasm originated in the nineteenth century with von Mikulicz, who thought that the cardiac sphincter was in spasm. However, in an anatomical study by Lendrum no real sphincter could be demonstrated. Nevertheless, the term and the concept of sphincter spasm have persisted to the present time. As early as 1888 Einhorn suggested another possibility concerning the pathogenesis of the disorder. He described a case in which he could pass the stomach tube without encountering resistance and concluded that the cardia probably failed to open reflexly during the act of swallowing. Rolleston, in 1896, made the same suggestion independently but it was not until Hurst introduced the term achalasia that the theory received attention.

Many other explanations have been given for cardiospasm. Some have to do with changes within the esophagus itself and others account for the difficulty through the influence of adjacent organs and tissues. Phrenospasm or preventriculosis, the name given to the condition by Chevalier Jackson, suggests that constriction of the lower end of the esophagus is caused by contraction of the diaphragm. The majority opinion, however, has been in favor of a neurogenic origin, that is, disease of the vagus nerve or of the myenteric plexus. In Lendrum's series, 10 of the 13 cases with adequate sections showed entirely normal vagus nerves. However, he did find a striking or complete absence of ganglion cells in the plexus and demonstrated that the loss was equally great in the undistended portion of the lower esophagus, which, he felt, argued against these changes being merely secondary to pressure. Therefore he favors Hurst's views that a failure of the sphincter to relax is the cause of the esophageal retention. Nevertheless, the prevailing opinion is that both loss of ganglion cells and ulceration of the esophagus are secondary rather than primary changes.

Comparatively little attention has been paid to psychic factors in the disorder in spite of the fact that the association of nervousness in patients with cardiospasm has always been recognized. Moschcowitz discussed cardiospasm in a study of the psychogenic origin of organic diseases and Winkelstein reported a group of patients with cardiospasm in whom psychic factors seemed to be the chief agents producing the disease. Kronfeld, quoted by Alexander, presented some evidence regarding the role of unconscious mental mechanisms in swallowing disorders.

We made an effort to study the emotional lives of patients with cardiospasm, to see if some meaning for the disorder could be found from the standpoint of behavior (Weiss 1944). All patients were referred to us for general medical study through the kindness of Dr. C. L. Jackson of the Bronchoscopic Department, Temple University Hospital. In all, 17 cases have been observed of which 9 permitted a fairly satisfactory psychosomatic study.

Clinical Picture.   There are three common important symptoms—difficulty in swallowing, pain and regurgitation of food. Food seems to stop before entering the stomach—it apparently sticks beneath the lower sternum. At first the swallowing difficulty may be intermittent with periods of relief of days or weeks. Later the cardiospasm becomes well established with a sense of pushing or forcing of food, with frequent attacks of distress or severe pain following meals. The patient often learns to regurgitate when he is especially distressed.

There is little difficulty in making the diagnosis of cardiospasm. The clinical picture is as a rule characteristic. Roentgen ray studies usually establish the diagnosis by the appearance of a dilated esophagus, with a smooth tapering point of occlusion. Jackson believes that esophagoscopy is essential to confirm the diagnosis, because he has found carcinoma in patients who have been reported by roentgen ray examination to have cardiospasm.

In the treatment of this disorder drugs have been of little use. The most successful measure has been some form of dilatation of the lower end of the esophagus. Since there is danger of perforation from the use of an ordinary bougie, special bougies have been devised for the purpose. These include Hurst's mercury-weighted tube and hydrostatic dilators.

Personality Study.   Cardiospasm is a psychosomatic disorder. It is important to emphasize that just as in other psychosomatic disorders connected with the vegetative nervous system, the psychic factor is not the whole problem. The very fact that this disorder has been described in children in the first few days of life definitely excludes the psychic factor as being present in all cases. There is undoubtedly an inherent tendency, a predisposition, to which the psychic factor is complementary, and it must be that both together, in the majority of cases, are necessary for the development of cardiospasm.

Cardiospasm usually is found to arise coincidentally with an emotional conflict, in many instances during puberty, in an individual whose early life gives evidence of personality difficulties. Other evidences of neurosis or other psychosomatic disorders are frequently present and are also common in other members of the family. As would be expected, parent-child and sibling relationships are seriously disturbed. At first cardiospasm often seems to manifest itself intermittently; later on, it may become permanently established. Exacerbations occur which frequently can be correlated with fresh psychic insults touching the particular complex of the individual.

We regard cardiospasm as an organ neurosis resembling conversion reaction but with elements of a vegetative neurosis. The physical disorder represents symbolically the unconscious conflict; it appears to be a compromise between the gratification of certain impulses and their rejection by another part of the personality. Superficially an important meaning of the disorder can often be stated in such simple terms as "I cannot swallow that situation." Therefore, this meaning can often be discovered by looking (psychologically) for the situation that the individual "cannot swallow." After the patient has been assured that no other cause can be found—cancer, for example—this kind of approach will often lead to a discussion of important emotional factors.

On a somewhat deeper level the disorder seems to represent another tendency, that is, an aggressive desire to incorporate some object with resultant spasm or inability to relax the lower end of the esophagus. The sexual, hostile and self-punitive aspects of this disorder are brought out in the various cases that are reported.

Whatever one believes regarding the etiological role of these mental forces, it must be apparent that to study patients with cardiospasm simply as physiological mechanisms, and treat them by mechanical measures without making some effort to understand the emotional make-up, is a very one-sided and inadequate method of dealing with the disorder. The above observations suggest the necessity for a combined physical and psychological study and treatment of the individual patient with cardiospasm. No one can deny the necessity for mechanical treatment in the established case of cardiospasm, but it seems possible that this additional psychic approach will help us deal with that group of patients who "do not tolerate the dilator well"; the patients who get no benefit from self treatment; a group which "tend to recur" or the group which "cannot be cured." Especially in regard to these groups we must consider the frequent observation that in a patient with a severe neurosis a physical disorder (such as cardiospasm) appears to be that patient's solution of his psychic conflict. The physical disorder, therefore, is necessary to the emotional life and until the psychic conflict is better solved, the particular disorder from which the patient suffers either must be maintained or must be replaced by another illness. In one case dilatation treatment was immediately followed by depression. Certainly, in an early case of cardiospasm, especially in a young person, psychologic study and treatment seem to us an essential part of the management. Indeed, we venture to suggest that the time is approaching when the physician will consider the neglect of psychological study just as serious an omission, in the total study of the patient with cardiospasm, as the failure to study such a patient with x-ray or the esophagoscope.

Treatment Problems.   Many of the above points were confirmed by McMahon, Braceland and Moersch who studied a group of 25 patients suffering from cardiospasm. Twenty-four patients had suffered from emotional trauma at the time of onset of symptoms. In general, symptoms were aggravated when the patient was nervous and upset, and were less severe or absent when things were going smoothly. In an experimental study of cardiospasm Wolf and Almy made repeated fluoroscopic observations of swallowed barium sulfate in 14 patients with well established cardiospasm. They found that the esophageal obstruction of cardiospasm was often associated with decided hypermotility of the lower two thirds of the esophagus. They also noted that exacerbations or remission of symptoms could be correlated with periods of stress or relative security in the lives of the patients. A discussion of emotionally charged topics was associated with hypermotility and obstruction in the esophagus, while relative security and relaxation were associated with diminution or disappearance of the phenomena of cardiospasm.

McMahon et al. suggest that if purely somatic treatment such as dilation or other operative procedure is used patients may have recurrence of symptoms; or, if the symptom was psychologically necessary, reaction to symptom removal may be pathological. In a surgical study from the Mayo Clinic 601 patients treated by dilation were observed by Olsen et al. over a 12-year period and the conclusion was reached that if satisfactory results are not obtained with two courses of hydrostatic dilations, additional treatment is likely to be of little avail, and the authors find that about 20 per cent of patients cannot be permanently relieved by dilation. For these they recommend surgical treatment but acknowledge that the late results are not favorable.

The following case illustrates the psychological background.

Case 30.   Cardiospasm

History and Symptoms.   A 55-year-old white man was referred through the kindness of Dr. C. L. Jackson from the bronchoscopic department of Temple University Hospital, with the diagnosis, established by esophagoscopy and roentgen ray, of cardiospasm. He was receiving treatments in the form of esophageal dilatations.

The patient gave the usual medical history of this condition. He stated that his illness began about eight or ten years before and had been progressive. He had consulted many physicians. Discouraged, he had invested a large sum of money with an osteopath who had promised cure; finally, very sick and without funds, he had come to the hospital. The previous medical history did not seem to bear upon this illness.

LIFE SITUATION

His life situation, however, was interesting. He had been "born into the drug business" and had never known anything except the long hours and tedious work of an underpaid pharmacy clerk. He maried young and five children came in rapid succession. It was a great financial struggle to look after them. While he was working very hard he had "some kind of a breakdown" during which there were nervous symptoms and he took bromides. His oldest and favorite son, then aged 20, had just obtained an excellent job which paid well. He gave his salary to his mother and the father was overjoyed with the finally achieved prospects of economic freedom. He had always pictured a great career for this able son and had looked forward to his financial aid to help him in his old age.

Marriage of Son. Without warning one morning shortly afterward he learned that this son had just secretly married. He said, "It was the greatest blow I ever received, not only because of the financial part of it but the way he did it" (that is, secretly). The patient went on to say, "I felt like a child crying until his heart would break" and he placed his hand on his epigastrium to show where he felt the blow.

He could not get over this disappointment and even considered having the marriage annulled on the basis that the boy was too young to marry. It was interesting to note, however, that he, himself, had married at the same age. He harbored a great deal of resentment toward the girl's parents who, he felt, had stolen his fine son from him. It was during this period that attacks of *swallowing difficulty* occurred and grew more pronounced and more frequent.

Further Aggravation. A short time later further aggravation occurred. He learned that his brother in England, whom he described as a ne'er-do-well, was cheating his mother of her small legacy. He went to England, brought his mother back and she then made her home with them. It seemed significant that the mother contributed her sole income to the upkeep of him and his family. In other words, while he accused his brother of having "bled his mother" he, himself, had already borrowed money from her and then took her weekly allowance for living expenses. His altruism in rescuing her from his ne'er-do-well brother seemed questionable.

The picture was that of a meek, submissive and dependent individual who had always worked hard without achieving success. He had strongly identified with his oldest son in whom he hoped to achieve the success denied himself. With his son's secret marriage came a tremendous disappointment from which he could not recover.

Experience with Osteopath. An interesting commentary in line with our thesis was his experience with the osteopath. He had consulted him, and was charged $1000, which his sons had to borrow, "for management of his case." It was interesting to consider why he felt like investing this great sum of money with the osteopath. He said, "The osteopath told me that my trouble was due to a spasm arising from a shock," and the patient went on to say, "he did not know about my son's marriage." He was much impressed by this diagnosis "because it was the first time that any doctor had suggested that shock and worry might be responsible for my trouble." He thereupon placed his entire confidence and all the money he could raise in the osteopath's hands.

The Meaning of the Illness. In the recital of his story, accompanied by great emotion, this poor druggist made the following significant and perhaps revealing statement, "My son's marriage was a bitter pill that I could not swallow." And who can say that that was not, at least, one meaning of the illness?

SUMMARY

A meek and dependent, middle-aged white man developed cardiospasm apparently in response to a life situation "which he could not swallow."

PEPTIC ULCER

It was previously stated that in the Mayo Clinic series of 15,000 cases of chronic dyspepsia more than 15 per cent had x-ray evidence pointing

to peptic ulcer as the cause. Thus peptic ulcer, especially of the duodenum, is the commonest organic lesion within the gastrointestinal tract
responsible for chronic dyspepsia. But it is not only because of its frequency that it is easily the most important psychosomatic problem encountered among the disorders of the gastrointestinal tract. The term
psychosomatic can be used without hesitation in connection with peptic
ulcer because today even the most organically minded physician recognizes the importance of "emotional factors" in ulcer cases.

To be sure, no one doubts the existence of a constitutional factor but,
as previously stated, it is impossible in the light of our present knowledge to delimit the role that the constitution plays from the influence
of environmental factors. Many instances have been reported of peptic
ulcer occurring in infancy and early childhood, certainly at a period
when the emotional conflicts, which we shall discuss later, could not
possibly enter (Guthrie-Donavan). This indicates only that the constitutional factor is dominant in these particular cases. But our point of
view in regard to etiology is that multiple factors usually are at work:
in some instances the constitutional element seems chiefly responsible;
in others the environmental influences seem more important, and among
these it is now recognized that emotional factors rank first.

Cushing, in a noteworthy paper which will be quoted again, observed
that all clinicians are familiar with these facts: (1) that highly strung
persons are particularly susceptible to nervous indigestion and associated ulcer; (2) that ulcers become symptomatically quiescent or even
tend to heal when patients are put mentally and physically at rest; and
(3) the symptoms are prone to recur as soon as the victim of the disorder resumes his former tasks and responsibilities. He concluded by
suggesting that highly strung (vagotonic) persons subjected to emotional
stress, and such other factors as irregular meals and excessive use of
tobacco, are prone to have chronic digestive disturbances often leading
to ulcer. This was as far as he felt that we could go, with the data at
hand, in interpreting the "neurogenic" origin of peptic ulcer and
explaining its existing prevalence.

Theories of Etiology.   There have been many theories regarding
the etiology of peptic ulcer: vascular, chemical or corrosive, gastric,
infectious, traumatic, mechanical, endocrine, vitamin deficiency, allergic
and neurogenic. Although some of these theories had their inception
almost a century ago—for example, that ulcer was dependent on vascular disease—and the other theories came along as new developments in
their respective fields suggested that this peculiar and baffling disease
might be explained on the basis of the newest etiological process, it goes
without saying that no one of them adequately explains peptic ulcer.

In appraising the various theories Eusterman stated that all noteworthy contributors agreed that ulcer is not the result of a single agent,
but is a product of the interaction of various agents; and that the constitutional or systemic factor is fundamentally essential. Hypersecretion
characterizes duodenal ulcer; decreased tissue resistance predominates
in gastric ulcer. Acid is indispensable to both processes but is not the
only factor. Twenty years ago Eusterman felt that the major facts of the

genesis and development of ulcer had been established, and that the causative factor which is operative in the vast majority of cases is the *psyche* mediated through the autonomic nervous system, producing a morbid physiological state conducive to the initiation, extension and chronicity of the lesion. To what extent inheritance or constitution acts in this group he could not say but he was perusaded that conscious and unconscious emotional factors which can be continuously operative are sufficient. Thus Eusterman was apparently most impressed by "neurogenic factors" in the etiology of peptic ulcer. We agree with his critical appraisal and would quarrel with him only concerning the use of the term *neurogenic*. Many authors apparently hesitate to use the term *psychogenic* and therefore all questions dealing with the nervous system, whether they be organic or emotional, are included in the term neurogenic. To this we object because the term psychogenic should be used for emotional factors if we are to respect them as causes of disease and deal with them courageously. Thus even from nonpsychological sources we are confronted with imposing evidence that psychic factors are of the greatest importance as a cause of peptic ulcer and so we have a clear-cut issue of psychosomatic medicine to discuss, namely, on the one hand a definite organic disease—peptic ulcer, which can be demonstrated by means of x-ray and surgery—and on the other hand, emotional factors which seem important from the standpoint of cause and treatment.

In order to replace the loose terminology "neurogenic factors" by the concept of psychogenesis in the etiology of peptic ulcer, let us begin by reviewing the work of Cushing, his associates, and others who have been interested in the connection between the central nervous system and peptic ulcers.

Clinical Observations. Cushing cited three instances of perforating lesions of the stomach, duodenum and esophagus following operations for cerebellar tumor and called attention to further instances of erosions of the gastric mucosa without perforation, after intracranial operations. He reported a case of pathologically verified chronic ulcer in a patient with cerebellar tumor and also cited the case of an individual having a roentgenologically demonstrable peptic ulcer with symptomatic and roentgen ray evidence of an organic lesion in the region of the third ventricle. He had frequently seen patients recovering from serious intracranial operations in whom during convalescence digestive disturbances strongly suggested incipient ulcer formation.

In an effort to explain these and other similar observations he reviewed the neurogenic aspects of ulcer pathogenesis and called attention to the first observations of that nature by Rokitansky, who believed that the cause of peptic ulcer was "a diseased innervation of the stomach, owing to a morbid condition of the vagus, and to extreme acidification of the gastric juice."

Experimental Observations. From his observations and the investigations of others Cushing undertook experimental studies which showed that intraventricular injections of pilocarpine or posterior pituitary extract caused, in man, an increase in gastric motility, hypertonus and hypersecretion leading to retching and vomiting which ultimately contained occult blood. Acting upon Cushing's observations his associates, Light, Bishop and Kendall, regularly produced peptic ulcers in animals with small intraventricular injections of pilocarpine and observed pathologically a local anemia of the stomach mucosa accompanied by surface hemorrhage and necrosis extending to the muscularis mucosae. Beattie showed in animals that direct electrical stimulation of the region of the tuberal centers in the infundibulum not only caused increased gastric peristalsis but also led to small hemorrhagic ulcers of the mucous membrane near the lesser curvature. After section of the vagi these gastric effects were not obtained. In a study primarily undertaken to investigate the heat regulating mechanism of the brain stem in cats, Keller produced bilateral lesions in the expectation of freeing the hypothalamus from its connections with the brain stem. Postmortem studies showed gastric lesions ranging from simple hyperemic areas to erosions extending through all the layers of the gut, and to punched-out perforating ulcers.

From these studies Cushing observed that the reaction of the stomach to intraventricular injections of either pilocarpine or pituitrin in man and to direct stimulation of the tuber or its descending fiber tracts in animals is *hypersecretion, hypermotility* and *hypertonicity,* especially marked in the pyloric segment. These are the effects commonly associated with chronic peptic ulcer in man. He believed that by the spasmodic contraction of the musculature, possibly supplemented by accompanying local spasms of the terminal blood vessels, small areas of ischemia or hemorrhagic infarction are produced, leaving the overlying stomach mucosa exposed to the digestive effects of its own hyperacid juices. This applies directly to the formation of chronic ulcer in man because Cushing agreed with many others that an erosion of the mucosa must be the primary stage in ulcer formation; "and since there is every reason to believe that acute erosions . . . are of common occurrence, any one of them may well enough be the precursor of a chronic lesion, should the original insult be sufficiently great or should a minor insult be continuous or frequently repeated at the same spot."

Notable contributions to the understanding of a relationship between the emotions and gastric response have been made in the past few years. Physical and emotional stresses associated with peptic ulcer can be mediated through a hormonal pathway entirely independent of the vagus nerve according to Gray and his associates. This hormonal pathway apparently leads from the hypothalamus to the pituitary and then to the adrenal, from which impulses are transmitted to the stomach. Injections of ACTH or cortisone increase gastric acidity, pepsin secretion and uropepsin excretion. This happens even in the vagotomized dog. Porter, Movius and French demonstrated a gastric secretory response to insulin hypoglycemia in the monkey and were able to resolve the curve of that secretory response into two components which could be related respectively to stimulation of the anterior and posterior hypothalamic area. Then Shay and Sun were able to show that in man, too, gastric secretion stimulated by insulin hypoglycemia showed an early peak of secretion dependent on intact vagi and a later peak dependent on the presence of the adrenals. Further work along these lines permitted a working hypothesis as follows: <u>Stress</u> acting on the posterior hypothalamic nuclei transmits the cholinergic and adrenergic neurohumoral agents to the pituitary stalk. From this point they reach the anterior pituitary by way of the portal circulation with the resultant release of ACTH to simulate the adrenal and then adrenocortical hormone stimulates the gastric secretion (Chart 4).

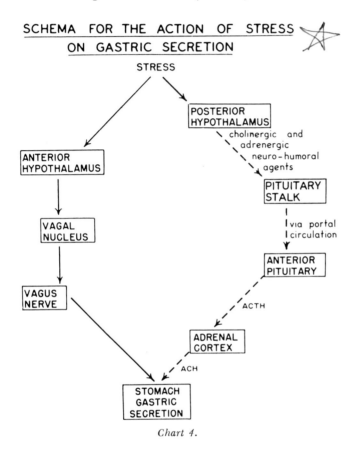

Chart 4.

Other links between the hypothalamus and gastroduodenal lesion, and further evidence of dual pathways of gastric secretion stimulation, have been shown by French. In cats, destruction of the <u>anterior hypothalamus</u> by electrocoagulation produced gastroduodenal hemorrhage, while similar damage to the posterior hypothalamus produced erosive lesions without hemorrhage. In monkeys, stimulation of the anterior hypothalamus increased the secretion of hydrochloric acid, an action blocked by section of the vagi. Stimulation of the posterior hypothalamus produced a later secretion of acid uninfluenced by cutting the vagi—but blocked by removal of the adrenals.

To investigate the effects of chronic stress, French implanted electrodes into the hypothalamus of monkeys and stimulated them several times daily for long periods of time. Gastrointestinal lesions developed in 8 of 19 animals that had received adequate stimulation.

Papez and MacLean have established the concept of the limbic system as a participant in emotional expression (see p. 62). This system, the great limbic lobe and the subcortical cell stations, is anatomically and physiologically a common denominator in all mammals. The limbic system is for the "body viscus" a visceral brain, that interprets and gives expression to its incoming information in terms of feeling rather than in terms of intellectualizing symbols.

Studies by Cleghorn and Heath give further evidence for an association between the circuits of the hypothalamic-endocrine system and the activities of the higher limbic lobe, so that little doubt remains that in the hypothalamic and endocrine systems mechanisms exist which explain some of the interrelations between physiological and psychological functions.

Conscious Emotional Factors.   For the purposes of the present discussion, it is noteworthy that von Bergmann in Germany and Alvarez in America have insisted upon the importance of nervous and emotional factors in their relation to ulcer formation. Alvarez called our attention to a certain type of individual who is particularly prone to develop peptic ulcer and referred to him as a keen, nervous, active, hard-living individual, upon whom surgeons are reluctant to operate because of the danger of recurrence of ulcer. He felt that arterial spasm may be one of the links between the emotions and ulcer formation and concluded that most ulcers are due basically to emotional factors and nervous tension. Alvarez has gone a definite step beyond the usual medical approach which is considered complete if it enumerates the physical and chemical data concerning the patient.

Wolff and his associates have made significant contributions to this subject. They had an opportunity to make very careful observations of a patient, Tom, with a gastric fistula and showed that day-to-day life situations which provoked certain patterns of emotional reaction induced hypersecretion in the stomach comparable to that which could be produced experimentally in animals from prolonged absorption of histamine, vagus stimulation and sham feeding. They discovered that:

1. Acid in small amounts was continuously elaborated in the subject under basal conditions.

2. Spontaneous transitory phases of accelerated secretion of acid occurred from time to time, and were accompanied by blushing of the mucous membrane and vigorous contractions of the stomach wall.

3. Emotions such as fear and sadness which involved a feeling of withdrawal were accompanied by pallor of the gastric mucosa, and by inhibition of acid secretion and contractions, a complex encountered infrequently in their subject.

4. Emotional conflict involving anxiety, hostility and resentment was accompanied by accelerated acid secretion, hypermotility, hyperemia, and engorgement of the gastric mucosa resembling "hypertrophic gastritis." (This series of events, much more commonly observed, was asso-

ciated with gastric complaints of the nature of heartburn and abdominal pain.)

5. Intense sustained anxiety, hostility and resentment were found to be accompanied by severe and prolonged engorgement, hypermotility and hypersecretion in the stomach. In this state mucosal erosions and hemorrhages were readily induced by even the most trifling traumas, and frequently bleeding points appeared spontaneously as a result of vigorous contractions of the stomach wall.

6. Contact of acid gastric juice with such a small eroded surface in the mucous membrane resulted in accelerated secretion of acid and further engorgement of the whole mucosa. Prolonged exposure of such a lesion to acid gastric juice resulted in the formation of a chronic ulcer.

7. The lining of the stomach was found to be protected from its secretions by an efficient insulation layer of mucus, enabling most of the small erosions to heal promptly (within a few hours). Lack of such a protective mechanism in the duodenal cap may explain the higher incidence of chronic ulceration in that region.

They conclude that it appears likely that the chain of events which begins with anxiety and conflict and their associated overactivity of the stomach, and ends with hemorrhage or perforation, is that which is involved in the natural history of peptic ulcer in human beings.

Unconscious Mental Forces in the Etiology of Peptic Ulcer. There are many patients with peptic ulcer in whom evidence of continued worry or emotional stress cannot be easily obtained, and clinicians interested in the "neurogenic" aspect of ulcer pathogenesis have been forced to stop at this point in their investigations. Although a distinctive psychosomatic pattern of hypersensitivity, hyperirritability and hyperactivity has been ascribed to peptic ulcer patients these characteristics are often so masked that there are no external manifestations of mental agitation.

The next step, and the one to which we particularly call attention, depends upon the necessity for understanding that forceful influences exist in the unconscious mental life and that these may play a part in causing peptic ulcer.

Draper, long a protagonist of disease as a "psysomatic" reaction, pointed the way to a deeper psychologic understanding of personality in relation to peptic ulcer by calling our attention to the unconscious mental life in his studies of patients with ulcer. But it was Alexander who developed the idea that permanent psychic stimuli from unconscious mental sources may be capable of stimulating the subcortical centers similarly to the direct irritations observed by Cushing and others. This constant psychic stimulation of subcortical centers apparently produces local functional disturbances in the upper digestive tract that may be followed by ulcer formation.

PSYCHOLOGICAL REGRESSION. Alexander informs us that in these patients psychoanalysis reveals a characteristic regression to the early stages of emotional life. In patients whom he has studied a strong desire for dependence on others was evidenced in the unconscious mental life but consciously the patient was dominated by ideas of independence, activity and success. Thus when unconscious passive-receptive oral cravings are not satisfied (as they can hardly be in an individual whose conscious life is devoted to activity and independence), they find their expression in this primitive way. The repressed wishes to be loved and taken care of find motor expression in the production of stomach symptoms.

This phenomenon depends upon infantile habit formations which serve as a pattern of behavior later in life. Alexander explains that the first form of being cared for and loved is nursing and the sensations of being loved and being fed become emotionally associated for the rest of life. If the wish to be loved, as one was by the mother, is denied gratification (repressed) the associated tendency for being nourished is energized.

While the personality of the ulcer patient is usually regarded as the efficient, go-getter type, Kapp working with Rosenbaum and Romano in a study of 20 men with peptic ulcer described two additional groups of persons according to their external personality characteristics, in addition to the "classic" ulcer personality type. Although all the patients showed intense, dependent unconscious strivings, in only 6 was the mechanism one of overcompensation marked by ambition and success.

A second group of 5 patients reacted by giving in partially to the dependent desires. As a result they appeared passive and shy with marked trends of feminine identification in their overt personalities.

The largest group of their patients, again with deep dependent cravings, utilized socially unacceptable means of dependency, such as chronic alcoholism and delinquency. They had little or no guilt, employed no socially acceptable defenses against selfish, demanding impulses, and were openly parasitic on their parents, wives or society. They took and grabbed continually and openly. Essentially this is the unweaned suckling type of personality whose oral needs appear to be insatiable.

Thus the majority of their patients with peptic ulcer either were outwardly passive and effeminate or openly acted out their deep oral desires. Ulcer symptoms developed as responses to frustration of these cravings when the various defense mechanisms which they used to handle such conflicts proved inadequate. Although the conflict situation is similar, the resulting personality façade may vary from exaggerated independence to parasitic dependence.

While formerly prevalent in women, peptic ulcer now occurs chiefly in men. There has been a remarkable shift in the sex incidence in the area of Western civilization during the past half century. A study of 25 women with peptic ulcer by Kezur, Kapp and Rosenbaum found that oral aggressive feelings played an important role and were often equated with denial of femininity. Frustration of dependent wishes was just as important among them as in men.

Wolf and Wolff from their studies of Tom attempted to relate manifest behavior and emotions to gastric function. Margolin in psychoanalytic and physiologic studies of his patient, Helen, suggested a relationship of gastric secretory activity to unconscious mental processes. He found the gastric response to conscious processes in Helen to be different from that noted in Tom. Tom's gastric secretion increased with anger and resentment while in Helen the opposite effect was noted when she displayed these feelings. Further contributions to the understanding of the relationship between the emotions and gastric activity were made by Engel, Reichsman and Segal in their studies on an infant girl with a gastric fistula. They demonstrated that the secretory rate was an intimate part of the total behavioral activity of the infant. The outgoing affective states, libidinal or aggressive, were associated with increased hydrochloric acid secretion while during depression-withdrawal reactions there was a marked decrease or even cessation of HCl secretion.

That there is not complete unanimity of opinion regarding the response of gastric secretion to the different emotions is shown in some interesting studies by Eichhorn and Tracktir on the effect of hypnotically induced emotions on gastric secretion of a group of students. Hypnotic studies showed that the volume of secretion and peptic activity rise during contentment and fall during fear and anger. Nor have the views of Alexander regarding frustration of oral wishes in the etiology of peptic ulcer gone unchallenged. Roth in a critical review of "The Peptic Ulcer Personality" surveyed the writings on this subject up to the year 1955 and concluded that neither the nature nor even the existence of a specific ulcer personality has been established.

By means of psychological testing (Rorschach test and Blacky Pictures) Streitfeld attempted to investigate the "theory of specific emotional conflict" in regard to peptic ulcer. Stating that a review of psychosomatic literature for the past two decades might give the impression that this theory is an established fact, Streitfeld investigated a group of 20 cases of peptic ulcer with a control group of 20 cases of psychosomatic disorders unrelated to the gastrointestinal tract in an attempt to find out whether strong oral conflicts are specific to peptic ulcer. He concluded that a strong oral-dependent conflict does not differentiate peptic ulcer from other psychosomatic disorders. He felt that the importance of frustrated oral-dependent needs in the etiology of ulcer formation has been overrated. Instead of being specific for ulcer he found this conflict in many other psychosomatic diseases and indeed concluded that it can be considered a typical emotional constellation in our culture. Nor did he feel that any special kind of defense system was present in the ulcer cases. Therefore he decided that his peptic ulcer patients did not differ from other psychosomatic cases in being frustrated in the gratification of their oral-dependent needs nor did they differ because of the overt personality they presented to the world. He found, however, that they did have a tendency to react with strong oral aggressive wishes to the frustration of their oral tendencies and in this way differed from other psychosomatic cases.

Nevertheless, the concept advanced by Alexander in 1934 is the most widely accepted formulation in psychosomatic medicine. Although it remains to be proved that frustration of oral needs is more frequent or more intense in an ulcer population than in a control group, it is a working hypothesis that has been helpful in dealing with ulcer patients.

THE PSYCHIC STIMULUS. Following the work by Shay and Sun, the same investigators with Dlin and Weiss undertook a study of a patient with a duodenal ulcer to see whether a relation between the emotions and the two phases of gastric secretion could be demonstrated. Twenty-four gastric secretory experiments were done on the patient within a period of 16 months. He was a frustrated, oral-dependent individual with phobic and compulsive tendencies. Psychological interviews were carried out in six experiments. Emotional stress produced an "early" and "late" response in gastric secretion similar to that produced by insulin hypo-glycemia. Both phases of gastric secretion could be blocked by drugs. No correlation was noted between overt behavior and the type of gastric response. Unconscious mental conflicts seemed to be more important in stimulating the "late" phase of gastric secretion. After several interviews with the psychiatrist a conditioned response of gastric secretion appeared and this response underwent extinction in approximately one month. The reintroduction of the psychiatrist into the experiment, even without an interview, stimulated an early phase of gastric secretion which seemed to be a manifestation of a hostile, frustrating transference relationship. The two phases of gastric secretion that can occur after emotional stress, the possibility of the development of a conditioned response, and the blocking effect of drugs on "emotional secretion" all must be considered in regard to treatment of ulcer.

A very interesting study by Weiner, Thaler, Reiser and Mirsky tested the hypothesis that individuals with a high pepsinogen secretion, as measured by blood levels, represent that segment of the population which is most likely to develop duodenal ulcer, given an exposure to certain psychic circumstances. The latter depend largely on the level of emotional maturity and the degree of life stress. In other words, it seems likely that there are three parameters which determine the pre-cipitation of duodenal ulcer, *viz.,* a physiological parameter which determines the susceptibility of the duodenum to ulceration, a psycho-logical parameter which determines the psychic conflict which induces psychic tension, and a social parameter which determines the environ-mental event which will prove noxious to the particular individual.

These investigators surveyed 2073 young men chosen at random while being processed for army induction prior to the stress of 16 weeks of basic training. Blood pepsinogen was routinely determined and each week the ten highest and lowest secretors were chosen for special psy-chological tests, gastrointestinal studies and x-ray examination. Without prior knowledge of the pepsinogen level or x-ray findings, the psycho-logical studies were evaluated to see if the hypersecretors could be differentiated from the hyposecretors and whether men with, or prone to, duodenal ulcer could be identified. These hypotheses were based on previous clinical observations which suggested that the hypersecretor, like the patient with duodenal ulcer, would exhibit on psychological tests evidences of intense infantile oral dependent wishes, marked im-maturity, tendencies to please and placate, and difficulties revolving particularly about the management of oral impulses and hostility. The findings indicated that persons with a high pepsinogen value in the blood are most prone to develop ulcer. Psychological studies showed that they were more "emotionally immature," and had a greater tendency to depression and denial of hostile feelings. Psychological tests alone—without knowledge from biochemical or x-ray study—made it possible to predict ulcers in 10 of 120 subjects studied, and ulcers were actually found in 7 of the 10. Of the three that did not have or did not develop an ulcer, two were correctly classed as hypersecretors.

In the 10 men selected as those most likely to develop an ulcer the psychological test material revealed that they belonged to the group of hypersecretors, and, in addition, showed evidences of intense needs to maintain relationships with others. Their anxieties centered around a fear of expressing hostility lest there be a loss of supplies for their needs and consequently they went out of their way to rationalize, deny and displace such feelings. The hostility was inferred to have been introjected with the consequent development of depression. The need to please and placate authority figures as potential sources of affection was particularly striking.

In summary, the studies reveal that neither a high concentration of pepsinogen in the blood (in other words, a high rate of gastric secretion) nor a specific psychodynamic constellation is independently responsible for the precipitation of duodenal ulcer under stressful environmental situations. Together, however, these two parameters appear to constitute the necessary essential determinants in the precipitation of duodenal ulcer on exposure to social situations which are noxious to the specific individual.

ULCER AND SURGERY.   Related to the question of the surgical treatment of peptic ulcer is the problem of the relief of symptoms of emotional origin. A large part of the physician's work is devoted to the relief of such symptoms by means of reassurance, medication of various kinds and, sometimes, surgery. The latter situation arises when pain continues in spite of medical treatment or when, for example, the healing of a peptic ulcer fails to take place. In such a case, nerves are sometimes cut or the ulcer area may be removed. The question then arises, if tension of emotional origin is responsible for the symptom or the persistence of the disease, what happens to that tension if we cut the pathways which transmit it? Does it cause other symptoms or disturb the organism in some other way?

Information bearing on this subject was furnished in a study of the new symptoms which develop following surgical treatment for duodenal ulcer. It has long been recognized that emotional factors enter into the problem of ulcer formation; the removal of the ulcer area by means of gastrectomy is a standard procedure for ulcer cure. Browning and Houseworth studied a group of patients and discovered that the surgically treated group had an increased number of psychosomatic and psychoneurotic symptoms after the removal of the ulcer area. The medically treated control group, in which ulcer symptoms were not significantly reduced in incidence or severity, revealed no such increase of symptoms following treatment.

Szasz made a psychiatric study of 25 ulcer patients who had undergone vagotomy. Twenty-two were men. There was roentgen evidence of ulcer before operation in all of the patients. Symptoms after vagotomy included severe diarrhea, persistent pain, addiction, depression, impairment of memory and a large group of miscellaneous symptoms. In two cases of addiction the symptom antedated the vagotomy by several years. Szasz notes that mild depressive episodes occur with great frequency in patients with peptic ulcer, but he encountered two moderately severe depressions that started very soon after the vagotomy. He concluded that when sufficient information is obtained about the patient his postoperative symptoms can usually be understood in terms of his preoperative personality structure. So far as psychodynamics in ulcer patients is concerned, Szasz feels that significant similarities between peptic ulcer patients are well established and refers to the characteristic psychodynamic conflict described by Alexander.

In their reaction to vagotomy, Szasz describes the psychologic characteristics of two types of cases: (1) the more the psychic energy is bound by the organic illness, that is, the more the ulcer symptoms and the therapy are of importance in the patient's psychic economy, the more likely will the result of vagotomy be unfavorable; and (2) the less the psychic energy is bound in this manner (i.e., little instinctual gratification being derived from being ill and from the medical regimen, and little secondary gain) the better is the prognosis.

The Psychiatric Aspects of the Postgastrectomy Syndrome. In the course of a study on the mechanism of the postgastrectomy syndrome (Adlersberg and Hammerschlag), it became apparent that almost all patients presented symptoms of psychoneurosis which in most instances had existed before the operation and even before the onset of ulcer symptoms. Several of these cases were studied psychiatrically to establish tentatively a connection between the personality structure of the patients, the development of peptic ulcer, the readiness to submit to surgery and the effect of the operation on the patient from a psychological viewpoint.

The analysis of the case histories led to the following conclusions: The psychiatric interviews conducted after the operations with the patients who had undergone medical and surgical treatment for peptic ulcer elicited material frequently not consciously known to the patient and therefore inaccessible to the physicians who had previously treated the patient. Repressed conflicts, discovered during the interviews, had produced chronic tension and guilt feelings which in turn had contributed to the ulcer formation. The readiness of the patient to submit to surgery was found to have been a neurotic escape or an atonement for unconscious guilt feelings. The surgical intervention thus played directly into the defense mechanisms of the patient in which the surgeon became the tool in the patient's unconscious scheme. The operation frequently created additional psychological and physiological discomfort. From these observations it was suggested that ulcer patients undergo psychiatric screening before an operation is considered.

The following case illustrates that, in some patients, only an understanding of unconscious mental mechanisms will permit an appreciation of the psychic forces that are important in a consideration of peptic ulcer.

Case 31.   Duodenal Ulcer

History and Symptoms.   A young white man fainted while at work, later had a black stool and was admitted to the hospital where a tentative diagnosis of bleeding peptic ulcer was made. This was later confirmed by x-ray which showed a typical ulcer deformity of the duodenum. He made good progress so that at the end of a month he was discharged from the hospital and then gradually returned to activity.

When first questioned he gave no history of any previous digestive trouble. He had had the usual childhood diseases but had never previously been seriously sick.

On further close questioning regarding gastrointestinal function he stated that his appetite, digestion and bowel function had always been excellent except that when he was worried about something or had had a quarrel with someone his appetite would leave him. Then he stated that for several months before the onset of his duodenal hemorrhage he had some slight indigestion. He recalled that on many occasions he ate more as a matter of habit than because of any real appetite, and that on some occasions he would have a heavy feeling in the epigastrium after eating.

The patient was a middle child of a family of five, two brothers and two sisters, all of whom were well. The father and mother were also living and well and there had been no digestive trouble in the family that he knew of.

Physical Examination and Laboratory Studies.   On admission to the hospital the physical examination showed a well-nourished young man with no abnormalities to be detected except a moderate degree of pallor. The pulse was rather rapid and the temperature was slightly elevated but both returned to normal within a short period of time. The hemoglobin was 60 per cent and the red blood cells were 3,000,000. X-ray examination was delayed until recovery was proceeding normally and then showed evidence of duodenal ulcer mentioned above. Improvement in blood count accompanied his general improvement and on discharge from the hospital the count was within normal limits.

LIFE SITUATION

The parents had been in humble circumstances and the patient had worked from an early age and by great effort had managed to put himself through school.

On superficial acquaintance he appeared to have a pleasant and affable disposition and always worked very hard to win the good opinion of his superiors. He had perfected himself as a machinist and held a responsible position.

Conflict over Marriage.   In the fall of the year preceding the onset of his trouble, he had met a young woman in whom he became much interested and in a very short time they became secretly engaged and planned elopement. He stated that his reasons for this were that the girl's parents objected because of his limited finances. On further conversation it developed that while it was true that he had paid marked attention to the girl, nevertheless he felt that he had been precipitated into an engagement and as a consequence became sleepless and worried a great deal about the responsibilities that he would have to assume and it was during this period of time that stomach symptoms developed. He had a premonition that he would get sick and, moreover, felt that it would be his stomach "that would go back on him." In spite of his engagement he did not have sexual relations because of moral scruples. To explain his hesitancy about marriage he suggested financial difficulty, the insecurity of his future and his inability to concentrate upon his work. He recognized that his mind was so occupied that he could not properly concentrate and hence felt that his work was suffering. During this period when he was so worried that he could not concentrate properly on his work he made a serious error which was discovered by his superior who humiliated him by taking certain responsibilities away. He felt the humiliation keenly. Then he became irritable and had a number of mild altercations with other people working in his department. These problems in turn seemed to worry him a great deal and then he would note that his digestion was particularly upset and that loss of appetite would persist until he was on friendly terms with his associates once more. He had always used cigarettes moderately but during these months smoked to excess, that is 25 to 30 cigarettes daily. He drank only occasionally and then not to excess. He became more and more indecisive about the marriage situation and especially about his financial responsibility and then occurred the digestive accident which resulted in his admission to the hospital.

TREATMENT

Certain medical measures had been instituted, that is, the withholding of food by mouth for the first forty-eight hours and then the principle of small, frequent feedings. Tobacco, of course, was not permitted and following his return to normal activity periodic rechecks of the duodenum by x-ray were made. The ulcer healed promptly and over a period of the succeeding five years never again showed any evidence of activity.

From the psychological standpoint it was explained to the patient that his conflict over the marriage situation had something to do with the precipitation of his illness and it was felt that so long as this conflict persisted it would be difficult if not impossible to bring about permanent cure. The patient himself readily grasped that this would be the case and hence felt that he must make up his mind either to marry or not to marry. He chose the latter and it would seem without perturbation because it was not long before his affections were engaged elsewhere. We did not believe nor did we persuade the patient that the psychological conflict was wholly responsible for his illness. It seemed rather to be only an activating factor in someone who, for unknown reasons, was predisposed to the development of a duodenal ulcer.

Follow-up.   The patient remained free of ulcer symptoms in spite of the fact that within a period of three years he had married another girl. On this occasion, however, he was financially in a much more secure position, had considerably more confidence in himself and, moreover, the engagement was one entirely of his own volition. He still suffered slight loss of appetite when working under stress or particularly when his sensitive nature was disturbed by criticism or altercation, but his functioning was close enough to normal so that he was satisfied with himself and we felt that he was likely to remain healthy.

The case is cited to illustrate that emotional problems frequently precede the onset of ulcer symptoms and especially sudden hemorrhage. Again and again in our patients with gastrointestinal hemorrhage of ulcer origin we have discovered evidence of a serious psychological conflict related to the particular personality structure of the patient which coincides with the time immediately preceding the onset of symptoms. We of course do not believe that there is a direct connection between psychological disturbance and ulcer formation but rather, as Alexander has stated, that the psychological difficulties may be responsible for changes in muscle tone and secretion which assist in disturbing the ulcer area.

Summary.   To summarize the discussion to this point it can be said that we have all been perfectly willing to recognize that the obvious emotional disturbances of life may have some effect upon the workings of the gastrointestinal tract but what we have been slow to recognize is that forces within us that are not so obvious have an even more pronounced effect.

Here, for example, was a patient who had a well defined ulcer of the duodenum which had been bleeding and therefore constituted a medical emergency. No question was raised about the psychological background of this problem when he was admitted; it was entirely a question of medical measures designed to improve the precarious state. But the question of the future then assumed importance and it therefore seemed that if we could understand him better as a person we would be better able to manage the illness. We need not go beyond that point at the moment. We sketched the life situation and the reaction of this young man as he tried to adjust and while there were some peculiarities, chiefly in the direction of exaggerations of normal trends, there was certainly no extraordinary departure from normal. And so it often proves to be in a patient like this. The material may be difficult to obtain and the application to the problem of the illness is likewise quite complex.

CONFLICT OVER MARRIAGE.   Now the point is that this patient had a deep conflict in his personality which manifested itself in regard to the problem of marriage. He did not recognize this, however; indeed, he refused to recognize it. His rationalization for not getting married seemed perfectly satisfactory to him. As Alexander pointed out, a certain drive or urge within him which he could not adequately express in action or words he apparently was trying to express through his stomach. The stomach apparently was disturbed in its function because he was trying to express certain cravings for love and affection, manifested by "hunger pains," instead of being able to obtain this affection in the usual way. This background has been described as the intimate relationship between the feeding process and the physical satisfaction of infancy. In the study of these adult patients with peptic ulcer and other so-called "functional" disturbances of the gastrointestinal tract we have been impressed that *bed and board in adult life are as indissolubly connected as sustenance and sensuality in infant life.* To put this in another way we can say that men with functional disturbances of the stomach have a very high incidence of marital difficulties. As we have tried to indicate, this is not easily analyzed and so we find many men who are very active, energetic and aggressive in their everyday social and business contacts who, nevertheless, have this infantile pattern deep down in their personality, of craving love and affection and expressing this craving by "hunger pains." Again the symbolism of the body language that we have discussed before will be recognized.

RELATION OF PSYCHIC FORCES TO ULCER FORMATION.   Alexander took pains to point out in the introduction to his studies that he did not consider that the phenomenon of a duodenal ulcer, as an end result of a long series of tissue changes, could be interpreted psychologically. In other words, the ulcer itself has no psychological significance whatever. What can be interpreted as direct effects of psychological factors are the disturbances in secretion and the change in the motor activity and possibly even the alteration in the blood supply of the stomach. It is not difficult to believe that in the presence of some additional constitutional or acquired factor an ulcer might be brought about.

Principles of Psychotherapy in Ulcer Patients.   Saul, formerly associated with Alexander, summarizes the psychological management as follows:

"In the first place, we shall concentrate upon the patient himself, and endeavor to discern the major motivations of his life and his relationships to his main feelings, conflicts and tensions. We shall be especially alert to his needs for love, ease, support, and dependence, and to all those desires which can be considered intaking in nature, i.e., of the same direction as the taking in of food. And we shall watch especially for any frustrations of these desires, whether by external circumstances or by the internal attitudes of the patient himself.

"The tempo of the interview is determined predominantly by the patient's personality make-up and by the intensity of his need for help. The physician can rarely force the issue. Rather his effort must be to get the patient to reveal himself. Sometimes, almost all one needs to do is listen. In other cases, the patient not only resists seeing the pertinent emotional forces, but it may even be dangerous to try to force him to do so.

"In the average case it is practicable to begin with a discussion of the physical symptoms. In general, first interviews begin very slowly. As the patient's confidence in the psychiatrist mounts and he feels that there is genuine interest and the possibility of being understood, the pertinent emotional material flows more freely. . . . The discussion of the physical condition usually can be led naturally to the emotional setting in which these began, and, once immersed in this discussion, the patient's deeper feelings usually emerge.

"If the patient is too resistant at this point, it is sometimes well to turn to the family background. In the end, one's aim is to elicit the patient's true major motivations and feelings, and how these developed from the emotional pressures of his childhood, on through to their relationship to his present symptoms. While it is impossible to present a list of the questions to ask, one must keep the patient talking, and bring out his feelings in childhood toward those who reared him, and how they shaped his present personality. One estimates the present emotional interplay and organization from his relationships to his family, friends, work, and recreation. One seeks for positive irritants and hardships, as well as for negative factors such as unsatisfied desires. There is no simple method for comprehending the core of the personality, or for estimating the intensity of the feelings and frustrations. This is a matter of psychological sense and psychiatric experience. It is remarkable how much one often learns by merely listening to the patient, while divesting oneself, so far as possible, of one's knowledge and preconceptions.

"Dreams are invaluable in many cases for penetrating rapidly and accurately to the major emotional forces within the person. It is inadvisable for the physician, inexperienced with dreams, to interpret them to the patient, but with a little interest and study he can often glean simply from the topics of the dreams what is central in the patient's mind: hostility, anxiety, desires for ease and escape, the pressure toward work and accomplishment, needs for superiority, etc. What the dreams tell is usually at least a helpful clue, but more often an invaluable aid in clarifying one's understanding of the fundamental emotional forces in the case. This understanding is the indispensable basis of rational treatment. In surgery, the cutting is the least; it is the understanding of the pathological physiology and anatomy, and the utilization of the surgical techniques for accomplishing a rational purpose. The analogy between rational psychiatry and surgery is a sound one. Psychiatric techniques, such as suggestion, reassurance, hypnosis, catharsis, and the like, are significant only when one understands the basic emotional situation and applies them rationally for well-defined purposes. Employed without this understanding, they are little more than a medieval laying-on of hands.

"We have already mentioned some of the therapeutic elements employed in the ordinary interview. The transference, or relationship to the physician, is always present and can be of great value as a means of emotional support. Neurosis is in essence the persistence of childhood desires and patterns. The patient coming to the physician tends unconsciously to adopt toward him the dependent, help-seeking attitude of a child to its parent. This gives the physician tremendous influence. The reaction is of great importance in the ulcer patients, in whom we deal so largely with needs to be fed emotionally. Usually it is not necessary to discuss the transference with the patient, but the physician must be constantly aware of it.

"Insight, properly used, is effective in the vast majority of cases. Like the interview, it must develop slowly and tactfully, at a tempo set by the patient. But where it can be imparted with reasonable completeness it is a powerful instrument, and makes the entire management much easier for the physician; for now the patient himself understands his problem, will himself have ideas for environmental changes, and in the favorable cases will endeavor, with real therapeutic urge, to alter his attitudes. Some patients, who typically are unable to accept anything freely and must be incessantly striving, can be mellowed noticeably in a very few interviews.

"In general, where one cannot relieve the patient through insight, changes in the environment, and relatively simple changes in attitude, one faces major surgery (psychotherapy), and it is necessary to call in the analytically-trained psychiatrist. This specialist is also effective for diagnosis and for brief causal treatment, in which he can often save much time. His contribution is *psychiatric accuracy*."

References

Adlersberg, D., and Hammerschlag, E.: J.A.M.A., *139:* 429, 1949.

Alexander, F.: Psychoanalyt. Quart., *3:* 501, 1934.

Alexander, F.: From Portis, S. A.: Diseases of the Digestive System. Lea and Febiger, Philadelphia, 1941, Ch. VI, p. 213.

Alvarez, W. C.: Am. J. Surg., *18:* 207, 1932.

Beattie, J.: Canad. M.A.J., *26:* 278, 1932.

Browning, J. S., and Houseworth, T. H.: Psychosom. Med., *15:* 328, 1953.

Cleghorn, R. A.: Psychosom. Med., *17:* 367, 1955.

Cushing, H.: Surg., Gynec. & Obst., *55:* 1, 1932.

Donavan, E. J., and Santulli, T. V.: Am. J. Dis. Child., *69:* 176, 1945.

Eichhorn, R., and Tracktir, J.: Gastroenterology, *29:* 432, 1955.

Einhorn, M.: Med. Record, *34:* 751, 1888.

Engel, G. L., Reishsman, F., and Segal, H. L.: Psychosom. Med., *18:* 374, 1956.

Eusterman, G. B.: J. M. Soc. New Jersey, *36:* 1, 1939.

French, J. D.: Psychosom. Med., to be published.

Gray, S. J., Ramsey, C., Reifenstein, R. W., and Benson, J. A.: Gastroenterology, *25:* 156, 1953.

Guthrie, K. J.: Arch. Dis. Childhood, *17:* 82, 1942.

Heath, R. G.: Psychosom. Med., *17:* 383, 1955.

Hurst, A. F. L.: J.A.M.A., *102:* 582, 1934.
Jackson, C.: Laryngoscope, *32:* 139, 1922.
Kapp, F. T., Rosenbaum, M., and Romano, J.: Amer. J. Psychiat., *103:* 700, 1947.
Keller, A. D., Hare, W. K., and D'Amour, M. C.: Proc. Soc. Exper. Biol. & Med., *30:* 772, 1932.
Kezur, E.: Kapp, F. G., and Rosenbaum, M.: Am. J. Psychiat., *108:* 368, 1951.
Lendrum, F. C.: Arch. Int. Med., *59:* 474, 1937.
Light, R. V., Bishop, C. C., and Kendall, L. G.: J. Pharmacol. & Exper. Ther., *45:* 227, 1932.
Lindemann, E.: Arch. Neurol. & Psychiat., *53:* 322, 1945.
MacLean, P. D.: Psychosom. Med., *17:* 335, 1955.
McMahon, J. M., Braceland, F. J., and Moersch, H. J.: Ann. Int. Med., *34:* 608, 1951.
Margolin, S. S.: Psychoanalyt. Quart., *20:* 349, 1951.
Moschcowitz, E.: New England J. Med., *212:* 603, 1935.
Olsen, A. M., Harrington, S. W., Moersch, H. J., and Andersen, H. A.: J. Thoracic Surg., *22:* 109, 1951.
Papez, J. W.: Arch. Neurol. & Psychiat., *28:* 725, 1937.
Porter, R. W., Movius, H. J., and French, J. D.: Surgery, *33:* 875, 1953.
Roth, J. T.: Arch. Int. Med., *96:* 32, 1955.
Saul, L. J.: Psychosom. Med., *8:* 204, 1946.
Shay, H., and Sun, D. C. H.: Am. J. M. Sc., *228:* 630, 1954.
Shay, H., Sun, D. C. H., Dlin, B., and Weiss, E.: To be published.
Sperling, M.: Psychoanalytic Study of Ulcerative Colitis in Children, Psychoanal. Quart., *15:* 302, 1946.
Ssasz, T. S.: Psychosom. Med., *11:* 187, 1949.
Stertfeld, H. S.: Psychosom. Med., *16:* 315, 1954.
Von Bergmann, G.: Berl. Klin. Wchnschr., *55:* 524, 1918.
Weiner, H., Thaler, M., Reiser, M. F., and Mirsky, I. A.: Psychosom. Med., *19:* 1, 1957.
Weiss, E.: Psychosom. Med., *6:* 58, 1944.
Willis, T.: Pharmaceutic Rationalis. London 1679, p. 23, taken from Major, Ralph H.: Classic Descriptions of Disease. Charles C Thomas, Springfield, 1932, p. 591.
Winkelstein, A.: Am. J. Surg., *12:* 135, 1931.
Wolf, S., and Almy, T. P.: Gastroenterology, *13:* 391, 1949.
Wolf, S., and Wolff, H. G.: J.A.M.A., *120:* 670, 1942.
Wolf, S., and Wolff, H. G.: Human Gastric Function. 2nd ed. Oxford University Press, New York, 1947.

Chapter X

Endocrine System
and Metabolism

THE RELATION OF DISORDERS OF THE THYROID GLAND TO THE EMOTIONS

It has been known for many years that emotional disturbances often accompany disorders of the thyroid gland. Certainly, it is not surprising to find emotional factors in a condition in which the clinical picture mimics the expression of fear and terror, and which has been described as "crystallized fright." There are the emotional disorders, neurotic and psychotic, which occur as a part of the clinical picture of hyperthyroidism; the autonomic imbalance and psychic shocks which often seem to precede hyperthyroidism; and lastly the anxiety states associated with thyroid enlargements without hyperthyroidism. The *emotionalism* of hyperthyroidism is well known and is not our special concern. It is equally well known that this emotionalism diminishes when recovery from the disease occurs. What we are especially interested in is whether personality disturbances of long standing may lead to an alteration of thyroid function, or, to put it another way, whether hyperthyroidism may represent a characteristic response of a special personality type to a specific psychic insult.

Differential Diagnosis.   One of the commonest problems in clinical medicine is the differential diagnosis of hyperthyroidism and anxiety neurosis. When a patient presents the clinical signs of hyperthyroidism and laboratory tests are confirmatory there is little question about the diagnosis. But it is the borderline case that causes trouble. Signs are absent, tests are equivocal, and the patient is nervous. If a history of long-standing emotional difficulties preceding the onset of symptoms and the other criteria (p. 73) for establishing a psychiatric diagnosis are present, one is justified in approaching the illness from an emotional standpoint. Certainly it is unwise in the face of such considerations to attempt surgery or the administration of radioactive iodine. Needless to add it is equally reprehensible to administer electroshock therapy to patients with hyperthyroidism in the mistaken belief that they are suffering from a mental disorder. It is reprehensible on two counts—(1) hyperthyroidism does not call for that kind of treatment and (2) neither does anxiety neurosis, which is often made much worse by electroshock treatments.

Preceding Emotional Disturbances.   Many observations have been made on the emotional disturbances that precede hyperthyroidism. In 1925, Nolan D. C. Lewis reviewed the literature and concluded that there was no generally accepted theory of the pathogenesis of exophthalmic goiter. That is still true today. Nevertheless, increasing attention has been paid to the incidence of emotional difficulties in the histories of patients with hyperthyroidism. Moschcowitz, Bram, and Hyman and Kessel are among the clinicians who have been impressed by such factors. Hyman and Kessel, who studied the problem of the relation of autonomic imbalance and hyperthyroidism, reported that "our patients almost without exception gave a history of psychic trauma preceding or associated with the development of the symptoms of exophthalmic goiter." But hints from life situations in series of cases compiled by clinicians and flashes of intuition by psychiatrists who have studied occasional cases are not enough to establish the importance of psychopathology in the etiology of hyperthyroidism. Felix Deutsch approached the problem psychoanalytically and postulated that a constitutional degenerative "Anlage" could be lighted up into exophthalmic goiter by nervous influences such as might arise in hysteria.

B. Mittelmann, in a discussion on the psychogenic factors in hyperthyroidism, felt that no work existed which used full modern psychopathological knowledge in its dynamic and descriptive aspects covering a large series of cases. Therese Benedek in the study and treatment of two cases thought that the increased activity of the gland helped to *release* the emotions of *anxiety* and *aggression* which in turn often gave rise to the clinical picture of mental depression. In a study of considerable importance 166 women and 34 men with hyperthyroidism were observed from a psychiatric standpoint by Conrad.

Psychosomatic Observations

Conrad began her examination with a careful check of the exact time and sequence of the appearance of symptoms of hyperthyroidism. This was followed by a review of the family situation. Particular attention was given to any alteration in any situation showing a time relation to exacerbation of symptoms and a constant watch was kept for signs of unexplained emotion. In this connection she called attention to a *flushing* of the neck and lower face which showed a high degree of specificity in leading one to the conflict over which the patient had "decompensated." If the patient was interviewed in a good light, this was frequently noted in mild form. The degree of severity showed some correlation with the elevation of the B.M.R. and also with the violence of the trauma recalled. The blushing extended from the upper chest to the middle of the cheeks and occasionally to the forehead, with the neck veins standing out and pulsations in the neck increasing in violence, so that in extreme cases the thyroid gland itself appeared to increase in size. This flushing was noted when specific sensitiveness of the individual to an emotional experience had been "touched off." In mild form, such a blush repeatedly established points leading to the patient's major unconscious conflict. Conrad remarked that once noted it was a signal for as much caution as the appearance of pain in palpating an acute abdomen. She was also impressed by the appearance of confusion when the patient was questioned about dates and a sequence of events focusing upon a traumatic situation.

It was increasingly evident that instead of long periods of worry and deprivation there was usually an *emotional conflict* at the time of onset of the first typical symptom of the disease. Many times a patient repeated a story of shock as the cause of illness and this later proved to have come after typical symptoms had been present for some time. Thus she emphasized the necessity for an exact study of the onset of the very first symptom and of the personal life situation at that time.

Disturbance in Mother-Child Relationship. Many hyperthyroid patients showed endocrine imbalance in their development and family history. The body form was often that of hypogonadal development. So far as the psychic situation was concerned some abnormality in the mother-child relation was usually obvious. Examination of the female patient often revealed anxiety at the time of onset of acute symptoms, which followed in the main two patterns: (1) a fear of loss of shelter and affection, often apparently equivalent to deprivation of the mother or loss of the mother's approval, and (2) a fear of the dangers of the mother role. Many of the patients had been subjected to a strain with a resulting sense of inadequacy in the "mother's care of child" relation which seemed to be badly tolerated by them. This kind of strain appeared to precipitate the syndrome or to bring about an exacerbation. A large number of patients had been deprived of their mothers at an early age and often the death was due to childbearing. These persons appeared to make desperate and lifelong struggles to win the mother's approval and to achieve likeness to her at the same time that they feared the responsibilities which she had. Worry over the mother's lot, however, was not limited to the dangers of pregnancy. It was often noted that the patient had been selected by the mother to share her anxiety and burdens even when there were older and stronger siblings. Even the male patients showed in a number of instances a disturbance in the mother-child relationship. Often there was conflict over partial identification with the mother. It was also noted that there was a tendency in a rather high percentage of cases to be dependent on the wife as a mother.

Previous Emotional Trends. Usually there was one or more previous episodes of nervousness or breakdown before the overt onset of the actual illness. Several cases who "never felt the same after the mother died" showed a typical sudden onset following another traumatic experience. Hysteria, anxiety, and paranoid and manic-depressive tendencies were often observed in these patients prior to the onset of their hyperthyroidism.

Anxiety Takes the Visceral Path. Therefore, Conrad suggested that the emotional pattern of these personalities may be explained by hypothesizing a pathological development, often a frustration, in the normal attempt to establish independence of the mother. She remarked that the classical neurotic symbolizes his conflict without somatic pathology—he suffers at a cortical level. In other words, instead of showing physical symptoms he presents disturbances in thinking and attitudes. But when conflicts in the personal life discharge energy into autonomic channels, pathological tension, congestion and imbalance of secretion may occur and may increase susceptibility to physical disease, precipitate it or cause an exacerbation of disease that is already present. As Deutsch suggested, Conrad also believed that this occurs in individuals with more or less hereditary weakness or acquired pathology. For anxiety to take the visceral path, there must also be an instability of integration for one's role in life, originating in the early formation of the personality, probably in the process of establishing independence of the mother. This pattern may be linked with a typical neurosis or occur without it. In the latter case the patient's relation with other people appears undisturbed while his attitude toward himself shows pathological insecurity.

Psychic Trauma.   So far as etiology of hyperthyroidism was concerned Conrad obtained a history of psychic trauma in 94 per cent of cases by a method of examination which stressed (1) the investigation of new developments in the life situation and personal relations at the time of onset of hyperthyroid symptoms; and (2) the evaluation of unconscious conflicts which were indicated by the appearance of a specific sign of emotion during history-taking.

All writers who have studied the problem from its dynamic aspects agree on a constitutional factor in the disease but there is also a remarkable unanimity of opinion regarding the psychological factors. Lidz and Whitehorn found that these patients react to a disruption or threat of disruption of the personal relationships upon which their security rests: the adolescent may be confronted with the loss of the more significant parent; a young woman is disturbed by the hurdle of marriage; an older person may be threatened by the loss of a child upon whom his security depends. In all of these situations it is seen that the patient is inordinately insecure. The attachment to a parent, usually the mother, is intense, and establishes a pattern for other relationships. To state the problem briefly, the authors describe a typical life situation, consisting of the disruption or threat of disruption of a dependent personal attachment, to which the vulnerable patient reacts intensely because dependency is necessary to fulfill a basic personality need.

In a detailed study of 24 cases Ham, Alexander and Carmichael also find the same basic personality factors and emphasize the struggle against underlying insecurity and dependency, illustrated, for example, by the manner in which such patients wish to take care of others, especially children. The specific dynamic pattern is outlined as follows: Frustration of dependent longings and persistent threats to security (exposure to death and other threatening experiences) in early life →unsuccessful premature attempts to identify with object of dependent cravings→continued effort toward premature self-sufficiency and to help others—→failure of strivings for self-sufficiency and taking care of others —→thyrotoxicosis.

Treatment Suggestions. (1) Increase the stability of autonomic function as, for example, by partial thyroidectomy or with radioactive iodine treatment and (2) psychotherapy aimed to increase the independence of the personality. To the extent that this is impossible of realization, the maximum of physical and emotional shelter becomes imperative.

Psychological Invalidism in Thyroidectomized Patients

Ruesch and his associates explored the problems of personality structure in relation to the onset of symptoms and recovery in 43 patients who had been subjected to subtotal thyroidectomy. There were 35 women and 8 men in the series; 32 had toxic and 11 nontoxic goiters.

The study indicated that patients afflicted with thyroid disease fall into two distinct entities as far as their sociopsychological aspects are concerned: the normal or almost normal girl (one third of the total) and the hysterical or anxious type (more than one half of the total). In the case of men it was a question of dependent personalities. Although surgical procedures were tolerated well by the normal girls, delayed recovery was pretty much the rule for anxious types and hysterical personalities.

Ruesch noted that the conformist attitude in these patients was outstanding. There was a great need for recognition and for dependence. Self-love and inability to express anger were the outstanding personality problems; overconformance to accepted ideals was the principal defense. In about half the cases a necessity to adjust to environmental changes was found at the time of onset of the disease. Because of their childhood pattern, the patients were poorly equipped to face these environmental changes; broken homes, for example, burdened them with premature responsibilities, producing feelings of insecurity. Ruesch recommends psychotherapy before and after this operation. His comprehensive article contains an appendix summarizing the sociopsychological aspects of patients with hyperthyroidism.

The following case represents a characteristic background of a typical case of hyperthyroidism.

Case 32. Hyperthyroidism

A white woman of 44 complained of nervousness and loss of weight. She said that she had always been nervous but that it had been worse in the last few months and that there had been a loss of about 10 pounds in weight in the last two months. Except for heart consciousness there were no other symptoms.

Past History. She had been married for fifteen years and had a son, aged 10, who was living and well. Prior to the birth of her child she had suffered from dysmenorrhea but that was no longer present. Nevertheless, she had had a long period of invalidism after the birth of the child—this she referred to as "a nervous breakdown."

The father had been a dreamy, incompetent person who had died suddenly from heart disease at the age of 50 and the mother, an accomplished and domineering woman, had been forced to earn a living for the family. The family consisted of three brothers and a sister. One brother, somewhat younger than the patient, suffered from manic-depressive psychosis and had been an inmate of institutions on numerous occasions. Still another brother was brilliant but erratic. Whereas the sister had enjoyed a college education and had married successfully, the patient had been saddled with responsibilities at home and denied educational opportunities.

Present Illness.   At first the patient was unable to find any emotional circumstance that coincided with the onset of her illness but after some discussion admitted that once more the family was torn with conflict over the question of the disposition of the manic-depressive brother. It always fell to the patient's lot to be responsible for him at such times as he was not in an institution. Just prior to the onset of this illness she had been faced with numerous responsibilities and suddenly was presented with the necessity of once more taking this brother into her home. She said, "I didn't know whether to mother him or smother him." Thus her conflict of maternal devotion and hostility was symbolized by this casual expression. Nevertheless, she took her brother, hardly recovered from a manic attack, into her home, felt great tension, smoked and drank to excess, and kept herself busy in order "not to have time to think."

Thus it was that increased "nervousness" and loss of weight became evident to her family and friends even before she herself noted it. Finally she was persuaded to seek medical attention and the classic picture of hyperthyroidism was found.

TREATMENT

The background out of which the hyperthyroidism seemed to arise was made clear to her and it was explained that the immediate problem could be met by surgery or radioactive iodine but that the emotional tensions of the past had to be dealt with differently in order for her to achieve permanent cure. She chose to be operated upon. The surgical removal of the major part of the gland was successful and she made a speedy recovery. Then with the help of medical advice she adopted a more realistic attitude toward her brother's illness, insisting that other members of the family assist in his care, and placed him permanently in an institution so that he would not prove to be so disruptive a force in the family situation.

The following cases represent various problems associated with or related to thyroid disease.

Case 33.   Nodular Goiter with Anxiety Symptoms

A young, married white woman complained of a lump in the neck and nervousness.

History and Symptoms.   She considered herself in fairly good health until about one year before, at which time she developed attacks of nervousness, especially in the morning, which were accompanied by a feeling of "a lump in the throat," tremors and nausea. They occurred frequently and especially about the time of the menstrual period. The attacks might last an hour or might last all day. She felt that they were often precipitated by emotional disturbance. She had had frequent nightmares so that she awakened with a start, was very frightened, and perspired freely. Following such attacks she was apt to have diarrhea. When she was nervous she had deep sighing respirations.

She was a premature baby and was considered a frail child, but had no serious illness. About four years ago in school it was noted that the thyroid gland was large. One year ago her father was operated upon for goiter after having had medical treatment without help for a long time. Following operation he did well, gained weight, and regained his health. It was about this time that the mother called the patient's attention to the fact that she also had a goiter.

Menses, established at the age of eleven, had always been painful and sometimes were accompanied by nausea. As stated above, the choking feeling in the throat was worse during the menstrual period.

Her family history other than the note mentioned regarding her father did not seem to have any bearing on this illness.

Physical Examination and Laboratory Studies.   Examination showed a small, thin girl with nodular enlargement of the left lobe of the thyroid gland. Other than this finding the physical examination was essentially negative. There were no objective evidences of hyperthyroidism. The urine examination was negative and the Wassermann was negative but the blood count showed leukocytes varying from 10,000 to 17,000 and the temperature chart showed that her temperature averaged about 99° or 99.2° F. with one elevation to 99.4° F. Pulse and respirations were not increased.

Basal metabolism tests had been plus 8, plus 14, and after a few days in the hospital plus 1 without any medication. The sedimentation rate was within normal limits. The gynecological examination was negative.

The patient was sent into the hospital first, to determine whether she had hyperthyroidism and secondly, to decide, even if she did not, whether to operate upon this enlarged gland. On the basis of the observations up to this point we concluded that there was no evidence of hyperthyroidism. The second question we will reserve for later discussion.

LIFE SITUATION

Unfortunately, terms for describing personality changes are not so precise as those for describing pulse or basal metabolic rates. But we have to do the best we can with close observation and description to make clear the pathological disturbance in the temperament of our patients and thus realize that this factor may be just as important as a very high basal metabolic rate.

Childhood. The mother died when the patient was born and she lived in an orphanage for three years, whereupon her father married again and she was taken home. Certainly three years in an orphan asylum was not the most auspicious way to begin life, even though this orphanage may have been an unusually good institution. A child placed in an orphanage is not likely to get the individual personal interest and love that a child obtains with his own parents. Even after she came to live with the family in her father's home she says she never knew until the age of fifteen that her stepmother was not her real mother. She had two older brothers but evidently the siblings weren't close enough to discuss such matters. When she found this out at fifteen she felt she understood why she had been neglected and why there had been a lack of personal warmth for her in the home. Of course it is common for children to feel neglected in *any* home but it may well have been that the stepmother was not able to feel the same interest in the patient as in her own child.

Marriage. She was married nine months before admission, to a man she had known for some time and liked very much. She had been very happy. At the same time anticipation of sexual relations disturbed her and during the first week of her marriage the idea of sexual intercourse was so distressing that her husband was not able to approach her. It took some time for her to become adjusted to the sexual relationship. Later, according to her statement, intercourse became quite satisfactory. We have learned that we cannot accept such a statement at face value in the beginning of psychotherapy. In fact we must not dwell too much upon the subject of sexual functioning. Later the importance of any disturbance in this field can be more easily discussed and understood.

Anxiety Attacks and Anxiety Dreams. In the past year and a half she had had what will be recognized as anxiety attacks, usually occurring at night, preceded by a dream in which something unpleasant was happening. Sometimes she was being pursued by animals or men. Sometimes in the dream she was falling from the roofs of houses and then would awaken in the anxiety state. Recently, she dreamed that a dog was biting her hand and she could not get away. She awoke crying, felt cold all over, and had palpitation. She had also dreams in which actual violence, such as a murder, had taken place.

Up to the time of the present illness this girl had done well in meeting her tasks as far as the casual observer could see. But fear and anxiety existed within and as a result of it she had begun to display symptoms and her efficiency had begun to fail.

Many patients with *social anxiety* do not develop anxiety attacks until much later in life than was the case with this patient. Fortunately, she had not developed a belief that she had a heart condition and was willing to listen to advice that could help her to understand her illness. She apparently was willing to believe that she did not have thyroid disease, although this had been suggested as the cause of her distress and she had been much impressed by the facts of her father's illness.

TREATMENT

The first question to be decided was whether this patient had hyperthyroidism and we came to the conclusion that she did not but that she did have a *simple goiter*. Then the question arose as to whether she should be operated upon anyhow and here a number of considerations entered. She was a young woman and the lump in the neck might be removed for cosmetic reasons if for no other. In addition there was always the possibility of further growth, of hyperthyroidism, and of the development of a cancer. Besides all that, and very important in this case, the patient had the knowledge of her father being treated for goiter for a long time without help and then the quick recovery following surgery. Then came the question of psychological preparation for surgery, which we consider one of the major questions in medicine. Surgeons are always so careful to prepare their patients physically for surgery; they would never think of performing a major operation without knowing that the cardiovascular-renal system had been surveyed but they almost never give any consideration to the kind of personality that exists in the individual who is about to be operated upon, how much anxiety is there, and what the effects of a surgical traumatic experience may be as far as the personality structure is concerned. We once had in the hospital ward an old woman who had a huge enlargement of the thyroid gland which was removed because it was pressing upon the trachea. She had some discomfort but not severe dyspnea. The anatomical problem loomed large in the clinical picture but the patient was very apprehensive prior to operation and after operation became completely psychotic. As it turned out we wonder whether perhaps she was not better off with the lump in her neck. Similar instances of how badly some patients react to surgery are dealt with elsewhere.

Therefore, the matter of preparation for operation especially interested us in this patient. We allowed about six weeks for seeing the patient once a week and getting acquainted with her problems. Here were some of the things we wanted to find out: Had many people noticed or commented upon the lump in her throat? How much would she like to have it removed? We tried to estimate from what she said just how important this lump was to her. Sometimes people are very sensitive in many other fields and yet the enlargement does not distress them or at least disturbs them very little. In that case one would not think of operating for cosmetic reasons alone. We tried to find out how much she feared an operation and how much of a shock she thought it would be to her. We put the question something like this, "How many people who have had operations do you know? Have they suffered from pain or distress during or after an operation? What do you fear? Is it pain or the effects of the anesthesia or the scar or discomfort connected with the scar?" Each time we talked to her about these things we tried to estimate what her reaction to operation would be.

Readiness for Operation.   We inquired about the lump in her neck and she reported that the swelling seemed more pronounced and caused a sense of pressure. She also felt that for cosmetic reasons she would like to have it removed. Her friends remarked about the lump and it embarrassed her to have attention called to it. As she was so extremely neat in her appearance it was understandable that this asymmetry of the neck would be a psychological problem for her. We discussed the matter of operation. We asked her how she would feel about the resulting scar upon the neck and her reply was that she thought she could endure the scar much better than the present lump. We warned her that an operation might not remove the sense of pressure of which she complained, at least not more than temporarily, since a sense of pressure in the neck was often of nervous origin and not due to pressure of a small growth such as she had. The patient felt that she would be willing to take this chance. At the end of two months the patient reported that her anxiety attacks had entirely disappeared. She was not busy at her place of work and therefore wanted to have the operation performed then. We felt that since her desire for operation had been consistent and that since her anxiety had subsided and she was making a better social adjustment, she was in a satisfactory emotional condition to meet the operation.

Operation.   The operation was successful and the patient was then sent to a convalescent home to recuperate. A small stitch abscess developed which she tolerated without a return of anxiety. This healed without producing a disfiguring scar and the patient felt well satisfied with the result. Her social adjustment has not been as satisfactory as we would like to see but there has been no return of anxiety attacks and it seems likely that further improvement will occur.

Therapy in Outpatient Department.   The patient reported to the psychiatric outpatient department one week after her discharge from the hospital. On this visit she was again informed that as a result of her study in the hospital, no cause of an organic nature had been found for her fatigue and her weakness. Her personality needs were put before her again and it was explained how important it would be for her to recognize these needs and so relate herself to people as to get some satisfaction for these needs. On this visit a maternal aunt had accompanied the patient. She seemed a kind and understanding person and so we explained to her in the patient's presence something of the latter's problem. This is a safe procedure when we are sure that the relative is really kind and understanding. In some cases a relative or friend may use such information to ridicule or harass the patient rather than to be helpful. But in this case we felt the aunt was sincerely interested in our patient and understood her problem. The result of this was to make the patient feel that she was not carrying the burden of her emotional problem entirely alone.

At the end of the first month the patient reported that her anxiety attacks were decreasing but might still occur in the presence of people when some incident of emotional significance occurred. In the next two weeks she reported that she was feeling still better and had had only one mild period of anxiety. This occurred when a new situation presented itself. She had her first altercation with one of the employees who tried to impose additional work upon her. On previous occasions our patient had always given in although there was inner rebellion. On this occasion she spoke up in defense of herself and declined to accept the additional work. The patient felt rather good about this in spite of her mild anxiety.

The next patient was at first treated for thyroid disease and later, for no better reason, for pituitary disease.

Case 34.   Severe Neurosis or Early Schizophrenia; Differential Diagnosis from Endocrine Disease

A single white woman, age 22, complained of a burning sensation in the stomach which extended "like a wave all the way to the genitals," attacks of palpitation, sweating and faintness.

History and Symptoms.   She had been well until one evening, in a motion picture theater, she had a feeling of oppression on the chest, palpitation, and sweating which caused her to leave the theater. On the street she felt faint, was taken to a nearby drug store and later to the office of a private physician. There the diagnosis of a *heart attack* was made. She was later treated for *thyroid disease*. Following this she was admitted to the Temple University Hospital for further investigation. The history at this time indicated that she had been short of breath since her "collapse" in August but that this had no relation to exertion. Palpitation occurred whenever she became nervous or excited. She observed that the hair of her arms was getting longer, blacker and coarser and that there was an abnormal growth of hair on her lip and chin and also upon the abdomen. About the same time she began to complain of a loss of appetite, a sensation of heat or a hot flash arising in the epigastrium and lasting several seconds to hours. This would extend like a wave down to the genitals. Since the beginning of the illness she had also complained of "fainty spells with a dizzy sensation." She became very weak and exhausted on walking and had to lie down.

She had measles and whooping cough as a child and at the age of 9 an incision and drainage of a thyroid abscess with a resulting sinus and fistula which took four years to heal. There had been no other illnesses. The menses had been regular up to the time of admission; they were profuse and the last two periods were associated with dysmenorrhea.

The family consisted of a father, 54, and mother, 55, who were living and well. There were two brothers and three sisters all of whom were well. A grandfather died of carcinoma of the stomach.

Physical Examination and Laboratory Studies.   On admission the temperature, pulse and respirations were normal. The blood pressure was 120/85. The skin of the face was rather coarse and oily and there was some excess hair on the upper lip and chin. There was a moderate amount of acne on the back. There was a small scar just at the right of the midline over the thyroid region but the thyroid seemed normal on palpation. The cardiovascular system seemed normal and the lungs were clear and resonant. The abdominal examination showed some striae atrophicae over the lower abdomen and hips, and there was some extension of pubic hair toward the umbilicus.

The urine and blood count were normal; a glucose tolerance test was slightly altered in the direction of diminished tolerance; the blood Wassermann was negative and basal metabolism was minus 3. Eyegrounds were normal and visual fields were normal. An x-ray of the skull was normal. The electrocardiogram was within normal limits. In spite of these negative findings it had been assumed that the patient had *pituitary basophilism* and she had been treated with irradiation to the pituitary gland. About the only change noted was that she missed a menstrual period. The same symptoms continued, she was then treated elsewhere with injections of glandular substance, and returned to the Temple University Hospital for further studies.

Second Hospital Admission.   The complaints were the same but on several occasions the blood pressure had been slightly elevated. Studies were repeated. This time the glucose tolerance test was normal and two basal metabolism tests were minus 5 and minus 6. Neurological examination was negative and the eyegrounds and fields were normal. Gynecological examination was negative. The general physical examination showed nothing different from before. The patient was normal in appearance except for the slight hair increase that we had already noted. She felt well when she was lying down but complained that after she was up and about she became very fatigued and had to lie down. Electrocardiograph studies in the recumbent and upright positions showed very slight evidence of postural circulatory changes. Slight flattening of the T wave occurred in the upright position. Pulse and blood pressure were practically unaffected.

LIFE SITUATION

Early Life and Family Background.   She had lived a very secluded life, entirely within her own family. As a child she was not allowed to play with the neighborhood children because the parents felt that she was superior to the others. This same attitude persisted throughout adolescence when she was not allowed to associate with the other young people of her town because they were not "the right kind." As a result this girl enjoyed no hobbies and no sports. She never learned to dance or to play cards. She had no special interest of any kind. She had never done a single day's work!

Her father was a Catholic and her mother a Protestant. About the age of 11 this girl became interested in the Catholic church (according to her statement because of a girl friend who became a Catholic) and she joined the church but had not kept up her interest. She did not seem much concerned about this and stated that the family was not concerned and it may be that this was true. Nevertheless, as we have discussed elsewhere, such a situation is often associated with conflict during adolescence.

Failure to Develop a Normal Personality.   A normal personality has been defined as one who is *free of symptoms, unhampered by mental conflict, has a satisfactory working capacity, and can love someone other than himself.* This girl deviated markedly from this definition. She had many symptoms. It is true that she displayed little obvious evidence of mental conflict, but she had no working capacity and was unable to love anyone but herself. The mental conflict was latent within this person, and was absorbed, so to speak, by the symptoms. Mental conflict would have been produced if she had been forced to live a normal existence. Never having learned to associate with other people, or to make friends, she would have had great anxiety if forced to take up these activities. Fatigue, one of her chief complaints, was due to the energy which she had to expend to maintain even her poor contact with reality. In the hospital she made friends with a few of the patients and said that she was happier here than she had ever been at any time of her life, and that she had made more friends than ever before. But even these few contacts proved too much for her, so that she remained fatigued most of the time.

Secondary Gain from Neurotic Illness.   The patient saw nothing particularly unusual in the way she had lived, and excused her lack of productive activity by the fact that she had not been feeling well. She believed herself to be seriously sick and to have a rare and unusual disease of the pituitary gland. Naturally any such diagnosis was eagerly seized upon by this girl who had been so poorly trained to meet life, and the diagnosis was used as an excuse for her invalidism. This case illustrated especially well the secondary gain of neurotic symptoms. We often see rather active, energetic people who have neurotic symptoms but the symptoms are only a handicap to them, not totally incapacitating. They do not give in completely to their symptoms, they continue to work, and continue to live a fairly normal existence. This girl never had any such ambition and through her symptoms she gained many of the things she was looking for, namely, the interest and attention of her family, especially the solicitude of her mother, the kind and thoughtful attention of nurses and doctors, and in the hospital she gained the opportunity of making some friends for the first time in her life. All these things were important, and in this case had been an obstacle to cure. However, a point which should be stressed is that *this secondary gain is by no means the cause of the illness*. We have heard it said in the past that neurotics have symptoms in order to gain attention and to seek refuge from life's difficulties. This is only part of the story because there must have been certain personality trends which brought on the symptoms in the first place. Then the symptoms, once under way, bring a secondary gain of variable importance to the patient, but this should in no sense be regarded as the cause of the illness itself.

The Nature of the Illness and the Diagnosis.   From the standpoint of *differential diagnosis* what had to be recognized here was the social anxiety and social prejudice, the extreme childlike dependency, the great poverty of ideation and affect about what her place in life should be at the age of 22, and finally the rather unshakable conviction that she was seriously organically ill. All this added together would indicate that this girl had an unusually severe neurosis, or was possibly in the hypochondriacal stage of *schizophrenia*. It is true that the clinical picture was not that of a well-developed psychosis. However, it must be remembered that schizophrenia is a disease which develops gradually, and that patients with this disorder who finally reach a psychiatric hospital have usually been seen during the developmental stage by the family physician or have spent some time in general hospital wards. From the standpoint of therapy it was encouraging that while this girl had led such a seclusive, unsocial life up to the time of admission to the hospital, she still had some capacity while in the hospital to make friends and be interested in other people.

Unlike patients we have seen who have been chronic invalids and led seclusive lives until middle age, we were more hopeful that this young woman could be rescued from invalidism by encouraging her to turn her attention *out* upon life instead of *in* upon her organs.

Follow-up.   A year later the patient reported that most of her symptoms had completely disappeared but that on occasions she had slight attacks of dizziness, nausea, and a burning sensation in the epigastrium. After the attack she felt a depressing weariness. However, she reported long periods of well-being between attacks during which time she was able to work and to attend movies, parties, and dances. She had gained 26 pounds in weight and altogether reported herself and her family as much pleased with her recovery.

SUMMARY

Here was a young woman who, aside from a slight excess of hair on the lip and chin, seemed quite normal on physical examination but who had been incapacitated for more than a year. The chief feature of the illness had been attacks of rapid beating of the heart, sweating and faintness with marked fatigue, and a sensation of heat in the abdomen. The laboratory studies showed nothing remarkable and yet this patient had been considered to have a disturbance of the endocrine system, probably pituitary basophilism, and had been treated with irradiation of the pituitary and injections of glandular extracts on that basis. Psychotherapy was successful in reducing anxiety.

THE ENDOCRINE SYSTEM AND THE PROBLEM OF CHRONIC FATIGUE

One of the commonest problems with which the internist and general physician have to deal is chronic fatigue. Often it is not the primary complaint or, at least, it does not emerge as the dominant complaint until after one has had some experience with the patient. At first the patient complains of something else, for example, pain in the heart region, palpitation and breathlessness, to mention one common group of symptoms (see cardiac neurosis p. 182). Or the patient may complain of headache, sleeplessness and irritability (see hypertension p. 225). Another important syndrome with which fatigue is associated has to do with gastrointestinal symptoms and depression of mood (see functional gastrointestinal disorder p. 265). Still another syndrome is characterized by generalized aches and pains, and sometimes a little fever, that is, up to but rarely beyond 100° (see psychogenic rheumatism p. 319).

The truth is that almost all neurotic and psychosomatic disorders are associated with fatigue and often fatigue is the outstanding symptom. This is so because emotional conflict uses up energy which is then no longer available for work and social purposes. After one gets to know the patient it becomes clear that underlying all of these syndromes is fatigue—chronic fatigue, unrelieved by rest, sometimes so pronounced that the patient leads a life of complete invalidism. Or his life is so impoverished that he can hardly work and social life is markedly restricted. Usually the patient has undergone considerable medical investigation and treatment, sometimes with long periods of hospital and sanatorium care. Various diagnoses have been arrived at—endocrine or metabolic disorder (hypo- or hyperthyroidism and the adrenal syndrome), obscure infection (chronic brucellosis and lupus erythematosus), malignant disease, menopause if the patient is anywhere near middle age, and, of course, nutritional difficulty (vitamin deficiency), hypoglycemia, anemia, low blood pressure, and such rare disease as myasthenia gravis.

In an effort to study this common problem, Allan compiled data on 300 consecutive cases from the Lahey Clinic in which weakness, fatigue or weak spells were the chief complaint. In only one case was vitamin deficiency held responsible for weakness. Anemia was found in only five cases. "Certain conditions, such as vitamin deficiency and glandular disorders, considered widespread causes of weakness by both the laity and the medical profession, were actually found to be rare, and not a single case of weakness due to liver trouble, poor elimination, or low blood pressure was encountered." The origin of the complaint was found to be physical disorder in only 20 per cent. In the remainder it was the result of a nervous state.

Diagnosis and Treatment.   People who are tired without exerting themselves, in whom fatigue often develops quickly in certain unpleasant social situations and, having done so, tends to recur in similar situations; people who inform us that they are just as tired when they get up in the morning as when they go to bed at night and who, above all, lose their fatigue when they are engaged in something which interests them—these are the people in whom we should suspect that fatigue is of emotional origin.

In approaching the patient from the standpoint of psychosomatic diagnosis, one must realize that in dealing with the emotions treatment cannot be separated from diagnosis and that from the moment of the initial contact with the patient the groundwork is being prepared for treatment. There can be no sharp division between the period of diagnosis and the period of beginning treatment.

Hypothyroidism.   Chronic fatigue is often attributed to hypothyroidism.

Desiccated thyroid gland is the oldest of the gland products, and the most widely used and abused. Almost any functional disturbance in women appears to be grounds for thyroid medication, which is not without danger. Patients are started on thyroid medication on the basis of a presumed thyroid deficiency, symptoms are not relieved, and the dose is increased. Since the thyroid substance is well tolerated it is continued for months and years. The patient consults another physician and an attempt is made to withdraw the thyroid medication. Then the patient presents additional symptoms, the basal metabolism is found to be low, it is assumed that the diagnosis of hypothyroidism is corroborated, and the patient and physician are persuaded to resume the medication. Part of the difficulty is that the continued use of thyroid substance depresses the function of the thyroid gland, and secondly the patient becomes dependent upon the thyroid substance. One could refer to this as *thyroid addiction*.

CONSTITUTIONAL INADEQUACY.   This leads to a consideration of "constitutional inadequacy," which we look upon as an unfortunate term. Most of these patients are not constitutionally inadequate. We must distinguish between pseudoheredity and pure heredity. If we look to the environment, to the family group especially, for the origin of these psychosomatic disturbances, we will often find emotional conflicts; by bringing the material to the surface and dealing with it in a more realistic way we can sometimes help these patients to become useful citizens again instead of labeling them constitutionally inadequate or burdening them with that other equally unsatisfactory term, neurocirculatory asthenia, which is usually just a name to cloak our ignorance of the life situation of the individual.

The same strictures apply to the various symptom diagnoses that are often made in the study of these patients and to which too much attention is paid, increasing the anxiety of the patient. In other words, the physician often becomes a pathogenic agent when he approaches these patients purely from an organic standpoint and stresses insignificant physical or physiological deviations.

VITAMIN DEFICIENCY.   Nowadays lack of energy is apt to be explained by lack of vitamins, but while these patients are sometimes too tired to eat and may not get an adequate diet, this is certainly not their primary problem. Indeed, they may eat too much in an effort to overcome "nervous hunger." What we must interest ourselves in is not so much a lack of vitamins as the lack of emotional satisfaction in their lives. There must be some kind of a balance to the emotional life; with too much expenditure on conflict and too little satisfaction coming in, the patient is headed for emotional bankruptcy.

THE FIBROSITIS SYNDROME OR PSYCHOGENIC RHEUMATISM (See page 522). These are the patients who complain of aches and pains in muscles and joints, who are "achy and stiff," but have no arthritis and do not develop it. Fatigue and sometimes slight fever are prominent symptoms. Physical examination and laboratory studies are usually negative. Many difficulties in diagnosis arise. Attention is often focused on the slight rise in temperature and the patient undergoes repeated studies from the standpoint of obscure infection. In addition to "fibrositis" and early arthritis, rheumatic fever and chronic brucellosis are frequently thought of.

In times past the patient with aches, pains, fatigue and slight fever was sometimes thought to have rheumatic fever and was often treated as a potential cardiac. This is no longer likely to happen but today he is apt to be labeled with a diagnosis even more difficult to disprove, namely chronic brucellosis. It is claimed by some advocates of chronic brucellosis, as an explanation for the syndrome under discussion, that negative laboratory tests do not necessarily exclude this possibility, and that since treatment is admittedly unsatisfactory it cannot be stated conclusively that chronic brucellosis is not the diagnosis. This position makes life difficult for the physician interested in the psychosomatic approach, for he assumes that if no evidence of physical disease is present, and there is positive evidence pointing to neurotic conflict of a nature and degree that would cause muscular aches and pains, and treatment along psychotherapeutic lines leads to improvement or cure, he has established the diagnosis of psychogenic rheumatism with a reasonable degree of accuracy. To make the problem even more difficult, chronic brucellosis and psychoneurosis admittedly may coexist. Frequently after an infectious disease, convalescence lingers and invalidism sets in. The belief is widespread that the organic disease produced the neurosis, whereas the actual mechanism is that the organic process has broken down the patient's psychological defenses, regression occurs, and an existing predisposition, determined by his personality structure, permits the neurosis to emerge.

However, in the majority of instances of this syndrome of "primary fibrositis" or psychogenic rheumatism one ought to be able to rule out chronic brucellosis and do it within a reasonable period of time. Otherwise the idea of an obscure infection becomes a fixation with the patient and it is difficult if not impossible to approach the illness from an emotional standpoint.

MENTAL DEPRESSION.   Again we must emphasize that thorough physical studies must be made but the personality and life situation must not be neglected. Particularly is it important to look for mood disturbances because so many of these patients with fatigue who have difficulty "getting going" in the morning, and who tend to improve toward evening, are suffering from mental depression. This is more marked in the morning and is accompanied by insomnia, early morning awakening, loss of appetite and weight, loss of sexual desire and impotence or frigidity, difficulty in concentration and decision.

Once we have excluded physical disease and done it expeditiously we can say to these patients that they have no evidence of organic disease. Often it is wise to add that neither do they have evidence of mental disease, because so often, with lay misconceptions regarding emotional problems, to suggest that the disorder is emotional means to the patient that it is mental and that he may be in danger of "losing his mind."

We always ask the patient toward the end of the study, "What have you thought about the cause of your illness?" One is often amazed at the extraordinary ideas entertained by these patients, some drawn from their reading or fantasies and some from the many medical examinations and investigations they have undergone. We can make no headway with these patients from a treatment standpoint until we have these first layers of anxiety out on the surface. As they are peeled off, new problems present themselves and these new problems will usually be found within the family group. Marital incompatibility and sexual difficulties are almost always present but the patients often hesitate to discuss them because they regard them as personal problems unrelated to their illness.

An explanation to these patients that their aches and pains and fatigue are due to the fact that they are always in a state of tension, that they do not know how to relax, even at night, and that because they are taut their muscles are crying out in protest, carries conviction and provides a stepping stone to ventilation of their emotional problems.

Instead of cautioning rest and more rest, which only permits the patient to "stew in his own juice," we recommend that he "carry on in spite of symptoms," and this he will often be able to do once he has divorced his pain from the fear of arthritis, heart disease, cancer or what not. Once neurotic pain is divorced from a fear of organic disease, it is remarkable how rapidly it will disappear or diminish. At the same time we advise him not to talk about his illness to his friends but try to cultivate the atmosphere of health by telling people that he is well no matter how badly he feels. As soon as possible we try to get him away from injections of vitamins and hormones, from sedatives and even physiotherapy, or if some of these measures are continued we make it clear to him that they are being used in a supplementary capacity and that the cure lies in emotional reeducation. It is of course sometimes necessary to make certain concessions to the previous organic miseducation that the patient has had. We cannot change our approach too quickly from disease to disorder, from the idea of doing something for the patient to having him do something for himself, from education along physical lines to the necessity for emotional growth. Many of these patients are emotionally quite ill and the efforts of the physician unversed in psychopathology to elicit material of importance will not only fail but may prove harmful. The essence of psychotherapy is to go no faster than the patient is prepared to go.

The following case is cited to illustrate the diagnostic problems that we have been discussing.

Case 35.   Chronic Fatigue

A young married woman complained of fatigue, pain in the joints and stiffness in the back. Her physician referred her for differential diagnosis of "a glandular disturbance of adrenal origin or Paget's disease."

She had had a child ten months before, just after moving into a new home. She was very busy "and kept going by driving herself." Her physician told her that she was suffering from nervous exhaustion and had her remain in bed for a week but when she got up her condition was unimproved. She was then given injections of vitamin B_1. Another physician suggested that an arthritic condition was developing but a consultant said that her trouble was functional, compared it to soldier's fatigue, and told her to keep a record of her temperature.

She said that "she had always been a tired person" but never seriously ill and that her mother "tried to make her less strong than she was."

The mother had always had "arthritis of the back and hands" ("is it inherited?") and her father had always been a "tired person." Although the mother was not crippled she had never been very active and spent part of every day resting. Like the father, she was always tired.

Four years before the present illness the patient had suffered from severe exhaustion for which she was studied in the hospital. A diagnosis of nervous exhaustion was made and rest was recommended.

The general physical examination showed a pleasant, smiling young woman with no evidence of organic disease. Routine laboratory studies were normal. The sedimentation rate was normal and tests for brucellosis showed no evidence of infection.

LIFE SITUATION

The patient was seen once every two weeks for four months and during this time continued to complain of being terribly exhausted and of pain and stiffness of the joints, although at no time was there any evidence of actual arthritis. In the interviews she dwelt continually on her symptoms and it was difficult to get her to talk about her life situation. She resented the suggestion that her feelings could have anything to do with her illness, because that would be a sign of weakness. Finally she mentioned that her husband had a bad family history in regard to mental illness and that "she had to spare him" because she feared a "breakdown" if he worried too much. She spoke of him as a failure, of their financial worries, and of the difficulties in their sexual adjustment.

Then for one week she felt better and "so relaxed that it seemed as though a weight had been lifed from her." Now she was able to say more about her husband, who was much older than she and who had never been successful. Because of his lack of success they could not have a child. Consequently "she grieved her heart out" and to this she attributed her previous state of nervous exhaustion. However, she went on to add that this could not be responsible for her trouble now because she had her child, "If only she could enjoy it."

Subsequent visits brought out the fact that now that she had her child she was greatly concerned because her husband was growing older and might not be able to provide adequately for them. Nor could her parents give her the security she wanted. They had left the business to their son and she could not bear to think of the possibility of some day being dependent upon her brother, whose wife she hated. "It would be awful to have to accept help from them." Moreover, the brother's wife had an independent income and lived on a lavish scale so that the patient was constantly reminded of her own inadequate income. Her mother was using up a small inheritance "running to doctors who dope her with phenobarbital" (using up the money that the patient ought to have). She had always resented her mother's invalidism and determined that she would not be such a neurotic person. She had been brought up as a "nice little girl," very polite and always eager to make a good impression on her elders, and completely unable to express her aggression.

She came back to the discussion of her husband; sex was not right; he was becoming more impotent. He was an impotent man who for so long could not provide her with a child which was "every woman's due," so she "grieved her heart out" and "nothing else mattered." Finally she had gone to work during the war period and earned enough money to afford a child. The husband had said that he would go crazy if he had financial worries and that threat was "all that she needed because of his bad history."

She had set her heart on having the baby as the answer to all of her emotional problems and then she discovered that many problems remained unanswered. Therefore, with the growing realization that things were not right, her discontent expressed itself in a constant state of tension. In spite of her conscious determination never to be a chronic complainer like her mother, she was "full of aches and pains." She presented a smiling exterior to her friends but her husband bore the brunt of her irritability while she suffered the constant aches of inner discontent.

As she ventilated her discontents and expressed some of her hostility she became less fatigued and had fewer aches and pains. While her recovery was far from complete she was rid of the idea of serious and disabling disease and was enabled to lead a fuller life. Followed for five years she maintained her improvement.

References

Allan, F. N.: New England J. Med., *231:* 414, 1944.

Benedek, T.: Psychoanalyt. Quart., *3:*153, 1934.

Bram, I.: Am. J. Psychiat., *92:* 1077, 1936.

Conrad, A.: J. Nerv. & Ment. Dis., *79:* 505 and 656, 1934.

Deutsch, E.: Med. Klin., *19:* 678, 1923.

Ham, G. C., Alexander, F., and Carmichael, H. T.: Psychosom. Med., *13:* 18, 1951.

Hyman, H. T., and Kessel, L.: J.A.M.A., (*a*) *85:* 1017, 1925; (*b*) *88:* 1478, 1927; (*c*) *96:* 2014, 1931.

Lewis, N. D. C.: M. J. & Rec., *122:* 121, 1925.

Lidz, T., and Whitehorn, J. C.: Psychosom. Med., *12:* 184, 1950.

Mittelmann, B.: J. Nerv. & Ment. Dis., *77:*465, 1933.

Moschcowitz, E.: Arch. Int. Med., *46:* 610, 1930.

Ruesch, J. Christiansen, C., Patterson, L. C., Dewees, S., and Jacobson, A.: Psychosom. Med., *9:* 77, 1947.

Chapter XI

Endocrine System
and Metabolism (Concluded)

ANOREXIA NERVOSA

One of the clinical syndromes perhaps most responsible for bringing the medical profession to believe that there may be a psychological background for certain physical diseases has been the condition called anorexia nervosa. Within recent years a number of excellent papers in which the psychological background is emphasized have appeared on this subject. Prior to this time the diagnosis of *Simmonds' disease* was almost invariably made whenever the syndrome of anorexia, emaciation and amenorrhea was encountered.

In 1874, Sir William Gull observed a disorder of young persons characterized by the following symptoms: emaciation, scaphoid abdomen, amenorrhea and the appearance of age. He noted the slow pulse and subnormal temperature, the equivalent of the depressed basal metabolism so frequently mentioned in case reports labeled Simmonds' disease. He made shrewd observations as to the psychic behavior of his patients. In particular, he noted their sense of well-being and their excessive activity in spite of extreme emaciation. He pointed out that this degree of activity would be impossible if the inanition were due to constitutional disease. After discussing hysteria, he chose the term anorexia nervosa as a name for the disease. He pointed out that all of the symptoms could be explained on the basis of the undernutrition which, in turn, was due to a "morbid mental state." This was a time when the function of the pituitary gland was unknown. It is remarkable that in spite of this clear description so much confusion still exists in regard to this disorder.

Simmonds' Disease.   At about this period of medical history many morbid states, which had been considered to be of psychological origin, came under the influence of the new cellular pathology with its structural orientation and from then on were considered of physical origin. Moreover, the rise of interest and activity in the field of endocrinology was a further reason for including this syndrome among the endocrine

Page 324

disorders. Simmonds in 1914 described the destruction of the anterior lobe of the pituitary gland which he observed at autopsy in certain cases of cachexia and reconstructed from the history the clinical picture of the disease that now bears his name. The syndrome is a chronic, progressive disorder characterized by loss of weight, asthenia, atrophy of the genital organs with decreased sexual function (in women, amenorrhea—in men, impotence), loss of the axillary and pubic hairs, changes in the skin, and decreased basal metabolic rate. Hypotonia, hypothermia, bradycardia, hypoglycemia, gastrointestinal disorders, anemia and achlorhydria may also appear. Cachexia is a late phase of the disease. The pathological changes besides those already mentioned are atrophy of the pituitary, skin, sexual glands, thyroid, parathyroids and adrenals. In advanced cases the internal organs are atrophied.

DIFFERENTIAL FEATURES. While the clinical picture of anorexia nervosa may reproduce all the symptoms of true Simmonds' disease the changes usually are not nearly so marked as in the true pituitary cachexia and autopsy observations prove that the pituitary is structurally intact. McCullough and Tuffer demonstrated an increased gonadotropic hormone excretion in some cases of anorexia nervosa, a finding inconsistent with severe pituitary failure.

Functional Pituitary Depression. From a psychological standpoint it has been said that "just as these patients are physically starved so are they emotionally starved." We would put that the other way around, because we must be very careful in the consideration of psychosomatic disorders not to put the cart before the horse. In other words, this condition differs from true pituitary disease because it is the psychological conflict which brings about the loss of appetite and undernutrition and, very likely, this in turn affects the pituitary function which is closely tied up with the cessation of menstruation and lowered basal metabolism. It seems that this is a true interference with the function of the anterior pituitary but the latter occurs as a result and not as a cause of the disorder. One piece of evidence to suggest that this is a functional depression is that, when the patients improve as a result of psychological management, their menses begin again and even pregnancies occur.

Psychic Traits. In all cases of this condition studied psychologically there have been serious neurotic traits and sometimes even psychotic manifestations. Most patients showed a noteworthy reticence in discussing themselves and particularly in discussing sexual topics. Masturbation was minimal or absent. In other words, there was a strong repudiation of sexuality and if sexual relations occurred they often had a marked traumatic effect upon the psyche. In fact, starvation, emaciation, and the resulting unattractive appearance in many instances made an excellent defense against establishing healthy social contacts with the opposite sex. Sometimes this state of undernutrition led to the breaking of a marriage engagement. Eating sometimes symbolized impregnation to these people and obesity represented pregnancy. Some of the other personality characteristics encountered were perfectionism, overconscientiousness, neatness, seclusiveness, shyness and dependence upon others. Such patients had difficulty in making friends and of necessity had a poor relation to parents. In many cases the parent had shown preoccupation with gastrointestinal functions and the patient as a child had been a "feeding problem."

A detailed study by Waller, Kaufman and Deutsch showed the symbolism of "eating as impregnation" in two patients whose personality structure was of the compulsive type. The whole syndrome represented an elaboration and acting out in the somatic sphere of a specific type of pregnancy fantasy. Secondary gain allowed the patients to obtain affection, to be the center of the family, to work out hostilities, and to provoke the environment to certain acts of punishment which would alleviate guilt.

Lorand likewise found that there was great immaturity in the personality development, which interfered with normal psychosexual development. In his patient, refusal of food also arose from fantasies of oral impregnation.

Clinical Findings. According to Nemiah, who made a psychiatric study of 14 patients with anorexia nervosa, the typical history is as follows: "A young girl, usually in her teens, stops eating. As the weeks go by she begins to lose weight, her periods cease and the patient, quite unperturbed by her changing habitus, will not heed the anxious urging of her family to eat. Indeed, she lies, hides food, or secretly disposes of it to avoid their vigilance, and despite her rapidly increasing cachexia, she indulges in all manner of vigorous activity to a degree startling in the face of her almost moribund appearance. At length, the threats and prayers of her family unheeded, she falls prey to an infection and succumbs, the victim of her 'perverted ego.'"

The clinical findings in addition to emaciation may be dry scaly skin, cold extremities, low temperature, slow pulse and amenorrhea. In some cases amenorrhea may precede the loss in weight, but return of menstrual flow usually follows improvement in nutrition without hormonal therapy. In fact, treatment with anterior pituitary lobe growth hormone or estrogenic hormone has not seemed to bring any permanent benefit to the cases of anorexia nervosa. Basal metabolism is usually low but this is due to inanition rather than to thyroid deficiency and attempted replacement therapy may be injurious instead of helpful. Insulin treatment may or may not add some weight but even if it does, such weight gain usually is only temporary and the persistence of the psychological conflict causes the added pounds to melt away again.

Principles of Treatment. Treatment, then, consists in making the patient aware of the nature of the mental conflicts underlying the condition, and at the same time trying to reeducate the patient to express himself in a more adult fashion than *by the rejection of food.*

While the fully developed syndrome of anorexia nervosa is a rare disorder, lesser degrees of poor appetite and inanition based upon the same psychological principles are exceedingly common. As we have pointed out before, the taking of food is the chief activity during the first year of life and continues for some time to be connected in an important way with the child's entire relation to life. If he is restless or tense he is fed and comforted by the mother. A mother who cannot understand the child's need for physical and emotional closeness to her may offer only food to the child. Parents often reward a child with something good to eat when some other reward would be more desirable psychologically (see p. 345). Thus it is that our relation to life starts through the feeding mechanism and may be continued almost exclusively through this channel. Appetite for food therefore becomes a substitute for and symbolic of an appetite for life activities. In all cases of anorexia nervosa we find the relation to life, usually expressed by enthusiasm for work, hobbies and friends, to be as inadequate as the appetite for food.

Johnson and associates, in a valuable study to which we will refer in the discussion of obesity, developed the concept that obesity and anorexia nervosa may be different phases in the response of a child to its family situation. It is not unusual for an obese adolescent to follow a dietary regimen until the fully developed picture of anorexia nervosa supervenes. Unconscious hostility on the part of a parent toward a child may be so marked that a child is repelled by food because of the parent's revengeful attitude toward eating. The mother of a patient with anorexia may consciously encourage, even implore, the child to eat and yet exhibit her unconscious hostility toward the child in countless ways, including the serving of food. Consciously the parent is well-meaning but her efforts are defeated by powerful unconscious forces. The child responds to the feelings of the mother rather than to the words that are used.

Thus we see that anorexia nervosa is a complex psychosomatic illness involving the whole personality, and that the treatment can never be limited to the administration of tonics or endocrine products.

Prognosis. Kay reported a follow-up study of 38 patients, including 34 women and 4 men, hospitalized at one time or another over a twenty-year period for symptoms of anorexia nervosa. He attempted to assess their present psychiatric status and to evaluate the long-range effects of treatment, particularly psychotherapy. Half the patients had been ill two years or longer, and 20 per cent for five years or more. He concluded that patients referred to psychiatric clinics with symptoms of marked aversion for food, loss of weight and amenorrhea tend to have a poor prognosis. When clear-cut psychotic features are not present from the outset, there is little tendency to develop psychosis. However, only 10 to 29 per cent recover to the stage of good adjustment, the majority continuing to show neurotic symptoms. Kay doubts that anorexia nervosa is a specific entity. "The term itself draws attention to only one aspect of certain psychologic disorders which center around the intake of food."

The following case illustrates many of the points that have been mentioned.

Case 36. Anorexia Nervosa

A white girl, aged 19, complained of loss of appetite and loss of weight, cessation of menstruation, and increasing irritability.

Present Illness. The patient had first consulted a physician two years ago because of a slight eruption on the face which was diagnosed as acne. She was advised to cut down on sugars and starches, which she did, and she blamed loss of weight upon this fact. The loss of weight began about a year later, at which time she weighed 105 pounds. Within a few months, her menstrual periods ceased, and for this she received "gland injections" from her attending physician. For a few months before admission she noted an increasing irritability and this she attributed to the fact that the family tried "to force her to eat." Her weight was finally reduced to about 74 pounds and because of the persuasion of her family and her physician she entered the hospital for study. It was not because she felt bad. As she stated, she was just as active as the rest of the girls in her group and would not have sought hospital care if her family had not insisted upon it.

Past History.   The systemic review did not reveal any additional information of importance and the past history was not significant except for an illness which was diagnosed as rheumatism shortly after she started school. Her mother stated that this was not rheumatic fever and that she was told that there was no evidence of heart involvement. She was a thin but healthy child.

The patient was the third in a family of four children. The mother and father were well and the other children were well and none had ever suffered from any serious physical disease.

She graduated from high school and had been employed as a secretary for about six months, when she lost her position, but not because of illness.

Physical Examination and Laboratory Studies.   Physical examination showed a small, thin girl who appeared alert and intelligent and seemed entirely comfortable and at ease in the ward. She had a few marks on her face of the previous acne eruption but they were entirely healed and not very noticeable. The body and limbs were very thin although the breasts were fairly well preserved. There was considerable hairy development on the arms and legs. The heart and lungs seemed entirely normal; the abdomen was scaphoid but otherwise there were no special findings. The temperature on admission was 97.5° F., the pulse 52 and regular, the respirations 14 and the blood pressure 94/56.

Routine laboratory studies—urine, blood count and serological tests—were all normal. Because the general physical examination and ordinary laboratory studies were normal we turned to the life situation of the patient before considering the question of differential diagnosis.

LIFE SITUATION

Family History.   The father of this patient was the owner of a store. He was described as a friendly person who had always been on good terms with the patient. The mother was also said to be a friendly person, interested in her children. The patient was the third in a family of four, the oldest a married sister who had no children. The brother, 20 years old, a college student, had been close to the patient and they discussed some of their life problems together. If we had accepted a superficial description of her she would have seemed to be what is called an extroverted person. She danced a great deal, went to movies and the theater, had many friends, and was socially popular. It is to be remembered, however, that there are no true extroverts or true introverts. Some apparently extroverted people are very sensitive, and because of this sensitivity avoid many things which go to make up a well rounded personality.

Adolescence.   It would appear that some external change in personality took place in this girl about the time of puberty. Previously affectionate, she became, as she termed it, "selfish and a snob." She became very interested in her appearance and in her clothes. She had a great desire to be liked and to associate with people whose appearance was very neat and striking in some way. She said, "I cannot endure people who are sloppy."

Attitude Toward Marriage.   She had never been able to tolerate any love-making of any kind. She was aware that many of her friends of both sexes indulged but she could not endure coming in too close contact with anyone. Not only was she unable to endure the idea of body intimacy but the idea of marrying and becoming a mother was unattractive to her. She felt that pregnancy and the nursing experience would spoil her appearance and be both painful and "messy." She thought that having children would spoil her figure, which in itself was a remarkable statement for one who presented the appearance of a scare-crow! When she pictured marriage at all it was only the social side —entertaining, travel and luxuries—which a man of means could provide. If she had children she would want to adopt them, obviously to avoid the responsibility, and what to her would be the unpleasant duty, of nursing and toilet training. She had no desire to prepare meals or take care of a house. She said, "I might if I loved someone." But she had never permitted herself to love anyone but herself. On two occasions she had felt emotionally and somewhat physically drawn to young men. This feeling seemed to disturb her, however, and she found a reason to break off these friendships. It was as if she sensed that to foster such a feeling would bring a sense of responsibility toward someone and hence change her position to that of being self-sacrificing and perhaps maternal instead of being able to enjoy the position of being the loved one herself.

Summary of Findings.   So here was a girl who was unable to give much to life but only wanted to receive. She realized that she was selfish and possibly had some desire to change, but so far she had found it difficult to do. At the age of 19 she should have been able to take some responsibility in relation to other people. She had not been emotionally educated to do so; instead she had been allowed to overemphasize appearance until this was her only source of satisfaction. And now she was becoming too thin, even in this age of slimnesss, to gain satisfaction.

It usually is true that people who have too much interest in themselves and too little for other people only end up by cheating themselves. Such was the case here. This girl's loss of weight, which was rightly regarded by her relatives as serious, was only an incident in the life of a person poorly adjusted to reality. She not only had starved herself physically but she first had starved herself emotionally. She had recently occasionally found herself crying without reason. This symptom plus irritability must be regarded as indications that this girl was unhappy and that her way of gaining satisfaction through over-attention to appearances was failing her. She sensed that something was lacking and that something was the satisfaction which comes from being able to have a warmer interest in others and to be able to express this interest.

THE MARRIAGE PROBLEM.   This girl had difficulty in regard to marriage. Her attitude was not quite what we would expect in a girl of her age. *So often physicians recommend marriage and childbearing as a short cut toward the solution of emotional problems.* Unfortunately people who are so immature as to find marriage an emotional hurdle which they cannot negotiate are the very kind of people who find difficulty in meeting the responsibilities of marriage. And then marriage serves not as a cure for but as a cause of the onset of many of their nervous symptoms. If such persons have not been brought up properly prepared for marriage it is much better for them to have a psychological preparation rather than to be forced or to force themselves into a marriage situation which may prove to be the cause rather than the cure for an illness. The same may be said for childbearing. To the person who is emotionally immature, having a child may increase rather than alleviate troubles. It is true that such persons are often very much better during the period of pregnancy (although this is by no means the rule) but it is after the child is born that trouble starts. Anxious mothers often make anxious children and thus we have an endless repetition of the neurotic problem.

TREATMENT.   In the question of treatment we must emphasize that simply adding a few pounds to this patient by means of forced feeding with perhaps the use of insulin would really be only a temporary measure, because as soon as she went home and met another emotional situation difficult to handle she would once more reject food just as she tried to reject life, and the added pounds would melt away. In other words, the only intelligent approach to this problem was to make an effort to reeducate this young woman in a new approach to life.

PROGNOSIS.   It appeared that this patient was fortunate in at least one respect. She was only 19, her illness had not lasted very long, and a correct diagnosis had been made and treatment started in the proper direction. Unlike patients who have reached mature years, who in other words have already lived their lives and for whom little can be done, and unlike patients who are so fixated in their invalidism that probably nothing can shake them loose from it, this patient was considered much more amenable to treatment because she was young and her psychological structure could perhaps be modified. In other words, it is much like the problem of tuberculosis. When the patients are far advanced in that disease there is little that we can do to restore them to normal, but when they come in because they have had a dramatic episode (*e. g.,* pulmonary hemorrhage) as the very first manifestation of the disease and we find on physical examination that there is only a small lesion in the lung, we are very hopeful that a cure can be brought about. This patient from a psychological standpoint seemed to be in the latter position.

TREATMENT

Treatment, therefore, consisted of attention to the personality. We tried to show her that no one can be complete in herself, that her interest in being admired was too great and would bring her increasing disappointment as she grew older. We tried to help her to be more tolerant toward people generally, and to see that virtues might exist in people who did not put so much emphasis on neatness as she did. Her marked antipathy to lack of neatness had come from an overscrupulous regimen during the period of *toilet training* as discussed in the chapter on psychopathology. Her training had been accomplished by the inculcation of an excessive disdain for anything which was not neat and clean. When such an attitude is taken in order to help accomplish toilet training and neatness the emotions spread away from excretions to include other things such as food, dress, environment, and even thinking itself.

On first entering the hospital the patient was unable to eat food from the regular house trays. When she was later put on a special diet, and extra care was given to the neatness of her trays in the diet kitchen, she was able to eat more. The food was the same but because it was more neatly served she found it more attractive and acceptable.

Discussion of a Plan for Living.   In treatment sessions with this patient a woman's appearance during pregnancy, her feelings over nursing, and the responsibility of toilet training were discussed with her. We tried to enable her to see that while these things had their unpleasant side they bring compensations which should far outweigh feelings of antipathy. We tried to show her that if she continued to avoid these necessary contacts with everyday life she would be missing emotional experiences that make life of value to most people. If it should actually turn out that this girl would want to renounce marriage completely, with its necessary intimate contacts with a man, then more emphasis would have to be put on some other kind of life work. She had vaguely thought of taking a course in accounting but as yet nothing had been done about it. She was drifting and hoped that some solution to her emotional needs would come without any definite plan. But we tried to show her that a girl must plan her life along one of the acceptable channels which will bring satisfaction. We tried to make her see the necessity of choosing either marriage or office work and of making a more definite preparation for one or the other. In some families an emotional preparation for family life takes place imperceptibly but thoroughly from childhood onward. In other families this is not the case and special attention has to be given to it later.

Tasting Life and Tasting Food.   We thought that as this patient learned to get into closer contact with people instead of remaining aloof and waiting to be admired she would lose her irritability and depression, and her desire to starve herself. An ability to taste life would probably mean that she could begin to taste food and her zest for life and zest for food would increase together. Superficially, anorexia had meant a wish to avoid any imperfections in appearance. It had meant avoiding food which did not seem entirely neat and clean, and it had meant avoiding responsibility. Finally it had meant something still deeper from the psychological standpoint and that was the rejection of people as well as food. To be in love or to like someone means a taking in of that person into one's thought and feeling. This is regarded unconsciously as a process which takes place by way of the gastrointestinal tract. The expression "my thoughts are full of you" means that the individual making this remark has taken something of the loved person inside himself. This girl had scrupulously avoided falling in love or emotionally taking anyone inside of herself. This attitude and her rejection of food definitely had something in common. To correct the rejection of food one must correct the attitude of rejecting love and its responsibilities. In other words, she must not be overscrupulous in regard to neatness and orderliness and even cleanliness, because to put it frankly there is a certain amount of dirt in the world that we have to learn to accept. Modern pediatricians are not afraid to allow children to come in contact with a little honest dirt and adults too must learn to accept reality. In other words, this immature young woman had to be helped to grow up emotionally. She had to be taught to behave differently toward people, and although this might stir up a little anxiety the physician had to occupy a position of confidence and authority so that he could allay this anxiety and thus permit a little more emotional growth.

Follow-up.   Treatment sessions were broken off after several visits to the psychiatrist but she continued under the care of her family physician who had a good understanding of the psychological background of the illness. No improvement was noted for many months but finally, for reasons that were not very apparent, she began to eat and gain weight, improved in her social relationships, got herself a job and at the end of a year was working steadily and again "tasting life just as she was tasting food."

DIABETES MELLITUS

Primitive man had to have a mechanism of homeostasis (Cannon) which would enable his endocrine-sympathetic nervous system quickly to prepare his body for fight or flight when his physical safety was threatened. In civilized man the same mechanism exists and apparently is called into action when man faces threats not necessarily to his physical self but to his security and prestige. One of the central factors of this homeostasis is a mobilization of the sugar in the blood leading to a hyperglycemia. It is strange that this mechanism has not been alluded to more frequently as a possible background for diabetes mellitus. It is true that emotional glycosuria and hyperglycemia, due to conscious fears or threats, are recognized but it would also seem that fears and threats of which the patient is not wholly aware could, by the very nature of their unconscious energy, act as a chronic stimulus to the insulin-producing mechanism and hence might have something to do with the development of true diabetes.

Dunbar summarized the studies of emotional glycosuria and hyperglycemia. She referred to the classic experiments of Cannon which demonstrated that cats, if excited or enraged, developed glycosuria. Sugar was found in the urine of football players after an exciting game and in students after a hard examination, and hyperglycemia occurred in aviators and in soldiers exposed to danger. The anxiety in some patients before operation has induced hyperglycemia. Suggestion under hypnosis has altered the blood sugar level.

Although some evidence (Mirsky) throws doubt on hyperglycemia as the responsible factor for the glycosuria which occurs with emotional stress and suggests that it must be attributed to a decrease in absorption of glucose from the kidney tubules, the clinical fact that emotional stress can produce a rapid rise in blood sugar concentration in diabetics, thus causing an exacerbation of the disorder, is generally recognized.

History.   Haagensen and Lloyd tell us that the beginning of our modern understanding of diabetes dates back to the opening year of the American Revolution, when Matthew Dobson, physician to the Liverpool Infirmary, discovered that the urine, which is passed in too great an abundance in this disease, contains sugar. This discovery led the way to attempts to control the disease by limiting the amount of sugar in the diet, a method which was not very successful. And so the matter stood for another hundred years, until in 1889 the experimental attack on diabetes was begun by a Russian physician, Oskar Minkowski, then a young assistant to Professor Naunyn at the University of Strasbourg. Minkowski removed the entire pancreas in a dog and discovered that severe diabetes at once developed which persisted until the animal succumbed a few weeks later; he also found the sugar content of the blood elevated. The next step was made in 1900 by Eugene L. Opie, at that time a young instructor in pathology at Johns Hopkins. Studying the microscopic sections of the pancreas of a little girl who had died of diabetes, Opie saw that the islands of Langerhans were so degenerated that they could not be identified. His observation led the English physiologist Sir Edward Schafer in 1916 to postulate the theory that these special pancreatic cells produced some form of internal secretion which controlled the metabolism of sugar. Shortly afterwards came the epochal observations of Banting culminating in the discovery of insulin.

We believe that psychological medicine also has important contributions to make to the subject of diabetes but, aside from a few excellent studies to which we shall refer, no concerted efforts have as yet been made to study the emotional component of this disease.

Emotional Factors.   There are very few references to emotional factors in the disease from the field of internal medicine but several have appeared from the field of psychological medicine. Of these, Daniels contributed a comprehensive review. The following material is taken from his study.

Daniels felt that the chief case against the importance of emotional factors in diabetes as reflected in the literature could be enumerated under the following heads: (1) studies showing heredity to be the determining factor; (2) military experience in which the evidence seemed to indicate that military life did not predispose to the development of diabetes; (3) the impression that nervous strain or shock does not lead to more diabetes or to any appreciable increase in hyperglycemia or glycosuria in those already having diabetes; (4) confusion between organic neurological changes and emotional tension which uses the autonomic system for discharge.

EXPERIMENTAL STUDIES.   Impetus was furnished to all branches of research in metabolism by the discovery of Houssay and Biasotti in 1930 that diabetes of depancreatized animals could be attenuated and their lives prolonged by extirpation of the anterior pituitary gland. Houssay's work and its consequences revolutionized theories of the mechanism of diabetes and led to the relinquishment of the simpler insulinogenic concept. This has broadened the base for the understanding of the influence of emotional factors. Evidence of implication of the hypothalamus in disturbed sugar metabolism, its importance as a center for the involuntary nervous system, and its participation in automatic emotional discharge make it a focal point in attempts to understand degrees of emotional participation in diabetes.

PERSONALITY STUDIES.   Studies of the hereditary factor in diabetes show quite conclusively the importance of a diabetic anlage and there is some evidence that this may be passed on as a recessive Mendelian trait. In evaluating the emotional factor in the etiology of the disease the constitutional predisposition should be taken into account. It seems unwarranted, however, to dismiss the importance of the psychic factor either on account of hereditary predisposition or on the evidence of the first World War that "shell-shock" is not an important etiological factor, because recent psychiatric contributions to the subject, though scattered, show an awakened interest with a new approach afforded by psychoanalytic insight. Emphasis is away from settling the whole question of psychogenesis in diabetes on the frequency of traumatic diabetes but is laid rather on the presence of anxiety, concealed or overt, which is unable to discharge through the conscious voluntary system and is forced through regressive changes to discharge at more primitive autonomic levels. It is well established that emotional changes can affect the blood sugar level. Up to the present time it has not been definitely proved whether or not it is possible to precipitate diabetes by such influences.

Cases in which emotional disturbances seemed of importance in the causation of diabetes were cited by Daniels, including the first report of a case of diabetes to be psychoanalytically investigated. The importance of attention to personality factors in the uncooperative case, as well as in those cases which react to emotional conflict with increased sugar, was stressed.

From the Psychiatric Field.   That neurotic manifestations occur frequently in association with diabetes is becoming increasingly clear as cases are studied systematically by observers trained in psychiatric methods. W. C. Menninger in two articles reviewed previous literature, reported on 30 cases of mental disorder associated with diabetes, and analyzed this material along with that of 93 cases of uncomplicated diabetes and 400 uncomplicated cases of mental disorder. Daniels, and Dunbar and associates, reported studies on successive diabetic admissions to a large general hospital which allowed them to contact cases that ordinarily would not be seen by the psychiatrist. Dunbar contrasted the diabetics studied with a parallel series of fracture and cardiovascular patients.

Menninger called attention to the present viewpoint of psychiatry that some of the most severe emotional conflicts are entirely unconscious to the patient, but with the exception of these authors there was no recognition of unconscious emotional conflicts. He listed 9 of a series of 30 cases studied by him as psychoneurotic. Five of his cases seemed to be the result of a psychological disturbance, appearing either with a mental disorder or during its course. These cases conformed to the following arbitrary requirements of such relationship: (1) Obvious psychopathology was evident prior to the development of the diabetic state. (2) The mental picture was quite different from the toxic state occasionally seen in either hyperglycemia or hypoglycemia. (3) The course of improvement of the mental picture was paralleled by the glycemic and glycosuric levels, with fluctuations in these as emotional upsets occurred in the psychic life. (4) The metabolic disorder was indicated by a persistent glycosuria (without dietary control or insulin), retarded glucose utilization curves of the blood sugar, and a response to dietary and, in some cases, insulin therapy. (5) With mental recovery, the diabetic condition cleared, requiring neither insulin nor dietary treatment. Menninger considered this the only such group described in the literature and gave abstracts of the cases in both of his articles. He stated that none of the cases lent themselves to psychoanalytic investigation so that the unconscious forces could not be determined. Actual psychotherapy was mentioned in only one case.

One of the questions which repeatedly occurs is whether or not there is any characteristic mental picture in diabetes. This has various aspects. The first is the question of toxic psychoses attributable to diabetes. Menninger reviewed the literature and came to the conclusion that "such a group of toxic cases represents a small percentage of the number of cases in which diabetes and mental disease are associated." He cited three such cases in his own series.

Depression is among the most frequent of the mental symptoms described, according to Menninger's summary of the literature. Daniels found depression to be an important complication in 10 cases of the 23 diabetic admissions studied, either from the history or while under observation. In 5 cases the depression was reactive to the loss of a love object prior to the onset of diabetes. When possible it is useful, in the case of depression, to make the distinction between a depression of a primary nature which might or might not be related to the diabetes, and a depression secondary to the diabetes. The knowledge by the individual that he is suffering from an incurable disease which, on account of the care necessary in treatment, sets him apart from the rest of his fellows in many cases explains the reaction. Much of the hypochondriacal self-observation which often accompanies such depressions can be explained in the same way. Because it is so natural, however, to conclude that such a patient is upset over his condition, it is possible to miss more fundamental neurotic reactions which may play a primary role. Cases of manic-depressive psychosis, appearing coincidentally or alternating with the diabetic picture, have been described.

ANXIETY.   Daniels stressed the factor of anxiety in his cases and thought the anxiety may have expressed itself through disturbed metabolism. He felt that since diabetics frequently have severe neurosis an opportunity is afforded to study the interaction of the two conditions. The fact that the diabetes might not be cured along with the neurotic symptoms does not prove that the neurosis may not have set the diabetes in action. We know too little about the problem of reversibility in organic disease and the point at which this is no longer possible because of structural changes. Daniels analyzed a case of diabetes and anxiety neurosis. Although the diabetes was not cured some interesting observations were made concerning the resemblance of the anxiety attacks and hyperinsulinism and the relation of hyperglycemia and glycosuria to emotional conflict.

The long-term observations by Hinkle and Wolf have demonstrated the importance of life stress on the course and management of diabetes. They found that major fluctuation in symptoms and insulin requirements frequently coincided with important episodes in the lives of their patients. In a girl of 15, who was followed by daily observation on urine glucose and ketones, ketonuria, thirst and polyuria appeared only at times of acute conflicts with the mother. To make certain that these changes were not the result of a willful manipulation of her insulin intake, she was admitted to the hospital for further study. There, under carefully controlled conditions, she was again exposed to conflict with her mother. Thirst, polyuria, ketonuria and dehydration promptly developed and continued for 48 hours. When the differences between the patient and her mother were reconciled, all the manifestations of ketosis disappeared, and the patient was restored to her former state of equilibrium, without use of additional insulin and without changes in fluid intake or diet.

FATIGUE AND DEPRIVATION.   Menninger found psychic trauma important in the precipitation of 2 of his 93 cases of uncomplicated diabetes. Dunbar found that such emotional traumata preceding diabetes occurred less frequently than in the cardiac and fracture patients, and that a long period of stress and strain was a more frequent occurrence. She pointed out, however, that such a period of stress and strain or definite emotional trauma immediately prior to illness is a frequent finding in numerous disease pictures and needs further evaluation. However, Dunbar felt that a *frequent pattern in diabetics was a steady grind of fatigue and deprivation with an increase in passive personality tendencies.* Resentment is called into play by daily life situations in contradistinction to the repressed unconscious hostility of hypertensive patients.

TYPE OF CONFLICT.   The essential feature would not seem to be the trauma, although this may play an important part, but the type of conflict measured in terms of tension and anxiety. Another important condition to have in mind is that it is not conscious emotional conflict, which has greater opportunity to discharge through the voluntary nervous system, that is most important but emotional tension that remains unconscious. This explains much of the seeming contradiction in the effect of transitory emotional upsets on the sugar level which has so confused diabetic specialists and led them to rule out the whole phenomenon as of little importance.

PSYCHIC CONDITIONING.   Daniels has pointed out that trauma which precipitates a neurosis has its effect because it impinges in many cases on an infantile neurosis which it reactivates, thus releasing more primitive anxiety patterns. Dunbar and associates in discussing diabetes stated that "from the psychosomatic point of view there is no more fundamental determinant of the organism's equilibrium together with its capacity to make adjustments than anxiety." In the diabetic and cardiovascular groups they found anxiety a prominent factor. In these groups the somatic and psychic conditioning and expression of anxiety presented a contrast with the fracture group. From the patients' subjective viewpoint there was a significant contrast because in the diabetic and cardiovascular groups the danger, as well as the handicap, was more diffuse and threatened from within, whereas in the fracture group the danger, as well as the damage produced, was concrete and seemed to come from without.

THE REFRACTORY PATIENT.   Rosen and Lidz studied a group of refractory diabetic patients who were repeatedly readmitted to the Johns Hopkins Hospital in diabetic acidosis. The refractoriness was in the attitude of the patients toward treatment rather than in metabolic eccentricities. All sorts of reasons were given by the patients: dietary indiscretions, changes in insulin intake, infections, but the real reasons were that they had sought to go into acidosis because of difficult situations. Rosen and Lidz detail some of the common features of the immature and poorly integrated personality structure of these patients.

The therapeutic problem consists of the difficult task of treating patients who are both diabetic and also psychotic or borderline psychotic.

While the difficulty in the refractory patient is largely in his personality it must not be forgotten that the personality of the physician is likewise important. Stearns reminds us that the manner in which the uncooperative reactions of the patient are approached by the physician is important in regard to success or failure of treatment. The patient often senses the physician's resentment even though a determined effort is made to appear friendly. Stearns refers to the exhortatory and inspirational techniques which may be effective at first but soon become ineffective; and the derogatory comparison of the patient's behavior with a mythical ideal patient, which only arouses resentment. The physician's threats, direct or implied, that failure to comply with the minute details of treatment will lead to disaster conjure up visions of amputation, coma and blindness and are often worse than useless.

Psychological Problems in Children.   In a study of diabetes in children Bruch, who has contributed so much to the study of the obese child (see p. 347), and has found common characteristics in these obese children which she could relate to the development of the obesity, has been unable to discover any uniform psychological picture in the diabetic children. However, since diabetes enforces a way of life to which the child and family must react according to preexisting patterns of behavior, the diabetes can be said to reenforce existing problems. A long-term study by Fischer and Dolger of 43 patients whose diabetes began in childhood called attention to the fact that diabetes is similar to other chronic illnesses in its effect on the psyche. Just as a hunchback or a cripple is always aware of his deformity, so the diabetic child is always conscious of his condition. He cannot escape the daily injection and is constantly reminded of his affliction by the discomfort produced by the needle as well as by the restriction in diet. Furthermore, there is always the fear of a possible hypoglycemic reaction. Good adjustment is possible, however, if there is understanding, harmony, and security in the home.

Bruch and Hewlett also reported on a psychologic investigation of a group of 21 diabetic children. In a third of the cases diabetes developed at the time of a disturbance in family relationship such as boarding out with relatives, divorce, deaths in the family, and so forth. Infection preceded the onset in less than a third of the cases. The first reaction of the families to the diagnosis was often one of great emotional disturbance and bewilderment. Frequently the mothers were responsible for dietary cheating because they could not bear to see the child deprived. Many children became adept at manipulating the diet and insulin so that before the next visit to the clinic a "clean" specimen could be produced. In emotionally disturbed families poor cooperation became the center of existing conflicts and was frequently associated with poor regulation. The authors shrewdly observed, however, that cooperation does not necessarily mean absence of neurotic conflicts. On the contrary, it may express a repressive, perfectionistic attitude toward the child, so that a more lenient medical regimen would sometimes help such families to accept diabetes with less guilt and anxiety, and thus offer the child a better opportunity for normal personality development.

Psychotherapy.   PSYCHOANALYSIS.   In addition to the patient analyzed by Daniels, a psychoanalytic study of two well-controlled cases of diabetes was reported by Meyer, Bollmeier and Alexander. Their method of observation was to correlate the psychoanalytic material with fluctuations of sugar output as determined by four to six daily quantitative urine examinations.

The first patient, a highly intelligent young man of 29, developed severe diabetes following an infection but during the course of serious psychologic conflict. He had been gravely ill as a young child and starved under a strict diet for almost a whole year because of a severe gastrointestinal disturbance. Apparently as a result he retained much of his infantile dependent and demanding attitude and was never able to accept the responsibilities of adult existence. He always felt frustrated and responded with hostilities because no one could gratify his demands for attention and love. These hostilities revived the old anxiety that he might lose love and security just as he was deprived of foods during the severe illness in early childhood. Emotional maturity was blocked by this anxiety and the patient never reached the psychosexual attitude of adult age. Diabetes developed at the height of emotional frustration which arose in relation to a sexual problem. A diagrammatic representation of sugar output showed that when his wishes to receive love and security were frustrated sugar levels were high, but when he escaped the conflict by turning to a neurotic solution characterized by depression and a withdrawal into self-pity lower sugar levels occurred.

Followed for six years after the completion of a successful analysis, he was well adjusted in his marital life, successful in his profession, and much attached to his child born a year after his marriage. He was in good physical health and the urine was free of sugar.

A second patient, a young woman, also developed diabetes under the strain of an emotional conflict of a striking similarity. The patient retained an infantile dependent and demanding attitude, and felt frustrated because her demands for attention and love were out of proportion to the reality situation of an adult and consequently were never adequately satisfied. To this frustration she reacted with hostility. Diabetes developed when these infantile wishes conflicted with the demands that were frustrated, and the sugar output decreased when her demanding attitude was temporarily renounced. Just as in the first case the sugar output was increased under the strain of this conflict, and decreased when the patient indulged in self-pity and passivity.

BRIEF PSYCHOTHERAPY.   Although psychoanalytic study gives the most thorough understanding of the personality structure and life situation of the diabetic patient, brief psychotherapy, based upon psychoanalytic understanding, is more available to the majority of diabetic patients. Commenting that diabetes is associated with almost every type of psychiatric disorder, with correspondingly varied personality structures, Daniels suggested that these personalities are frequently under "forced draft" from endogenous or exogenous chemical substances associated with the disease or its treatment, so that repressed aspects of the personality or neurosis become highlighted. This emotionally as well as chemically charged atmosphere makes brief psychotherapy as important for regulation in some patients as diet or additional insulin.

In the majority of patients help was asked by the medical service because of a tendency of the patient to shock easily or because of confusion in distinguishing between true insulin shock and a clinical picture which resembles shock with normal or even high blood sugar (p. 342).

Reporting on 8 young patients, Daniels found that conflict between parental dominance and repressed hostility was present in all cases, and a direct relationship between this and sexual conflict was most marked in the females.

In passing, Daniels commented that one important therapeutic element which should not be ignored is the effect of group classes on diabetics, now employed in many clinics while patients are learning the necessary dietary and other regimens. These frequently act as a form of group therapy by showing the patients that they are not the only ones afflicted with the disease, giving them the opportunity to exchange experiences, and furnishing the encouragement and support of the doctors and dietitians. This established class instruction should furnish a valuable guide for further development of group therapy.

Discussing a test based upon the urine sugar output, which was used to differentiate between emotional glycosuria and stabilized diabetes mellitus, Bollmeier and Meyer felt that psychotherapy has great therapeutic possibilities in the first group of patients—indeed, that it may prevent some from becoming true diabetics.

Mirsky insists that the physician should treat the urine less and the patient more. "He should be concerned with the amount of calories the patient retains rather than the amount that the patient eats or excretes. The proper use of insulin permits this on a normal diet. Even with the free diet the physician cannot shirk his responsibility since giving a patient freedom insofar as choice of food is concerned is of little avail unless, at the same time, the patient is handled sympathetically. Given an opportunity to mature emotionally, the diabetic patient will confront his wishes and his frustrations and make such compromises as are more consistent with both his chronologic age and social milieu. Then, he will act and eat as a normal individual and neither harm himself nor his evironment."

The important observations of Hinkle and Wolf, previously referred to, conclude with the following statement: "Knowledge that various forms of life stress may have an important effect on the course of diabetes does not necessarily simplify the treatment of the disease, but in some cases it provides one with another tool for dealing with recurrent episodes of ketosis or hypoglycemia. By studying the patient as a person and obtaining a reasonable understanding of his life history and present life situation, the physician can discover without great difficulty those aspects of his private life which are stressful to him. Sometimes, by discussion with the patient, he can so change his attitude toward persons or situations that events which formerly seemed threatening to him cease to seem so. Sometimes the physician can help the patient to modify his life situation by his own actions or by changes in his behavior. Sometimes he can persuade other persons in the patient's environment to alter their attitudes and behavior for the patient's benefit."

The following case is one of many that we have studied indicating the kind of life situation that frequently is found in diabetic patients. It lends point to Dunbar's observations regarding the *steady grind of fatigue and deprivation with an increase in passive personality tendencies as the psychological background of many cases of diabetes.* However, we are not concerned to try to prove that emotional factors are responsible for diabetes. What we are interested in is to show that the emotional part of the problem of diabetes has been neglected and that it is an important phase of the problem with which we must concern ourselves.

Case 37.   Diabetes Mellitus; Passive Personality; Fatigue and Deprivation

The patient was a young white man, studied at the Jefferson Hospital. The diabetes was discovered following loss of weight which was noticed by friends. On his second admission an observation was made by one of the physicians that excitement caused a rise in his blood sugar. His diabetic condition always responded well to treatment, but he was very careless about insulin after he left the hospital. His fourth admission to the hospital was for *coma* which came on during the night. Recovery was prompt and thereafter he promised to take better care of himself.

LIFE SITUATION

The *mother*, to whom the patient was greatly attached and whom he described as "sweet and altruisic," died at the age of 55 when the patient was 20. She had been sick about a year with carcinoma of the stomach and had been invalided for several months. During the latter part of the illness the patient took care of his mother at night.

The *father*, whom the patient always hated and whom he described as "selfish and mean," died at the age of 72, of pneumonia after being sick only a few days. He had previously always been well. The patient was at his father's bedside after an absence of ten or twelve years. During that night he sat in a nearby room and "searched his memory for traces of love for his father" but he could find none.

The *patient*, 28 years old, was the youngest of a family of six children, two brothers and three sisters. The oldest sister was operated upon three years before for tumor of the stomach and had been well since.

Childhood.   The patient was a fairly healthy youngster always deeply attached to his mother. As long as he could remember he knew that his father was mean to his mother. The father would frequently leave home and about three or four years before the mother's death definitely separated from her. The father contributed very little to the support of the family so that his mother from the earliest days of the patient's childhood was forced to work (domestic service). One of the patient's earliest memories was of being thrown out of the house by his father on the occasion of the birth of his sister's baby.

He attended high school for two years and then quit to go to work at the age of 15. For a time while working he went to a preparatory school in the evening thinking that he would later study pharmacy. About the age of 18, he worked for his brother for two years in the paper business, which he did not like (the father was once in that business).

Mother's Death.   The mother, by hard work and great saving, had managed to purchase a small home. It was placed in the name of the brother. During her last illness she said in the presence of the brother and the patient that she expected the brother (six years older than the patient) to look after the patient. The patient looked upon this as a "verbal will" and considered that he would share one half of the estate. He looked after his mother very tenderly during her final illness. The brother was also very good to the mother but "not so demonstrative in his affection."

The patient took the mother's death very hard. He was unconsolable, despondent, seclusive, and tortured with suicide thoughts. According to their religious custom they continued to live in the house for thirty days and then he and his brother went to his sister's home. The first night away from his old home he woke up with a choking sensation and this happened again a day or two later. A physician treated him and referred to it as a nervous affection of the throat. A month later he left town to visit the oldest sister. He stayed for six months, had a job, and because he felt that "nothing mattered" he had an affair with a married woman ten or twelve years older than himself. This was his only sexual experience. His explanation of this episode was that he "just didn't care what happened."

Quarrels with Brother. He returned to Philadelphia in order to dedicate a stone for his mother's grave and then he, with his brother, continued to live with a married sister. During these two years the mother's house was rented and the patient took it for granted that eventually he would get his share. At the end of two years the estate came up for settlement and the brother broke "the verbal will" and refused to give the patient his share. A terrible scene followed in which he felt like killing the brother. Thereafter for about three or four years there was constant tension and much quarreling with the brother about his share of the estate. Each time that he saw him a quarrel would follow in which the patient would always come off second best because he would get so angry and excited that he was unable to express himself. Furthermore, he would deliberately "hold himself back" so as not to prolong the quarrel. At the end of about two years the brother married and found further justification for keeping the estate. He brought his wife to live in the same house with the sister and after about six months the patient left to live with a younger sister to avoid so much quarreling. He lived there about two years and then took a room by himself because he desired to be "independent" and a month later he was admitted to Jefferson Hospital, his diabetes having been discovered.

The interviews with the patient would leave him nervous and excited and interfere with his sleep. After the last interview his hands were cold and damp and he complained that the left hand, that is, all of the fingers and the thumb, felt numb and it was observed by the physician that the middle and ring fingers of the left hand were paler than those on the right. The patient called this condition "neuritis" and said that he had had it ever since his coma attack. Apparently, however, it was of *vasospastic* origin.

SUMMARY

A soft, effeminate, passive young man with marked attachments to mother and hatred of father transferred the hatred to a brother when the latter took from the mother something which belonged to the patient. Constant quarreling with the brother for a period of three or four years preceded the discovery of diabetes. Between hospital admissions he received only indifferent attention to his diabetes and occasionally let up on dieting and insulin.

After the attack of coma he promised to do better but frequently expressed the wish that he had not recovered. The patient himself was of the opinion that constant quarreling may have had something to do with his illness. His passive personality was long subjected to the steady grind of fatigue and deprivation.

SPONTANEOUS HYPOGLYCEMIA (HYPERINSULINISM)

Still another aspect of carbohydrate metabolism which has not been sufficiently dwelt upon is the confusion which exists between the clinical condition known as functional hyperinsulinism—a form of spontaneous hypoglycemia—and the anxiety state. This same confusion occurs in diabetics when it is suspected that an overdose of insulin has been given. Both occurrences are frequent. Repeatedly patients with anxiety neurosis and anxiety attacks are said to be suffering from hyperinsulinism and the diagnosis is thought to be confirmed if the blood sugar, taken at the time of the attack, is found to be low. Even if the blood sugar is not low, so great is the confusion in regard to this subject that the term *dysinsulinism* is frequently applied simply because organic medicine will adopt almost any subterfuge rather than use the term anxiety neurosis. We do not deny that there is such a clinical state as spontaneous hypoglycemia due to hyperinsulinism. Indeed a number of cases have been proved to be due to pancreatic adenomata and after their removal the patient has recovered. But a great many patients labeled *functional hyperinsulinism* are suffering from *anxiety neurosis* and the differential diagnosis is not difficult if one will just take time to make fasting blood sugar tests as well as a study of the personality and life situation of the patient before jumping to a hasty conclusion. So-called functional hyperinsulinism is not associated with low levels of the fasting blood sugar (Conn).

Further studies by Conn and Seltzer emphasized that spontaneous hypoglycemia and hyperinsulinism are not synonymous terms. The former is the generic term. It includes all clinical situations in which the blood sugar may fall to abnormally low levels spontaneously. The term hyperinsulinism is confined to those types of spontaneous hypoglycemia in which an absolute increase in the production of endogenous insulin is believed to occur. These authors regard functional hyperinsulinism as the common form of spontaneous hypoglycemia, accounting for 70 per cent of all cases. The hypoglycemia is postprandial and never occurs in the fasting state. The manifestations are not progressive as in organic hyperinsulinism. The fasting blood sugar is normal but the response to glucose tolerance is pathognomonic. Levels below 40 mg. per cent must be demonstrated to make the test diagnostic.

In the course of a study of the emotional status of a group of diabetic patients, Musser and his associates found a striking association between the symptoms of hypoglycemia reactions and excessive anxiety. The patients reacted to hyperventilation with typical symptoms of "insulin reaction." They conclude that when the hyperventilation syndrome occurs in an anxious diabetic patient, symptoms occur which can be mistaken for a true insulin reaction. Appropriate psychotherapy assures more successful management.

Breidahl and associates feel that the term "hyperinsulinism" should be reserved for patients in whom tumor of the islets of Langerhans has been demonstrated or for people who have received an injection of an excessive amount of insulin. Thus they differentiate between hyperinsulinism and so-called "functional" or "spontaneous hypoglycemia." In 76 of 91 cases an actual tumor of the islets of the pancreas was found. The attacks must be associated with exercise or fasting, blood sugar level during an attack must be less than 50 mg. per 100 cc., and the attack must be relieved by the administration of sugar. Fasting up to 72 hours is a valuable diagnostic test and has replaced the glucose tolerance test. They found the results of the glucose tolerance test too variable and difficult to interpret and feel that nervous patients with vague symptoms should not be diagnosed as having hyperinsulinism simply because varying degrees of hypoglycemia develop some hours after the injection of glucose.

A clinical point utilized in supporting the diagnosis of spontaneous hypoglycemia is the tendency for patients who suffer from weakness and feelings of anxiety to carry candy or to eat some other food when they feel an anxiety attack coming on. It is presumed that the body chemistry is calling for carbohydrate. This presumption does not, however, take account of the psychological needs of the organism which can also be satisfied by swallowing. Referring to our discussion of the association between gastrointestinal function and anxiety (p. 21) we will recall that the anxious and irritable infant is soothed by swallowing milk and the pattern is established so that the anxious and irritable adult unconsciously seeks to comfort himself in the same way. The implications for obesity will be discussed later (p. 344).

Psychic Manifestations.　　The psychic manifestations of spontaneous and induced hypoglycemia are well known, the latter particularly because of the wide use of insulin. In general, these symptoms consist of anxiety, irritability, excitement, confusion, and finally complete loss of consciousness (hypoglycemic coma).

Case 38.　　Diabetes with Anxiety Attacks, Thought to be Hypoglycemic

A young white man with a neuropathic background was first seen because of indigestion which was proved to be of functional origin. Prompt recovery followed. In spite of his obvious neurotic tendencies he was an efficient and capable business man and shortly after he came under our observation was elevated to an important position in the concern for which he worked. On his next visit to us, at which time he again complained of indigestion and buzzing in the ear, which we also thought was functional, he reported that his responsibilities were great and "that the person who had previously occupied his position had died of overwork."

The pressure of meeting these responsibilities seemed to weigh heavily upon him and within the following six months he developed glycosuria which at first was transient and later became permanent with an elevated blood sugar. Control of diet and insulin was begun and he got along satisfactorily for the next few years. Then he developed acute appendicitis and during his hospital stay, while recovering from the operation, he was very apprehensive about "complications," and frequently showed anxiety symptoms that he felt were due to overdosage of insulin, but on each occasion it was found that his blood sugar was normal or beyond the normal. Again and again it was necessary to prove to him that these so-called hypoglycemia attacks were in reality anxiety attacks.

Case 39.　　Functional Hypoglycemia

A white man of 34 complained of fatigue and exhaustion, abdominal discomfort, a sense of pressure in the head, and occasional sharp pains in the head followed by palpitation and sweating.

History and Symptoms.　　At first he stated that his trouble had begun in the previous spring when he began to feel fatigued in the early afternoon. Then came an exhausted feeling in his legs. The exhaustion became more general and more pronounced and was followed by poor digestion and loose bowel movements. In spite of frequent eating he had lost about 10 pounds in the last year.

The sharp pains in the head occurred only rarely and were associated with dizziness, palpitation and sweating.

On close questioning he stated that he really had not been well since the age of 19. At that time he had begun to have pains in the back and in the legs and later suffered from indigestion.

Following a glucose tolerance test the patient was told that he had spontaneous hypoglycemia and was encouraged to eat frequently.

The father had died suddenly in his sleep at the age of 73. Previous to this he had suffered from a mental depression, and the patient felt that he resembled his father. Otherwise, the family history did not seem important.

Physical Examination and Laboratory Studies. The patient was an alert and intelligent young man, who was obviously quite apprehensive about himself. He was fairly well nourished, in spite of the loss of about 10 pounds during the previous year, and the general physical examination disclosed no evidence of organic disease. He was then referred to the hospital for special study.

A glucose tolerance test was done with the following results: Fasting sugar 82 mg. followed by a curve of 100, 62, 60 and 55. This was repeated with a slightly better response: fasting sugar 80 mg. followed by a curve of 131, 133, 90 and 57. The temperature in the hospital fluctuated between 97 and 98.6, in other words, there was a tendency toward hypothermia. Basal metabolism was found within normal limits and there was no evidence of adrenal dysfunction. Sedimentation rate was within normal limits and other ordinary laboratory studies were normal.

LIFE SITUATION

The patient was born and brought up in a small community in the Middle West. He described his father as a successful and important member of the community who was very religious, strongly opinionated, and a strict disciplinarian in the rearing of his children. In spite of his devotion to the church the patient had never felt that the father had any real affection for him. The patient felt that perfection was demanded of him and he was fired with ambition to get ahead. He tried very hard to excel in regard to both studies and athletic endeavors. Although not gifted intellectually and small for his age, he exerted himself to compete in scholarship and in athletics and made fair success at considerable effort. He had his heart set on a professional career but the father lost considerable money in 1929 and thereafter became depressed, and the patient was advised by his mother to take a position with his uncle (the mother's brother) who was a storekeeper in another town. After he had formed this connection at the age of 19 he became ill and, as before stated, he had never felt right since.

Shortly after moving to the new community he married and his wife had three children in rapid succession. All during the years he worked faithfully but received no advancement and, as a consequence, had a difficult time getting along on the small salary of a clerk and "was never out of debt." He felt very strongly that his work was not appreciated and during the last spring he had made some ineffectual efforts to find another position after concluding that the work was monotonous, that he was in a rut, and that he could never "find his way out."

Explanation of Illness. After giving this picture of driving energy and throttled ambition the patient was told that all studies were negative for evidence of organic disease and that the low blood sugar was probably of functional origin, in other words, very likely due to the excessive production of insulin—functional hyperinsulinism. It was also suggested that perhaps throttled energy, which could not find an outlet along normal aggressive channels, might have something to do with the excessive secretion of insulin— that his pancreas was being driven to too much activity. He became very excited at this suggestion that energy for driving ahead had been dammed up in him and was seeking a way out by disturbing the function of his organs. He insisted that he had always known that he could never get well so long as he was in his uncle's store and that in order to recover, he must get out and be "on his own." It seemed very reasonable to him that his dammed-up energy was trying to find a way out by means of excessive pancreatic function. We suggested that perhaps the satisfaction which he craved was the cause of his abdominal discomfort—that here was a displacement of his craving for recognition, forming a void which he was trying to fill by frequent eating.

We discussed this problem of his eating between meals and suggested that perhaps he really was not so hungry but that it was just an attempt to satisfy this craving which represented something else, that is, in early life the need for recognition that he had been so eager to achieve in the eyes of his father and, later, the need for recognition of his real worth by the uncle.

It occurred to him that the pressure in his head might also be due to throttled energy —"like steam under pressure trying to find a way out." The patient was cautioned not to make any impetuous decisions until he had had time soberly to review his feelings.

On a subsequent occasion he informed us that he had had a talk with his wife about the material that we had discussed and then had a talk with his uncle, whom he found "surprisingly understanding." He had served notice on his uncle rather indirectly that he might have to leave the business in order to get well and the uncle assured him that this was not necessary, that he would receive some immediate recognition, and that his future was assured—that when his uncle retired he would become the manager of the business.

Follow-up.   The patient improved immediately, and within a period of about two months he had lost most of his symptoms, and "for the first time, was really enjoying life."

SUMMARY

A young white man presented symptoms of exhaustion and anxiety which were attributed to spontaneous hypoglycemia. It was true that he had a hypoglycemic reaction to the glucose tolerance test but it was felt that this was functional and secondary to his anxiety state. The life situation showed evidence of long-time frustration and when it was suggested that this dammed-up energy was finding a way out by means of excessive secretion of insulin, the patient seized upon the suggestion with a great deal of avidity, unburdened himself of some of his anxiety and aggression, and made an excellent recovery.

To have called the illness spontaneous hypoglycemia or hyperinsulinism, to have encouraged frequent eating, and not to have made an effort to find out the nature of the anxiety which stood behind his functional hyperinsulinism, would not have helped this patient.

OBESITY

With the widespread adoption of the psychosomatic point of view more and more attention is being paid to emotional factors in obesity. It is not strange that this should be so. Next to the state of the weather, there is hardly a topic of conversation mentioned as frequently as weight loss or gain. This applies not only to women but to men as well, particularly in recent decades when the obesity problem has been stressed from a health standpoint as well as for appearance's sake. It is recognized that the latter factor is not confined to women.

Excessive weight brings people into conflict for several reasons. First, overweight makes people look older and less attractive from the standpoint of our national ideal of good looks. Secondly, many people are aware that obesity may have something to do with the development of such diseases as diabetes, hypertension and heart disease. Then, of course, conflict occurs when they attempt to do something about it, for they would like to maintain an attractive figure without foregoing the pleasure of eating. To avoid the unpleasantness of dieting, patients often resort to harmful drugs or injure themselves by overexercise. A condition which was looked upon as a question of glands and calories is now regarded as a complicated problem in which family background, which refers to attitude as well as constitutional factors, is important. In other words, while obesity may run in families, habits are just as important as genes.

Intake of Food.   Exercise and the functioning of the ductless glands have something to do with the problem of weight gain but the most important factor is food *intake*. As stated in the section on psychopathology there is a great deal of sensual pleasure associated with the function of the mouth. The lips and tongue are well supplied with nerve end organs highly sensitive to food and drink. The greatest

JUNIOR PSYCHOSOMATIC MEDICINE

EXAMINATION

Answer 4 out of the 5 questions listed below.

1. You have just finished taking history from a 35 year old woman
    who has been married for 12 years, who has not been able to
    conceive a pregnancy despite the fact that she and her husband
    have never used contraceptives and want to have a child. She
    has sought medical consultation with you because of her wish for
    another medical evaluation of her supposed sterility. List as
    many contributing factors as you can which might have come up
    in the clinical historical examination which you would want to
    investigate further either by physical, laboratory or clinical
    psychological examinations.

2. In no more than 50 words, discuss the psychosomatic aspects
    of "hypothyroidism."

3. In 50 words or less, discuss briefly the psychosomatic aspects
    of "low blood pressure."

4. Outline the medical and psychological work up of a 46 year old
    man with pylorospasm accompanied by elevated gastric acidity
    but no ulcer formation or tumor mass and discuss briefly the
    management of the emotional aspects of this syndrome.

✓ 5. Discuss briefly the management of a 14 month old child brought
    to you for consultation by its mother because he is a stubborn
    child when it comes to eating and is frequently refusing or
    regurgitating food to such a degree that both the mother and
    the child are upset.

pleasure to the human being during the first year of life comes through this mouth area in the acts of nursing, eating and drinking. As the months go by other pleasure stimuli should enter his range of vision or feeling and should be incorporated in his developing personality.

EMPHASIS ON EATING. However, whether or not this is so depends largely upon the family background of the child. Some families are quite "oral" in their orientation to life. The parents pride themselves upon having good food. The mother says, "Whether we have enough of other things or not we'll have good things to eat." A treat for such a family will be a good meal rather than creative work or play. They talk about food and the various ways it should be cooked and other interests in life suffer proportionately. If a child grows up in such a family he is almost certain to place an overvaluation on food and eating. When the child goes to school or camp the mother voices her fear that he may not have enough to eat. The impression is gained that if he does not eat well something dangerous will happen to him. Everything about the offering and receiving of food is endowed with a high emotional value.

In a paper devoted to food and allergies Kaufman pointed out that foods can be classified according to their emotional significance to the individual.

"Most of us have at one time or another used certain foods in larger amounts than usual when we felt some special need to have emotional security. These are the 'security' foods. For example, in times of severe stress many persons unconsciously find it necessary to increase their intake of milk and milk products. Such persons often rationalize their need for milk as eating 'lightly,' that is, not putting too great a load on their stomachs. But milk used in this way often symbolizes a strong desire to regress to the days when major decisions were made by the parents.

"We also have certain specific foods which serve us as 'reward' foods. If we are thwarted and frustrated, or if we feel that others have not appreciated sufficiently achievements which we accomplished through great effort; or if others fail to commiserate with us sufficiently on our failures, we tend unconsciously to eat 'reward' or 'party' foods. We are good to ourselves by eating more chocolate, more ice cream, more nuts, more hot dogs, more cake—or perhaps we indulge ourselves in a tin of caviar.

"Certain foods seem to be used as 'fetish' foods—these are the ones which we think we can't do without. Some persons feel that unless they have red meat in their diet, they won't have the strength to carry on with their daily work; and others feel the same way about bread, the 'staff of life.' It is quite common for people to feel that if they diet they will become weak and often when they succeed in losing a few pounds, some 'kind friend' puts a stop to the effort by telling them how 'awful' they look.

"Then there are the 'pleasurable association' foods. Sometimes, we eat certain foods because they remind us of happy circumstances. Then, we have the 'grown-up' or 'maturity' foods like coffee, tea, beer, etc., which were 'for adults only' when most of us were children. Many individuals deprived of these foods as children, make overdetermined use of the 'grown-up' foods later when they become grown up chronologically.

"On the other hand, we have our private list of foods with which we have *unpleasant associations*. There are foods to which we develop aversions through religious training or through cultural upbringing. We have taboos against eating nutritious and wholesome foods which we consider culturally as coming from filthy sources. In addition, we develop certain aversions because we associate certain foods with the onset of some acute illness that we experienced in the past. Foods pleasurable in one form may be unpleasurable in another form. Then, we develop certain aversions to foods that have built-in conflict and anxiety associated with them. 'You must eat spinach,' when not to eat spinach is to defy parental authority, and to eat spinach is 'knuckling under.' Some aversions to wholesome foods operate on this infantile level—and some husband-wife conflicts are touched off when the wife serves spinach and urges her husband to eat it.

"Each individual has developed very early in his life conditioned responses to eating and to certain foods. His conditioned patterns of reacting are his individual integration of behavior he has learned from his culture, his relation to his parents (particularly the mother), and from his own life experience.

"The whole eating process is, moreover, a special training process by which the growing infant learns to accept various restraints and to live by certain conventions; 'baby must eat his meat before he can have his ice cream.' Food is used as a reward for achieving certain desired behavior patterns in the learning process. It is also used punitively and hostilely. Mother righteously tries to feed the child a food that she knows he despises— and then spanks him for not eating it, compounding the punishment. Eating, restraining of personal liberty, and punishment are frequent associations which are so strong in the lives of some people that they have an aversion to all food, and eat merely to sustain life and regard the eating procedure as ugly and unpleasant, to be gotten over with as rapidly as possible. Those who have received kindly and understanding food training by a patient mother can derive special enjoyment from eating—the pleasurable associations of early training outweigh the restraints and punishments."*

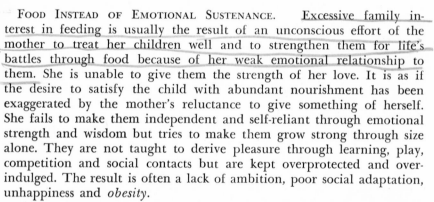

FOOD INSTEAD OF EMOTIONAL SUSTENANCE.   Excessive family interest in feeding is usually the result of an unconscious effort of the mother to treat her children well and to strengthen them for life's battles through food because of her weak emotional relationship to them. She is unable to give them the strength of her love. It is as if the desire to satisfy the child with abundant nourishment has been exaggerated by the mother's reluctance to give something of herself. She fails to make them independent and self-reliant through emotional strength and wisdom but tries to make them grow strong through size alone. They are not taught to derive pleasure through learning, play, competition and social contacts but are kept overprotected and over-indulged. The result is often a lack of ambition, poor social adaptation, unhappiness and *obesity*.

Endocrine Glands.   It may be that the endocrines play a part but that part may be a secondary functional disturbance as a result of the psychological situation. For example, when menstrual irregularities occur in obesity, they appear to be secondary because the menstrual cycle can often be restored simply by getting rid of the fat. At any rate it should be obvious that the interrelation of personality, social situation and glandular function is a highly complex one.

Richardson reported that obesity which is demonstrably of endocrine origin is rare even in an endocrine clinic, whereas fat people constitute a large section of the general population. Moreover, in ordinary obesity he found little evidence of endocrine disturbance; the obese woman has normal skeletal and sexual characteristics. "It often happens, of course, that an obese patient receives an endocrine preparation of some sort and loses weight. But this is no evidence that the preparation has any biological action on the fat apart from its psychotherapeutic effects. When the emotions are involved, as they usually are in any deviation from good health, it is enough that the patient should believe in the remedy to produce a psychological effect on the disease. If endocrine prepara-

* From Kaufman, W.: Psychosom. Med., *16:* 10, 1954.

tions were not available for the treatment of obesity the patient would probably be equally benefited by some other form of medication."

We do not deny the importance of the endocrine glands in the problem of obesity; we only urge psychosomatic consideration in every instance of this disorder.

Personality Studies.   Some of the above observations were made by Bruch in an important study of 140 obese children and their parents. Marked delay in ability and willingness to take care of themselves was noted in three fourths of the group. A concurrent evidence of *immaturity* in emotional development was shown by the symptom of *enuresis* which occurred in 40 per cent of those studied.

PHYSICAL INACTION.   Entrance into school marked the first opportunity for social contact in these children. About two thirds of the group were considered physically inactive. Few of them made use of the opportunities for muscular exercise provided by the school playground. They remained isolated and without playmates. Even in recreational activities involving other than muscular exercise there was little indication of creative self-expression. The majority of them sought the "made" entertainment of movies and radio. Only a small number of parents had encouraged activity or initiative in other ways. In fact, their overprotection of the child was extreme, sometimes to the point of wanting to accompany the child to school and even to the classroom door to help him remove his outer clothing. It is small wonder that these children expected that everything would be done for them. Slow and awkward movements were thought to be due to lack of training games and other activities rather than to any abnormality in the mechanism of transformation of energy.

FAMILY SETTING.   Although obesity apparently often "runs in families" this fact does not exclude more than one mechanism. Richardson emphasized that transmission can take place in one of two ways, or both of them at once: by genetic inheritance, or through the medium of the family life and its social and cultural setting.

In a study with Grace Touraine in relation to the family setting from which obese children come, Bruch observed that in such families the amount of money spent for food was disproportionately large. The obesity was rarely a matter of concern to the parents although concern over minor physical ailments was excessive. Many of the fathers were weak, unaggressive people with little drive or ambition. The mothers had suffered from poverty and insecurity in their own childhood. In only a few families was there marital happiness. At times there was open fighting and frequently contempt was expressed for the father by a domineering mother. The families were usually small in size. Seventy per cent of the children studied were either an only child or the youngest child. One half of the children were admittedly unwanted. Sometimes hostility was openly expressed by cruel punishment or shown through unreasonable and severe discipline. But the most conspicuous feature in the attitude to the obese children was *inconsistency*. Most prominent was an open display of protectiveness. But this seeming manifestation of devotion and affection was frequently like a thin veneer that barely covered the underlying insecurity in relation to the child. *The fundamental rejection was compensated for by overprotection and excessive feeding.* These contradictions were more frequently observed in mothers than in fathers.

PSYCHIC CONDITIONING.   Muscular activity had been associated with the idea of danger in these fat children. Hence the lack of muscular activity and excessive intake of food were both factors in obesity, to which social and emotional adjustment were intimately related. Of course, all obesity does not have its beginning in childhood. It may come on at any age. What that age will be is determined in many cases by the same factors that cause the onset of any neurotic symptom. When insecurity or need for affection and attention becomes more pronounced than the maturity of the personality can cope with, anxiety appears. If the pattern of that personality has been set up so that oral gratification through eating allays anxiety, then obesity is likely to result. If this conditioning to excessive eating is great enough, obesity may occur in childhood. If the conditioning is only latent in the framework of the personality, indulgence in overeating may not occur until some stress makes itself felt later in life. For example, an adolescent moves to a new neighborhood or enters a new school. He fails to get off to a good start in making friends and entering into social activities. Denied such pleasures he regresses to oral gratification, eats excessively, withdraws to himself, further limits his muscular activities, and as a consequence gets fat. More than likely the obesity will be blamed on "glands."

A married woman of about 42, a large, soft, dependent and passive creature, took care of her husband and his business as a mother would and had little of the pleasures, satisfactions and responsibilities of a wife. After several visits to us she volunteered the information that some six or eight years ago she discovered that her husband was having an extra-marital affair and that thereafter "she had let herself go." That is, she had given up trying to dress attractively and had eaten as she pleased. As a consequence she gained a great deal of weight. It was obvious that when she was denied certain satisfactions in life she regressed to oral satisfaction and as a result she became very heavy and, of course, even less attractive to her husband. It was not too difficult to point this out and to hold out as the incentive for a strict reduction diet, the possibility of regaining her interests in life and regaining her husband's interest in her.

Psychological Aspects of the Treatment of Obesity.   Therefore, whether the endocrine factor is large, small or nonexistent, it is necessary in approaching the obesity problem to study the emotional life. We should elicit a history concerning the parents and siblings which will show the influence of the family situation in the development of the patient's personality. Was the mother herself a deprived and insecure person? Bruch and Touraine noted that not only could common factors in the background of mothers of obese children be found in the actual events of their lives, but that even more important aspects were reflected in their responses to them, in their self-pitying attitude towards the past.

Resentful submissions, incessant preoccupation with their misfortunes, and condemnation of others for their frustration manifested itself in their words as well as their behavior.

MOTHER'S ATTITUDE.   What was the mother's attitude toward the patient during his gestation and at birth and in his developmental years? What was her attitude toward food in general and toward the feeding of the patient in particular? Did she encourage play and exercise, stimulate initiative and imagination? Was she overprotective in her attitude and strict in her discipline or was she friendly and tolerant? Were her mother and father compatible, and what was the father's role in discipline and in the inspiration of the patient? Were food, drinks, and candy used as rewards for good behavior or were rewards less related to oral gratification?

In a discussion of the compliance factor in the development of specific emotional difficulties, Johnson and associates (Frazier et al.) emphasize that children reflect the conflicts of their parents as well as their constructive attitudes. In the families in which children have neurotic, psychosomatic, psychotic or antisocial problems, there are mixed feelings of affection, mistrust, anger and respect between the spouses and toward the children. The marital relationship is unsatisfactory, and many of the frustrations thus arising are deflected in specific fashion to each child. The scapegoat child is the one who receives the brunt of a particular parental conflict; there are frequently several scapegoat children in a neurotic family, each reflecting a different parental conflict. On this basis they describe five types of neurotic difficulties exhibited by the children: (1) family obesity, (2) clinical obesity, (3) skinniness, (4) certain ulcer problems and (5) anorexia nervosa. In each family there is parental ambivalence toward the child, the intensity of the hostile component increasing from types 1 to 5.

ATTITUDE TOWARD REDUCTION.   A patient can consciously desire to reduce and unconsciously cheat on his resolve. He may consciously want to limit his food intake but another part of his personality fears deprivation. It is quite common for such patients to feel that disease may attack a thin body. In fact, when we get into more deeply unconscious ideas we find that some are even more bizarre. For instance, the very woman who consciously wants to diet to lose weight and become more attractive has at the same time a marked anxiety about becoming more attractive. She is afraid she will fall into sexual temptation or if she is single she is afraid some man will really ask her to marry him and she will be drawn into responsibilities which she is afraid to face. Obesity in some women has the unconscious significance of pregnancy because of the primitive belief that impregnation occurs through eating.

OBESITY AS A MANIFESTATION OF NEUROSIS.   Richardson reported in detail a case of obesity in a woman which began before the age of 10. The central psychological features were deprivation by the parents in childhood, for which she blamed chiefly her mother, and an atmosphere of severe sexual repression. She early relinquished the expectation of affectionate care and understanding from the mother and regarded herself as a waif. She longed for a family and children but was strongly inhibited and rejected men. To a large extent eating took the place of affection but she also invested it with the symbolic meaning of impregnation following the childish idea of gastrointestinal pregnancy and parturition.

"Examples could be multiplied to show neurotic symptoms in the obese: the destructive effects of the obesity; anxiety, guilt, self-depreciation, depression, and a compulsive type of eating analogous to alcoholism or a drug addiction. That the neurosis affords a psychological gain is indicated partly by the fear of losing weight. Fat is used as a barrier against men and marriage and against other affectionate relationships of adult life."

NERVOUS HUNGER.   Patients do not present themselves for psychological study because of obesity. But treatment of patients for other conditions has revealed valuable information regarding the matter of overweight. Either sex may use the *eating* process to *allay anxiety* or to gratify pleasure cravings which should be satisfied in other ways, as for instance through a better sexual and social adjustment. A nagging, intolerable sensation in the epigastrium often referred to as "nervous hunger" is symbolic of the emptiness of the emotional life. The effort to fill this void with food instead of emotional sustenance is a frequent cause of obesity.

It is not surprising that feeding and feelings should be related. Anyone who has observed an infant recognizes that he feels out the world with his mouth and that everything that he can lay his hands on goes into that aperture. Moreover, the feeding process of infancy becomes closely connected with the attitude of the mother or nurse. If the feeding process is associated with love, affection and security the child is apt to be content and the digestive processes normal, whereas if there are tensions, insecurity and anger associated with the feeding process, disturbed patterns of gastrointestinal behavior are apt to be established which reassert themselves later in life when the individual meets life situations which reawaken old associations. So foods and eating are associated with high emotional values.

A woman who had been married twelve years, childless, and twenty pounds overweight, reported that whenever she felt unhappy or depressed she felt that she must have a good meal. She would describe the meal in great detail, how good the food was, and how kind and friendly the waitresses were. Psychological study showed that she had a strong need to be loved but an even stronger need to hate, to criticize, and to be unreasonable and disagreeable. After she was permitted to express a great deal of her hostility she was finally able to be friendly and tolerant. Then she made up her mind to reduce. She said, "I guess I felt so mean I didn't care whether anyone liked me or not." A deeper study of her unconscious mental processes showed that her fat abdomen symbolized a pregnancy. When she was able consciously to bear the idea of a child the normal way she wanted to get rid of her fat. Naturally all of this material was not disclosed at one time. She would get discouraged occasionally and then eat too much. But as treatment continued, dieting became easier. She said, "I didn't realize how much I nibbled all day long. I didn't know I was eating much when really I was eating most of the time. It was like having company to eat a little something. Now I'm on a diet and I feel I have enough. It's really easy when you have a definite purpose and nothing pulling you the other way."

Psychotherapy. All kinds of worries, tensions and frustrations may lead to overeating and sometimes the psychological disturbance is so severe that the eating is like an obsession, indeed, very much like addiction to alcohol. Patients often explain that they cannot restrain themselves from stuffing themselves with food in spite of the fact that they suffer the most severe guilt reaction afterwards. Such people, in whom it is obvious that powerful unconscious mental factors are at work, had better be referred to psychiatrists for help. The lesser problems can be handled by the general physician if he utilizes the psychosomatic approach. If the nervous disturbance is of a temporary nature, reassurance, sedation and discussion of current problems may be sufficient to overcome it. When the emotional tension is due to deeper and stronger influences, more effort must be made to understand the family relationships in an effort to determine the cause of the increased desire for food.

The effect of psychotherapy without the use of calculated diets was studied by Nicholson. Ninety-three patients were divided into the following four groups:

1. Thirty-eight patients were treated by superficial psychotherapy without calculated diets and without medication; the patients were offered a simple explanation of energy exchange and the caloric value of foods.

2. Thirty-five patients were given a calculated diet of 800 calories. An experienced dietitian explained the diet and, when desired, further instructions were given on return visits. There was no medication, nor was any effort at psychotherapy attempted.

3. Ten patients were given 5 mg. of amphetamine sulfate three times a day. No psychotherapy was attempted and no calculated diet was offered.

4. Ten patients were handled as in Group 3 except that thyroid substance was administered instead of amphetamine.

All obese patients studied were found to have some type of psychoneurosis in varying degrees. Psychotherapy resulted in a higher percentage of successful results than was obtained from the other methods of attempted reduction. Nicholson concluded that both psychotherapy and the reestablishment of proper dietary habits are essential for permanent weight reduction.

Kotkov discussed the application of group psychotherapy to the obese. Group psychotherapy sessions with obese adults of both sexes are described. Although no unusual over-all weight loss occurred, group psychotherapy served as an invaluable experience for the maintenance of weight loss in 48 per cent of the patients who had not succeeded with other methods.

PREADOLESCENT HYPOGONADISM

Concern over the development of small, fat boys is one of the common problems presented to the pediatrician and general practitioner interested in endocrinology. Such boys, who will usually develop in normal fashion if they are given the opportunity, are frequently regarded as instances of dystrophia adiposogenitalis and treated with testosterone. Since the distribution of fat resembles that found in women and adult eunuchs, the physician is inclined to make a diagnosis of obesity due to hypogonadism, particularly since the genitalia appear small. The apparent hypogonadism is due to the fact that the penis is usually embedded in suprapubic fat. When the fat pad is pushed back and the penis and testes are measured, it is evident that the genitalia are within the range of normal when compared with previously established standards. From a study of 1500 males Schonfeld established such standards of development by correlating measurements of penis and testes with the degree of maturation of the secondary sex characteristics. Schonfeld believes that the actual size of the genitalia is of physiologic significance only after pubescence and that "a great deal of therapeutic confusion has been created in the literature by the failure to appreciate the range of normal variation of genital measurements, age of onset of pubescence, and the characteristics of growth of the various types of body configurations (somatotypes). Many of these normal boys have been subjected to prolonged endocrine treatment with the induction of pubescence, and their normal development is fallaciously attributed to endocrine therapy. An accurate evaluation of the existing status and future prognosis is essential for the proper management of the prepubescent and pubescent boy." Schonfeld described a test to prognosticate whether a boy will have spontaneous pubescence. The test is based on the ability of the testes to respond to stimulation by chorionic gonadotropins of human pregnancy urine.

When hypogonadism actually exists the physical and psychological consequences are, of course, disastrous. Boys who in early childhood were active, healthy, husky children suddenly discover at adolescence that they are different from other boys, who make fun of them. Kasanin and Biskind discussed the change in personality that followed specific treatment in seven cases. Their patients had remained adolescent. They showed an abnormal body contour, retained a highpitched voice, and showed no growth of genitalia. Doubt regarding themselves "leads to a great deal of resentment mixed with the feeling of rage and frustration, which is usually repressed, and the only thing evident on the surface is a feeling of bitterness and hostility. . . . The most important change effected by successful treatment is a better relationship to the world." All of their patients became more affectionate, less hostile, less jealous, not so bitter, and did not shrink from people any more. They met men and women on an equal basis, and were not afraid to compete.

References

Bollmeier, L. N., and Meyer, A.: J. Arkansas Med. Soc., *41:* 121, 1944.
Breidhal, H. D., Priestley, J. T., and Rynearson, E. H.: J.A.M.A., *160:* 198, 1956.

Bruch, H.: Am. J. Dis. Child., (a) *59:* 739, 1940; (b) *60:* 1082, 1940.

Bruch, H.: Psychosom. Med., *11:* 200, 1949.

Bruch, H., and Hewlett, I.: Psychosom. Med., *9:* 205, 1947.

Bruch, H., and Touraine, G.: Psychosom. Med., *2:* 141, 1940.

Conn, J. W.: J.A.M.A., *115:* 1669, 1940.

Conn, J. W., and Seltzer, H. S.: Am. J. Med., *19:* 460, 1955.

Daniels, G. E.: Am. J. Psychiat., *93:* 711, 1936; Psychoanalyt. Quart., *5:* 513, 1936.

Daniels, G. E.: Psychiatry, 7: 121, 1944.

Dunbar, H. F.: J. Nerv. & Ment. Dis., *86:* 712, 1937.

Fischer, A. E., and Dolger, H.: Arch. Int. Med., *78:* 711, 1946.

Frazier, S. H., Jr., Fanbion, M. H., Giffin, M. E., and Johnson, A. M.: Proc. Mayo Clinic, *30:* 227, 1955.

Gull, W. W.: Tr. Clin. Soc. London, 7: 22, 1874.

Haagensen, C. D., and Lloyd, Wyndham, E. B.: A Hundred Years of Medicine, Sheridan House, Inc., New York, 1943.

Hinkle, Jr., L. E., and Wolf, S.: J.A.M.A., *148:* 513, 1952.

Houssay, B. A.: New England J. Med., *214:* 971, 1936.

Houssay, B. A., and Biasotti, A.: Endocrinology, *15:* 511, 1931.

Kasanin, J., and Biskind, G. R.: J.A.M.A., *121:* 1318, 1943.

Kaufman, W.: (a) Ann. Allergy, *10:* 308, 1952; (b) Psychosom. Med., *16:* 10, 1954; (c) Acta Psychotherapeutica, suppl., *3:* 162, 1955.

Kay, D. W. K.: Proc. Roy. Soc. Med., *46:* 669, 1953.

Kolkov, B.: Psychosom. Med., *15:* 243, 1953.

Lorand, S.: Psychosom. Med., *5:* 282, 1943.

McCullough, E. P., and Tuffer, R.: Ann. Int. Med., *14:* 817, 1940.

Menninger, W. C.: (a) J. Nerv. & Ment. Dis., *81:* 1, 1935; (b) J. Ment. Sci., *81:* 332, 1935.

Meyer, A., Bollmeier, L. N., and Alexander, F.: Psychosom. Med., 7: 335, 1945.

Mirsky, I. Arthur: (a) The Biology of Diabetes Mellitus in Man, Institute on Psychosomatics, University of Nebraska, February 11, 1948. (b) Emotional Factors in the Patient with Diabetes Mellitus, presented before Section on Nervous and Mental Diseases, Ohio State Medical Association, April 1, 1948, Cincinnati, Ohio.

Musser, M. J., Lorenz, T. H. and Derus, G. J.: J.A.M.A., *152:*1113, 1953.

Nemiah, J. C.: Medicine, *29:* 225, 1950.

Nicholson, W. M.: Am. J. Med. Sc., *211:* 443, 1946.

Richardson, H. B.: Psychiat. Quart., *20:* 400, 1946.

Richardson, H. B.: M. Clin. North America, p. 1187, Sept., 1946.

Rosen, H., and Lidz, T.: Psychosom. Med., *11:* 211, 1949.

Schonfeld, W. A.: J.A.M.A., *121:* 177, 1943.

Simmonds, M.: Deutsche med. Wchnschr., *40:* 322, 1914.

Stearns, S.: New England J. Med., *249:* 471, 1953.

Waller, J. V., Kaufman, M. R., and Deutsch, F.: Psychosom. Med., *2:* 3, 1940.

Chapter XII

The Genitourinary System and
Sexual Function in the Female

DIFFERENCES IN PSYCHOSEXUAL DEVELOPMENT

Psychosexual development has already been discussed in Chapter II, but there are certain differences in the psychosexual development of the female from that of the male that should be pointed out in a chapter devoted exclusively to the genitourinary and sexual functioning of the female.

The nursing experience in males and females is probably a similar procedure. A variable, however, may be the mother's attitude toward the sex of the child born to her. She may be rejecting of any child born to her or she may be rejecting of males only or females only. She may be accepting of females until two or three have been born to her, then her own wishes and the pressure of husband or relatives may cause her to be rejecting of the next child should it be a girl. A rejected girl child may and probably will have her own maternal function interfered with. A woman who has not known the pleasures of being touched, mothered and cuddled in infancy will have her own problems when her turn comes to do so—no matter how much she may be taught about it by her doctor or in the books she reads.

Toilet Training. It is possible that in toilet training mothers may insist upon higher standards of cleanliness and neatness for the female child than for the male. This seems logical in view of the fact that women seem to be so much more sensitive to the appearance and order of their homes or offices than are men. It seems safe to say that most men are more accepting of disorder, disarray and drabness than women. Most women want some color, beauty, order and cleanliness in their lives and concern themselves about it more than men. Perhaps this is in the interest of society's division of labor, but Freud indicated that it was connected with sublimations of toilet training experiences and with this we would agree.

Masturbation. Statistically, females masturbate less than males in a ratio of roughly six to ten. This may be due to some neurophysiological differences in the sexes but we suspect the fastidiousness of mothers results in more inhibition of masturbation in females than in males. Certainly there is no reason from the standpoint of anatomy why masturbation would be any less pleasurable in the female than in the male. As yet we have no studies to indicate that the female has any fewer nerve endings in her phallic structure than the male. It seems likely that stimulation in and around the moist body aperture in this region carries meanings that are disturbing to mothers, making masturbation less reprehensible in the male child than in the female child. Moreover, it must not be forgotten that there is a longstanding cultural acceptance of the male as being a more excitable animal sexually. It is not only safer for him to be so but there is less taboo about it. This must certainly enter into the incidence of masturbation.

Studies of sexual behavior during psychosexual growth seem to point to the fact that early sexual arousal genitally has a direct relationship to later sexual interest. These findings would seem to support those who believe that early sex arousal leads to later sexual immorality, but there is more to sexual behavior than an immoral use of it. There is need for a greater sexual similarity in rhythm and compatibility between men and women in order to enhance marital harmony. This would, in many instances, prevent extramarital sexual activity with its inherent problems. In short, the sexual function is complex and many-sided and it cannot be disposed of by saying "suppress all sex interest in the child and there will be no problem." The powerful sex energies have many good avenues of expression and great social usefulness and we need to give their presence in the personality the wisest acceptance that we can.

Penis Envy. One of Freud's most hotly contested concepts is that females suffer from penis envy. Yet observations show that females emerge from their psychosexual growth with different values than men. These differences seem to increase rather than diminish with the passage of time. The differences in appearance genitally make much more difference in female psychology than is commonly recognized. For instance, the female child notices the absence of the male genital and feels inadequate and dissatisfied with her lot. She feels she has been cheated out of a useful and visible portion of anatomy. She is envious of the male and the freedom and variety of his life which seems to go along with his having a penis. Such an initial conclusion may be heightened and exaggerated by her observation of family life. Moreover, rarely is the girl told that her sexual organ can give pleasure to a man in addition to conceiving children. If such ideas ever cross her mental horizon they come too late to be incorporated into her psyche and do her much good. She is forced to try to make a virtue of her unawakened sexuality and to look down upon the male for his sexual aggression. Hence she spends much of her life frustrating him sexually and comforting herself that she is morally of finer fiber, with greater discipline and will power and a higher cultural and aesthetic sense than he. Actually, she is unwilling or fearful of accepting her feminine role and seeks to outdo or compete with men.

During puberty and adolescence she attempts to accept menstruation and other signs of development with the best grace she can. It is unfortunate that society cannot yet be frank with its boys and girls—its young men and women—and teach them more precisely what it means to be men and women. At its best, a marriage in which a man and woman do all they can to help, comfort, support each other, meet the sexual needs of each other, help each other develop mentally, is civilization at its finest. Conversely, when a man and woman marry and do not understand or meet each other's needs, when they create tension, frustration and hostility in each other, then marriage is a socially destructive unit and a breeding ground for personality maladjustment, mental disease and psychosomatic illness.

MENARCHE

All races have shown guilt over menstruation and according to their folklore they have needed some impersonal or plausible way to explain its occurrence. To account for the onset of menstruation at puberty there was an early belief that some snake or wild animal had injured the girl, or that the spirit of an ancestor had had intercourse with her. The idea grew that the monthly flow of blood in the woman was accompanied by cruel and hostile wishes within her, and, as a result, women were dangerous at this period and needed special taboos erected against them, and some degree of seclusion from others, lest harm arise from contact with them.

Menstrual Taboos.   It is important to consider these old beliefs and superstitions because, as we know, such beliefs die out slowly in mankind. Many centuries of education and enlightenment are necessary for the individual to be entirely rid of their influence. We must admit that the girl of today, while not told exactly the same things as her sister of a thousand years ago, is nevertheless placed under certain restrictions and taboos just the same, and many superstitions are established for her concerning the menstrual function. In our society it is common for a man to regard a menstruating woman as dirty and disgusting, and so she often regards herself, and this may be in part responsible for fear or anxiety on the part of one or the other, or both. Some groups of people have menstrual taboos which are intended to protect the man against the dangers of the menstruating woman. In these groups the menstruating woman, her bed, and her clothes are dangerous to the man and should not be touched until eight days after the cessation of the menstrual period, and until after the woman has completely immersed herself in water.

Anxiety and Superstition.   Women, likewise, have anxieties, suspicions and superstitions relating to menstruation. They often refer to themselves as "being ill" during the time of the menstrual period. They often do not dare to bathe during this time and only wash themselves to the waist. Many women prefer to remain in bed for a day or two because they were taught to do so by their mothers or some other woman, lest the bleeding become too profuse or stop completely if they go about their work in the usual manner. Among certain people menstruating women are forbidden to sew, to knead bread, to handle cut flowers, to preserve fruit, or to water young plants. A menstruating woman's touch is considered capable of blighting crops, withering gardens, bringing fruit from trees, killing saplings, turning wine to vinegar, or causing mares to miscarry. If we ask why the menstruating woman is regarded as so dangerous to growing things, the following answer has been suggested: In primitive tribes menstruation was regarded as a sign of sexual excitement. As culture changed, the sexually excitable woman was regarded as a danger to the stability of the home, and to the legitimacy of the heir. This original connection of sexual excitement and menstruation has been lost and there remains the taboo against menstruation itself. Nevertheless, many civilized women still exhibit considerably increased sexual excitement around the time of the menstrual period.

Many people of both sexes regard menstruation as unpleasant or dirty because they associate the menstrual flow with urine or with feces, in short, an unpleasant excretion which cannot be controlled. They feel that a discharge from that portion of the body must be regarded as dirty or contaminated. In both sexes, menstruation arouses some anxiety because the bleeding stirs up some childhood fantasy that an injury has been done to the female and this *same* injury could occur to the male. Some women regard menstruation as a repeated confirmation *each* month of a belief that they have injured themselves through masturbation.

Effect on Children. It is important to consider that the child is subject, year after year, to the effect of a periodically recurring indisposition of the mother at the time of the menstrual period. At these times she may be irritable, self-centered, often depressed, and may remain in bed a day or two. At the same time, children, because of their curiosity or because of the carelessness of the mother, become aware that bleeding is taking place. Rarely is any explanation given and the child is left to draw its own conclusions, which are often bizarre but fairly certain to include the idea of injury and pain. Menstrual bleeding stirs up anxiety and fear of *genital mutilation* in the minds of both the little girl and the little boy. At the onset of menstruation the girl is often treated unkindly and unsympathetically, is not enlightened by the mother, and hence concludes that she has some unspeakable condition for which she feels unpopular and cast out. The girl realizes that she is experiencing something about which people just cannot express themselves. She feels the hostility of everyone for being in this state. She regards herself as unclean and unwanted by her parents, her brothers and sisters, and society in general. At this time activities and pleasures have to be curtailed, or at least she is too often told that this should be the case. With all of this taking place in the mind of the child at puberty, not to mention what takes place afterward, it is small wonder that women grow morose and irritable as this phenomenon recurs each month.

In the female child who may have been envious of the privileges of masculinity and who still had the hope of some day growing into a boy, these hopes are blasted when menstruation begins at puberty. The bleeding is a very definite evidence of the need to accept the feminine role, and if the advantages of the latter have not been portrayed to her, this realization may have a very saddening effect. Furthermore, many girls approach puberty and menstruation with some hope that when menstruation begins they will be accepted by the mother and the sisters and other women into a greater intimacy and friendship. They often find that this does not take place since the whole subject is one with which women generally associate little dignity or prestige. Hence the girl finds that she has all the discomforts of menstruation and none of the advantages of her growing maturity. Thus we see this phenomenon of menstruation as one which, each time it occurs, stirs up fantasies of hostility toward both sexes—toward women because the mother let her be born that way, and toward men because of envy of the freedom to which their organs seem to entitle them.

More Education Needed.   Surely a more widespread and sensible education of the growing girl about menstruation is needed. It is important to teach every young girl the facts of menstruation in a realistic and kindly fashion. What are the important facts that she needs to integrate into her mind? That she as a woman can expect a flow of blood from the vagina monthly from the age of 12 to 45 approximately. This prepares the inside of the uterus for the growth of a baby if conditions are right for its conception. This bleeding is neither harmful nor dangerous. It generally lasts from three to five days. It is a universal fact of nature. It is to be accepted. It need not interfere with normal living.

When the facts of menstruation are discussed questions about conception and pregnancy are very likely to arise. They also should be discussed. There are numerous ways to do this and numerous pamphlets and books are widely available. Yet a conspiracy of silence still holds between many mothers and daughters. The medical profession has an obligation to help women understand the meaning of sex and the important role it plays in their lives. It has a far-reaching impact on their self-esteem, their freedom from anxiety, their marital happiness and their function as mothers.

THE SEXUAL ACT

Definition of Orgasm.   Because of anxiety and prudishness the subject of orgasm is a difficult one to deal with in women. First, our language alone hardly suffices for getting at the real truth. The physician can start by asking a married patient, "Is your sexual life congenial?" The patient may say only "Yes," or elaborate further. But this question at least starts thinking in this area. Then the physician may ask, "Do you achieve orgasm in your sexual relations?" Few women will be able to answer accurately. Some will answer affirmatively just to bring the discussion to an end. Others do not know what the word means. For the physician to be at all sure that he is getting accurate information he will have to describe what occurs during orgasm. He must speak somewhat as follows: "Does your sexual excitement reach a point of greatly heightened pleasure? Do you reach a climax? Is it accompanied by a muscular tension generally and involuntary movements of the pelvis with increased breathing and heart beat, and after a few seconds does it subside with a great feeling of relaxation?"

These things at least must be present as a part of full orgasm. About one third of women rarely if ever have this experience. Another third have it about half the time and another third have it most but not every time a sexual act is consummated. Only a small two per cent or thereabouts have orgasm with the frequency of a man who has it practically every time he enters into sexual union with his wife.

Frigidity and Impotence.   The inability to function normally with the genital organs either for procreative purposes or for pleasure is fairly common. This condition, called *frigidity* in the woman, is much more common than its counterpart, *impotence* in the male. The proportion of adult women who are unable to achieve complete sexual satisfaction is more than 50 per cent. There is a large number of women who never achieve orgasm at any time in their lives. Others have sexual satisfaction for a period of from one to five years after marriage and then the capacity for achieving satisfaction is gradually lost. Others do not begin to have orgasm until six months or a year have elapsed after marriage. Then they enjoy sexual pleasure for a time and once again lose the capacity for satisfactory sexual relations. Some women enjoy love-making before marriage, have an active erotic fantasy life and imagine that they have considerable sexual feeling, but in the marriage relationship are disturbed to find that actual sexual relations mean very little to them. Many women will enjoy sexual relations when on a holiday or vacation away from home but with the responsibilities of everyday life they derive little romance or pleasure from the sexual act.

THWARTED SEXUAL DEVELOPMENT.   It is not surprising that capacity for sexual feeling is poorly developed in the female. Too often in the past, and even quite commonly now, a great deal of pressure has been exerted upon the female which tends to thwart psychosexual development. She is usually kept in ignorance of sexuality as long as possible, and when grudgingly permitted to know anything about sex she is often told that the sexual relation for the woman is "not nice, degrading, wicked, dirty, disgusting, impure, shameful, dangerous." She is told that no "nice" woman has sexual desires, and that such desires lead to impulsive, uncontrollable sexual behavior resulting in disease, pregnancy and social ostracism.

MARRIAGE AND THE SEXUAL FUNCTION.   The reader already knows that when a human being has been taught to hate or fear some idea or act long enough and intensely enough it is with great difficulty that he can change his point of view. When this point of view is acted out by an organ of the body, that organ can be stubbornly obedient to the old prohibition long after a need for change has taken place. Marriage does not change points of view regarding sexual behavior. Marriage gives only legal and religious sanctions. The capacity to make full and wholesome use of these sanctions must be present in the personality through sensible and friendly education. A girl cannot be taught to hate and fear sexual relations for twenty years and then overnight accept them as correct, dignified and pleasurable. Hence it is important for the growing girl to have *enlightenment as she asks for it* concerning the functions of the genital organs and the sensations associated with them. It has long ago been proved that information about sexuality does not lead to vicious and immoral behavior. When children are given credit for common sense and restraint in their sexual lives they will behave better than if it is assumed that they have no intelligence or average consideration or will power. At the same time they will develop the feelings in the sexual organs so necessary to a happy, well-regulated sex life in marriage. As Menninger reminds us, sexual feeling does not arise in the prostate gland or the uterus, even though these organs are often indicted in impotence and frigidity and treated by manipulation and surgery.

The capacity for sexual feeling is present in every healthy man and woman. But whether those feelings are permitted to be felt in the sexual organs depends upon whether acceptable ideas and emotions concerning sexual functioning have been allowed to develop during the growth of the personality, or whether these ideas and feelings have been smothered by fear, guilt, shame, disgust, and hatred for anything and everything sexual.

PSYCHOSOMATIC BACKGROUND OF IMPOTENCE AND FRIGIDITY. We recognize that not all cases of impotence and frigidity are psychological in origin. In rare instances certain organic diseases of the nervous system such as multiple sclerosis, transverse myelitis, tabes dorsalis, anterior poliomyelitis, and others, may cause this condition. We recognize also that acute financial problems, grief, overwork and other circumstances that induce emotional stress may temporarily reduce or abolish sexual desire. But we do wish to emphasize that the physically and emotionally healthy man and woman should have a capacity in the marital relationship for sexual function *with pleasure* if the ideas and emotions in relation to this function are rational and well integrated.

Even though many husbands pay too little attention to achievement of orgasm in the female (often referred to as "having a climax") the common saying, "There is no such thing as a frigid woman—it is only the man who is clumsy" is not true. Women too must share the responsibility for inadequate sexual expression. The man or even the woman herself often concludes that she is "probably cold by nature" or that "women weren't meant to feel the same way in sexual relations as men." On the contrary it is quite important that the woman share equally in the pleasure of intercourse. Just as the husband wants his wife to share his vacation pleasures or sit at the same table and enjoy his food with him, or share the beauty and sensual pleasure of a painting or sunset, so he should want her even more to share this most meaningful experience of all. There is no human relationship in which so much can be shared, so much of emotional and spiritual value given as in the sexual relationship, if the attitude toward each other as man and wife is normal.

ORGASTIC PLEASURE. There is considerable variation in the time taken in coitus for both parties to achieve orgasm. It is a well-accepted fact that the female, because of her nature and training in these matters, is slower to come to the point of sexual excitement and orgasm than the man. It is important that before coitus is undertaken the man should attempt to bring the woman to a state of sexual excitement by kisses, caresses and fondling of the breasts and genitals. Preliminary sex play of this kind should last for a number of minutes in order that the woman become interested for actual coitus to begin. The period of time during which the genitals are united may vary from two or three to fifteen or twenty minutes. It is not easy for many women to achieve orgasm in less than two minutes of genital union and coital movements. Ejaculation in the male occurring before this time is likely to result in disappointment in the female and chagrin in the male, particularly if the latter has any feeling whatever for his partner's pleasure.

Relative Degrees of Severity of Impotence and Frigidity

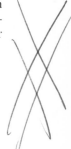

Male	Female	
1. Potent but coitus lacks pleasure	1. Occasional failure to obtain orgasm	
2. Potent but has coitus under protest	2. Only occasional orgasm	
3. Interested in coitus but cannot always have erection when desired	3. Mild pleasure in coitus but without orgasm	Usually accompanied by some lack of vaginal secretion
4. Inadequate or partial erection	4. Vaginal anesthesia with no special aversion to coitus	
5. Premature ejaculation	5. Vaginal anesthesia with aversion to coitus	
6. Impotence complete but interest retained in coitus	6. Dyspareunia and vaginismus	
7. Impotence complete with no interest in coitus		

VAGINAL ANESTHESIA WITH AVERSION TO COITUS. Women in this group derive no pleasure from sexual intercourse and in addition resent it. They feel that they are being exploited, imposed upon, degraded, and made to suffer unnecessarily. They often utilize the fear of pregnancy in order to avoid intercourse. Sometimes they pretend to be menstruating in order to escape participation in the sexual act and they may either distrust contraceptives or deliberately say they do in order to avoid intercourse. In discussing contraception (p. 367) we shall have something to say regarding women who learn the method but fail to continue to use it. Many such women belong to this group.

DYSPAREUNIA AND VAGINISMUS. In some women intercourse is always painful. The pain may be so pronounced as to prevent the insertion of the penis. If the penis can be inserted, pain may be felt only at the beginning or sometimes during the entire act. As one might suppose, abundant and pronounced early life fantasies of the sex act as a horrible, painful and harmful experience are to be found in the psychological study of these women.

Any interference with a free flow of psychic energy into the sexual act may cut down the secretion of the mucous glands of the vagina which is intended to facilitate the act of coitus. In other words, the woman may consciously permit intercourse but unconsciously try to deny entrance to the penis by failing to provide secretion.

Causes of Frigidity and Impotence

1. *Fear of disapproval or punishment*
    (*a*) Fear of criticism or ridicule.
    (*b*) Fear of bodily injury from some disapproving person other than the partner.
    (*c*) Fear of pregnancy.
2. *Hostility toward the partner*
    (*a*) A general resentment toward the opposite sex with desire to do them harm.
    (*b*) The woman resents what she considers domination by the man.
    (*c*) The man is envious of the woman and her role in life and refuses to give her pleasure because of this envy.
    (*d*) A fear of one of the partners of injuring the genital organs of the other.
3. *Conflicting loves* (usually unconscious)
    (*a*) Man loves some other woman and is unconscious of it (mother, sister); or woman loves some other man (father, brother) and cannot accept husband sexually.
    (*b*) Latent homosexuality; *i. e.,* persons of the same sex are loved rather than persons of the opposite sex.
    (*c*) *Too much self-love.* Love of another person is an overflow from self-love. In these cases there is no love left for the sexual partner.

Fear of Disapproval or Punishment.   It has already been pointed out that criticism and ridicule regarding matters pertaining to sex are too often exerted upon the child and adolescent. Masturbation is the first genital sexual act which is indulged in, and this is often severely criticized or ridiculed. Later the same child may be criticized or ridiculed for his attempts to come in contact with the opposite sex in normally acceptable social relations. Through such unfortunate attitudes he comes to associate so much that is shameful or harmful with sexual behavior or with advances toward the opposite sex that it is very difficult to overcome these attitudes after marriage has taken place. The married person still feels that disapproval, criticism or ridicule is bound to come from some source because of a normal interest in sexual pleasure, and this may prove to be an important factor in determining the onset of impotence or frigidity. Some people never get over a longstanding threat that they will be punished for sexual activities.

Young married couples who have to live in the same home with the parents of one partner may be greatly inhibited in sexual relations, fearing they will be overheard, or fearing that the act of intercourse will be assumed and they will meet with disapproval the following day. In more than one instance we have seen the inability to achieve orgasm cured merely by the young people moving out of the parents' home and taking an apartment of their own. The sense of freedom obtained in this manner was sufficient to remove an inhibiting fear of censure. Sometimes the fantasies in the minds of these young married couples are poorly understood by persons uninstructed in the evils attached to such unfortunate early attitudes as we have just discussed. We have known many a newly married man living in the home of the father or father-in-law who has had the feeling that each morning when he came downstairs he would be soundly thrashed for having had intercourse with his own wife. In the same way the newly married woman meets her parents the next day with the fear that she will be scolded and put out of the house for having had intercourse with her husband.

Fear of Pregnancy. This is one of the most common inhibitors of free sexual expression. It is for this reason that contraceptive advice is so helpful in removing some of the anxiety and hence some of the in-hibiting influences connected with sexual intercourse. It goes without saying that this is only one of the more superficial rationalizations of inability to perform normal intercourse and therefore contraceptive ad-vice cannot cure deep-seated inhibitions. On the other hand, there is still a belief common among many women that if they do not become sexually excited and do not have orgasm they will not become pregnant. While there may be a very remote relationship between the orgasm of a woman and the possibility of becoming pregnant it is an everyday occur-rence for completely frigid women to become pregnant. In other words, for practical clinical purposes there is no relationship between frigidity and the ability to conceive.

Hostility Toward the Partner. Unconscious hostility is one of the common causes of frigidity and impotence. Many men have suffered so much at the hands of their mothers that they never overcome an intense hostility toward women in general. A man so affected may see many de-sirable qualities in his wife and wish to treat her kindly, but the accumu-lated unconscious hatred does not permit him to do so. He may have a strong unconscious desire to hurt, punish or soil her with his penis—a desire so strong that the result is a reaction in quite the opposite direc-tion and he becomes completely impotent. In the same way there is the woman whose relations with her father and brothers have been of such an unfriendly nature that she finds it very difficult to love another man or make him happy with her body. She will not give him the gift of an orgasm nor allow him to make *her* happy. In some cases the woman will actually taunt the man for being unable to arouse her and condemn him for a weakness which is really her own. Some women have grown up so deprived in their own lives and yet seen the advantages accorded to their brothers, that they learn to hate the male genital organ, which seemed to them to be the one reason why brothers had been granted so many privileges which had been denied them. As a result they have no pride in their own sexual organs, feel inferior, and in their envy of the male role are unable to have sexual pleasure.

Just as some women are envious of the prerogatives of men there are men who have the same feeling about women. Some men envy women the opportunity to stay at home, to wear pretty clothes, to bear children, and their role of passivity in the sexual act. They resent the attention which women receive. These men are reluctant to give the women sexual pleasure or to give them a child. They resent having to take care of the woman and child, and unconsciously wish to be taken care of as children themselves. When these passive trends are strong impotence may be the result.

Sadistic Concepts.   Some individuals have been brought up with a sadistic concept of sexual relations, fearing that sexual intercourse will result in some harm to themselves or to their partner. Many women have the idea that to participate in sexual relations means to be hurt by the man's sexual organ. Some carry into adulthood a childish fear that the penis is so much larger than the vagina that they will be torn and injured. One patient said, "I know it's foolish but each time I am faced with sex relations I feel I am going to be pierced with a sword." Even if the woman does not have definite fantasies of injury it is likely she may feel that the sexual act is humiliating and degrading and is an act which no man with any kindness and consideration would perpetrate upon a woman. In the same way that women fear injury by the male organ, men fear injury at the hands of the woman. Many stories are told among boys and young men of how the vagina may contract and constrict the penis so that in some cases an operation on the penis has been necessary in order to bring about separation of the couple. While many boys and young men hear these stories and pay little attention to them others take them quite seriously and *never* lose the fear that such an occurrence *could* take place. Of course no such possibility has any basis in fact, but the idea that the vagina is a mysterious organ with possibilities of harm latent within it may have sufficient force to inhibit erection. Further, the fear that the woman may have a venereal disease which will cause the man much pain and incapacity is quite common, and it is well known that this belief is often based on warnings uttered by the parents, intended to keep young people continent, in place of giving a well-rounded, wholesome sexual education.

Just as the partners may fear harm coming from each other, so may they also fear *doing* harm. The fear of injuring the partner in the sexual act may be just as strong and just as inhibiting to satisfactory relations as the fear of being harmed one's self. Of course, just as with many irrational fears, underlying the fear of doing harm to the partner, there is implied some degree of a wish to do this very thing.

Conflicting Loves (Usually Unconscious).   Anyone who has been at all observant knows of cases in which a man has such a strong attachment to his mother that he has very little interest in any other women. Of course, such an attachment with a sister could also take place, or even with some more remote relative who had played an important role in the man's life. Should he become interested in marrying, his early emotional attachment may be so strong as to prevent him from functioning sexually with his wife. Such men will often say, "My wife is a wonderful woman, very capable and very important to me, but I just can't seem to love her in an intimate sexual way." The same conflict in sexual love can take place in the woman who has an overstrong attachment to some man with whom she has been closely related during her developing years. This is most often the father but may be a brother or an uncle. She has never realized the sexual component of this emotional bond and feels that she is in love with her husband until the sex relationship demonstrates the emotional barrier between them. Such women will say, "My marriage seems like that of all my women friends until my husband wants to make love with me physically—then I feel he is an alien, an outsider, as if he were someone I never could know well enough for that."

LATENT HOMOSEXUALITY.   There are some individuals who have never developed enough emotionally to be able to love intimately a person of the opposite sex. Their interests and emotional satisfactions lie with those of the same sex, and sexual relationships with those of the opposite sex seem meaningless. The latently homosexual woman remains frigid and the latently homosexual man is likely to be completely or partially impotent.

Bearing on this question are the important studies by Kinsey, who finds "that something between a quarter and a half of all males have demonstrated their capacity to respond to homosexual stimuli; that the picture is one of endless intergradation between every combination of homosexuality and heterosexuality; that it is impossible to distinguish so-called acquired, latent, and congenital types; and that there is every gradation between so-called 'actives' and 'passives' in a homosexual relation."

Taking issue with theories of homosexuality based on urinary hormone findings Kinsey asserts "any hormonal or other explanation of the homosexual must allow for the fact that both homosexual and heterosexual activities may occur coincidentally in a single period in the life of an individual; and that exclusive activities of any one type may be exchanged, in the brief span of a few days or a few weeks, for an exclusive pattern of the other type, or into a combination pattern which embraces the two types.

"Any explanation of the homosexual must recognize that a large portion of the younger adolescents demonstrate the capacity to react to both homosexual and heterosexual stimuli; that there is a fair number of adults who show this same capacity; and that there is only a gradual development of the exclusively homosexual or exclusively heterosexual patterns which predominate among older adults."

SELF-LOVE.   Again there are some individuals with such great self-love that they have little emotion free with which to love other people. They have difficulty in sharing even time and effort with anyone else, let alone having that amount of energy directed toward others which is necessary for sexual relationship. Such a state of affairs is frequently seen in the severely neurotic and the latently psychotic. They are entirely absorbed in concern with their aches and pains or their bizarre ideas about themselves or the outside world, and they have no thought or interest in sexual functioning. However, as we leave this extremely pathological group we come to some people in the ordinary walks of life who may be doing a fairly good piece of work, all of whose available energy is channeled into this activity. For instance, a man may have a work project which means a great deal to him. He works and dreams of the success and acclaim which will be his, and is so preoccupied with his work and his dreams that he has no interest or energy for sexual functioning with a woman. Certain artistic temperaments fall into this group.

There are women who may be doing good work but the interest they center upon themselves in relation to their work and the prestige obtained through it, or their interest in clothes, jewelry and the appearance they make or the social success they can achieve, occupy them to such an extent that they have no emotion left over for loving a man in a sexual way and giving him anything so personal and intimate of themselves as sexual feelings. Some women can extend their feelings of self-love to cover their children and take great pride in the children and their appearance and the children's success as though the children were part of themselves. To these women a sex relationship with a man is only a means to an end, and it does not enter their thinking to share with him a feeling of pleasure during the sexual act.

Effect on Spouse. These people who try to be so complete within themselves and will not permit themselves to be dependent upon their marital partners for the emotional satisfaction which the sexual relation affords are often very baffling to their spouses, who feel left out, and eventually inferior. Such self-absorption on the part of a woman often drives the man to a house of prostitution or to a mistress who gives him something which the wife never does, namely something of herself emotionally. When the husband is of this self-loving and self-contained type the wife is usually in a somewhat more difficult position. It is not so easy for women to seek extramarital relationships, and they often suffer in silence, become hostile and develop neurotic symptoms.

Psychosomatic Problems of Frigidity. It is easily understandable that the effect of frigidity on the woman is different from that of impotence on the man. Whereas an impotent man is incapacitated in regard to the act of intercourse, a frigid woman submits to the wishes of her husband and the lack of enjoyment leads to indifference, resentment, or even disgust. Growing out of these reactions are various physical problems. Ruesch and his associates, in a monograph devoted to a study of chronic disease and psychological invalidism, discussed some of these problems. The life histories of the frigid women in their series resembled each other closely. They were characterized by a high rate of marriages, marriages at an early age, greater than average divorce rate, and a large number of medical experiences and operations. There was a great lack of love and security in their childhood. Marriage often served the purpose of breaking away from home at an early age, looking for security and love, and to prove that they were grown-up people.

SEXUAL ADJUSTMENT

Premarital Examination. Many women seek a premarital examination wanting a variety of information. They wonder if they are generally healthy, of course, and then want to know if there is any impediment to a satisfactory sex life with their future husbands. If an impediment such as an unyielding hymen exists, the woman would, with the concurrence of her fiancé, prefer to have this condition corrected before marriage. She would want to make sure that her husband-to-be was sufficiently well informed to appreciate the importance of this and not think that an intact hymen and bleeding on the first night were important evidences of virginity. The woman would want to know that her pelvic measurements were satisfactory for normal delivery of a child. If a non-Catholic she might well want to discuss contraception and if the diaphragm and jelly were the method agreed upon be given some instruction as to its use.

A woman having a premarital examination may have questions she would like to ask and the physician should provide time and create the proper, unhurried rapport for asking them. For instance, she may want to know how frequently one should have intercourse. Here she can be told a wide variation exists and that since sex relations are beneficial and not harmful she and her husband must be guided by what is mutually most satisfactory to them. She may want to discuss some old fear she has had that masturbation earlier in her life will interfere with her sexual life in marriage. She can be reassured that it will not. She may want to know whether the use of contraceptives can be harmful. Certainly, the commonly used ones such as the condom or diaphragm and jelly are not harmful. She may want to know if first intercourse will be painful. In short, the physician who begins to appreciate the sexual ignorance yet the curiosity to know, the accumulation of fears and old wives' tales in the mind of the average woman will, in a friendly, understanding way, make the premarital examination a helpful visit and one that can be the cornerstone of a constructive doctor-patient relationship in the years to come.

Contraception. One of the common problems which soon presents itself in discussing any difficulty in sexual adjustment is the matter of contraception. As physicians, we want to know whether contraception is being used and if the method is satisfactory. Is it comfortable, is it reliable, and is there any conflict over its use? It must be admitted that no absolutely reliable contraceptive exists today, short of the removal of the uterus or both ovaries. The contraceptive techniques commonly used are withdrawal, vaginal douches, observance of the so-called safe periods, or the use of some mechanical device. Neither withdrawal nor vaginal douches are very reliable, nor is the safe period at all reliable for women with irregularity in the menstrual cycle. The mechanical devices most commonly used are rubber or fishskin protective sheaths, vaginal rubber diaphragms, cervical caps of metal or hard rubber, jellies, foam tablets, suppositories, sponges, or combinations of these devices. All of these methods are safe as far as the patient's health is concerned when used according to proper instructions by the physician, but they vary as to reliability. While most vaginal devices are harmless when properly used, intracervical or intrauterine appliances, on the other hand, may be harmful. Foreign bodies placed in the cervix or within the uterine cavity may cause an infection, or may set up an irritation which might be a factor in starting neoplastic growths. Consequently, if the responsibility of contraception is assumed by the woman it should be by means of some intravaginal procedure.

THE RUBBER DIAPHRAGM AS A CONTRACEPTIVE DEVICE.   The contraceptive technique which utilizes a flexible rubber diaphragm plus a spermicidal jelly which can be inserted by the woman herself before each coitus, has now been quite generally accepted as the most satisfactory means of contraception. The rubber diaphragm covers the cervix of the uterus, and combined with spermicidal jelly the safety factor is nearly 100 per cent. When we say this we mean that studies of many women over a period of many years have demonstrated its great value when used intelligently. The cases which appear to be failures have been traced to faulty insertion of the diaphragm, or failure to use the contraceptive jelly, or to some carelessness on the part of the couple themselves. The woman must be given a diaphragm of the proper size and be taught how to insert it correctly. Usually she is made to practice the procedure a few days and then return and demonstrate to the physician that she can perform the manipulation correctly. The diaphragm is left in place for eight hours after coitus, at which time a douche of plain water is used and the diaphragm removed, dried and kept in a clean place until used again.

CONTRACEPTION AND ANXIETY.   There can no longer be any question regarding the necessity for planned parenthood. This makes it important that a satisfactory contraceptive method be made available and this in turn will give married people freedom from what may be termed normal anxiety in their sexual relations. It is true that some people have scruples against the use of contraception, but these scruples seem to be diminishing each year as the importance of human health and happiness are given a more prominent place in our thinking.

There are some women who do not want to use a diaphragm and jelly for contraception because they regard the procedure as too messy, or because they claim that they feel uncomfortable when retaining the diaphragm after coitus. Some women feel that the responsibility for contraception should be assumed by the man through the use of condoms or by withdrawal. They feel that to assume the responsibility of contraception lowers their dignity and makes them appear too interested in the sexual act. Some women claim that they just cannot trust such a contraceptive device. Naturally we have to suspect the motives of these women; they usually have long-standing prejudices against the sexual act itself, and their expressed reasons against contraception are excuses or rationalizations because they wish to do nothing to facilitate intercourse.

These attitudes are only present in women with some frigidity, and rather than try to convince them about the faulty attitude toward contraception one must take up the more fundamental question of the frigidity itself. Many subtle problems arise. A woman may have strong religious scruples against the use of contraception but overcome them sufficiently to try to use the method. Failure may result from a "deliberate accident." She is either deliberately or unconsciously careless in the use of the method because she cannot circumvent the anxiety resulting from a conflict over a deviation from her life-long beliefs.

The diaphragm and jelly is usually a much more satisfactory contraceptive device for both the man and the woman than the use of a condom. A much smaller surface of foreign material is introduced between the sexual organs, thereby giving both parties more capacity for pleasure.

THE PRACTICE OF WITHDRAWAL.   Withdrawal is an unsatisfactory method of contraception from the standpoint of sexual pleasure and because it is not easy to control, pregnancy may occur. Withdrawal causes a separation of the genital organs at a time when the greatest emotional exchange between the partners should be taking place and therefore often does not permit sufficient sexual excitement in the woman to bring about orgasm. It may produce a feeling of unrest and anxiety in either or both parties, and lead to a state of general dissatisfaction. It is widely practiced but must be condemned.

Some cases of frigidity due to a fear of pregnancy, and without deeper and more complicated psychological background, can be cured by the use of a contraceptive method which the patient can trust. We believe the number of cases in which this can take place is relatively small, but forms, nevertheless, a definite group.

Contraceptive instruction should be a part of every medical school curriculum and a birth control clinic a part of its associated hospital work.

While physicians as individuals have become more liberal in regard to imparting contraceptive advice the medical profession as a whole remains conservative to the point of refusing to recommend contraception except in cases of serious organic disease.

DISTURBANCES OF MENSTRUATION

Amenorrhea.   Few studies have been done on this subject by those working in psychosomatic medicine. One reason has been that amenorrhea, to a great extent, has been assumed to be caused by a defect in the endocrine system and endocrine threapy has been prescribed. The second reason is that amenorrhea is not a particularly distressing or incapacitating symptom, and hence study has not been so urgently demanded. Nevertheless, Dunbar gives a number of references to observations which European observers have made on this subject. They felt that a large number of cases of amenorrhea seen during the war were due more to the lack of men than lack of nourishment. The condition was found in well-nourished women as well as in the undernourished, and often disappeared as soon as opportunities for sexual relations with men were restored, even though coitus did not actually take place.

Some very interesting observations on the subject of amenorrhea were made in an internment camp in the Philippines during World War II. Among 1042 women of menstrual age (American or British) Whitacre and Barrera found 125 patients with amenorrhea which had developed since the outbreak of the war. Of 60 nurses who had been through the campaigns of Bataan or Corregidor, 50 per cent exhibited menstrual disturbances; amenorrhea was present in 23 per cent. In many of these patients the menses stopped abruptly after the first bombing of Manila, or soon after internment and before a food deficiency could have had any affect. The physiologic amenorrhea of pregnancy, or the fear of it, was ruled out as a cause, and patients with chronic diseases were omitted. It seemed clear that emotional shock was responsible. In spite of the difficulties under which they worked an effort was made to study ovarian and anterior-pituitary-like gonadotropic excretion. In two selected patients estrogen was absent from the urine while gonadotropin was present, probably in increased amount. The investigators felt that worry and fear, acting through the autonomic nervous system, had caused a complete suppression of ovarian function. Most of the women overcame the difficulty within a few months and the good results were probably due to psychological influences.

In a study of amenorrhea to which further reference will be made, Paschkis, Rakoff and Cantarow reported one patient in whom it was possible to follow the progressive improvement in the endocrine mechanism in the course of psychotherapy. In this young woman failure to menstruate developed promptly after a quarrel between the patient and her mother when the latter learned the girl has been dating surreptitiously. During the argument the mother fainted. The girl thought she had died and became hysterical. Thereafter she did not menstruate for a year at which time she was studied in the endocrine clinic. No other cause for the failure to menstruate could be found. Psychotherapy was begun, including several interviews with the mother, which helped to develop considerable understanding and cooperation. During the course of the psychotherapy there was a sudden change in the excretion of hormone followed shortly thereafter by menstruation which then continued in a normal fashion.

Kelley, Daniels and associates investigated 26 women between the ages of 18 and 35 referred from the Sloane Endocrine Clinic, New York, who had complained of secondary amenorrhea of at least six months' duration and of "unknown origin." The term "unknown origin" referred to the fact that organic disease had been excluded. As controls, women who had never experienced secondary amenorrhea were also studied. The most striking facts elicited by the investigation were the high degree of psychosexual immaturity, the presence of psychological conflicts arising in the earliest period of infantile development, and attitudes and thinking often more closely related to psychosis than to neurosis. These women functioned both physiologically and psychologically as if they had never reached puberty. The authors felt that psychiatric help was often imperative in these cases but also cautioned that a psychotic breakdown during treatment was a real hazard, the possibility of which had to be taken into account.

UNCONSCIOUS INFLUENCES.   It is well known that the wish to be pregnant may result in amenorrhea and distention of the abdomen. On the other hand, fear of an unwanted pregnancy may cause cessation of the mentrual flow for a month or longer. That is to say, the menstrual flow, while linked up with ovarian function and tending to follow a definite cycle, nevertheless seems to be under the control of the emotions in the same way, if not to the same extent, as the secretion of tears, saliva and perspiration. Emotions quite profoundly regulate the discharge or retention of secretions, and in the case of the menstrual flow may have as powerful an effect as the endocrine regulatory mechanism itself.

Dysmenorrhea. Dysmenorrhea is a symptom rather than a disease. It occurs with great frequency. In a study of a large group of student nurses dysmenorrhea occurred in 52 per cent. It may be due to pelvic disease but usually occurs in the absence of any recognizable cause and is then spoken of as functional dysmenorrhea. Even when pelvic lesions exist caution must be exercised in attributing menstrual pain to the disease process, for example a displacement of the uterus or a simple cyst of the ovary, which may have little effect in the production of dysmenorrhea. The mere existence of some abnormality in the pelvis is not positive proof that it is the cause of menstrual pain. That is the reason why careful study, prolonged observation, and the psychosomatic approach are important before surgical measures are tried.

CLINICAL ASPECTS. In addition to pain various other symptoms are frequently encountered such as general lassitude, headache, gastrointestinal disturbances, mental depression and emotional instability. The explanations that are usually advanced for menstrual pain are mechanical obstruction of the cervical canal, hypoplasia of the pelvic organs, congestion, and other vascular disturbances, constitutional defects such as structural or physiological inadequacies, endocrine disturbances, allergy and psychogenic factors. It is usually stated that no one theory adequately explains all cases and, like many other psychosomatic problems that we have discussed, in the majority of instances there is probably more than one cause. It is probable that a structural or physiological problem plus a psychological factor may be in the background of a large number of cases.

A GENERAL PROBLEM. Therefore, so-called *functional dysmenorrhea* presents a general rather than simply a pelvic problem, and a general survey rather than just a pelvic examination is essential before treatment can be instituted. A general physical examination not only may reveal organic disease but gives information concerning general nutrition, constitutional defects, endocrine abnormalities and neurological disturbances. Examination of the pelvis may reveal evidence of genital hypoplasia, such as poorly developed external genitalia, short interior vaginal wall, shallow posterior fornix, infantile-like cervix and acute pathologic anteflexion of the uterus. Psychological study often reveals emotional instability and a background of psychoneurotic tendencies such as we shall discuss shortly. In the majority of instances of functional dysmenorrhea we deal with young unmarried women, and emphasis upon mild anatomic or developmental anomalies of pelvic organs, persistent and ill-advised local or surgical treatment, or a long series of injections of questionable value may give temporary benefit but in the long run are distinctly harmful. In this connection let us refer once more to the statement made by Clifford Allbutt in 1884 regarding a neuralgic woman (p. 8). Dysmenorrhea may occur, like many other neurotic symptoms, in women who do not "appear" nervous. The fact that a patient appears calm and poised does not exclude a psychogenic cause for this symptom.

PSYCHOLOGICAL STUDY.   In personality studies on patients with dysmenorrhea Wittkower and Wilson found that many patients suffering from dysmenorrhea had been either unusually aggressive and boisterous tomboys resenting their feminine role or ailing, complaining children unwilling or unable to give up their childish dependence on their parents and possessing strong needs or cravings for sympathy and protection. As adults the dysmenorrhea patients were deeply resentful of their feminine role or obviously immature physically and either shy and shut-in or chronically anxious and complaining.

Others have noted the physical masculine attributes—voice, hair, bones —that coexist with distinct masculine attitudes and aversions against the female role. This is by no means the rule, however, and often an absolutely female habitus exists along with the same emotional conflicts.

Karen Horney noted that dysmenorrhea usually starts, if not at puberty, at the time when the patient comes in contact with adult sex problems. In patients suffering from this condition there are unconscious fantasies of the sex act as something cruel, bloody and painful. One of her patients felt sexually aroused whenever she heard or read of cruelty. She described the pain which she had at the time of menstruation "as if her insides were being torn out." As a child she had the idea that in intercourse the man tore something out from the body of the woman. In her dysmenorrhea she emotionally acted out these fantasies.

While the subject is far from solved there is enough evidence to suggest that the psychosomatic approach is essential in the study of functional dysmenorrhea and certainly should precede any attempts to cure the condition by surgical means.

Leukorrhea.   Here again, as in the subject of amenorrhea, the majority of studies along psychological lines have been made by Europeans. Dunbar has collected the observations of the outstanding authorities. E. Graefenberg stated that the psychogenic component of leukorrhea is little disputed. Psychogenic leukorrhea is particularly resistant to the customary gynecological treatment, and for this reason patients often go from physician to physician until the psychological background of the condition has been recognized. One case was reported by Bunneman in which the patient's leukorrhea had stubbornly persisted for twelve years in spite of all gynecological procedures. It was cured by hypnosis. After a year's time the leukorrhea began again following sexual excitement. It again disappeared in response to hypnotic suggestion and remained absent for six months. In order to convince himself that the cessation of the symptom could not possibly have been an accidental coincidence Bunneman brought it back again by suggestion.

Naussauer termed leukorrhea the "headache" of the lower abdomen, thus indicating that it develops without disease of the genital organs. Mayer felt that unconscious sexual ideas led to hyperemia and hypersecretion in the genital region with a decrease in tonus of the smooth musculature.

PSYCHOLOGICAL FACTORS.   Two cases of leukorrhea in which psychological factors seemed important have been observed by one of us. In the first the symptom was precipitated by constant sexual excitement from much erotic fantasy occuring each day. Treatment was not sought for this symptom alone, even though it was rather annoying at times. Inquiry revealed that following marriage and satisfactory sexual adjustment and the living out of the sexual fantasies and erotic desires, the leukorrhea disappeared.

Another case was observed in a quite different type of personality. This patient was single, 21 years of age, and came from a very happy home. As a result of large quantities of repressed hostility she had frequent cramps and diarrhea which would last for days at a time. She had been treated as a case of colitis. After months of intensive psychiatric treatment and readjustment of the personality the colitis was cured. In the course of treatment, however, it was observed that when diarrhea was controlled there was a leukorrheal discharge. Both of these symptoms cleared up simultaneously and it seemed that the leukorrhea, like the diarrhea, was a production from the body of something unpleasant, one purpose of which was to vent repressed ill-feelings upon the environment.

From the accumulating evidence it surely is a physician's duty in a case of leukorrhea in which disease or infection does not seem responsible, to inquire of the patient what ideas are associated with the discharge, and to acquaint the patient with the existing knowledge of what such a discharge may mean from the standpoint of behavior.

Functional Bleeding.   There are some women in whom the rhythm of uterine bleeding does not conform to the average pattern. They bleed overlong when the period should have ended. They begin bleeding again at times after two or three weeks when their usual rhythm is 28 days. In short, they bleed irregularly when no ascertainable cause is to be found. It is, of course, easy to assume that there must be some endocrine imbalance but endocrine therapy does not always cure the condition. It is thought that a personality factor is involved. Women have been observed frequently to bleed when they are being faced with an unwanted sexual experience with a male—or at least when faced with a sexual experience they have considerable conflict about, for example, on the wedding night—even though menstruation is not expected.

Moreover, in some women such unpredictability and irregularity and lack of rhythmic control physiologically seems to correspond to some weakness in coping with problems, and the bleeding is an attempted solution. Just as it solves a sexual conflict it may also say, "You see, I am not well. You must excuse me from the duties of a robust existence." It seems to represent a personality defect not unlike that of enuresis—an incontinence of the uterus.

Premenstrual Tension.   It is well known to every physician that women are prone to undergo certain emotional changes for a varying period preceding menstruation, sometimes terminating when the menstrual flow begins, and sometimes continuing until the menstrual flow has ceased. The term *premenstrual tension* has been applied to this syndrome. Important symptoms are a varying degree of depression of spirits and irritability, headache, insomnia, outbursts of crying, physical unrest, a sensation of the entire body described as "being jittery" or a feeling that "they would like to jump out of their skin." This syndrome is usually attributed to menstruation by the patient and is often explained by the physician on the basis of dysfunction of the endocrine glands. Many glandular preparations have been used in its treatment. Medical writers, in discussing this syndrome, often refer to the 40 or more per cent of *normal women* who suffer from this condition. There are others, however, who disagree with the point of view that these are normal women. They regard these symptoms as being evidences of an underlying neurosis and hence due to the expression of unconscious fantasies. They believe that if endocrine imbalances or deficiencies exist, they are either secondary to the underlying psychological disturbance, or just another phase of the disturbed psychosomatic make-up. Hence, it would be understandable that endocrine therapy might produce temporary alleviation of symptoms, either by substitution or through the effect of suggestion, but in neither case would the deeper cause of the condition be eradicated.

Symptoms of premenstrual tension cannot be accounted for on the basis of generalized water retention alone. Lamb and associates felt that some correlations might be established by simultaneous physiological and psychiatric observations on a group of persons with premenstrual tension and on a group of controls. A questionnaire study was made of 127 student nurses, ranging in age from 18 to 35. From this group 10 subjects were selected for careful study. Five were controls and the other five had symptoms of premenstrual tension. The study covered at least two menstrual cycles. There was no indication that the behavioral manifestations of premenstrual tension reflect alterations in the cerebral neurophysiology. Endocrine activity was within normal limits in all subjects, with no demonstrable distinction between subjects with premenstrual tension and controls. Although they found no evidence to substantiate the theory of psychogenic etiology for premenstrual tension, there were some differences in the behavior, other than the premenstrual manifestations, differentiating the two groups. The subjects with premenstrual tension showed greater emotional instability throughout their cycles, and in general they were less assertive.

PSYCHOPATHOLOGY. Premenstrual tension is a common condition known to many women but perhaps even better known to their husbands and children because they are the victims of the personality change. Some of these women cannot fully accept their feminine role. They protest consciously or unconsciously about being women and they hate menstruation as a symbol of femininity. They often say, "I did not realize my period was due until I began to be tense and irritable." But the mind knows and the mind has a time consciousness and it feels threatened by the hormonal changes that are about to bring on another bleeding period—a vivid reminder of the castrated state. Psychotherapy that deals successfully with these deeper conflicts may result in relieving premenstrual tension.

The Menopausal Syndrome.   One of the most important disorders met with in relation to the endocrine glands is the menopausal syndrome. It is estimated that at or about the time of the cessation of menstruation, 80 per cent of women experience a variety of unpleasant symptoms, but only 10 to 15 per cent require treatment. The *vasomotor disturbances* manifested by "hot flushes" and "cold shivers" are accompanied by emotional instability, insomnia, depression of spirits, irritability, anxiety attacks, palpitation, headaches, giddiness, nausea, fatigue, dyspnea, sweating, "tingling" in the skin and extremities, and sometimes obesity. The anxiety and depression of spirits may be of such severity that the patient can no longer carry on her daily tasks, rest comfortably, eat, or control her thoughts and actions. In some instances removal to a mental hospital may be necessary. However, a relatively small percentage of women who have been reported as suffering from menopausal symptoms develop frank psychoses.

THE MENOPAUSE AND THE CLIMACTERIC.   If a woman is "nervous" or presents symptoms of obscure origin she is almost certain to be told that it is the menopause or the "beginning of the menopause." Hardly is she through her twenties before she begins to think in such terms, often, we regret to say, with the assistance of her physician. From then on until ten years after the menses cease, this shortcut to an involved psychosomatic problem is called upon for an easy explanation, and the injudicious resort to estrogen therapy. It is well to remember that the vasomotor phenomena which are alone characteristic of the climacterium are rarely pronounced in the woman who is still menstruating regularly.

Some observers make a distinction between "menopause" and the "climacteric." They believe that menopause should be used to mean simply cessation of the menses, whereas the term climacteric, which is derived from the Greek and means "rung of the ladder," should be used according to its original meaning to signify a critical epoch of life. These epochs were supposed to occur every nine years, the important ones occurring at eighteen and sixty-three, the latter being called the "grand climacteric."

From a psychosomatic standpoint the epochs of "changes of life" are indeed important. Life is constantly changing and many periods necessitate emotional and ideational adjustment. The menopause is only one such period. Puberty, adolescence, leaving the parental roof, engagements, marriage, parenthood, are all changes which require readjustment. This adjustment process often fails and neuroses and psychoses appear as a result. Hence, we should be careful not to attribute much more importance to either the cessation of the menses or to this particular epoch than to these other epochs. "Nervous symptoms," so-called, occurring at the time of the menopause are frequently treated quite casually by the physician. He says, "Oh, of course. The change of life," or "This was to be expected," and prescribes some glandular preparation. The majority of physicians believe that most of the menopausal symptoms can be controlled by the administration of estrogenic products. The element of suggestion in such treatment is rarely considered.

It is also important to point out that in attributing all symptoms to the menopause equally tragic mistakes are made in overlooking physical diseases. We must emphasize once more that the psychosomatic concept means no less study of the soma than of the psyche. Just as too great an absorption in endocrine matters leads to serious errors in regard to emotional matters so, as shown by Stoddard, many serious physical diseases are overlooked because all symptoms are attributed to endocrine dysfunction.

PSYCHOLOGICAL IMPLICATIONS OF THE MENOPAUSE.   Nature has undoubtedly been wise in bringing about a cessation of menstruation at the age of 45, or thereabouts. For after 45, woman's strength usually begins to wane, health and security become more precarious and it is better that her capacity for childbearing ceases. Most women have as many children as they want by this time and are glad to have nature bring an end to this particular responsibility.

However, women are not prone, by any means, to regard the cessation of menstruation as an unmixed blessing. It has many psychological implications and most of them are tinged with morbid rather than wholesome attitudes.

While women may have mixed feelings about the value of menstruation, they nevertheless regard it as a sign of vitality and when menstruation ceases, they feel a certain vitality has gone. They feel they are advancing from middle age to old age. They feel they have joined the ranks of "older women." Further, they are prone at this time to become more conscious of certain periods in their lives which have not measured up to their earlier hopes, dreams and aspirations. For instance, they feel they are getting older and have not achieved the social status they wished, or have not had as many children or as much romance and, possibly, erotic adventure as they would have liked. They feel that now life is moving on and they must relinquish some of these desires.

We live in a society where a great premium is placed on youth, beauty, vitality and sexuality. With the climacteric and the cessation of menstruation, women are prone to feel less valuable in these competitive areas. Some women become unduly afraid that their husbands will turn their attention to younger and more physically attractive women. Others are under the mistaken conception that sexual desire and sexual interest will disappear with the cessation of the activity of the sexual glands. This, of course, is not true. The capacity for sexual enjoyment is determined in very small measure by glandular activity.

All of these problems cause a loss of self-esteem and depression of spirits. Anxiety is aroused and the future seems more insecure and unfriendly. Often enough, tension arises to produce insomnia. Irritability, which is a common symptom, may be due to a great lack of satisfaction with the self. It is as if the woman is attempting, by her irritability and anger, to make things right again and thus reestablish the old order. Some women at this time may have an increased sexual interest and activity, as if through this they can make a final bid for erotic and romantic adventure. Some of them become increasingly interested in cosmetics, fashions and other womanly things to enhance a feminine attractiveness which they feel to be fading. Some shrink from social life as an answer to their feeling of inferiority, while others increase their activity and make excessive demands for attention from their families and the community.

PREVIOUS PERSONALITY DISTURBANCES.   Careful study has shown that patients who develop menopausal neuroses and psychoses have had personality disturbances of long duration. The syndrome occurs especially in people who have lived narrow lives of intolerance and prejudice and who have been worrisome, parsimonious, pedantic, sexually frigid, and poor mixers socially. They have taken little from life and given little. They may have been full of romantic fantasies but lacked the drive to create a life that was romantically satisfying. They have not been able to relax and enjoy life's pleasures but instead have held themselves rigidly to a code of duty.

It is small wonder that when the menstrual bleeding, which is the symbol of femininity, motherhood, sexuality and all the ideas that go with these concepts, is about to disappear, the woman who has led an empty life becomes anxious and panicky. *Injections* into the body of one so tortured in mind often create the feeling that a deficiency is being supplied—that the force which enables a woman to achieve romance, happiness, love, children and prestige is being put back into her. Unfortunately that force has been there within her for a long time and she has not had the personality equipment with which to take advantage of it. The energy of life, as represented by glandular activity, did its best from the age of puberty onward to tell her that she was a woman and that a certain kind of behavior on her part would make her happy. But a bulwark had been erected in her mind built of fear, prudishness, intolerance and hate, against which the glandular activity was powerless. The secretion of the glands could not coordinate harmoniously with ideas and emotions of loving and being loved, of sexual intercourse with pleasure, or with a desire for pregnancy and motherhood, and as a result the woman has reached the menopause emotionally unfulfilled as well as glandularly deficient.

ESTROGENIC TREATMENT.   In discussing a paper on estrogenic treatment for the menopausal syndrome, Pratt stated: "It seems increasingly difficult to know what symptoms to attribute to the menopause. A group in Chicago reporting on 1000 women found that 85 per cent had no interruption of daily routine at the time of the menopause and only 15 per cent showed symptoms. If all these symptoms mentioned are due to interruption of ovarian function, it seems strange that the symptoms are so widely different in various individuals and so frequently entirely absent.

"In our own hospital when some physician has made a diagnosis of menopausal symptoms, I ask him to observe the patient carefully and then send her to me for therapy. I will not tell him what therapy is to be employed. I have a preparation of theelin in oil and the same kind of oil without theelin sterilized and ready for injection. Just as much improvement has been noted with the oil without the theelin as there is with the theelin in the oil. I am not the observer, for the physician who refers the patient is the one who makes the notes on the change of symptoms."

Novak states that the only clear-cut symptoms of ovarian failure, and hence the only indications for replacement therapy, are hot flushes involving the head, neck and upper thorax, with or without sweating in these areas, and the less troublesome hot flashes or hot tingling sensations involving the entire body. These may be aggravated by emotional stress. Other symptoms associated with menopause, such as headache, vertigo, fatigue, arthralgia, nervousness and irritability, are probably functional and not due to estrogen deprivation. In those patients in whom the symptoms are severe enough to warrant some sort of treatment, it is necessary, as already stated, to make sure that the symptoms are due to the menopause. In any case the patient should be assured that she does not have a disease, that the menopause is not attended by dire consequences, and that it will not persist indefinitely. In many patients this is all that is required, but, if the patient is inclined to be high-strung, mild sedation may be prescribed.

It is also recommended that if a hormonal agent must be given, it should be a long-acting drug that when given by mouth will inhibit pituitary activity without producing unpleasant side-effects. Novak feels that administration of estrogens other than by mouth is rarely indicated. To this the general physician often answers that he can utilize psychotherapy in a systematic way only if he can persuade the patient to return for regular visits by giving injections of estrogen (McFarland). By giving the patient time, and the feeling that someone is interested in her and her problems, the patient derives benefits in addition to the injection.

This is a frequent problem when the non-psychiatrist attempts to administer psychotherapy. He cannot persuade the patient to return "just to talk" unless he uses medicine which may or may not be necessary. An injection is the most persuasive form of therapy to bring the patient back, but often the injection is delegated to the office nurse and the only communication between the patient and the physician is a brief greeting, a pat on the back, or a prescription for another "placebo."

TREATMENT SUGGESTIONS. Swooning, tight corsets and excessive modesty went out with the "mauve decade" but repression of sexuality is still a part of our culture. If girls can be taught to look upon menstruation as a normal physiological function and as an evidence of "growing up" that makes their parents proud of them, menstruation will be accepted as a part of living rather than a "curse." And it must not be forgotten that a healthy approach to the menstrual life is good insurance against a stormy menopause.

Girls should be better informed about romance, wifehood and motherhood, so that they can appreciate each in turn as they come. They should know more about their own psychology at an early age, as well as that of the opposite sex, so they can build a happier, more satisfying marriage, or, if they are single, a more satisfying work and social life. They should know more about childbearing so that they can enjoy their children, rather than worry so much about them. Young women should be taught to cultivate versatility in early life, so that they can enjoy a social life, participate in community interests, keep up with current events, plan varying vacation activities, cultivate hobbies, and achieve a sense of usefulness and acceptance to buffer them against any morbid thoughts which center around "growing old and being unwanted." The woman who has enjoyed life as she goes along and has a reasonable sense of her own self-esteem, who has been conscious of her hopes and aspirations and has been courageous in working them out, should not mind the "change of life" which, as the name implies, is merely a rung in the ladder of life, an epoch a woman must pass through.

For the woman who has not been well adjusted or who has not planned her life well, or for the woman who has not been able to achieve satisfaction, psychotherapeutic help is one of the most effective tools for combating the symptoms of this age period. The patient must be helped to talk out her frustrations, her disappointments, her conflicts, her morbid ideas about her own body, or her apprehensions about the future. Psychotherapy will enable her to see wherein some of these ideas are either exaggerated or entirely incorrect. It can show her how to widen her mental horizons and take on new interests, even though her life hitherto has been limited. There is no guarantee the patient will enjoy doing new things, but, fortunately, many women are able to do more, feel more and enjoy more when given new ideas and the encouragement to carry them out.

In other words, we do not believe that the answer to the treatment of the menopausal syndrome lies in replacement therapy alone. In this connection it is interesting to observe that at the present time psychiatry is going through a phase of "shock therapies." Various theories have been advanced to explain the improvements noted from "shocks" in emotional illness. Chemical, physiological and metabolic changes of a temporary nature are supposed to be induced. It is well known that major psychological shocks have a profound effect upon the thoughts and the emotional trends of man. The effects of artificially induced shocks upon the psyche need further study. The human body is a complex machine, taking in energy in one form and putting it out in another. Everything which is introduced has an effect upon emotion and ideation as well as upon somatic function. If an injection is given or an electric current is introduced, it affects the feeling and ideas of the person so treated as well as his metabolism. One might say that there is an emotional and ideational metabolism as well as a physical metabolism.

NEED FOR FURTHER STUDY. In many cases attempted "replacement therapy" has had no beneficial effect, in fact, has increased the symptoms. But here, as in the cases that have apparently been benefited, both physical and psychological observations are lacking. Studies similar to those by Benedek and Rubenstein, in which psychological changes in the patient are observed *simultaneously* and *independently*, along with glandular therapy, will help us to understand this complicated psychosomatic problem. In regard to this matter, however, Bennett and Te-

Linde find that while it is true that most symptomatic menopausal women have vaginal smears suggesting estrogen deficiency and, under the influence of implanted estrone, the smears become of the estrogenic type, they also have frequently noted relief from symptoms without any changes in the vaginal smear and are inclined to believe that the dosage necessary to relieve the symptoms in many women is less than that required to alter the vaginal epithelium.

What are the fantasies of the patient concerning the material that is injected into him? To the mind of the average layman a hypodermic injection means that a "strong" drug is being introduced. Moreover, it is introduced in a way that is known to bring quick and often miraculous results. Sometimes it is regarded as a "strengthening" form of therapy. The active principles of the sex glands of both men and women are looked upon as "rejuvenating," "giving new life," and "giving new energy." So in some cases hypodermic injections of such a potent "force" may well stimulate a latent belief within the mind of the patient. Certainly this would seem to be true in those cases in which a neutral solution was injected with such good results. However, the real point is that until more psychosomatic studies have been made simultaneously and independently by the endocrinologist and psychiatrist, neither of them is in a good position to be too positive in his opinion of the causal factor in the menopausal syndrome.

Case 40.   Psychic Factors in the Menopausal Syndrome

History and Symptoms.   A woman of 44 complained of "indigestion" with difficulty in swallowing, distress after meals, belching of gas, constipation, "spells" of nervous agitation with palpitation of the heart, weakness, marked insomnia, hot flushes, and dull headaches. She had been given injections of estrogenic material for three months without effect.

LIFE SITUATION

Her personal history was as follows: She had been the third sibling but the first girl in a family of five children. Her mother was a very strict and rigid woman who made it a point to keep her children as ignorant as possible of the world outside the home. Although they lived on a farm, the patient was not allowed to play freely around the place but was urged to be "in the house" winter and summer. The patient and her sister were taught to regard the farm hands—in fact, any strange man—as "undisciplined cavemen or sex fiends." The patient was given no information on sex matters. She received no instruction regarding menstruation and there was great fright and anxiety when she first discovered the bleeding. During her teens the patient was not allowed to go to dances or parties and any girl who did so was talked about by the mother in a most disparaging way.

Marriage.   Finally at the age of 21 the patient left home to study music. She met a young man who was very attentive to her and with whom she fell in love. He embraced and kissed her but she felt so stirred emotionally that she refused to see him any more lest her sensual desire lead her to do something wicked, although what this was she did not fully realize at the time. He proposed marriage by letter but the patient did not dare to come in contact with him again. She thought of him "day and night" but steadfastly refused to see him. Finally at 23 she was wooed with great persistence by a simple, unimaginative man, untalented and uninspiring. She finally consented to marry him but she "never knew why."

Children.   She became the mother of two daughters. For a time after marriage she continued to get satisfaction out of her music but finally she had to give this up because she felt so anxious and uncomfortable when asked to perform. She had enjoyed music and the prestige and praise it brought but now she denied herself this source of satisfaction. Her sexual relations were always without feeling. She curtailed her social relations to a considerable extent because of a fear that she might feel the need to go to the toilet and would be too embarrassed to do this. So this imaginative woman found that because of anxieties placed in her by her mother over ordinary physiological functions she lived a very narrow life devoid of emotional satisfaction. In turn, she disciplined her two daughters in much the same way that she had been disciplined and worried that in spite of her precautions one of them "might do something foolish." Her symptoms were greatly exaggerated when her oldest daughter would have a date with a young man. She would be sleepless, have "anxious spells," and attacks of indigestion.

Psychic Problems.   Here were problems of a psychological nature which could not be solved solely by injections of glandular extract. It was necessary to try in a series of psychiatric interviews to show this woman, first, how her way of life had left her dissatisfied and resentful, and second, how to find some substitute satisfactions as well as substitute glandular preparations. She was shown how she had cut herself off from the man she loved, from sexual gratification, from the prestige and satisfaction her music would have afforded and that her lack was more in the emotional than in the glandular sphere. Again we must emphasize that one must be careful to go slowly and to win the patient's good will and acceptance before pointing out the personal failures and subsequent resentment against those responsible for deprivations. If the patient does not have confidence in the physician such efforts will result in the release of more aggression than the patient can handle, anxiety will be increased instead of decreased and often, quite unexpectedly, treatment will be broken off. However, if the patient seems sincere and willing to be taught then she can be shown what has been lacking in her life and she can be encouraged to make such amends as are still possible.

TREATMENT

In the present case we allowed her to express some of her dissatisfaction with her husband and then enabled her to view his foibles with more tolerance and to see that he was not very different from the husbands of her friends. We succeeded in getting her to take up music again after expressing her just resentment against her own early deprivation. She was able to see that her oldest daughter had some rights to a life of her own about which the patient must not be too jealous. As a result of helping her to see things in her life as sources of conflict and hence to attack them as problems to be solved, the patient began to take a new interest in life as a wife and mother instead of living as an introspective recluse. Spells of anxiety and "shakiness" diminished and she began to sleep better, eat better, and thus gained strength to resume her social life. This required twelve sessions of one hour each over a period of twelve weeks. A certain innate "love of life" had remained alive in this patient in spite of her impoverished social existence and contributed greatly to so much improvement in so short a time. We do not say that the glandular therapy which she received was of no value but we are trying to show that personality modification must be accorded at least equal standing with replacement therapy.

WAITING TOO LONG FOR HELP.   It is regrettable that so many women wait until the menopause acts as the precipitating factor to make them seriously ill before they seek help along emotional lines. By this time they often are so fixed in their way of life that modification is difficult, if not impossible. Since they have not made satisfactory emotional investments, their personalities become bankrupt. This is especially true if they lack the intelligence and inner resources to permit reeducation and substitute satisfactions. *One of the tragedies of practice is the woman of middle age who has led an impoverished emotional life but has escaped serious neurotic illness (usually by means of repeated pregnancies, often recommended by her physician) and then for the first time at the menopause finally breaks down.* Certainly for some such women it would be better if the breakdown came sooner so that they would seek help when they were in a better position to be helped. To draw an analogy along more physical lines, it is often to the advantage of a tuberculous patient if his disease is made known early in life by some dramatic occurrence, such as a pulmonary hemorrhage, which forces him to get proper treatment then, instead of pursuing a subclinical course with slow destruction of pulmonary tissue and discovery of an advanced tuberculous process late in life when little can be done.

Physicians should stress more psychological preparation for the menopause. Slowly American women are learning that the menopause offers no dangers to the body or mind if reasonably healthy physical, mental and emotional life has preceded this period.

PSYCHOLOGY OF PREGNANCY

Psychology of Labor and the Puerperium.   Fear of giving birth to a child is almost universal. Ideas from childhood or even later life which concern themselves with the notion of great pain and suffering, being cut open, being torn, being split apart or dying at the time of childbirth cause great anxiety. Many women are not consciously aware of such ideas but suffer anxiety during pregnancy which increases as the time for childbirth arrives. The patient hears from other women, "You are never the same after having a child"; "The loss of blood makes you weak and sometimes you never get your strength back." Many women feel that "they have given their all" when they have had a child, in return for which they should be adored and pampered the rest of their lives. This kind of thinking is related to that which was described as failure to recover from illness or operation. It is responsible for a state of passive dependency that may last much longer than it normally should. With good prenatal and postnatal care childbearing is a normal experience from which there should be quick and easy recovery and no unpleasant after-effects.

TREATMENT.   Proper mental hygiene concerning pregnancy and childbirth should be given to female children and carried on in the school system.

The physician should be aware of the anxieties which may attend pregnancy and childbirth and should encourage the patient to talk about her fears. He should frankly explain the processes of pregnancy and delivery in a truthful but reassuring way. Just as we discussed with regard to illness and operations, physicians should be careful in their use of terms and not emphasize to their patients that they have had a "hard" or "difficult" labor. This is especially true for certain personalities.

Vomiting of Pregnancy.   A frequently encountered psychosomatic problem is the vomiting of pregnancy. Physical factors are undoubtedly concerned but there is also a large psychogenic component in the vomiting of pregnancy. As we have pointed out before, there are many women who for various reasons do not want to become pregnant. This wish may be quite conscious or quite unconscious. If the latter, it may be masked by conscious ideas of wanting a child but this is the kind of patient in whom the vomiting of pregnancy is especially apt to occur.

Such patients unconsciously feel that being pregnant indicates that some sin has been committed, or they feel that pregnancy may spoil their figure, interfere with their pleasure or add some unpleasant responsibility to their lives. Consequently, quite unconsciously of course, they would like to rid themselves of the offending fetus. Their childhood fantasies suggest that pregnancy has taken place by way of the gastrointestinal tract and they conceive of the expulsion of the fetus in the same way. The education of later life on the anatomy of the internal organs does not change their vague, childish concepts of babies growing in the stomach and, therefore, unconscious mental forces vainly attempt to get rid of the baby by vomiting.

It is impossible to say to what extent the vomiting of pregnancy is due to a physical (hormonal) factor or how much is due to a psychological cause. As in so many other psychosomatic problems both factors probably operate in most cases, their relative proportion depending upon the psychosomatic structure of the individual. Kroger and DeLee report using hypnosis successfully in 17 of 19 cases of nausea and vomiting of pregnancy, in which little or no relief had followed a wide variety of symptomatic treatments.

TREATMENT.   The psychological aspect of the vomiting of pregnancy can be approached as follows:

Prophylaxis

1. Healthy emotional development for children.
2. Proper sexual instruction of children, including emphasis on the dignity of pregnancy and motherhood.
3. Sexual hygiene and marriage courses in schools and colleges.
4. Avoidance of the concept of morning sickness or any other gastrointestinal upset as an inevitable complication of pregnancy.

Immediate Treatment

1. If the vomiting of pregnancy is severe the patient should be put to bed in a quiet room, with nursing care, and relatives and friends excluded.
2. Present the problem to the patient as one of resistance to the pregnant state. Explain the mental mechanisms detailed above. Do this even though it is felt that other factors are playing a role. To regard vomiting in pregnancy as a physical ailment and to neglect it as a problem in behavior is to fail to do justice to the patient.

Pseudocyesis.   False pregnancy is a relatively rare condition but its very existence shows us the powerful effect of ideas and emotions upon the body physiology.

The classic case usually involves a neurotic woman, near the menopause, who has had no children and strongly desires a child. Other cases occur in younger women who have had illicit intercourse and, fearing pregnancy, are convinced that they are pregnant. In addition to the amenorrhea and enlarged abdomen, the patients present all the symptoms suggestive of pregnancy, including morning nausea and vomiting, enlargement and tingling of the breasts, areolar pigmentation, and even milk secretion. Sometimes the symptom complex is carried through so convincingly that the patient apparently comes to term and the error is not realized until labor is unproductive.

A study of three cases by Steinberg and associates indicates that not only is pseudocyesis accompanied by subjective and superficial appearances of true pregnancy but that the urinary excretion of gonadotropins and estrogens is increased in this condition as it is in normal pregnancy. Although the output of gonadotropins and estrogens was far above normal, it was not sufficient to result in a positive Friedman test. After the patients manifesting pseudocyesis had been convinced of the nature of their condition, the signs and symptoms disappeared and the excretion of hormones returned to normal level.

The authors conclude that in view of the absence of pregnancy or abnormality of the pituitary or ovary, it appears that this increased hormonal output must be attributed to the influence of the psyche on the endocrine system.

Fried, Rakoff and associates reported 27 patients with this condition who presented themselves as pregnant with the usual signs and symptoms. The most common symptom was a menstrual disturbance but breast changes with secretion occurred in 22. In 11 there was softening of the cervix and some enlargement of the uterus. In each case the pelvic examination was normal. Hormonal studies indicated changes that were thought to be due to primary stimulation of the anterior pituitary gland by psychic factors.

It has been said that this syndrome does not occur in the Negro, but in the group reported they were greatly in the majority (23:4). All patients were considered neurotic, 6 to a severe degree. The basic psychologic mechanism appeared to be anxiety arising from conflict between: (1) strong sexual drives and life situations favoring pregnancy, and (2) early teaching, experiences, and folklore which had negatively conditioned these women in regard to reproduction. Superficial psychotherapy often produced a complete reversal of attitudes but occasionally other therapies were combined to give objective "proof" of the nongravid state. Effective therapy relieved the syndrome so that there was a return to a normal cycle of menses and hormonal pattern, and pregnancy occurred in 4 of the 8 previously infertile women.

Spontaneous Abortion.   There are many factors that enter into the premature expulsion of the embryo but emotional factors must be included. This is so in spite of the fact that there are hundreds of women who carry an unwanted pregnancy to term. We see many instances of the woman's ambivalence concerning motherhood. These present themselves in infanticide, in suicide where the mother kills her child and herself, in dreams where the mother kills her child or her child dies while she is powerless to rescue it. We hear women state their hostility toward children and express their distaste for motherhood. We see many women with a conscious wish for motherhood adopt a child and then destroy their child's happiness with unloving and sadistic behavior. And when we consider the body's obedience to a fantasy such as in pseudocyesis, we have to conclude that the psychotic patterns may exert themselves through the reproductive mechanism to produce a spontaneous abortion.

From the other point of view we see patients who have not conceived or who have had abortions become able to carry a pregnancy through successfully after intensive psychotherapy. The same thing has occurred when maternal feelings have been activated by adoption.

We have already pointed out that the effects of emotions exerted through the endocrine system are slower and, if anything, more significant than those which, for instance, produce stage fright. But they are nonetheless important and while they may be more unwieldy therapeutically they must nevertheless be part of the physician's knowledge and philosophy as he treats sick people. Even if he cannot always change quickly something he recognizes, he can at least avoid giving harmful diagnoses or entering into unwarranted therapies.

Prenatal Care.   Women can generally use some guidance in prenatal care. Some women overprotect themselves and are afraid to exercise properly or engage in social life to the degree that is healthy for them. Others go to the other extreme and do not get the proper rest. Some eat and drink excessively and gain more weight than they should. Some do not keep to the check-up schedule recommended by the doctor. Some are ashamed of being pregnant or are angry at being pregnant and show this by a lack of care of themselves and a lack of concern for the unborn fetus. Pregnancy should be a matter of concern to the patient and when she is too indifferent, too fearful, too careless or shows any extreme attitude it should be tactfully investigated.

Psychological Preparation for Labor and Delivery.   Some preparation of the woman for delivery of her child is highly desirable. This is carried to a high degree in the Grantly Dick Read method. This method is intended, among other things, to counteract the difficulties which may complicate labor in women who lead lonely lives and take insufficient exercise. It is also aimed to counteract the effects of ignorance of the childbearing process and to neutralize feelings of guilt and shame. Patients attend antenatal classes and are instructed in the physiology of labor and relaxation so that they can be cooperative members of the team when labor begins. Read feels that fear and other emotions give rise to additional emotional tension at the time of delivery. The emotional tensions create muscular tensions and the tensions in turn produce pain and more fear. Relatively few obstetricians follow Read's method totally but his presentation of the method to the medical profession has made many more aware of the importance of attitudes in childbirth.

Many physicians are aware of the need to prepare the patient to some degree emotionally for what is about to happen. They know it is important to seek her cooperation in harmonizing her body tensions with the rhythm of uterine contractions and to have her aware that the obstetrical team is there to help her with a procedure of considerable personal significance to her. Nurses and interns need to be kept conscious of the fact that every delivery is an event of tremendous personal significance to the mother and to the father as well. A quiet, serious consideration and a cooperative kindly approach are essential. The woman will surely "labor" more effectively for those she has come to trust and appreciate.

The subject of pain should be discussed and the physician can say something like the following: "As you know, this is not a painless procedure. We will do our best to keep your pain at a minimum and it will not be too distressing if we all work together." This gives the patient an opportunity to express herself about pain. Some women demand that there be no pain at all. Others actually want no anesthesia or analgesic. But some discussion will enable the physician to plan his approach. A woman who feels she has had some say in what happens at this time will, other things being equal, be a more satisfied, relaxed and cooperative patient during the puerperium. There is an increasing trend to have the husband present during delivery, which doubtless has its merits if patient, husband and physician are all in agreement about its desirability. If one of the three is reluctant the possible benefit of a shared experience of such an intense nature may be vitiated.

It has been suggested that emotional conflict has some relationship to uterine inertia and hence good psychological preparation should act as a prevention. The same holds true for hemorrhage.

The Importance of Nursing.   It is recommended that, when possible, infants should be nursed at the breast for about eight months. Aside from the question of any virtue which may be in mother's milk, this is an important procedure from the standpoint of emotional adjustment and personality structure. To be held close to the mother, to feel her warmth and to have the oral satisfaction of nursing on a human rather than an artificial nipple, establishes emotional security for the infant during crucial months of his development. Such an experience may pave the way for later health and happiness.

If the nursing experience has been satisfactory a gradual change from the breast to other feedings will offer little difficulty. It is the insecure, anxious child who fears what is new and different and may rebel at changing from breast to bottle. If he does rebel, tact, patience and a calm, soothing manner will help in time. The mother who quickly grows pessimistic about the ability of her child to make the normal transition, and who runs to the phone to call the physician at the slightest sign that the child does not wish to conform, adds to the problem.

Rooming In.   All that has been said about the desirability of close contact between mother and child can be facilitated by having mother and baby in the same room in the hospital rather than placing the infant in a nursery removed from the mother except at feeding time. This, to be successful, must be something the obstetrician, pediatrician and family doctor believe in and also something the patient can be educated to accept—unless she already wants it. It is a facet of what we believe to be positive mental health philosophy. Placing the newborn child with the mother postnatally need not be overfatiguing, as some argue, because, actually, when the mother realizes the needs of the newborn child for the security of her presence she becomes more relaxed, is more content and rests better.

INFERTILITY

More attention is being paid to possible psychogenic factors in infertility. There are five million childless couples in the United States, most of whom, it is estimated, are childless from infertility and not from choice.

How much of all sterility is "functional" depends on whether a clinic or private practice is being surveyed. The incidence seems to be much higher in private patients, but it is safe to say that about one third of all cases have no evidence of organic disease to account for the sterility. Mental and emotional strain seem to be the chief factors in producing it. Certainly frigidity is a common and sterility is not an uncommon result of the deep-seated neurotic anxiety which pervades our culture.

Is there a connection between the symptoms of frigidity, vaginismus (vaginal spasm) and dyspareunia (painful intercourse) on the one hand and sterility on the other? The incidence of frigidity is much greater than that of sterility so that there is no absolute relationship, but the question remains whether the same factors that influence frigidity may also lower fertility. A lack of total orgasm, which goes with frigidity, might possibly impair the involuntary part played by the pelvic apparatus in insemination. We are not sure of this because while there are certain animals, especially the rabbit, in which ovulation occurs as a result of coitus, there is no evidence that this occurs in the human nor can we prove that orgasm facilitates insemination in any other way. However, lack of proper orgasm might cause secondary local congestion and thus lead to impaired function in the pelvis. Many gynecologists believe that pelvic congestion may result from sexual excitement not discharged in orgasm.

The psychosomatic point of view suggests that the tensions of day-to-day living affect our normal physiological functions, including those of reproduction. Such problems as sharing an apartment with in-laws, financial insecurity, husband entering military service, ideas of infidelity, and so on, seem to affect the ability to conceive while peace of mind and relaxation apparently promote fertility. Just as the fatigue of everyday living, with its tensions and responsibilities, leads to lessened desire and less frequent intercourse, so do vacations with freedom from responsibilities often lead to greater potency, less frigidity, more frequent intercourse and, in turn, conception.

It has been noted in sterility clinics that the act of seeking medical advice often leads to conception before studies have even begun. It is presumed that the very fact that the couple have made up their minds to do something about their problem somehow promotes fertility.

It is important to emphasize, however, that although the psychological factor is undoubtedly important in relation to conception, it is only one of the multiple factors that enter into the question of sterility. In other words, fertility is a relative problem to which husband and wife each may contribute in varying degrees. Moreover, both physical and emotional factors may exist in husband and wife to lower fertility and fertility is enhanced as these various factors are dealt with. It is really a percentage-wise proposition in which the chances for conception increase as one after another of the various physical and emotional problems are solved.

A contributing factor may be the attempt to determine ovulation time by temperature recording—the anxiety produced by the necessity for performing coitus at a particular time may cause tension in both husband and wife. This has been called "temperature chart phobia." A young couple who had been trying to have a child for three years was still faithfully recording temperature and attempting coitus at ovulation time. The wife had suffered from both endocrine disturbances and pelvic infection. When these were cleared up the husband, a rather passive and dependent person, would lose his desire as ovulation time approached because he felt it his duty to perform coitus. Each time that his wife failed to conceive he regarded his failure to impregnate her as a reflection on his manhood. The wife in turn became so tense that it was difficult for her to relax at the time of coitus and her tension continued each month as she waited to see if pregnancy had occurred. When the rigidity of this schedule was relaxed conception promptly occurred and after this the husband was able to perform with more pleasure because "the goal was no longer conception" and the wife, too, was able to relax and achieve more pleasure in intercourse.

Mechanisms in Functional Sterility.　　The question arises as to how psychological factors actually produce sterility. Here we have had much speculation but until very recently not much scientific evidence. Spasm of the fallopian tubes has often been held responsible. Since it is well known that tension of emotional origin may express itself by spasm in various other parts of the body and since we also know that tubal spasm does occur, it is quite natural to assume that this is an important mechanism in functional sterility. Then, too, we have always known that emotional factors may influence the menstrual function and hence ovulation, so that here again is a mechanism by which emotional factors can produce sterility. Interesting scientific evidence in this regard has been established by Pashkis, Rakoff and Cantarow. They made endocrine studies of patients whose failure to menstruate was attributed to various causes. Among 85 such young women there were 23 in whom the disturbance in ovarian function occurred after marked psychological stress, such as sudden death in the family, infidelity in the husband, incompatibility and violent quarreling, or the sudden departure of the husband to war service. The previous menstrual history had been normal and there was no evidence of organic disease to account for the ovarian dysfunction. Laboratory studies indicated failure of ovulation in all cases with evidence of deficiency in the estrogen hormone.

Although failure to menstruate was the most common manifestation of a disturbance in ovarian function in their patients, the authors emphasize that this was a selective group in which the psychological stress was acute and the resulting disturbance quite obvious. They suggest that in many patients less marked disturbances of psyche and sexual function may permit menstruation to continue but ovulation does not occur.

Utilizing the stress gage to record human nongravid uterine contractions Bickers demonstrated that the emotions may affect uterine physiology and in this way play an important role in infertility. He reported a patient of 27 with a history of nine years' infertility. Sterility survey of husband and wife revealed no organic or physiological explanation for the infertile mating. The patient was hypersensitive and reacted in an exaggerated way to all the vicissitudes of life. She was subject to recurrent episodes of exhilaration and depression and was obsessed with an overwhelming desire for motherhood. The uterogram suggested a normal pattern of contractions for Day 19 of the cycle. It was run for

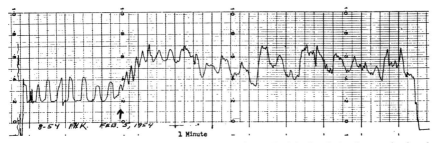

Figure 7. Uterogram in a patient who was obsessed with the desire for motherhood and had a long history of infertility. The uterus showed a relatively normal pattern of motility until, at the point indicated, patient was told that, on the basis of this study and those previously made, pregnancy for her was highly improbable. Hypermotility with arrhythmia followed immediately and persisted for the duration of the experiment, something over 7 minutes. (Bickers, W.: in Fertility and Sterility, vol. 7, 1956.)

some 18 minutes in order to be certain that it represented the intrinsic physiologic pattern of the uterus. At the point indicated she was told that, on the basis of this study and those previously made, pregnancy for her was highly improbable. The emotional reaction and its effect upon the uterus are readily apparent (Fig. 7). Hypertonic, dysrhythmic contractions appear on the uterogram. "Perhaps it is not stretching the imagination to concede that a uterus reacting in such a manner is one in which sperm migration is likely to be impeded. The intrauterine pressure here is 240 mm. of water, whereas the normal pressure at the height of contraction rarely exceeds 60 mm. of water."

The Psychology of Functional Sterility. Various suggestions have been made regarding the psychological problems of sterility. Conception occurring after adoption and conception after the first medical consultation have been mentioned as indicative of the psychological factor. Then there is the pregnancy which occurs in career women after they have decided to give up their work. Various social factors such as the fear of being seen or overheard during coitus when living in the home of in-laws are certainly common deterrents to conception.

Douching "for cleanliness" immediately after coitus, of course, interferes with conception and is probably due to the advertising of "feminine hygiene," a misunderstanding on the part of many women in regard to sterility.

Many couples believe that sterility is "natural" or "God's will" and if they were meant to have a child it would happen. Hence, they fail to seek proper help. In one such couple, both husband and wife had been reared in strict, Puritanical homes. The husband was sterile. They finally overcame their scruples about "interfering with the laws of nature" and the wife submitted to artificial insemination which proved successful. She gave birth to a healthy child which, shortly afterward, developed a slight illness. Then the wife became ill with symptoms that proved to be psychosomatic. Investigation showed that she harbored the belief that because she had "tampered with God's will" she would be punished by losing her child. The anxiety arising from the child's illness made her sick. More will be said about the emotional problems of artificial insemination later (p. 393).

The husband is much less likely to consult a physician for a sterility problem than the wife. Often he fears that if he is found defective it would be a reflection on his manhood. Therefore, his wife may have difficulty persuading him to seek help. Fortunately, his sperm can be examined without his actual presence in the consulting room but, needless to say, his active cooperation in the study is much to be desired.

In spite of protestations to the contrary an aggressive, dominant woman who assumes the masculine role in her marriage is likely to have psychogenic barriers to conception; the last thing that she wants is pregnancy. In reviewing basal body temperature charts with infertile women, some gynecologists have suspected that part of the attraction of keeping the record month after month is the assurance that pregnancy has *not* occurred. Sometimes these women seem very pleased when they are told that the sperm analysis of the husband has disclosed the cause for the sterility.

Some recent studies of the personalities of women with functional sterility have given additional information regarding these problems. Ford, Forman and associates have conducted a joint investigation of patients with infertility in which gynecologists and psychiatrists cooperated in making detailed independent physical and psychological studies. In the group of functionally infertile were placed the patients who had no demonstrable mechanical, chemical or endocrinologic reason to explain their failure to conceive, and whose husbands were found to have adequate sperm analyses. The psychiatric survey was conducted under five headings:

Personality Survey

1. Motivation for pregnancy; basic question asked:
    (a) What does it mean that she cannot get pregnant?
    (b) Why does she want a baby?
2. Marital history.
3. Menstrual and reproductive history.
4. Family background.
    (a) Stability of home.

(b) Relation to brothers and sisters.

(c) Socio-cultural level.

5. Role of parental identifications. Person(s) from whom she believes she gained significant attitudes, particularly regarding life role, work, marriage, sex and reproduction.

In those with functional infertility the following was obtained:

1. Motivation for Pregnancy. Thirty-two patients were seen in the Infertility Clinic; an obvious conclusion would be that they genuinely desired pregnancy. However, in answering the two basic questions they all gave one or more of the following answers to explain their desire for pregnancy: (1) to satisfy husband's demands, (2) to patch up a shaky marriage, (3) to be like other women, (4) to have something of their very own—*someone to love them*, (5) to show their mother how to raise a child, i.e., the baby's rearing was intended as a rebuke to their mother. Exploration of these typical answers showed that they arose from neurotic conflicts rather than the normal attitudes of fulfillment through motherhood. In fact, before the study was far advanced many patients realized that they actually did *not* want to have a baby, and that pregnancy would precipitate real neurotic anxiety.

2. Marital History. The following themes predominated: Early impulsive marriage frequently based on guilt over illicit sexual relationships, belief in pregnancy or rarely actual pregnancy, frequent marital discord, threatened or actual separation, divorce or abandonment and bad sexual adjustment.

3. Menstrual and Reproductive History. There were preponderant references to attitudes denying their sexual, menstrual and reproductive role, with many instances of genital and menstrual disturbances, i.e., vaginismus (vaginal spasm), frigidity, sexual avoidance, painful menstruation, irregular cycles, bleeding disorders, etc. There were several references to "abortions" of a believed pregnancy, with the themes of unconscious guilt over it.

4. Family Background. There was high incidence of the following circumstances, singly or combined: (1) maternal harshness, rigid unloving discipline particularly regarding feeding, weaning and toilet training with imposition of adult standard of performance from earliest infancy; (2) early imposed maternal responsibility for younger siblings (enforced maternal role); and (3) death or abandonment by one or both parents early in life with frequent shifting parental surrogates. In private cases socio-cultural background was upper middle class or better; in clinic cases it was lower or middle class. This is emphasized to indicate that emotional rather than material security seems the crucial factor for the fate of the personality.

5. Role of Parental Identifications: Specific Attitude Countermanding Pregnancy. Two special personality trends were outlined:

(1) DENIAL OF THE MOTHER IMAGE. Five showed mixed feelings toward the mother with intense yearning blocked by hateful or revengeful attitudes. Everything mother stands for is rejected, particularly her reproductive role. The patients felt grossly deprived by their mothers, believed they gave them not love but things and had rejected them because they were females. The usual situation showed that the mother herself had rejected motherhood, had been aggressive and dominant, trying to emulate the male role, and had bowed to pregnancy as inevitable while longing for a male child as a solace. The mother's repudiation of the daughter and her femaleness both seemed responsible for much trouble; the daughter learned that breast feeding was a nuisance, something begrudged; she learned to hate her budding female biology so that the onset of menstruation was a disaster, menses dirty or a curse, marital sexuality an imposition, childbirth an inescapable burden. She developed attitudes corresponding to the mother's, but often of greater severity.

(2) IMITATION OF MALE ROLE. Four patients presented typical aggressive masculine protest personalities. All were insecure in the female role; their ideal was to prove themselves better than any male. Three were career women who escaped into marriage when they sensed the imminent failure of their masculine role; the fourth married a passive male and dominated him. There were strong drives toward masculine activity with the wish to gain affection in this way. There was great hostility to men with wishes to ridicule them vocationally and sexually. Overt anxiety was more prominent in this group than in the first where it was expressed more through mood changes (depression predominantly), physical symptoms and personality distortions.

Surprisingly enough Ford and his associates concluded that a psychogenic factor was present in *most* of their infertile patients, whether organic pathology was present or not. To what degree it was responsible for the infertility in the organic group is questionable, but this does suggest that among the generally accepted criteria for the diagnosis of functional sterility, as is true of so many other medical problems, psychological and physical factors both enter in varying degrees and that one cannot make a sharp separation between the organic and functional condition but must consider both aspects of the problem in every instance of the disorder.

Therefore the authors indicate that whether the problem is one of failure to ovulate due to hormonal disturbance or spasm of the tubes due to psychological tension, the demarcation between organic and psychogenic sterility becomes indefinite if we consider in addition such things as defects in the lining membrane of the uterus, "hostile" cervical secretions and faulty sperm production as possible psychological effects.

The authors conclude that a more rational approach to the study of infertility would be to incorporate the psychological study in the routine investigation rather than including it after all possible organic causes have been eliminated and the diagnosis of psychogenic infertility has been suggested by exclusion of organic disease.

Treatment.   It may seem strange to say that the psychological treatment of functional sterility should begin in childhood but it is probably clear from what has been said up to now that this is so. Proper sex education contributing to proper psychosexual adjustment and a happy home with mature parents are the best background for the development of children who will later marry and want to become parents. We are becoming more enlightened and better educated in this regard and the parents of today are more liberal in their attitude toward sexual problems. If children can grow up with healthy attitudes toward menses, sexual intercourse, masturbation, pregnancy and the menopause, much good can be accomplished and perhaps some of these functional sterility problems avoided. Thus the preventive aspect of the management of sterility not only involves the physician and the psychiatrist, but more especially the family, the school and the church.

All physical treatments of sterility must be carefully evaluated because it is recognized that about a third of all sterility patients will get pregnant regardless of the treatment used, probably in response to suggestion. The close attention, the patience and the personal interest of the physician probably have much to do with this.

Psychotherapy is of course the treatment of choice for psychogenic sterility, but since the sources of the disturbance have their origin in the early period of the patient's life it can hardly be expected that a few interviews will be successful in all cases. Often much more intensive psychotherapy may be necessary; but even the superficial psychotherapy which any physician can employ may be very helpful and this, of course, consists of encouraging the patient to ventilate her feelings in the hope of reducing anxiety and tension. But we must not forget that the husband too may require psychotherapy just as he may require physical treatment for his defective sperm.

Psychological Aspects of Artificial Insemination. Although the majority of sterile matings show responsibility divided between the two partners, each of whom contributes some degree of infertility, it has been estimated that in about 10 per cent of cases the fault lies wholly, and in another 20 per cent chiefly, on the male side. Since treatment of the male is largely unsatisfactory, a possible solution to the problem exists in the form of artificial insemination with semen from an outside donor. Considerable attention is now being given to the legal, moral and ethical aspects of this procedure.

Lamson and associates discuss the problem somewhat as follows. Donor insemination is not illegal, nor is it considered to be immoral except by minority groups. But since it involves the invasion of a woman's body for purposes of reproduction by a man not her husband, it does overstep the bounds of the conventional social mores. On that account certain special emotional reactions may be expected over and above those that occur in ordinary cases of involuntary sterility.

A wife denied the full emotional experience of motherhood because of the infertility of her husband is bound to develop special reactions and attitudes toward him. Some degree of resentment is inevitable, together with a devaluation of his masculinity. These feelings may increase to the point of becoming intolerable to both partners, particularly if the man is deficient in sexual potency as well as in fertility. More frequently the wife succeeds in making an adjustment to the situation. Three sorts of reactions occur singly or in combination: first, the masculine-aggressive woman insists on having a child of her own body, cost what it may. She is a ready though rarely an ideal candidate for donor insemination, sometimes obtaining her husband's reluctant consent by a species of emotional blackmail. Second, there is the wife who accepts childlessness and lives on good terms with her sterile husband but demands from him constant proof of his masculinity in the way of achievement and material success. And, third, the truly motherly woman compensates for the lack of children by directing her motherliness toward other persons or objects, real or symbolic.

Feminine psychology is not intrinsically antipathetic to donor insemination. No doubt large numbers of women would gladly receive this sort of help were it not for other deterrent influences. The procedure is new, strange and radical. It is vaguely associated with suggestions of legal and moral irregularity. Results once obtained are irrevocable and must be accepted for better or worse. But apparently what makes wives hesitate more than anything else is the fear, sometimes well founded, that their husbands will not be able to make both the immediate and the long-term adjustments necessary for the happy working out of the project. In general, the renunciation of children is less traumatic to husbands than to wives. In the case of male sterility, however, special emotional factors affect the husband. He knows that he is responsible not only for his own disappointment but also for the frustration of his wife's yearnings and as a result he is beset by feelings of inadequacy, inferiority and guilt. As a rule, similar feelings do not greatly trouble sterile wives of fertile husbands. But the traditionally proud lord of creation, finding himself unable to create a baby, is likely to develop a strong sense of personal devaluation.

As regards their attitudes toward donor insemination, sterile husbands may be broadly classified in three groups: First, there are the men, often tending to be neurotic, who are so constituted psychologically that the whole idea is unacceptable. Such a man considers the performance of the operation as scarcely less offensive than adultery. The wife's pregnancy aggravates by contrast his own feeling of biologic infertility. Jealousy of the unknown donor may develop. The child is likely to be more resented than loved. In these circumstances insemination would simply invite emotional and social disaster. Since most men of this type never come to discuss their problem, it is hard to estimate how common they are, but one suspects that the total number is considerable. The second group is the direct opposite of the first in that the attitude of its members toward insemination is basically simple and unaffected. The idea of another man's intrusion does not disturb the husband. He shares with his wife in the emotional satisfaction of pregnancy, welcomes the child and soon identifies himself in the role of father.

The majority of men who request donor insemination for their wife belong to a third group, intermediate between the two just described. Such a husband is obliged at the outset to overcome some degree of reluctance and hesitation, but this he manages to do, impelled by one or another of several motives: To make his wife happy, to obtain a child that he himself desires, to discharge his guilt feelings or to conceal his sterility. If he succeeds in making a really satisfactory adjustment, all will be well; often he becomes as eager as his wife to have the operation carried out. But no type of case requires more careful psychological evaluation, since it is always possible that the man's attitude, however sincerely he believes in it at first, may prove to be unstable and transitory. In some future emotional crisis he might even react so strongly as to develop feelings of resentment, hate and disgust toward the whole situation.

Because of these considerations the formula for accomplishing the most good together with the least harm is careful study of all applicants with refusal on the part of the physician to accept unsuitable cases.

GYNECOLOGICAL SURGERY

Although we will discuss psychological factors in general surgery (p. 495), something must be said at this point regarding gynecological surgery.

It should be kept in mind that surgery of the female sexual organs has special meaning to the patient. This is not to assume that she will always be emotionally disturbed over an operation in these areas but certainly even in the most stable woman careful psychological consideration is necessary.

Hysterectomy. The removal of the uterus means the end of the childbearing capacity. When occurring at the menopause or after it should not create too much tension or conflict. But we have pointed out the fact that many women greatly resent the climacteric as a misfortune. "Time," the enemy, has attacked them and robbed them of some of their sexuality. So even at the menopause, or after, the woman may resent, consciously or unconsciously, the removal of her uterus. Some feel this may interfere with their capacity to function sexually—or be satisfactory sexual partners. Some believe that removal of the uterus means that they have cancer and have not been told. To others it may mean they have been robbed of youth and put in a class of older women.

The more a hysterectomy antedates the menopause the more likelihood there is of intensification of the foregoing fears and conflicts.

What then shall one do? Know these possibilities and discuss them and give the patient an opportunity to ventilate her feelings beforehand. This is a great safeguard! Patients appreciate being told—being prepared. How often we hear the patient cry, "I wasn't told." To some patients this is a repetition of parental breach of faith suffered in childhood. But whatever its root, it is easier to deal with an informed, cooperative patient who has been given a chance to express her feelings and who knows at least a little of what the organ she is losing means to her. Not only does the preoperative preparation make a calmer patient but it will make it easier to discuss any postoperative qualms she may have.

Mastectomy.   A removal of the breast unilaterally or bilaterally may be much more disturbing than a hysterectomy. At least the knowledge of the loss of the uterus may be restricted to the patient and the surgeon who did it. But a mastectomy cannot be so easily concealed. Women are especially proud of their breasts and hate to have any alteration made in the contour of their bodies. This may connote being changed into a man. Women fear they will be less attractive to their husbands. They fear discovery while undressing. And even though a prosthesis may meet the world's demands aesthetically they have to live with their own image of their altered body contour. Here again preparation before the operation and a little time to contemplate the result before it happens is a great help. To see that the surgeon has some awareness and sympathy for what he has to do to her helps the patient to cooperate postoperatively and meet changed conditions.

Therapeutic Abortion.   A therapeutic abortion may create many conflicts for a woman. First, she may actually want the child very much, as does her husband. But even if such is not the case she may feel she should want the child and hence will assume guilt over the procedure even though her physician and a consultant say the abortion is mandatory. In such a situation she would need help to go over some of her earliest attitudes about motherhood, her home and religious teaching in order that she could understand the present reality and not remain caught up in teachings and values that were valid when she was younger and healthier but which no longer hold in the presence of disease. A signature of consent from the patient and husband may be only a small part of the total consent which will give them, especially the woman later, peace of mind for this sometimes legal but unconventional operation.

Tubal Ligation.   Tubal ligation is an operation which carries some of the psychological overtones of hysterectomy as well as some of those for therapeutic abortion. Tubal ligation is an operation that theoretically and sometimes actually is a reversible procedure. But a surgeon might hesitate to guarantee its reversibility. So we have to consider what a tubal ligation is for its significance to the patient and her total life situation including age, marital status, number of children and personality make-up.

If the operation is done because conditions of health preclude children one should make sure the woman can understand this and does not criticize herself for evasion of maternal responsibility. To tie the tubes means barrenness and sterility and this may seem very negative to a woman whose self-esteem is already a little shaky. If she is young and thinks she has all the children she wants, she still has to consider the possibility that disaster might take one or more of her children and she might want to become pregnant again. Conceivably she might lose her husband, marry again and want to reproduce.

Examination and Diagnostic Procedures.   It is not only with the more serious gynecological operations that one needs to be sensitive to the psychology of women. For many women the simplest pelvic examination is construed unconsciously as partly an attack, partly a seduction. It takes time for the medical student, intern and even young physician to acquire a wholesome and sensitive understanding of a part of the body so highly charged emotionally as are the female sex organs. Some refuse to recognize the sensitivity of women and cover their lack of rapport with undue bluntness and directness, with humor, with sarcasm, or with an extreme detachment that makes the patient feel like a window mannikin with a number. To gain some awareness of a woman's psychology the physician needs to be interested, to listen, to ask questions and supplement what he hears and learns from the patient with occasional readings in dynamic psychology.

References

Beckers, W.: Fertil. & Steril., 7: 268, 1956.
Bennett, H. G., Jr., and TeLinde, R. W.: J.A.M.A., 118: 1341, 1942.
Dunbar, F.: Emotions and Bodily Changes. 2nd Ed. New York, Columbia University Press, 1938.
Ford, E. S. C., Forman, I., Willson, R., Char, W., Nixson, W. T., and Scholz, C.: Fertil. & Steril., 4: 456, 1953.
Fried, P. H., Rakoff, A. E., Schopbach, R. R., and Kaplan, A. J.: J.A.M.A., 145: 1329, 1951.
Kelley, K., Daniels, G. E., Poe, J., Easser, R., and Monroe, R.: Psychosom. Med., 16: 129, 1954.
Kinsey, A. C.: J. Clin. Endocrinol., 1: 424, 1941.
Kroger, W. S., and DeLee, S. T.: Am. J. Obst. & Gynec., 51: 544, 1946.
Lamb, W. M., Ulett, G. A., Masters, W. H., and Robinson, D. W.: Am. J. Psychiat., 109: 840, 1953.
Lamson, H. D., Pinard, W. J., and Meaker, S. R.: J.A.M.A., 145: 1062, 1951.
McFarland, J. E.: J.A.M.A., 156: 1273, 1954.
Novak, E. R.: J.A.M.A., 156: 575, 1954.

Paschkis, K. E., Rakoff, A. E., and Cantarow, A.: Clinical Endocrinology. New York, Paul B. Hoeber, 1954.

Perloff, W. H.: J. Clin. Endocrinol., *10:* 447, 1950.

Pratt, J. P.: Am. J. Obst. & Gynec., *31:* 782, 1936.

Read, Grantly D.: Childbirth Without Fear. 2nd Ed. Harper & Bros., New York, 1953.

Reusch, J., et al.: Chronic Disease and Psychological Invalidism. Psychosomatic Medicine Monograph. New York, Paul B. Hoeber, Inc., 1946, p. 126.

Steinberg, A., Pator, N., Winheld, E. B., Segal, H. I., Schecter, F. R., and Coulton, N. H.: Psychosom. Med., *8:* 176, 1946.

Stoddard, F. J.: J.A.M.A., *129:* 508, 1945.

Chapter XIII

The Genitourinary System and
the Sexual Function in the Male

INSTINCTUAL FORCES

There are two main instinctual drives which are always asserting themselves in the individual who is trying to make an adaptation in a busy and none too friendly world. These are the aggressive drive, leading toward a mastery of the environment, and a sexual drive, leading toward reproduction. Through the first, man seeks to gain sustenance, comfort, possessions and prestige. He must learn to control the aggressive force skillfully lest it show harmful and destructive tendencies which will either bring punishment upon him and alienate him from those who could help him or will turn back upon him in the form of disease or accident. Through the sexual impulse—broadly speaking, an instinctual drive for sensual gratification—man seeks to give and receive pleasure in close physical contacts. Through the contact of the genital organs, man reproduces himself. Through gratification of the senses, through food, warmth, kind words, sweets, etc., children learn to feel love for those who treat them well, and become willing and able to feel the same for others—their playmates, friends, sweethearts, marital partners, and finally their own children.

GENITAL FUNCTIONING

This process seems a natural and harmless one, and yet it must be admitted that there is a great deal of social condemnation of genital functioning as a whole without consideration of the fact that there is a right time and place for this kind of behavior. Rarely is there any intelligent consideration on the part of parents and teachers of the purpose and importance of genital function. As a result the genital tract as a body system falls most directly in the path of a deluge of human emotions of a most unfortunate character.

The genital organs have their own physiological functions to perform as well as being the most important organs of love-making and the *only* organs of procreation. As a result they fall heir to many taboos, feelings

Page 398

of disgust, shame, fear, anxiety, and even hate. *None* of these feelings *should* be associated with the reproductive organs. It has been definitely shown that with intelligent information and the development of love and good will associated with sexual functioning, human beings will conduct themselves in a highly satisfactory fashion; but that fears, taboos and prejudices, on the other hand, may lead to crippling of the behavior.

EDUCATION IN SEXUALITY

In this chapter considerable material will be presented concerning the sexual function and the emotional problems concerned with satisfactory sexual relations. The relation of the sexual function to health has not been adequately dealt with in medical teaching. The study of medicine is to a certain degree a sublimation of the desire to know more about the human body and its functions, of which the sexual function is by no means the least important. Medical students are eager to know more of this subject, and rightly so, for they feel that the more they know of this vital factor the better they will understand human behavior in general and therefore the better physicians they will become.

There is a greater freedom in our society for the growing male to express himself sexually than there is for the female. He urinates with greater freedom, there is less taboo associated with the act of urination and he is given a wider latitude in his male role than is the female. This may seem obvious and insignificant but it does presage a different attitude in the casualness attached to sexual genital functioning.

The female can play her role in sexuality if she acquiesces. Whether she takes pleasure or not in doing this is not a matter which young people of either sex consider very seriously before marriage—although they should. It is the male who has to worry about his ability to perform. In beginning his sexual activity he faces a great crisis. Can he achieve an erection and be a man or does he face the humiliation of not being able to play his part in the sexual act? If we are realistic and realize that roughly 85 per cent of males have intercourse before marriage, then we must accept the fact that many of these contacts are with prostitutes or girls of experience in sexual matters. In connection with prostitutes, there is the fear of infection. With the non-prostitute, the male additionally has to contend with the fear of impregnation, with its responsibilities and loss of prestige if pregnancy occurs, and the fear of harm to a girl for whom virginity has a value. It seems important, then, to understand how anxiety regarding the sexual function develops.

TYPES OF POTENCY DISTURBANCE

Potent But Coitus Lacks Pleasure. There is a group of men who are able to achieve erection when desired and are interested in the sexual act but for whom, when it actually takes place, there is always something lacking in the achievement of the anticipated pleasure. Some of these men seem to take more pleasure in boasting of the number of their sexual conquests than they take in the sexual act itself. Their pleasure is not so much in the company of women as in discussing their sexual feats with other men. One cannot actually say that they achieve no pleasure at the height of orgasm; rather the pleasure is not what is anticipated. When such a sexual difficulty occurs in the marriage relationship it discourages them from frequent attempts at intercourse.

The physiological apparatus of these men works well but they do not love women very much. They may find a thrill in courting the woman and getting her to yield sexually. The man may get some sense of achievement that he has possessed her but he does not care to spend much time with her, does not enjoy her company, is not made happy in sharing her thoughts in mutual activities other than sex. Such men are most likely to be promiscuous. Hence they are not as likely to complain of their sexual make-up or attitude as the wife, although this psychology may gradually lead to a more definite physical impotence.

Potent But Has Coitus Under Protest.   There are some men who have little difficulty in achieving erection and having intercourse. However, they believe that intercourse is harmful and saps the energy and strength from a man, leaving him tired, exhausted, and unfit for his work the following day. In marriage such a man has intercourse infrequently, or if the wife's sexual desire causes him to have coitus more frequently than he desires, he acquiesces under protest.

These men are often responsible for a marriage problem when married to an actively sexed woman. While it is usually the frigid woman who has a limited interest in sexual activity, here the situation is reversed. These patients believe too much of what they have read of the devitalizing effect of sexual intercourse and the discharge of semen. If they have any physical impairments or illness the problem is even greater, since this serves to justify their neurotic attitudes. They believe that intercourse makes the illness worse. They need a great deal of insight into the nature and origin of their misunderstanding and much encouragement to give of themselves and their semen in sexual relations. Modesty often prevents wives from complaining to their physician about the situation. When the difficulty on the part of the husband is successfully treated, however, the strength of the marriage bond may greatly improve. Health, of course, will improve because of a better sexual adjustment.

Interested in Coitus But Cannot Always Have Erection When Desired. In this group of men coitus has considerable attraction at all times, but when the opportunity for intercourse arises the capacity for erection disappears. This group has a high degree of unconscious fear of harm or criticism which may follow sexual activity. Added to this is anxiety about "involving" themselves, "injuring" themselves, "losing" themselves in a love relationship. (See Treatment.)

Inadequate or Partial Erection.   Some men who are interested in coitus and are consciously eager to satisfy the woman sexually are unable to obtain a vigorous erection. Only a partial erection is achieved so that it is difficult to enter the vagina, or if the vagina is entered, the man is unable to be sufficiently forceful or vigorous in his movements to bring satisfaction to the woman.

Such a man has the same psychological problems as those discussed above. The inadequate erection is the somatic compliance of the man who does not wish or dare to firmly or vigorously penetrate the woman as part of an intimate love relation.

Premature Ejaculation.   This is the most frequent disturbance of sexual functioning in men, causing them frequent humiliation and feelings of inferiority, and producing a lack of sexual gratification in the female. In some cases ejaculation of semen takes place before the male has actually inserted the penis within the vagina. In other cases ejaculation takes place almost simultaneously with entrance into the vagina or a few seconds later, entirely too soon for the woman to have received any stimulation from the penis which would aid her in achieving orgasm. In some married couples premature ejaculation is the cause for an inability in the female to achieve orgasm. In some men this symptom is looked upon as a personal peculiarity rather than a symptom, and hence they do not consult a physician. Often neither party regards this condition as anything unusual since neither has obtained information which makes comparison with others possible.

DEFECT IN EMOTIONAL DEVELOPMENT.   In many cases of premature ejaculation the male is too embarrassed to consult a physician for his difficulty, and the woman has too much consideration for him to force him to do anything about it, and a long-standing sexual disharmony results. Sometimes, unfortunately, when the patient has consulted a physician who knows little about the subject, the condition is treated casually or even jokingly and he comes away worse than before. The patient should at least be informed that he suffers from a defect in his emotional development which has interfered with his ability to exercise control over ejaculation and that such a condition is amenable to psychotherapy, rather than being made to feel that he suffers from some organic defect or glandular deficiency which has to be treated by injections, manipulations or surgery.

Impotence Complete But Interest is Retained in Coitus.   There are cases in which the ability to achieve erection is lost and yet emotionally the man is interested in women and interested in functioning sexually with them. Inasmuch as a capacity for erection depends so much upon psychological factors, it is of some importance to distinguish this group from the next group of those having *complete impotence with no interest in coitus.*

The man who is impotent and has no interest in coitus is likely to have many more inhibitions and a more severe neurosis underlying his symptoms. Other things being equal, it would take a longer period of treatment in such a case because those factors which were interfering with his interest in sexual functioning would have to be dealt with before getting at the factors which were merely interfering with erection itself.

AWARENESS OF WOMEN'S SEXUALITY

Occasional Failure to Achieve Orgasm.   Women have many fantasies of which they are not aware regarding sexual functioning, and are more sensitive in matters of love and sexuality than men, so that it is not unusual for them to have an occasional failure in achieving orgasm during intercourse. However, it is important to pay some attention to these occasional failures lest they gradually become more than occasional and mark the beginning of a definite problem of frigidity. If the husband neglects or is unable to be ardent in his love-making before intercourse is begun, or if the woman is under special stress (for example, unusual concern with the children) enough psychic energy may be lacking to result in a failure to achieve orgasm. If this happens too frequently, however, it should not be looked upon as something natural but as a defect in the woman's capacity to function normally in the sexual sphere.

Effect of Frigidity on Wife.   It is easily understandable that the effect of frigidity on the woman is different from that of impotence on the man. Whereas an impotent man is incapacitated in regard to the act of intercourse, a frigid woman submits to the wishes of her husband and the lack of enjoyment leads to indifference, resentment, or even disgust. This attitude in a woman can contribute to the impotence of the man.

FUNCTIONAL URINARY DISTURBANCES

It is quite well recognized in medicine that functional disturbances of urination may depend upon emotional factors. Nocturia in a medical history does not necessarily mean kidney or prostatic disease but may indicate a functional disorder. The bladder, like the stomach, may register emotional disturbances. The difficulty has been, as with so many problems in psychosomatic medicine, in having some practical approach which the patient could understand and which could be of actual value to him in the control of his symptoms.

A Substitute for Sexuality.   The function of urination from the physiological standpoint is periodically to relieve the discomfort of accumulated urine within the bladder. However, this function may serve different psychological ends. It has a pleasurable erotic component in children, as urination is the first excitement and source of gratification associated with the genital organs. It is the forerunner, so to speak, of later orgastic pleasure in coitus. Bedwetting is succeeded by masturbation and nocturnal emissions and the prohibitions of the toilet are succeeded by the prohibitions of society against sexuality. Hence just as various sexual acts may be resorted to surreptitiously for sources of gratification, so urinary symptoms may represent at a more unconscious level a substitute for sexual activity. It is quite common for women to have frequency of urination when thrown in company with the opposite sex. Children and adolescents will often have an erotic dream and awaken to find that they have urinated in bed. Adults will often dream of urination accompanied by highly pleasurable sensations and men may awaken to find that there has been a seminal emission.

Aggressive Component.   The aggressive component in urination is well shown in our coarser vituperative language since expressions referring to urinating or defecating upon the victim or the hated person are so common. Such ideas date back to early childhood when the child discovers that the contents of the body can be used to express hostility.

Children and adults often urinate with marked frequency, the idea expressed to those in authority being, "Since you want me to behave properly and not wet myself *or anyone else* you must let me go to the toilet any time I like." This may be a very time-consuming and wasteful gesture in a group of workers. They capitalize in an aggressive way upon a necessity which cannot be refused. Finally, frequency of urination may be used to punish one's self in that it leads to great inconvenience and the necessity of curtailing social life. A reduction of usefulness takes place just as in phobic behavior or in the compulsion neuroses.

Lack of Emotional Control. In short, a persisting defect in sphincter control means a lack in emotional control either in the erotic or aggressive parts of the personality or both. These need to be uncovered and the patient helped to work them out in other ways.

The problems of sphincter control in the male almost always center around (*a*) enuresis that has persisted into adulthood and (*b*) inhibition of sphincter release in the presence of others so that the patient cannot urinate in public toilets. This of course excepts some incontinence in the aged senile.

A male of 19 suffered from enuresis while attending college. He came from a home with an oversolicitous mother and an overstrict and severe father. He was unpopular with his classmates for being so aggressive, arrogant and argumentative with them. He was only a fair student and had unrealistic daydreams of success without effort. The enuresis seemed to be a combination of two things in his personality: (1) an insensitivity to the expectations of others, (2) a refusal to conform which pervaded both consciousness and unconsciousness. Weekly psychotherapeutic interviews over a four-month period reduced his symptom considerably.

A male of 34 sought treatment for (*a*) inability to enjoy life and (*b*) inability to urinate in any public toilet. The first symptom was quite serious but the second was no less so. Few men who do not have this difficulty can appreciate the acute discomfort and apprehension attendant upon the inability to urinate in a public toilet. A few types of work give the protection of privacy but many jobs, including life in the armed forces, make this symptom a most distressing complaint. This man had a harsh, threatening, domineering father. He had a warmer mother but her efforts did not help the patient much since she permitted herself to be as intimidated by the father as the children were. This patient felt that as a child (*a*) he had no right to urinate, (*b*) this like any other act was a defiance of the father, and that (*c*) deep underneath his intimidation of his father was a desire to destroy his hated father (or any male for that matter) with his penis, his urine and any of the weapons his penis and urine symbolized. As a result of many hours in psychotherapy, and understanding the meaning of urination as an act of defiance and a struggle for competition with other men, he came to feel more comfortable in their presence and could relax the sphincter and urinate when it became necessary. Occasionally he would still have some difficulty, even after several months of treatment, and he did not become the happy-go-lucky man he wanted to be. He was satisfied to find life and work bearable and to be able to give up his suicidal tendencies and despair.

THE MALE CLIMACTERIC

With the increased interest of the medical profession in endocrinology and the exploitation of this interest by pharmaceutical houses in marketing endocrine products, a flood of literature has crossed the physician's desk on what is termed the male climacteric, or even less aptly the male menopause. This syndrome is said to occur in the middle or late forties and to be characterized by nocturnal urinary frequency, fatigue, indecision, hot flushes, decreased libido and "impending" impotence. Other symptoms such as vertigo, excessive perspiration, mood changes, headaches, impaired mental concentration, numbness, tingling, tachycardia, palpitation, weakness, lack of endurance, a feeling of inadequacy in undertaking new duties, and a tendency to seclusion are sometimes included as a part of the syndrome.

An Ill-defined Syndrome.   Most of these symptoms have been conspicuous in the psychoneuroses, particularly neurasthenia, and were described as far back as 1869 by Beard. Certainly such symptoms often arise from emotional conflict, and can be effectively treated by psychotherapy. We believe that the syndrome spoken of as the male climacteric or male menopause is even less well defined than the menopausal syndrome in the female and consequently that there is less justification for organotherapy, to the exclusion of psychotherapy, in the management of nervous symptoms that appear during this period.

Heller and Meyers, utilizing gonadotropic excretion as well as testicular biopsy specimens in a careful study of 38 cases, tried to find the answer to the following questions:

1. Is there an organic basis to justify the claim that the male climacteric is a true clinical entity?

2. Is it possible to distinguish between the male climacteric and psychoneurosis or psychogenic impotence either clinically, by laboratory methods, or both?

3. If the syndrome exists, what therapy is advisable?

4. Is the male climacteric a normal accompaniment of the aging process or is it a pathological problem?

Commenting that no objective evidence has been brought forward to prove that the male climacteric is an actual clinical entity or to differentiate it conclusively from psychoneurosis or psychogenic impotence, they say, "Ordinary clinical experience arouses considerable skepticism as to the existence of the male climacteric because of (a) the similarity between symptoms attributed to this syndrome and those referable to psychoneurosis, (b) the retention of fertility by most men well into old age, (c) the absence of regressive changes in secondary sexual characteristics of most elderly men comparable to those which customarily occur in women after menopause. In most elderly women there are unmistakable signs of ovarian failure, namely atrophy of the uterus, vagina, external genitalia and breasts, a deepening of the voice, a tendency toward hirsutism and a loss of feminine bodily contours. In contrast, most elderly men exhibit no physical signs of testicular failure; genitalia and secondary sexual characteristics show no regressive changes; beard and bodily hair remain intact, and bodily contours remain masculine."

The diagnosis of the male climacteric was established in 23 cases by the finding of pronounced elevation in gonadotropic hormone excretion, comparable quantitatively to that occurring in castrates. This was corroborated in all of 8 cases subjected to biopsy, by histologic evidences of testicular atrophy and degeneration. The diagnosis was further supported in all of 20 cases treated by specific response to a therapeutic test with androgens. A clear-cut differentiation of the male climacteric from psychogenic impotence was made by the urine gonadotropic assays, which were decidedly elevated in the former group and normal in the latter.

Since laboratory procedures which will positively differentiate climacteric from psychoneurotic patients are usually not available for clinical practice, the authors recommend the following therapeutic test: Administer 25 mg. of testosterone propionate by intramuscular injection five days weekly for a period of two weeks. Evaluate the clinical status at that time, noting the effect on symptoms and sexual potency. If at the end of the two weeks trial of therapy the patient has shown no improvement, either of two conclusions may be justifiable: (1) The patient is not experiencing the male climacteric or (2) he will need such an excessively large daily dosage of testosterone that treatment is financially unpractical. If the patient does respond it may be necessary to determine whether the improvement is actually due to specific relief of testicular failure or whether it is merely due to suggestion. Withdrawal of therapy until symptoms return and then reinstitution of therapy with placebos may be required to settle the question. Most therapeutic studies have not been adequately controlled. Proper control requires the use of placebos and, preferably, that a double-blind technique be used when a series of patients are being studied. Testosterone therapy is not without its hazards: sodium retention leading to cardiac failure in older men; pituitary inhibition with azoospermia in younger men; and, if a prostatic carcinoma exists, unsuspected or not, possible increase in its activity. The last is important in view of the frequency of dormant prostatic cancer in elderly men.

Heller and Meyers observe that the average male will not experience the climacteric. Their clinical observations and laboratory studies indicate that both the germinal and the hormonal functions of the testes are preserved well into senility in the average man. It is true that reduction of function occurs, but there is fairly adequate maintenance in most cases.

So they conclude that *whereas in the female the menopause is an invariable and physiological accompaniment of the aging process, in the male the climacteric is an infrequent and pathological accompaniment of that process.*

Need for Psychotherapy. When some method will enable us to say which symptoms are due to gonadal deficiency and which are due to emotional conflict, we will be in a better position to combine endocrine therapy and psychotherapy. Meanwhile we emphasize the necessity for scientific psychotherapy rather than empirical organotherapy.

In a case study of the sex hormones and psychic conflict Tauber and Daniels found that the male sex hormone stimulated a special aspect only of sexual functioning. Frequency and strength of erections were increased in the beginning. Priapism or penile response resembling priapism was seen following the *injection of androgenic substances.* These erections were not always accompanied by pleasurable increases of tension or desire for intercourse. In fact with the erection the patient might remain emotionally unmoved. The investigators felt that the sex hormone assists in preparing the individual for sexual activity. Yet the hormone can be utilized to advantage only if, over and above the physiological effect, there is a wish to participate in the sexual relationship. Although the administration of the male sex hormone temporarily produced a period of sexual rejuvenation, probably capable of repetition, it became evident that the patient's most effective psychic equilibrium was maintained after the discontinuance of hormonal therapy.

A Period of Adjustment. In discussing the menopause in women we pointed out that between the ages of forty and fifty years there were many social and personal adjustments to make. The same is true with men. Many increasing family and business responsibilities are met with. The final realization that one has gone as far as he can go, that youthful ambitions will not be realized, is a common and important problem in this period. It is a decade fraught with much emotional conflict. Frustrations arouse latent hostilities; the life situation itself, plus a special susceptibility, may well produce irritability, tenseness, mental depression, decreased interest in expressing love genitally, feelings of inadequacy, a tendency to seclusion, headaches and palpitation, without the necessity for a primary defect in glandular function. Whether the psychological factors can, in themselves, give rise to secondary glandular dysfunction is a question that we will reserve for later discussion. Middle-aged men fearing impotence often laughingly ask, "Could this be the change of life, doctor?" Sometimes the question has been prompted by an accusation on the part of the wife and the patient informs the physician that his wife "has been kidding him about the change of life." Some of the feelings underlying these statements can be easily inferred —joking and kidding have been hiding a good deal of anxiety.

Seeking Quick Cure. There always has been a tendency in medicine to seek a quick cure for mental symptoms—a cure which need not call into consciousness the emotions of the patient or of the physician. Three of the most important magical tools for this effort have been: (1) some appliance through which electricity could be given, (2) manipulation and massage, (3) the hypodermic syringe. The first and second have long been favorites in the treatment of impotence of psychological origin and now the third enters in the cloak of science to "replace the strength of declining manhood." The lurid literature of certain of the drug firms has been in part responsible for this new method of exploiting neurotics. We do not mean to say that some form of replacement therapy for gonadal deficiency does not have its place, but, just as in the female menopause, we deplore its use as a panacea for the multitude of complaints included under the syndrome of the male climacteric. The psychiatrist rarely sees a patient suffering from neurasthenia who has not been treated over a number of months or even years with tonics, sedatives, glandular injections, and still other methods which have given only temporary relief. The case of mild depression which will respond to replacement therapy will respond more surely to psychotherapy and stands a better chance of remaining well, because one must not forget that the suggestive effect of glandular injections is short lived.

Psychosomatic Observations.   It is always unfortunate for the cause of science when an illness of psychological origin yields to the suggestive effect of another method of treatment. The element of suggestion is not evaluated and a false therapeutic claim is established which provides another hurdle for the cause of psychosomatic medicine. However, better observations are being made. Rosenzweig and Hoskins carefully administered a variety of endocrine preparations to a male homosexual for six months and at the same time studied him psychologically without being able to detect any modification of personality.

The study by Tauber and Daniels, already referred to, combined replacement therapy and psychological observations on a male castrate. In the beginning, treatment with androgenic substance increased sexual desire, but this was followed by a subsequent decline in potency which was influenced only by psychotherapy. Study of the emotional life revealed that there was a homosexual trend, i.e., a wish to play the feminine sexual role. At the same time, there was a conscious rejection of this wish. The patient showed marked hostility toward those people representing father and authority. Castration had actually taken place at the hands of a man (surgeon) and the patient had been made more effeminate. This increased the patient's passive personality trends. Since passivity was a challenge to the patient's security as well as to the cultural tradition of being virile, it naturally produced an aggressive response, in this case directed toward the physicians who treated him. The authors here made the point that inasmuch as castration introduced a greater feminine component into the personality, the patient's sexual conflicts were intensified. Having been made more feminine through castration, he had to struggle emotionally against his passive tendencies. Because of this psychological conflict he was unable to cope adequately with the sexual tension induced by hormones. Thus it became clear that after castration, hormonal therapy might operate to interfere with effective sexuality. Consequently the lesson may be drawn that it is important to study the personality before hormones are administered; otherwise the success of treatment by replacement therapy may be jeopardized.

Just as we have made the point before, it is not a question of either hormonal replacement therapy or psychotherapy but rather the necessity for a psychosomatic study of the individual to be treated, in order to determine whether one or the other or both will be necessary.

Case 41.   The Male Climacteric?

History and Symptoms.   R. K., a white man of 53, complained of tension and fatigue. He had always been a teacher in a small town and had one son, who had referred the patient to us.

He said that he had been working hard, smoking moderately, and taking an occasional drink. For the last two or three years there had been a gradual diminution in his sex desires—"it had never meant much to him."

Physical Examination.   The physical examination was negative except for slight elevation of the blood pressure which had not been noted five years previously. There was slight tremor and on further questioning the patient stated that he had become a little more intolerant to heat and somewhat irritable. Ordinary laboratory studies were negative and basal metabolism was within normal limits.

In a note of that visit we observed the following familiar, differential diagnostic problem with which we were concerned at the time, namely, anxiety neurosis, so-called neurocirculatory asthenia, mild hyperthyroidism and, in relation to the whole problem, the question of the male climacteric.

LIFE SITUATION

The son told us that his father had been getting more irritable during the past year and suggested that he was worried about the future. On that basis we began the discussion using the illustration of "body language"—that dizziness and vertigo may be the body's physical expression of insecurity. He said that since the new governor had come into office a bill had been passed forcing the retirement of teachers at the age of 62 and in his case this would provide only a small pension which would be insufficient for him and his wife to live on. He had invested all of his money in his son's education and wondered whether the son would be willing and able to take care of them. As he discussed this problem he became very emotional and it was obvious that this was the point that was disturbing him. We spoke about the son's future and the fact that he wouldn't let his father down and then reassured him as to the absence of organic disease.

He remained well for more than three years. Then he began to lose weight, and became worried and fretful. The physical examination showed frequent irregularity in the heart rate, and the electrocardiogram indicated early evidence of myocardial disease. Otherwise the examination was negative and basal metabolism was still within normal limits. The patient was smoking heavily. His wife's illness and the necessity for looking after her himself "had been too much for him." But his son had entered the service and this had reactivated his insecurity.

SUMMARY

Here was an average man reacting to stress and strain by presenting some of the psychic, sexual and vasomotor disturbances that are sometimes associated at this period of life and are now often referred to as the male climacteric. Whether they should be is not so much the question except in so far as it bears upon treatment. In general it may be said that too much is apt to be blamed on the menopause and just as in the woman, treatment is apt to be restricted to endocrine products. In this case very simple psychotherapy did a great deal. It was the kind of psychotherapy that any physician should administer and it does not have to be called psychotherapy. It is simply a normal part of the physician-patient relationship but it depends upon a knowledge of psychopathology. Here too we see the necessity for equal attention to tissue pathology as we watch this middle-aged man developing degenerative heart disease which of course will also enter into the question of his emotional problems to produce indissoluble psychosomatic relationships.

TREATMENT OF GENITOURINARY AND SEXUAL PROBLEMS

Disturbances of Sexual Functioning

As stated in the introduction the sexual function is almost invariably impaired in the various neuroses and psychosomatic states. So true is this that the degree of sexual impairment often serves as a crude index to the degree of neurotic disturbance. In other words it is one phase of the disturbed personality development and as such demands treatment. Some cases will need more attention to the sexual life than others. Naturally in a neurosis in which actual frigidity or impotence is present, every effort should be made to bring about a cure of this condition because, while not in itself the cause of the neurosis, it may constitute the most serious symptom or may add to the total problem of treatment. When a personality disturbance is interfering with sexual functioning it means that one of the important means of drawing emotional sustenance from the environment is cut off and therefore needs treatment along with other aspects of the personality problem, in order to strengthen the emotional resources of that patient. Hence it should be made clear to the patient that impotence and frigidity are not personal peculiarities which must be kept hidden but are fairly common conditions which can be treated psychologically. Even though impotence and frigidity are only two of the many symptoms that may occur in a neurosis, it seemed best, because of their special importance, to discuss their treatment here rather than in the chapters devoted to the general aspects of treatment.

Eliciting History. We suggest the following procedure for eliciting the psychopathology which underlies these conditions:

Obtain complete life history of the patient according to the personality outline (p. 78) but with special emphasis on the following topics:

1. Did the parents seem to be in love with each other?
2. Were they affectionate with each other and tolerant of a demonstration of affection in others?
3. Did the patient receive any sexual education and if so, when?
4. What was the attitude of the parents toward sex matters? [Three general attitudes commonly found in parents: Sexual expression was (*a*) accepted; (*b*) condemned; (*c*) ignored—worst of all!]
5. Were sexual matters regarded as disgusting? Why?
6. Was any care taken in sexual education to separate sexual functioning from the excretory function?
7. Was there any religious attitude in the home which made sexual pleasure incompatible with ethical standards?
8. Were love of the opposite sex and sexual expression associated or not?
9. Were fears cultivated over sexual expression, such, for example, as the evil results of masturbation, the pain of venereal disease, or the shame and disgrace of illegitimate pregnancy?
10. Was sexual indulgence pictured as mean or hateful, disgraceful, or frivolous?
11. Was there any excessive emotional attachment to either parent?
12. Were the social and procreative roles of man and woman, respectively, clearly outlined during the period of psychosexual growth?
13. What evidences are there from scrutiny of the patient's history of social behavior to indicate homosexual love or too much self-love?

14. Was there much or any masturbation, during adolescence and prior to marriage? If not, what was the reason for its absence?
15. Was there much spontaneous genital feeling aroused through the reading of romantic stories, petting, dancing, or as a result of daydreams about the opposite sex? If not, what reason is given?

Summary

1. What wrong attitudes and feelings exist in the patient which must be changed?
2. What new attitudes and feelings must be learned in order to create the proper attitudes for sexual functioning?

Physician's Attitudes. It is very important that the physician who intends to assist patients in a better sexual adjustment should believe in the importance of a good sexual adjustment for good emotional health. At the same time he himself must not have too many prejudices or condemnations concerning sexual behavior. Otherwise the patient will sense the physician's prejudices or condemnation and will be unable to tell the real truth about himself.

Psychotherapy. In the modification of the deep prejudices and fears which surround the sexual function the physician, to do effective therapy, must have good insight into the effects of faulty sexual teaching in childhood and be able to undo, educate, reeducate and inspire new attitudes and behavior. He needs a philosophy of life which gives wholesome sex activity its proper place. If he has this and sees the problem when elicited in the history, change in the patient begins in the first interview. Patients often ask as their problem is being analyzed, "What do I do?" This question should not baffle the physician who can answer: "After you have seen the problem, ideas and attitudes will begin to rearrange themselves in your mind automatically. Then make up your mind what you want to do and we will see what keeps you from doing it."

A simple realistic formulation of normal, logical living may be very helpful. For instance, many a man does not know what to do about his wife's frigidity. He sulks, he complains, he gets drunk, he tries a mistress and still does not solve the problem. He could be shown how to set a suitable time and place for a discussion and say to his wife: "We married to share each other's lives and to take care of each other and if possible make each other happy. I am more interested in sex relations than you. But you can have sex relations more often, I am sure, if you will realize that it is important and meaningful to me. It is not wrong or wicked, it is not harmful to you. Quite the contrary. Why should we be angry, reproach each other, have scenes and discord because of something we could make work out well if we accepted and practiced the vows we made when we married? I will try to make you happy in as many ways as I can and surely you can try to make me happy in this way."

A talk with sincerity and common sense as its basis, held soon after trouble begins, might not solve all sexual maladjustment of this sort but it could start the solution of a great many problems. If a husband lacks the common sense or courage for this approach the physician can give it to him. If a man overlooks such an approach because of its simplicity, remind him that a simple, sincere, forthright approach, applied with good will, solves many problems, including sexual ones.

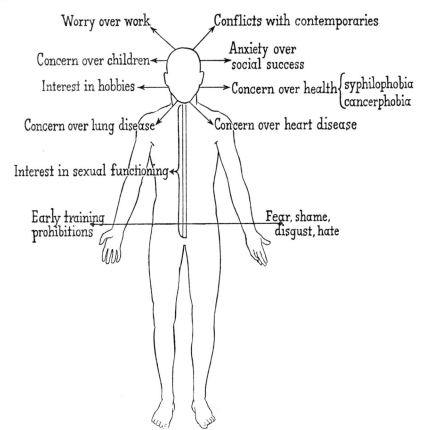

Worry over work

Conflicts with contemporaries

Concern over children

Anxiety over social success

Interest in hobbies

Concern over health { syphilophobia, cancerphobia

Concern over lung disease

Concern over heart disease

Interest in sexual functioning

Early training prohibitions

Fear, shame, disgust, hate

Figure 8. This diagram is an attempt to show graphically how certain factors may cause impotence and frigidity. Early educational prohibitions to the personality are sufficiently strong to prevent psychic energy from finding its way into the genital function, and this energy is expended to excess in many other channels. To effect a cure, redistribution of psychological energy is necessary. Anxiety and false beliefs must be relieved so that energy can be withdrawn from an area where it is being needlessly expended, such as worry over heart disease or worry over work, and allowed to flow into the genital region.

Sometimes men in middle life experience an occasional sexual difficulty and worry about a premature decline or loss in potency. This is often due to too great a preoccupation with business and other responsibilities. Solving problems takes an intense output of aggressive energy. Life is a competitive struggle. Fighting and loving are antithetical. A woman once said of her husband, "He has worked so hard at solving problems that he has lost the desire to love a woman." She was right. Men do this and their sexual potency declines because of it. They should have this factor pointed out to them and be advised to make the necessary changes to compensate for it. It may be overambition which is making them work too hard, or it may be guilt at the thought of playing. The same thing, of course, applies to women but their aggressive pre-occupation is more often one of running the house, keeping it clean, and rearing the children. But with the increasing number of women who are working the same problems arise in them, so that both sexes are having difficulty in enjoying each other as much as would be desirable.

Most sex problems between men and women are not difficult to understand. What is difficult is to get them to pause, and think calmly about what the place of sex should be and could be in their lives if they were kind to each other. To these problems the physician has to give time, understanding, wisdom, and the ability to relate the phenomena of psychosexual growth to the presenting problem. Then his job is to reeducate his patients along these lines.

Psychological Factors in Urological Disorders

Some years ago Menninger discussed psychological factors in urological disease. He introduced the subject by suggesting that even the idea that psychic factors were important might seem presumptuous since the existing knowledge of anatomy, bacteriology and immunology in this field was so much more complete than the knowledge of psychology. Moreover, thousands of urologically afflicted people are being successfully treated every day without any particular consideration of psychological factors. Nevertheless, he felt that a discussion of the psychological factors had a very practical value. He remarked then, and it is still true, that few psychiatrists are competent to make urological examinations, while few urologists are interested in making psychological examinations. The urologist examines the patient's genitalia, and the psychiatrist examines the patient's emotions, and each comes to his own conclusions. Menninger suggested examining more carefully the respective findings and theories of the urologists and the psychiatrists with respect to the symptoms of importance. He discussed the problem somewhat as follows:

The Urologist's Point of View. The urologists have made certain observations concerning the organs involved in impotence which cannot be disputed. They find, with some degree of regularity, that many patients complaining of impotence show definite congestion and inflammation of the posterior urethra, especially of the verumontanum, and tenderness, enlargement, and congestion of the prostate, either with or without evidence suggesting infection. The interpretation generally given these data by the urologists is something as follows: The prostate becomes the site of a local infection owing to a combination of factors—for example, masturbatory congestion plus infection, or local injury plus streptococcal localization. The resulting inflammatory reaction impairs functional activity (impotence). The impotence causes the patient mortification and anxiety—he is driven by this distress to seek medical treatment and comes to the urologist. The urologist treats the local condition (by massage, irrigation, endoscopy, chemotherapy, and so on) and it shows improvement. The impotence then (sometimes) disappears, and the theory is substantiated. However, the persistence of both inflammation and impotence may be regarded as evidence for the theory of an organic lesion which resists efforts toward removal.

The Psychiatric Point of View. Psychiatrists find that many patients suffering from impotence prove upon examination to have a definite psychological need for this symptom, in spite of their distress about it. In other words, they have unconsciously *wanted* to be impotent in order to satisfy certain unconscious emotional needs. We have already referred to some of the specific emotions which, though they exist only in the unconscious, exert a contrary and prohibiting effect upon the sexual function. These consist in one or more of the following: (1) fears, especially of punishment or of injury; (2) hostilities toward the love object; (3) conflicting loves, particularly parental and homosexual fixations; (4) rejection of the masculine (or feminine) role with its responsibilities.

Associated with and dependent upon these emotions is a great sense of guilt, and experience has shown that the relief of this sense of guilt by any one of several devices will frequently serve to free the patient from his fears and thus from his inhibitions. Psychiatrists therefore are willing to believe that urological treatment occasionally cures impotence even when it is of psychological origin, but they ascribe the cure not to the structural changes effected by the treatment but to the gratification of the need for suffering always associated with the sense of guilt—for example, guilt over masturbation. The urologist finds the prostate enlarged, pus cells in the secretion, states emphatically that "prostatitis" is responsible for the impotence and treats the patient by prostatic massage and topical applications to the deep urethra. The patient has confidence in the urologist but also pays in time, effort, money and actual physical suffering. Thus guilt over his earlier sexual "offense" is relieved.

Prostatitis. Burning on urination, a sense of pressure in the perineum and in the rectum, and even pain in the lower back are often attributed to "prostatitis." Examination may find the prostate slightly enlarged and, whether enlarged or not, massage will sometimes produce a few pus cells. While pyogenic bacteria are rarely found, a diagnosis of "prostatitis" is usually made and treatment with prostatic massage is recommended.

For some patients prostatic massage, although painful, seems to yield certain satisfactions, and they are willing to keep it up indefinitely. Others, of course, find it tedious, time-consuming and painful, and eventually seek relief elsewhere.

Pain, pressure and discomfort in the perineal area are common under certain stressful circumstances of life, and even if the prostate is slightly enlarged and produces a few pus cells, it may not be the cause of discomfort. It is not difficult to create an "addict" to prostatic massage out of a guilt-ridden male worried about his genital apparatus.

Inquiry into the patient's thinking about disease in that area is indicated. He should be given an opportunity to discuss his psychosexual development—including his attitude toward masturbation, premarital and extramarital sexual experience. Any urethral discharge he may have had and *what was said about it* should be investigated. Worries should be ventilated and he should be reassured that his genital tract is healthy. This plan of procedure, (1) history, (2) examination, (3) discussion of special points and (4) reassurance, should settle the problem in most cases. If a second or third discussion and ventilation of worry do not suffice, consultation with a psychiatrist should be suggested.

References

Heller, C. G., and Meyers, G. B.: J.A.M.A., *126:* 472, 1944.
Menninger, K. A.: J. Urol., *34:* 166, 1935.
Rosenzweig, S., and Hoskins, R. G.: Psychosom. Med., *3:* 87, 1941.
Tauber, E. S., and Daniels, G. E.: Psychosom. Med., *3:* 72, 1941.

Chapter XIV

The Respiratory System

THE EFFECT OF EMOTIONS ON BREATHING

The respiratory system, like the gastrointestinal and cardiovascular systems, is profoundly influenced by the emotions. "Sighing respirations" are well known in general medicine, and while they are frequently referred to as "shortness of breath" it is generally recognized that they accompany functional illness. When we are frightened we "catch our breath," and under certain other emotional circumstances we breathe deeply. A feeling of "a weight on the chest" is a frequent symbolic representation that the patient has a "load on his mind" which he would like to get rid of by talking to someone about his troubles. "Smothered feelings" also often represent a conversion of repressed emotion which the patient has had no opportunity to talk about. "Ventilating" our feelings often allows us to breathe easier and feel better. A weight on the chest is a frequent symptom accompanying the nocturnal anxiety attack. Many nocturnal attacks of bronchial asthma are preceded by an anxiety dream. Textbooks of medicine are beginning to consider the "mental aspects" of pulmonary tuberculosis, and included in the case histories of this disease are events of emotional significance which have occurred coincidentally with the onset of symptoms. No attempt is made to regard this as a direct cause and effect relation, but physicians are beginning to suspect that some kind of relation does exist. More will be said on this subject shortly.

Analogy to Gastrointestinal Tract.   Binger, in an excellent article on "The Psychobiology of Breathing," points out that the respiratory apparatus is genetically and structurally related to the gastrointestinal tract, and that in many ways they seem to function similarly. Embryologically, the pulmonary respiratory apparatus develops from the hind part of the ventral wall of the head gut. He further points out that both systems are concerned with the incorporation of certain substances of the external environment, with the transport of these substances to the tissue cells, and with the excretion of certain products of tissue metabolism. He indicates how both digestive and respiratory systems can be susceptible to similar derangements such as spasms and secretory changes, and that both may act as pathways for the entrance

Page 415

of infectious organisms. He observes that if Alexander is correct in his assumption that the gastrointestinal tract may act out certain emotional trends having to do with ingestion, retention and elimination, it is conceivable that an organ system so closely parallel embryologically and functionally can exhibit similar responses. Indeed Alexander and Saul analyzed respiratory tracings with special reference to psychological correlations and felt that there was suggestive evidence of a relation between intaking and eliminating tendencies, observable in the mental life, and certain characteristics of the spirograms.

Neurosis and Respiratory Tracings.   Christie several years before had made a somewhat similar study in an effort to see whether there was any relation between the type of respiration and the type of neurosis. In speaking of the anxiety neuroses he referred to the fact that *effort syndrome,* while usually classified as a cardiac neurosis, is essentially

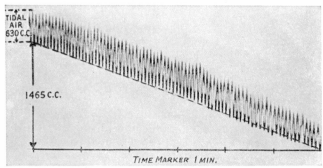

Figure 9.   Respiratory tracing from a normal individual. (Christie: Quart. J. Med., vol. 4.)

respiratory and that the invariable symptom is breathlessness, although most patients also complain of palpitation, giddiness, sweating and precordial pain, all exaggerated by exercise. He remarked that the breathlessness is reflected by a tendency to rapid and shallow breathing rather than a true hyperpnea. By inspection of the thorax in a case of effort syndrome he pointed out that it is possible to say that the breathing is rapid and shallow, but a respiratory tracing brings out several points which he believes to be even more characteristic of this condition: (*a*) an irregularity of the respiratory level; (*b*) an irregularity of respiratory depth; (*c*) a less marked irregularity of respiratory rate. Some of the examples of respiratory tracings taken from his article are reproduced. He does not, of course, believe that all cases of respiratory neurosis will give a typical respiratory tracing. But he does feel that the respiratory irregularity, if sufficiently pronounced, is diagnostic of a respiratory neurosis. A study of the respiratory curve as observed in the ordinary basal metabolic test will often furnish a clue in regard to these matters.

In a pneumographic study of 22 patients (15 with asthma and 7 with anxiety states) Stevenson and Ripley also found that respiratory patterns vary with the emotional state. Recordings were made while the subject was interviewed by the physician who discussed various topics and attitudes known to be of relevance to his life and illness. Respiratory symptoms were evoked in more than half of the patients, and the symptoms were related to changes in the respiratory pattern.

Sighing Respirations in Anxiety States. One of the commonest complaints of the neurotic patient is shortness of breath. When pressed for an explanation such a patient will frequently place his hand over the lower sternum and illustrate by a deep, sighing respiration that he "cannot get enough air." Whether he takes a great number of shallow breaths, or a smaller number of deep breaths, he exposes himself to the dangers of hyperventilation and alkalosis, and even tetany and uncon-

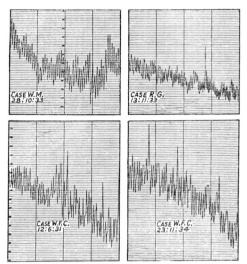

Figure 10. Respiratory tracings from cases of effort syndrome. (Christie: Quart. J. Med., vol. 4.)

sciousness, as eventual results. There are patients with severe anxiety states who sometimes fear that their breath may be cut off, and they are thrown into a panic. Misinterpretations on the part of the physician increase the patient's fear of heart disease, inability to breathe, and so forth; on the other hand a simple explanation of the mechanics of ventilation and reassurance regarding the absence of disease may accomplish a great deal.

In an analysis of a large number of spirograms Finesinger showed that the incidence of sighing respirations was highest in the group with anxiety states—60 per cent, as contrasted with 21 per cent for normal control subjects. Other neurotic and psychotic disturbances fell in between.

Physiological Mechanisms. After noting the observations by Christie and calling attention to Finesinger's studies that "unpleasant thoughts" are associated with increased depth and rate of respiration, Wolf and Wolff (in a paper previously referred to) made some deductions on this subject from their own observations:

1. That the hyperventilation observed under these circumstances is probably not the result of an increased CO_2 content of the blood.

2. Parenchymal engorgement of the lung is not a factor in the production of hyperventilation in these studies.

3. The production of hyperventilation, or at least its instigation, involves nervous mechanisms. The experiments of Wolf and Wolff suggested ". . . how the contractile state of skeletal muscle in posture and bodily movement associated with various emotional states may be linked with respiration. For example, if a discouraged, dejected individual listlessly approaches a task of lifting a weight or climbing stairs, the act is done so awkwardly that many more than the usual proprioceptive end organs are stimulated, and hyperventilation results. This barrage of afferent impulses may then, directly or indirectly, exert an influence upon the respiratory center. That this is not alone the result of a greater oxygen requirement for muscles inefficiently used was demonstrated by the fact that the oxygen consumption was not increased in proportion to the increased ventilation in these experiments."

4. Increased oxygen requirement in association with disturbing emotions may act indirectly in the production of dyspnea.

Engel and his associates studied the clinical aspects of hyperventilation, which they regard as psychogenic in origin in most instances. They divide the symptoms into those related to reduction in consciousness and those related to tetany. Reduction in consciousness correlates with the degree of slowing in the electroencephalogram while tetany is unrelated to changes in the E.E.G. Reduction in consciousness is associated with giddiness, faintness, lightheadedness, fullness in the head, blurring of vision, and other signs, while tetany appears after much longer periods of hyperventilation and is much less frequent.

Finally, in regard to such mechanisms, Faulkner observed that in a man being bronchoscoped, suggestions which produced feelings of insecurity caused the lumen of the bronchi to become smaller in diameter.

FUNCTIONAL RESPIRATORY DISORDERS

Case 42.   *Neurotic Dyspnea*

History and Symptoms.   A young white woman complained of "a smothering feeling and an inability to get the proper amount of air." She also said that her appetite was poor, on occasions she vomited, and there had been some loss of weight and strength.

The trouble had begun at the age of 18 just after she had finished high school. For some time she had been aware of enlargement of the neck but now she became nervous, suffered from smothering and choking sensations and a diagnosis of toxic goiter was made. She was admitted to a hospital, was studied for some time, and finally a thyroidectomy was done, but the symptoms grew worse instead of better and she was taken to a large clinic, where her family was told that there was no organic basis for her difficulties and that there was no point in being concerned about her shortness of breath. She then came east to make her home with her married brother but symptoms became so pronounced that she was finally brought to Philadelphia and tracheotomy was performed with the insertion of a tube. For the succeeding two or three years she considered herself pretty well but then once more suffered from exhaustion and a feeling that she was not getting enough air. It was at this time that she first came to our attention.

There was nothing remarkable about her previous health except that she had always been underweight and that the menstrual period had been established late and had been irregular and quite painful.

Patient was the middle child in a family of four sisters and a brother. The mother and father were both living and well. One sister had chronic arthritis and another had successfully been operated upon for goiter in a large clinic.

Physical Examination. Patient was an undernourished young white woman, who wore an expression of sullen suffering. The blood pressure was normal. There was some evidence of acne on the back and face, and the hands were cold and sweaty. There were no signs of hyperthyroidism. Examination of the mouth and throat showed nothing definite but the patient gagged easily. The breathing space of the nares seemed satisfactory. Aside from the scar of the goiter operation and the presence of a tracheotomy tube, the examination of the neck showed nothing abnormal. Heart and lungs were normal. The abdominal examination showed some generalized tenderness but this seemed a part of the general nervous reaction of the patient because there was no rigidity and no organs or masses were palpable. Knee jerks were excessive but the extremities were otherwise negative. We concluded that there was no gross evidence of disease and that we were dealing with a vagotonic type of individual.

LIFE SITUATION

The patient had been born and brought up in a small town in the far west. The father was very strict in the upbringing of his daughters and would not allow them to go to parties and dances like other girls of their age. Consequently there was often much quarreling in the home because the mother was much more lenient and sympathetic.

After she graduated from high school there was some question as to whether she should remain at home or go away to school as some of the other children had, and it was during this period that her attention was centered on the thyroid gland and the "toxic symptoms." After her admission to the local hospital her brother and his wife who lived in the east came home for a vacation and the decision was left to them whether she should be operated upon by a local surgeon or sent to a nearby large clinic.

Operations. In spite of the fact that the father could well afford to send her away to a more experienced surgeon the brother decided that it would be satisfactory for the operation to proceed and consequently it was done. As stated above, immediately afterward she became worse and then it was that she came east with this brother and his wife to make her home with them. On the way they stopped off at a large clinic where, according to the patient, the brother was told that it "was all nerves." As a consequence when she developed attacks of breathing difficulty in his home she was treated very unsympathetically and finally at the end of about six months she came to Philadelphia to make her home with an aunt. Then it was that the *tracheotomy* was performed and a tube inserted.

Marriage. Following our examination in 1934, when the patient was reassured about herself, she remained in fairly good health and subsequently married a man "who was very kind and considerate" and constantly solicitous about her health. She remained fairly well until about 1939 when symptoms returned and grew progressively worse. She became convinced that she needed a larger tube "to let more air in" and this was done but her symptoms continued.

Once more she was examined but again no evidence of organic disease was found. Now it was possible to learn a little more about her as a person.

Hostility. She very much resented the implication that there was no organic disease. In spite of her passive and docile exterior she would look at the examiner sharply and say angrily, "Well, what then *is* causing my breathing difficulty?" It became clear that she blamed the trouble on the "terrible operation" that was originally done on her neck and the scar tissue which she imagined was contracting and displacing the tube to one side.

She also had a great deal of resentment for the clinic where it had been said that her condition was "all mental" and she particularly held her brother responsible for the whole disastrous occurrence that had so wrecked her life. It was only by cautiously introducing the subject of her brother and his responsibility into the conversation that her resentment for him and particularly for his wife came out. She really felt that it was the wife who had influenced the brother to have her operated upon by the local surgeon so that "their vacation would not be interfered with." It was obvious from her conduct that she harbored a great deal of resentment. Slowly it was made clear to her that her principal symptom was *exhaustion* rather than shortness of breath and that the latter was related to the former. Then it was pointed out that her intense resentment and hostility which she had nursed over this great period of years was largely responsible for her exhaustion because it had sapped her energy. The explanation seemed a satisfactory one because as she *aired her hostility* she was able to breathe better; in other words, she was able to "let more air in" and at the same time she had more energy.

The occurrence which had been responsible for the return of symptoms seemed to be the fact that her brother had ceased to communicate with her and on one occasion she learned that he had been in her vicinity and had not even troubled to call her up. This inflamed her already great resentment.

SUMMARY

A young white woman suffered from exhaustion and breathlessness. She had been operated upon for goiter and then because of shortness of breath tracheotomy had been done and a tube inserted. Later symptoms returned and she felt that the tube was too small to allow enough air to enter but a new, larger tube failed to help her. Physical examination showed no organic reason for the dyspnea and the patient's attention was directed to the exhaustion instead, and the explanation was then given that emotional conflict stood in the background of the exhaustion. The emotional conflict surrounded a great deal of repressed hostility for a brother whom she held responsible for her misfortune, and when she was able to give expression to her hostility her symptoms diminished, that is, she was able to give herself better ventilation. The problem was an interesting one chiefly because of the complicated psychosomatic situation.

Case 43.   *Anxiety Attacks; Hyperventilation*

History and Symptoms.   A colored woman, married, aged 30, complained of attacks of breathlessness, weakness and palpitation. The first attacks had occurred a little more than two years ago. She was then free of attacks and perfectly well for about a year and then they recurred on three or four occasions during the past year. She also complained of frequent vomiting during the last few months.

The first attack occurred at night. She woke up with what she described as tremendous shortness of breath and pounding of the heart. She was sleeping on the first floor next to a window; she jumped out and ran up the street, feeling sure that she was about to die. The subsequent attacks occurred chiefly at night. She had been examined on several occasions during or immediately after an attack and attention directed to her heart as a possible cause. Previous medical history threw no light on these attacks. Her father was asthmatic; otherwise, the family history was negative.

Clinical and Laboratory Studies.   The intern on receiving ward suggested *hypoglycemia* as a cause, but although the initial fasting blood sugar was low subsequent tolerance tests failed to confirm this suggestion. The cardiac department suggested from their study that the patient might have suffered a *coronary occlusion* but there was nothing in the clinical picture to confirm this diagnosis. The gynecologist thought she might be *pregnant* but this was ruled out. General physical examination demonstrated no abnormalities. The blood pressure was 110/70. The temperature remained normal throughout her stay in the hospital. The urine was repeatedly negative; the blood count good; the Wassermann negative. X-ray studies demonstrated a normal chest and a completely normal gastrointestinal tract including the cholecystogram. The basal metabolic rate was minus 2. The vital capacity was 78 per cent. Neurological examination was negative and the eyeground study was normal. Thus, it was felt that we could safely rule out any evidence of organic disease.

LIFE SITUATION

Study of the emotional life revealed the following facts. At about the age of 14 or 15 the patient had a long illness during which she suffered from severe pains in the head. Many physicians were consulted but they failed to relieve her. She was finally taken to an "herb" doctor who informed her that someone had "poisoned" her by doing something to a lock of her hair and that was the reason that she had pains in her head. (She recalled that a man, working in the same factory, had removed some hair from her comb.) The cure prescribed was too tie the belly of a live frog against her forehead overnight! The following morning the frog was to be taken to the front door and if he hopped away he would carry her "misery" with him. She was very much upset by the process and very frightened; nevertheless, the frog behaved well and the "misery," so she states, left her, never to return. When 16 she married but continued to have sexual relations with another man and was frigid with her husband. He accused her of her infidelity and she finally left him, whereupon he said to her, "As long as you do not live with me, you'll never do any good." She tried her best to banish this thought from her mind, but, as we shall see, without success.

Powerful Effect of Superstition.   The first attack, as described above, occurred one night after she had had sexual intercourse with her lover and it seems reasonable to suppose that this furnished a situation to call forth the curse or "poison" that her former husband had put upon her. The reason that we suggest this is that after complete physical and laboratory investigations had been made upon this patient, we informed her that we could find no evidence of organic disease. She thereupon volunteered that this "bad nigger," her former husband, must have "poisoned" her. Asked why she hadn't suggested this idea before, she intimated that she had taken refuge in the thought that various doctors had suggested that she really had heart disease and also that the idea of being "poisoned" was so intolerable to her that she had done her best to keep it out of her mind.

A dream suggested some thoughts of unconscious origin to confirm our suspicions. She very often dreamed of snakes. Recently a dream occurred in which she was swinging over a pit where there were many snakes with black tops and white bottoms. To these snakes she associated enemies and "her husband, who hates her." Apparently the dangerous snakes symbolized the husband's "poison" that threatened her. Later she stated that on occasions she had also seen visions and heard voices.

Effect of Spinal Puncture.   We did not hope for success in the psychotherapeutic management of this patient but during the course of her study a spinal puncture was done which she concluded had "drained the poison off" and she left the hospital much improved.

It is of course noteworthy that not only in suggestible people do such physical measures often bring about temporary help. We have discussed this problem in other connections. The point is that so long as the underlying psychological origin of the anxiety is untouched, the symptom will return or something else will take its place.

The potency of the *taboo* in primitive thinking as a cause for anxiety probably occurs more often than we have been led to imagine is possible in our present-day civilization. Certainly it was well illustrated in this young colored woman, who must be considered as an early schizophrenic.

EMOTIONAL FACTORS IN COMMON COLDS

While it is generally agreed that colds are due to infection, there remains the suspicion that other factors are involved, particularly in the patient who develops colds too frequently. Some patients say they "have a cold all the time," or they "get over one cold, only to get another," or they "have a cold from the beginning of the winter until late spring." Stories like the following are frequently heard. A shy party guest finds himself sitting in a draft and knows that this may cause a cold, yet he is afraid to move lest he call attention to himself, or feels he would be imposing upon his host to ask to have the window closed, or for some other reason continues to remain in a position which endangers his health. Then there is the young woman who rides in an open car on a cold day and wears her most fetching clothes, but at the same time, clothes which are neither comfortable nor suitable for the weather. It is more important for her to make a pleasing impression upon someone than to think of the danger to her health.

These are rather superficial matters and might come under the heading of plain carelessness or foolhardiness. Nevertheless, they indicate that inquiry into the habits of living is necessary in cases of the common cold. The shy, anxious person who dares not move away from a drafty window can be reassured that he will not be despised or laughed at if he seeks to protect his health. The vain person can be shown other ways of gaining favor and prestige than courting a respiratory infection by unnecessary exposure.

More Complex Psychological Problems.   When we consider the people who seem to have repeated colds in spite of anything they do, and who may, in fact, be taking excellent care of themselves under all situations, we may find more complex psychological problems related to their indisposition.

Saul and his colleagues reported a study of 15 patients, treated psychoanalytically for other reasons, who were subject to unusually frequent colds and sore throats. Following treatment every one of these patients had been either entirely free from colds, or had them with conspicuous rarity. No treatment other than psychoanalysis had been employed in any of them.

CLINICAL FINDINGS.   Some of the clinical findings follow: A middle-aged man had a very passive personality which had resulted from spoiling in childhood by an overindulgent mother. This passive component of his personality was, of course, unconscious, and to keep it concealed, the patient made a great show of independence. When his expectation of receiving what he wanted from others was thwarted in his daily life, he reacted with dreams of attacking people with his mouth. His wife noted that his dreams and restlessness were accompanied by severe grinding of the teeth. As a result of these activities his throat, gums and jaws would be sore in the mornings. At the same time he would react with nasal congestion and secretion. If the thwarting of his desires was severe enough there would be coryza, mild depression of spirits, nausea, constipation, headache and fatigue. The symptoms would disappear almost immediately following insight into the unconscious mechanisms of his demands on those around him and his rage at being thwarted. For two years following the analysis of this patient there were no more colds, something the patient had never experienced before. Moreover, he was free from a mild soreness of the pharynx which had been persistent for many years.

Another patient who had severe colds all winter had anxiety, restlessness, and hypochondriacal fears of tuberculosis, accompanying each cold. A low-grade fever was almost invariably present. In this case, just as in the man previously mentioned, the colds occurred whenever the patient became distressed and panicky because her intense demands for attention and affection were thwarted.

In some patients *leukorrhea*, diagnosed by the gynecologist as a catarrhal vaginitis, often accompanied the cold. It was felt that the emotional stimuli might be the same for both a nasopharyngeal catarrhal secretion and a vaginal catarrhal secretion. This is an interesting connection when one thinks of the similarity of the lining mucosa and the presence of erectile tissue in both the genital and nasal regions.

ANXIETY AND DEPRESSION.   Saul and his coworkers believe that the general feeling of fatigue, loss of energy, malaise, and so forth, so frequently seen in colds, might be the manifestations of a mild depression of spirits and anxiety accompanying the cold rather than the toxic manifestations of the local inflammation.

"FEEDING A COLD."   The relation of this type of cold to allergy, rather than to infection, was mentioned but it was thought that whether the cause was a germ, a virus, changes in temperature, allergy, or a combination of factors, the emotional situation was the main etiological factor. These workers thought that the old saying, "Feed a cold—starve a fever," may have arisen because of the fact that these people who had been emotionally thwarted had some of their longings satisfied through eating, and that the eating process, therefore, did more than supply necessary nourishment. The conclusion of this study was that while one must recognize other factors than emotional conflicts in common colds, nevertheless, there may be cases which will be resistant to treatment until some deep personality problem is readjusted.

Relation to Allergy.   It is unfortunate that more psychological studies are not available of the common condition, *vasomotor rhinitis*, which is a kind of perennial hay fever. Elsewhere reference will be made to the general problem of the relation of the emotions to allergy and again the studies of Saul and his co-workers will be quoted. Probably many of their observations concerning hay fever apply equally well to this condition.

Usually vasomotor rhinitis is regarded as a purely allergic problem but its relation to sinusitis is important. Formerly it was often regarded as *sinusitis* and numerous operations were performed, usually without benefit. Now it is recognized that vasomotor rhinitis frequently precedes sinusitis. By blocking of the nasal passages drainage is interfered with and sinusitis may follow. What is not recognized is that emotional factors are just as important as allergic factors in its etiology (p. 486). This is a subject to which Wolff and his associates have devoted considerable attention.

EMOTIONAL FACTORS IN PULMONARY TUBERCULOSIS

Anyone who has carefully studied pulmonary tuberculosis realizes that there is more to the etiology of this disease than a constitutional factor and the presence of the tubercle bacillus. Two additional factors are undernourishment and fatigue. It has not been sufficiently stressed that there are emotional patterns which are related to eating habits, appetite and nutrition, and that these may be responsible for the underweight with which many cases of pulmonary tuberculosis begin. Furthermore, anxiety may prevent adequate sleep and rest. Finally, the shallow respiratory excursion seen in certain anxious personalities may play some role in this disease. These and other emotional factors should be considered in the etiology of pulmonary tuberculosis.

High Incidence of Neurosis.   It has been frequently observed by physicians and nurses working in tuberculosis sanatoria that there is a high incidence of neurosis in persons suffering from this disease. So often the neurosis is attributed to the disease but, as suggested above, the neurotic constitution may be present before the disease starts and indeed may be a factor in the etiology. In other words, neurotic symptoms during the course of tuberculosis are the result of neurotic trends present in the personality previous to the disease and only accentuated by it. The restrictions imposed by sanatorium life and the experiences of chronic illness, of course, add their complications. Intensive psychiatric treatment of the neurosis accompanying many cases of incipient tuberculosis would do much to hasten cure and to insure that the cure lasted, by bringing about a more efficient utilization of the patient's psychic energy.

A strong need for love and protection seems to be present in some of the cases which have been studied, the same trend which has been found in cases of disease of the upper gastrointestinal tract. One patient may have been overworking in order to obtain satisfaction for this emotional need, meanwhile taking poor care himself, while another patient may have reacted much more passively, readily submitting to the slightest indisposition, but in either case the relation of this emotional need to the total picture of the disease must be given more attention by general medicine. Certain aspects of this problem are understood and brilliantly described by Thomas Mann in *The Magic Mountain*.

Psychopathology.   A study of 785 patients by Wittkower, observed over a period of two and one-half years, provides much useful information concerning the role of emotional factors in tuberculosis. Wittkower made an attempt to explain the basis and the common features of the precipitating mental upsets.

He found that an inordinate need for affection is a common feature of the premorbid personality of tuberculosis patients. This need for affection may be openly expressed, thinly disguised, well concealed or flatly denied. Situations which arouse aggressiveness or endanger the delicately poised security system of the patients often precede the onset of symptoms of tuberculosis. In other words, he felt that individuals who develop tuberculosis seem to have in common an inability to deal adequately with their aggressive impulses and are prone, though for varying reasons and in different ways, to turn them against themselves.

A study by Benjamin, Coleman and Horndein demonstrated the high incidence of psychopathology in hospitalized patients with tuberculosis and showed the importance of personality factors in the onset and course of the disease and therefore the necessity for psychiatric orientation in treatment and handling. However, no pretuberculosis personality features common to a large majority of the patients were found. Dependency problems were of prime importance but this, the authors pointed out, might be a result of tuberculosis rather than its cause. In half of the cases, severe emotional conflicts, precipitated by actual life situations, were present at or shortly before the onset of the clinical tuberculosis. The authors felt, however, that the data were inadequate to draw conclusions as to any specific relationships. The same was true regarding emotional factors during the course of the disease. Hostility, as found by Wittkower, seemed to be of particular importance, or rather the status of it. Apparently unconscious hostility, which is inhibited, exerts an unfavorable influence, while the capacity to express conscious hostility is favorable.

Social Readaptation.　　Coleman and his associates were impressed with the relationship between personality trends and prognosis. Discussing all phases of the care and management of the tuberculous patient, they emphasize that medical care should include:

1. orientation of the patient to his illness,
2. evaluation of organic and psychologic factors and their interaction,
3. a plan of treatment to include organic and psychosocial factors,
4. a period of social readaptation, with regard for psychosocial as well as organic limitations. They look upon psychiatric insight not as an occasional need but as of continuous importance in any program of comprehensive care in tuberculosis.

Social Work and Tuberculosis.　　Largely through her work in tuberculosis the social worker has become recognized as an indispensable member of the medical team. Her position was securely established as a result of the broader approach to illness and disease achieved through the medical experiences of World War II. Where tuberculosis is concerned she enters into every phase of treatment, hospital admission and home care. Spencer explains that "family problems may arise during hospitalization which are harassing to the sick person and may impede his recovery. It is the [case] worker's responsibility to deal with these problems, frequently in cooperation with some other agency. Such situations may be due to the following causes: the lack of continuous correspondence from the family, the lack of a regular allowance, fears based on poor familial relationships, the threat which the illness presents to the patient in relation to his status in his home and community, and guilt arising from the inability to be a provider. In addition there are more deep-seated motivations, such as: realization of an unconscious drive to be sick in order to abandon family, job and community responsibilities; hostility toward a member of the family, who may be imagined as an instrumental agent in the inception of the illness; and restlessness as a result of the enforced relinquishment of normal social outlets and experiences with the family.

"The same or opposite reactions in the family picture may be noted and dealt with by the community [social] worker: anxiety caused by illness of one of its members; fears of infection of another individual of the group, generated by a knowledge of the disease and enhanced by the necessity for a checkup of every other group member; hostility towards the patient for having brought the disease into the home; acknowledgement, conscious or otherwise, by mother, father or siblings that they may have been in some way responsible for the patient's breakdown; rejection of the patient as a cause or result of the disease and bringing into consciousness of this rejection by the necessity for hospitalization; overcompensation for relief at the removal of the patient, expressing itself either in the attitude of being unwilling to face separation or in the anxiety manifested regarding the patient's progress."

Speaking of the service in a tuberculosis hospital, Spencer concludes that a comprehensive social service and vocational therapy department is an important factor, not only in the arrest or cure of the tuberculosis, but also in the stabilization of the personality to the end that the patient may remain well.

In a later paper from the same institution Axelrad emphasizes that the social worker's approach must be integrated with the total plans formulated jointly by the physicians, social worker and guidance counselor. She calls attention to the fact that staff members specifically trained to deal with the psychological difficulties of the patient need good medical orientation and the reverse is equally true; that is, staff members responsible for the physical care of the patient must have a psychological orientation.

Excessive fear of tuberculosis is a common clinical problem. It occurs both in those who have never had the disease and in those who have recovered from it.

Case 44.   Tuberculophobia—Fatigue and Slight Fever

History and Symptoms.   A young woman complained of fatigue and slight fever. She had been told that there was "something suspicious in her lung," whereupon she consulted a specialist who examined her thoroughly and told her that he did not *think* that she had tuberculosis. Nevertheless, the slight fever continued, and with the conviction of tuberculosis still present, she remained at rest in bed for one year. During that period she complained chiefly of fatigue and occasional mild diarrhea with a good deal of mucus in the bowel movements.

Physical examination and x-ray studies failed to disclose evidence of organic disease, and discussion brought out the following story.

LIFE SITUATION

During the winter prior to her illness she was keeping company with a young man and the townspeople took it for granted that they were engaged. The following summer, while she was considering the question of the marriage date, she became irritable, lost weight and felt ill. In September she had what she called "an attack of ptomaine poisoning" following a dietary indiscretion. It was during this attack that the fever was discovered and the suspicion arose that the lungs were affected.

Rest in Bed.   She then gave up her work and spent practically a year in bed. During this period the young man remained as attentive as ever, but she told herself that it was not fair to him to continue her engagement. She argued with herself in the following fashion: In view of her continued illness, she felt that it would be better to give him up; that she would not be strong enough to marry, to have children or to do housework. She had many more "reasons" why she should not marry. For one thing, both a brother and a sister had been unhappily married and were divorced. She also felt that her mother needed her, that she was happy at home, and did not like to leave. She informed us that her husband-to-be did not have enough money to marry but, on further discussion, there seemed no question that he would adequately support her.

TREATMENT

It seemed to us that a different approach to her problem was indicated. Instead of agreeing with her that she must exercise caution and that it would be better for her to put marriage out of her mind "until she was well," she was told that there was no physical evidence to indicate organic disease; that her slight fever was due not to any lung trouble but simply to a slight bowel disturbance which, in turn, was very closely associated with the worry and stress incident to the problem of marriage. We carefully avoided the term "colitis."

Then she was told that her illness represented an unconscious effort on her part to escape the responsibilities of marriage, and that all the points she raised about not getting married were simply self-deceptive rationalizations to assist her in escaping this responsibility. She then admitted that shortly after her engagement "she had a premonition that she would get sick." She was told that it was necessary for her to face the fact that she must either marry or not marry, and that she could not go on as she was going. Shortly afterward she announced that she would decide upon a marriage date. Following this resolution she became worse than ever. Her menses became irregular, she was fatigued all the time, had pain in the back, and became upset if there was any variation from her usual routine. Finally she forced herself to marry. Adjustment to marriage was difficult but at the end of a year she reported that she was fairly well. She still had considerable fatigue but did not worry about tuberculosis and no longer took her temperature.

This did not mean that all her troubles were over. Often there are grave problems ahead for the emotionally immature person who marries. This phase of the problem has been discussed earlier.

SUMMARY

A young white woman, following a slight bowel disturbance, discovered that she had fever. Suspicion was aroused that she might have tuberculosis and she spent a year in bed. Conflict over marriage stood in the background of the illness and partial recovery followed her marriage.

References

Alexander, F.: Psychoanalyt. Quart., *3:* 501, 1934.
Alexander, F., and Saul, L. J.: Psychosom. Med., *2:* 110, 1940.
Axelrad, R. K.: News Letter, Am. Assoc. Psychiatric Social Workers, *15:* 4, 1946.
Benjamin, J. D., Coleman, J. V., and Horndein, R.: Am. J. Orthopsychiat., *18:* 704, 1948.
Binger, C.: Ann. Int. Med., *11:* 195, 1937.
Christie, R. V.: Quart. J. Med., *4:* 427, 1935.
Coleman, J. V., Hurst, A., and Hornstein, R.: J.A.M.A., *135:* 699, 1947.
Engel, G. L., Ferris, E. B., and Logan, M.: Ann. Int. Med., *27:* 693, 1947.
Faulkner, W. B.: Northwest Med. J., *40:* 367, 1941.
Finesinger, J. E.: Am. J. Psychiat. (*a*) *100:* 159, 1943. (*b*) *100:* 659, 1944.
Holmes, T., Goodell, H., Wolf, S. G., and Wolff, H. G.: The Nose. Charles C Thomas, Springfield, Ill., 1949, Ref. 1, p. 590.
Saul, L. J. et al.: Internat. J. Psycho-Analysis, *19:* 451, 1938.
Spencer, E. C.: Jewish Social Service Quart., *19:* 307, 1943.
Stevenson, I., and Ripley, H. S.: Psychosom. Med. *14:* 476, 1952.
Wittkower, E.: A Psychiatrist Looks at Tuberculosis. London, The National Association for the Prevention of Tuberculosis, 1949.

Chapter XV

The Respiratory
System (Concluded)

BRONCHIAL ASTHMA

Asthma is a well-defined clinical condition that has been recognized since the days of antiquity. Thomas Willis described the disorder in detail in 1679 and stated that "the Ancients allowed the cause of it to be only obstruction of the bronchi," but he himself referred to "the default partly of the lungs and partly of the nerves appertaining to the breathing parts" (Major). In fact he held that every inveterate case of asthma was a mixed affection due to a combination of the two causes.

Diagnosis. The diagnosis of bronchial asthma is seldom difficult. Nevertheless, if we listened as carefully to the things that patients say as we do to the noises that their organs make we might learn a great deal more about the illness. With our stethoscopes we hear the patient with asthma wheeze but if he can talk and we give him a chance to be heard, he will tell us about other symptoms besides shortness of breath and, deliberately or unconsciously, will reveal much about himself as a person. That is, his feelings and his attitudes may give us as much information about his illness as the sounds that we hear or the tests that we do.

Emotional Factors in Bronchial Asthma. In the past twenty years or more many observations have been made and articles written on the relation of the emotions to bronchial asthma. Neurotic trends were recognized but, as in other "organ neuroses," were generally held to be due to the disease rather than causally related to it. It was noted that the sufferer from asthma often seems to make the most of his attack by drawing attention to himself and, by his distress, disturbing those around him to the utmost. Now, however, we recognize that the gain through such behavior is only secondary. The psychological factors that are important lie far deeper in the unconscious mental life, have no such thinly disguised purpose, and reveal themselves only after patient study.

McDermot and Cobb, in a clinical survey of 50 cases of bronchial asthma, studied each case from a psychiatric standpoint. They summarize their study as follows:

1. Thirty-seven of the 50 cases studied seemed to have an emotional component in the asthmatic attacks.

2. The 13 "nonemotional" were predominantly young males.

3. Twenty patients reported that the first attack was emotionally precipitated.

4. Thirty-one reported that later attacks were often emotionally precipitated.

5. Thirty patients showed neurotic traits other than asthmatic, usually of a compulsive nature.

6. Only 20 per cent of the "emotional group" were benefited by somatic therapy, while 54 per cent of the "nonemotional group" were benefited. Likewise in the "neurotic group" only about 20 per cent were helped by drugs and biological products, while 50 per cent of the "non-neurotic group" were helped.

Personality Structure of Children Suffering from Asthma. British investigators have been keenly interested in the psychological study of asthmatic patients. Strauss studied the psychogenic factor in asthmatic children and felt that a very large percentage were both overanxious and insecure. This anxiety often reflected the personality of the parents, who, in many cases, were themselves overanxious and insecure, and therefore would be expected to arouse a similar response in the children. He felt that the asthmatic children fell into two groups. The first were children who had been very much wanted by their parents, such as an only child or the first boy to be born in a family of girls, or vice versa; while the other group were definitely unwanted children whose parents were overcompensating for their unconscious hostility toward the child.

Rogerson, Hardcastle and Duguid also worked predominantly with children who presented the "asthma-eczema-prurigo syndrome." They report that out of 23 "no less than 17 of the children were fussed over and overprotected by their parents to a pathological degree. This was not just a slight abnormality of parental attitude, it was pathological to a degree which made one feel that if these children had not been brought to the hospital with asthma or prurigo they might easily have been referred on account of the nervousness engendered in them by this situation."

ATTITUDE OF PARENTS. This overprotective attitude of the parents was due to varying causes. In one case the overprotectiveness on the part of the mother was understandable, owing to the fact that she had lost several children and the patient was the only surviving boy. In several cases the children were born very soon after marriage; in two cases they were incident to forced marriages. In such cases the conscientious mothers were torn between a desire to love and cherish the children and a feeling of not really wanting them, which latter feeling, however, was so repugnant to their social ideals of maternity that they found great difficulty in bringing it to conscious expression. As a result of this ambivalence the mothers attempted to cherish and protect the children all the more strongly in order to overcome the feelings of guilt which the real attitude toward the child tended to produce.

THE ASTHMA-PRURIGO PERSONALITY. These authors conclude: "In

fact, if we might be permitted to generalize from this small group of cases we might speak of an asthma-prurigo personality. The characteristic of this 'asthma-prurigo' personality which our patients have shown may be summarized as follows: high intelligence on verbal tests with a poorer performance ability, marked overanxiety and lack of self-confidence, considerable latent aggressiveness and egocentricity."

PSYCHIC CONDITIONING.   The authors raise the question, which they leave partially unanswered, as to how far some of these characteristics may be "the result of difficulties produced by the disease itself in the patient's relationships with others." It would seem quite possible that the excessive anxiety of these children and their parents' overprotective attitudes may be in part a reaction to the disability caused by illness. A severe asthma attack with its acute threat of suffocation is obviously a terrifying experience to both the child and its parents and it is not surprising that children who suffer from asthma should develop feelings of helpless anxiety and insecurity and a tendency to cling to their parents, nor that the parents should develop an overprotective attitude toward them merely as a reaction to the fear of the asthma attacks themselves. On the other hand, the examples cited above make it plain that in a number of the cases reported in this study the overprotective attitude of the parents existed prior to the onset of the asthma and had also a deeper motivation, such as need to overcompensate for not really wanting the child or the fear of losing the only surviving child after several other children had died.

RORSCHACH STUDIES.   There is some evidence from Rorschach studies on asthmatic patients which suggests that the personality disturbance existed before the onset of the disorder. The Rorschach method (see p. 107), a projection test of the personality, has been widely used in recent years and seems to be one of the oustanding methods of personality evaluation. Schatia, who analyzed the Rorschach records of 40 patients suffering from bronchial asthma, confirmed an impression gained by a number of analytical workers that asthmatics tend to have compulsive personalities without evidence of phobia or compulsion. Dunbar called attention to this fact in 1938, and Felix Deutsch made similar observations from psychoanalytic study.

THERAPEUTIC EFFORTS.   That the overprotective attitudes of the parents and the excessive anxiety of the children probably also have some part in the causation or at least in the aggravation of the asthma itself is indicated by the results of Rogerson's therapeutic efforts, which were directed primarily to encourage greater independence in the child and a less inhibiting and overprotecting attitude in the parents. In accordance with their concept of the personality disorders associated with asthma, they attempted by psychotherapy to modify the attitudes of both the child and the parents. They tried on the one hand to induce the parents to adopt a less solicitous attitude toward their children and to allow a greater degree of independence; on the other hand they attempted to diminish the anxiety of the child and to encourage the child itself to adopt more independent attitudes. In a considerable proportion of the cases, the effects of this sort of treatment were very satisfactory even when the child remained in the home environment in which the asthma attacks had been severe.

The Site of Selection for Organ Neuroses. Gillespie, also of London, expressed his belief that "an idea may become the affective stimulus which elicits the asthmatic response just as much as pollen or horsehair." He believes that asthma furnishes a striking test of what needs to be emphasized in the education of the medical student: that the body and mind are one, or at least that their interaction is so close that no examination of a patient should neglect some consideration of what is going on in his mind. He felt that not only could psychological factors in the shape of emotions or ideas elicit individual attacks, but that these factors could also act in a continuous fashion to produce a state of tension which every now and then would reach the stage of explosion expressed by a paroxysm of asthma. Why the organism should choose asthma as a special mode of expressing mental unrest, he thought, depended upon constitution, a preexisting fear of lung disease, a preexisting disease of the lungs, a conception of breathlessness, or an imitation of asthmatic attacks which the patient had witnessed. Felix Deutsch has also been interested in the choice of organ in organ neuroses. He suggests that many affections of the respiratory tract in childhood, coinciding with excessive emotional dependence upon the mother, formed a combination which might result in asthma. Thus the early affections of the respiratory tract plus its use for the expression of conflicting tendencies throughout childhood would create a personality of a specific structure. The mothers in these cases usually encourage the dependence and at the same time suppress the aggressive tendencies in such children; hence, the conflicts underlying this interaction between mother and child form the background for asthma.

Further Psychoanalytic Observations. The most comprehensive work on this subject has been carried out at the Institute for Psychoanalysis in Chicago. The work was first reported in a paper by French, which later appeared in monograph form. Twenty-seven cases were studied. The cases chosen were nearly all patients in whom *allergic hypersensitivity* had been previously demonstrated by means of allergic history and skin tests, this work having been judged by an experienced allergist.

Variability in Personality Traits. When the cases were reviewed from a psychological point of view, the first impression was that the sufferers from asthma varied considerably both in their personality traits and in the type of emotional disturbance for which they sought treatment. A number of the patients had been particularly good children and in adult life their behavior was characterized by an urge to help and give to others. Some of the children, on the other hand, were brought to treatment because of their particularly aggressive behavior. In one of the adult patients and in one of the children the picture was that of a compulsive personality with mild compulsive neurotic symptoms. An asthmatic man sought treatment originally on account of conscious homosexual impulses.

Common Features. However, in spite of these differences, the cases showed certain common features. In several it was found that the patient would have an attack when he was exposed to a situation which might estrange him from a parental figure, usually the mother. This might occur in an actual life situation or might be portrayed by dreams. The attack of asthma occurred at the point where the defenses failed and the patient was suddenly exposed to the conflict between an actual life situation and the fear of losing the mother's love. These emotions would become transferred to the physician in the course of treatment, and the patient's fear of losing the good will of his physician took the place of his original fear of losing the mother's love. Over and over again these patients would become blocked just at the point where the unconscious material was leading up to a confession, which represented an attempt at reconciliation with the mother figure. They would be afraid to confess and would develop an attack of asthma. As long as the technique of winning reconciliation with the mother by confession was successful, the patients appeared to be protected from asthmatic attacks. When the confession got "choked in the throat" an asthmatic attack occurred in its place.

Relation to Crying. There was much to suggest that the asthma attack is really a sort of equivalent of a cry of anxiety or rage which has been inhibited and repressed. For some reason, in the situations which provoked asthma attacks the child was unable to cry. Some of the patients stated they had not cried for years, and others boasted they had never been afraid. In some of the treated cases it was observed that as the asthma attacks ceased, attacks of crying appeared in their stead. Such replacement of asthma attacks by crying was particularly apt to occur as insight was gained into the cause of the attacks.

Threatened Loss of Mother's Love. The fear of temptation, and the loss of love threatened by yielding to the temptation, seemed to occur particularly in relation to the mother. Frequently, in the family histories, it was noted that the mother was overprotective to the child and bound the child to her in a dependent relationship but at the same time rejected the first signs of the child's genital interest. This created a situation in which the first early strivings of genital sexuality became a temptation which threatened to deprive the child of the mother's love, upon which it was so dependent. It was striking with what frequency the mothers of these patients played the double role of being at one and the same time seductive and prohibitive. Four of 6 adult male patients had continued to sleep with their mothers until the age of puberty or even later.

Aggression. The situation which threatened loss of the mother's love did not arise out of sexual temptation in every case. Pregnancy in the mother or the birth of other children seemed to play a role in precipitating asthma attacks. The possibility of another child, or the actual presence of another child, was a definite threat of the loss of the mother's love, and this in turn stirred up aggressive impulses, both toward the mother and toward the younger child.

Other Defenses. Defenses other than confession were utilized by the patients. Some were overobedient, seeking to avoid rejection in this way.

Still others utilized sickness and suffering for gaining sympathy and affection. It was noted that symptoms such as rheumatic pains or headaches would tend to protect the patient from an attack of asthma. In the case of a male patient, an attack of asthma resulted in his being taken into his mother's bed. It was noted that many asthma patients were particularly prone to attacks of asthma at times when they were in conflict as to whether or not to leave some mother figure. Similarly, during psychological treatment, it was observed that asthma attacks tended to occur predominantly on weekends or during the periods just preceding some separation from the physician.

Summary.   To summarize this material concerning the emotional background of attacks of asthma, French concluded that asthmatic attacks tend to be precipitated by situations that threaten to separate the patient from some mother figure. The separation feared may be actual physical separation; more frequently it is the danger of estrangement from the parental figure due to some temptation to which the patient is exposed. In such a situation the asthma attacks seem to have the significance of a suppressed cry.

In this connection Alexander added that in some asthma histories we learn of the peculiar, childish habit of breath-holding. To be sure this habit may occur also in nonasthmatic children. The background of breath-holding, however, seems to be always the same: A spiteful protest against the environment, something like a hunger strike; "If I do not get the protection I want, I will not breathe." Alexander continues, "The other emotional factor in the asthma attack expresses just the opposite tendency. The patient suppresses an expiratory function, crying, by which he would express his protection-seeking attitude toward the mother. This suppression of crying represents the opposite tendency, the wish not to give in to the dependent attachment to the mother.

"Thus, the asthma attacks, like a hysterical conversion symptom, express both opposing tendencies: the protest against separation and the protest against wanting to reestablish a dependent relationship to the mother by crying. This conflict seems to be the deepest and most primitive substratum of the asthma attack."

PSYCHIC AND ALLERGIC FACTORS COMPLEMENTARY.   Finally French and his colleagues concluded that *psychological* and *allergic* factors probably stand in a somewhat complementary relationship to each other in the etiology of bronchial asthma; that in some cases asthma attacks may be precipitated by allergic factors alone, in others by emotional factors alone, and in still others the combination of allergic and emotional factors seems necessary to bring about an attack.

The following case is cited in detail to show the interplay of complex factors in the pathogenesis of bronchial asthma and to indicate certain treatment problems.

Case 45.   Lifelong Asthma; Recovery Following Psychoanalysis

History and Symptoms.   A healthy-appearing, young white woman was first seen in June 1946. She reported that she had had severe asthma since early childhood and that in the more than twenty years that she suffered from this disorder she had known only a few periods of real freedom. These were the periods during which she was away at school, and her two pregnancies. She also had eczema as a child and on a few occasions since, and vasomotor rhinitis which had been quite bothersome in recent years.

The mother suffered from migraine and had asthma in her early years, and a brother had hay fever. The father had died of "heart disease" in 1942.

The patient reported that eczema began in early infancy and that asthma occurred at about the age of 2; this was confirmed by the mother. When the asthma became quite severe about the age of 7 she was studied in a large hospital where allergic tests were made for the first time. These tests were repeated frequently afterward, the last time three years ago in the course of a complete study at a well-known clinic. Certain foods were denied the patient which she says she eats with impunity during the periods when she is free of asthma.

Physical Examination and Laboratory Studies. Physical examination showed a robust young woman with no evidence of eczema, rhinitis or asthma at the time of examination. She appeared to be in good health, and no evidence of organic disease was detected. Routine laboratory studies were negative.

LIFE SITUATION

She was an obedient child who was taught cleanliness early. Brought up in a small community where the parents were in comfortable circumstances, she enjoyed all of the material possessions that a child could want. In fact she reported that her father, a tense, nervous and domineering person, "gave gifts instead of understanding." He demanded exacting obedience and the patient resented his treament of her as well as of the mother. The father was so emphatic in his instructions to the young girl regarding men that she was constantly warned about the dangers of murder and rape. Pity for the mother, the mother's air of martyrdom and her threats of withholding love, forced the child into a submissive attitude. She tried to make up to the mother for the way the husband treated her.

Disturbed Relationship to Mother. She looked to the mother for approval, was very dependent upon her and yet, as she reached later childhood, found difficulty in accepting gifts from her. She felt that there was something wrong about doing so and this feeling has continued to the present time. Apparently accepting a gift was an indication of the dependence against which she struggled. When she went away to school, for the first time she became free of asthma for a long period and the asthma would recur only when she returned home at vacation time. In the junior year she was assailed with doubt regarding her choice of career but was afraid to change because of the mother. In order to solve the problem she became engaged, married the following year, and immediately became pregnant, "in order not to have to finish school." She was well during the pregnancy but a few weeks after the birth of the child asthma began again, and she then decided to leave home and move to Philadelphia. The father objected but she left anyhow. Shortly afterward he died of "heart disease." She felt no grief, "only a slight guilty feeling," and merely expressed the thought that "if she had not left this might not have happened."

Emotional Factors. Sexual intercourse, which had been painful before the birth of the child, continued to be unsatisfactory. She became concerned about the frigidity and decided to consult a physician but again asthma interfered. After another period of hospital observation failed to help the patient, she and her husband decided to move south. She did not, however, do well there and they ran into great difficulties, with the husband trying to earn a living and take care of the sick mother and child. The patient came north to visit the mother, who had remarried, so that she would no longer have to worry about the mother "being alone," but the asthma continued. When her child was three she decided that because she had been well during pregnancy another pregnancy would be helpful. True enough she again felt completely well during the second pregnancy but again developed severe asthma shortly afterward. Now the husband's difficulties were redoubled because he not only had to work harder to earn a living but had a very sick wife and *two* young children to look after.

The patient went from doctor to doctor until finally one of them suggested that emotional factors must have something to do with her illness. For the first time she began to think of her illness from that standpoint and, recalling that during her school days she was entirely comfortable away from home and sick as soon as she got home, she concluded that her relationship to her mother must be the reason.

Self-Analysis.   Now, as the patient "thought the problem out for herself," she went through a very bad period. She was sleepless and despondent, had a "terrible, queer, detached feeling"—as if she were in another world; suffered from dizziness, pressure on the head, blurred vision; had fears that she would lose her mind or commit suicide and was unable to be alone with the children for fear that she might harm them. Her physician was in constant attendance and she poured out to him many of the thoughts regarding her life and her relationship to her parents, husband and children. She spoke of resentment against the father, of her hated dependence upon her mother, and of a nameless resentment against the husband "as though she would like to throw a knife at him." At the same time she admitted that he was an extremely able person and an excellent husband. If anything "he was too good" to her. She decided that she had been escaping from life and that with the doctor's help she would learn to face things. Now her black moods came and went and at times she felt exhilarated. For the first time she was able to achieve orgasm in intercourse. She felt like a different person: as if "a new personality was emerging." She described this new person as more adult, possessing a great deal of self-confidence. For several weeks she continued in this mood and was quite free of asthma but then, for reasons that she did not understand, her chest tightened up again and she became as ill as before. The couple decided to leave Florida and on the way north by automobile she was very ill, causing the husband a great deal of distress and effort as he looked after her and the family.

Conflict of Love and Hate.   After establishing herself in Philadelphia she very quickly improved as she was encouraged to talk about her life situation. Almost her whole conversation centered on the topic of her relationship with her mother and just as she described her life up to this year as one of affection and devotion to the mother, now her sentiments were just the reverse. She could find almost nothing good to say about the mother. In an interview with the mother we did not gain the impression that she was mean or malicious but it was apparent that because the mother had been deprived of love as well as material things in childhood she was determined to see that her own child was loved, protected and denied nothing. Thus she overprotected the child, confided in her regarding her loveless marriage, and made the girl too dependent upon her by threatening her with loss of love. These were the conclusions that the patient had reached in her self-analysis.

She described the mother as an infantile person who had encouraged the child's dependence, overprotected the daughter to satisfy her own emotional needs, dominated her by threatening loss of love and by an attitude of martyrdom, withheld help when it was necessary, and gave gifts that were not wanted.

The patient had some insight, however, because she spoke of desiring a better relationship to the mother with neither the affection she had felt before nor the hostility which she now feels. The mother would call on the telephone and say that she was going to visit the patient and the patient would develop an attack of asthma immediately upon hanging up the receiver. The mother would send gifts that the patient found impossible to accept, or if she did accept them she promptly lost them. On one occasion she lost a valuable piece of jewelry and felt no remorse. This quixotic behavior was not confined to the mother, however, because on one occasion the husband gave her a twenty-dollar bill which disappeared the next instant and was found in the baby's play-pen. The husband recovered it and handed it back to her, telling her to be careful, and the next moment it was gone again. This time it was found in the waste basket.

Dreams.   Her dreams dealt with frustration (for example, being tied up in a car that could not get up a hill, or in a plane that could not reach its destination). About the time that she was trying very hard to get established in a home she had a dream of "buying a house with a fence around it. In order to get the house she had to take the fence." In the face of this very obvious symbol she was asked what fenced her in and her reply was her illness, her mother, and housework. She was trapped in her adult life as well as in her childhood by the dependent relationship upon her mother, which she hated but from which she could not escape. It seems significant, however, that all the time that she was freely expressing her hostility for the mother she was free from asthma except for very minor attacks occurring in direct connection with the mother's visits, presents or telephone calls. The husband observed that when the mother visited them the patient "withdrew from him, not only sexually but in every way."

PSYCHOANALYSIS

However, the patient was not satisfied with herself. As she explained, "My symptoms were changed into feelings but I couldn't live with them either." So in 1949 she was referred for more intensive psychotherapy.

The analyst reported that she spoke of her "peculiar dependency on doctors" which had begun very early in life. She had a feeling of great personal loss when discontinuing treatment with her various physicians. She spoke of the father's elation when her brother was born and her own love for that brother which was only akin to her love for her son. She straightened out her relationships to men through her work with the analyst. She came to realize that an adequate expression of emotions protected her from asthma. In other words if she was able to express strong feelings then there would be no asthma.

As she improved she was able to take a summer job working in a girl's camp where she was reliable, thoughtful and understanding and achieved a good deal of recognition.

Suddenly the mother died of a cerebral vascular accident and although "everybody expected her to be sick," the patient remained well. She was able to express the normal amount of grief but adjusted well and for the first time she experienced feelings of missing her father. In 1951 she appeared at a psychosomatic conference and was proud to be able to say that she had been free of asthma, or any other serious symptoms, and was able to function well.

As she worked out her feelings of hate and love and became more certain of her feminine identity, she found that her conflicts in relation to father and brother had been displaced to the many physicians in her life. She also saw that the same problems came up at home and involved her son and her husband. For the first time she achieved emancipation from inhibitions in regard to these important people so that she was able to live more comfortably with them. She has now been well for more than five years. She is not only free from asthma but has become a much happier and more capable person and leads a full life. Because she had expressed her feelings so well in a number of letters she was encouraged to write her life story.* Some excerpts from it may be interesting in getting a patient's reaction to psychiatric treatment and to illustrate points of importance in the management of such patients.

First some comment about her attitude toward psychiatry:

"As the attack eased up, and I was able to rest more comfortably, I thought how just a few years before I had condemned psychiatry. I had felt that it excused people and took away from them all responsibility for their own acts and behavior by placing the blame on their parents or environment. Now I knew how much that was a distortion of the truth. True, I was what I was because of my parents. But they could not have acted differently, for they too were products of their environment. And I was no more responsible for the unconscious childish reactions that were making me sick than I was for the color of my hair or eyes. In turn my children would suffer for my immaturity. Nothing could be done until I had recognized the fact that there was a connection between my feelings and my illness. But once I was made aware of that, then the responsibility and moral obligation became mine, to do something about it, to help myself. I could not do it by blaming my parents, but rather by understanding them, and what wrong attitudes and values were fostered by my reaction to them.

"Indeed, rather than take away responsibility from me, psychiatry made mine much greater. The comfort that I used to have, of being able to blame my attacks on the climate, or diet, or dust in the house, was no longer mine. The turning point in this long search for health began when I could no longer look to an external excuse for my illness, but had to look to myself to find out what it was I was running away from. I had to learn to face myself."

Then some comments about her childhood:

"My mother often related how she could control me by threatening not to love me.

* To be published as "My Inward Journey" by Lorraine Picker, Westminster Press, Philadelphia.

She had no idea how potent and dangerous was her weapon, for she would never knowingly have hurt me. So at a very early age began the pattern of behavior that was to repeat itself many times unconsciously through the years.

"When I was almost five, a baby brother appeared, for which I had no preparation. It was the biggest event in our lives. A party for a boy! And a diamond bracelet for the wife who bore a son! It was the only time in my life that I can remember my father's getting drunk. Life in the house revolved around the baby—and I loved him most of all. I never felt jealous for a minute, and devotedly took care of him and worried about him as if he were my baby. But during the next year my asthmatic attacks became more frequent and severe. Our family doctor suggested to my parents that they take me to a large medical center for a better examination than the small town offered. Days of testing and study at the hospital convinced these specialists that I was an extremely allergic child, sensitive to many things, who would need constant treatment over the years. They recommended that we return to the town from which we came, to a graduate of their institution who had just started practice there.

"We went back to this doctor who was to take care of me for the next fifteen years. He began a series of tests that consisted of small scratches on my skin. Eggs, chocolates, and nuts were the biggest offenders in food. The doctor warned that even a tiny particle of egg in a piece of cake could bring trouble. Other substances such as pollen and cold germs were made up into vaccines for injections. All pets would have to go, pillows and mattresses would have to be changed, rugs and drapes and all dust catchers removed from my bedroom. I think it took years for my brother to forgive me for not being allowed to have a dog. I'm sure had the choice been up to him, he would have chosen a dog over his sister.

"Getting the injections did not present a problem. I went three times a week, and when I was about seven or eight I was able to go without my mother. The doctor was warm and friendly, and often during the years that I went so regularly, the nurse would beckon to me to come ahead of the other patients into the fascinating inner office and laboratory. There he would let me look through his microscope, or use his typewriter. Often he would send out for cokes, and talk to me about school and my friends, and there was always an affectionate hug when I left. I began to look forward to those visits with him. Twenty-five years later when the jig-saw pieces of my life began to fall into place, I understood that I received far more than just the injections—I received affection and acceptance, and a relationship that I did not have at home with my father. There would have to be a long period of analysis and introspection before I would perceive that among all the other feelings that my illness masked, were these means of getting and retaining this relationship. Without asthma, I would not have been able to see the doctor so much."

SUMMARY

A young woman suffered from asthma which began at the age of 2. Eczema preceded the asthma and vasomotor rhinitis occurred in recent years. There was a family history of migraine, asthma and hay fever. Allergic factors apparently were not important in relation to the patient's illness; psychological factors seemed to be. Such was her dependency upon the mother's love and her fear of estrangement from the mother that she married and became pregnant in order to solve a conflict in regard to finishing school rather than confess to the mother her inability to pursue a course which she no longer wanted.

When for the first time, at the age of 26, it was suggested to her that emotional factors might have something to do with her asthma, she went through a period of self-analysis which apparently precipitated a near-psychotic reaction. The self-analysis brought into consciousness a deeply submerged *hostility to the mother* so that the patient, who had previously felt only affection and respect, now could hardly abide the mother. But whereas in the period of conscious devotion (and repressed hostility) she suffered almost constantly from asthma, in the period in which she expressed her hostile feelings she was comparatively well. However, as she stated, "she could not live with her feelings" and was therefore referred for psychoanalysis. Following successful psychoanalysis she has remained free of asthma for a period of more than five years and is healthy and happy in all other respects.

Lessons to Be Learned.　　　What lessons can we learn from this psychosomatic presentation of an allergic patient with lifelong chronic bronchial asthma who, following successful psychoanalysis, has now been free of trouble for nearly five years? First of all, we think we should say that as far as the asthma is concerned we do not know that it is cured, although this is the longest period of freedom she has ever had. It may be that the threshold of tolerance has been raised and that only for that reason is she free of asthma. However, the greater maturity that she has achieved and the improvement in all aspects of her personality suggest a more fundamental change. Nevertheless, we think one must agree that when the removal of an allergen or a hyposensitization process "cures" the patient it proves only that one factor has been removed and the morbid chain of events interrupted. The same reasoning may be applied to psychological factors.

This patient had clumsy psychotherapy, superficial psychotherapy and deep psychotherapy in turn. Lindemann once said, "Clumsy psychotherapy is just as dangerous to the social life as clumsy surgery is to the physical life." When this patient was suddenly confronted with the idea that her relationship to her mother might be the cause of her asthma she went through a very bad period. She was sleepless and despondent, had a "terrible, queer, detached feeling," and had fears that she would lose her mind or commit suicide. She was unable to be alone with her children for fear that she might harm them. Fortunately she had enough stability to come through this period without catastrophe.

So, a word of caution must be sounded in respect to the psychological treatment of the patient with bronchial asthma. Asthma, like ulcerative colitis, often seems more closely related to psychosis than neurosis and sometimes clumsy psychotherapy may remove the symptom but permit psychosis to emerge. There is suggestive clinical evidence in this regard in patients who sometimes alternate between psychosis and asthma, and it has also been observed that the incidence of bronchial asthma (as well as other psychosomatic disorders) is less in mental institutions than in the general population, suggesting that the disorder protects the individual from developing a psychosis. Moreover, we must remember that sometimes with the use of cortisone and ACTH certain mental effects are observed. Instead of exhibiting euphoria some patients become depressed and others actually psychotic. This must be borne in mind in relation to the use of these drugs in patients with bronchial asthma.

Following the period of "self-analysis" the patient entered upon a course of superficial psychotherapy which helped get rid of the symptom, that is, the asthma, but produced no fundamental change in her personality and permitted a disturbance in her feelings that was just as difficult to live with as the asthma. When serious emotional disturbances exist in the individual one must do more than just relieve symptoms. Otherwise the necessity for symptom formation remains and another manifestation of emotional tension, which may be more painful than the original symptom, occurs.

The doctor-patient relationship is illustrated by the conditioning which she had in her childhood relationship to her physician when, as she later realized, the asthma permitted her to cultivate an emotional attachment which she missed in her relationship to her own father. Apparently this prototype determined many of her reactions to physicians later in life. This is an important lesson for every physician to learn. Anything that can throw light on the doctor-patient relationship is of great importance to the practice of medicine.

References

Alexander, F.: Psychosom. Med. Monograph IV, 1941.

Deutsch, F.: Internat. J. Psycho-Analysis, *20:* 1, 1939.

Dunbar, H. F.: Psychoanalyt. Quart., *7:* 25, 1938.

French, T. M.: Am. J. Psychiat., *96:* 87, 1939.

French, T. M., and Alexander, F.: Psychosom. Med. Monograph IV, 1941.

Gillespie, R. D.: Brit. M. J., *1:* 1285, 1936.

Major, R. H.: Classic Description of Disease. P. 540. Charles C Thomas, Springfield, Ill., 1932.

McDermott, N. T., and Cobb, S.: Psychosom. Med., *1:* 203, 1939.

Picker, Lorraine: My Inward Journey. Westminster Press, Philadelphia, to be published.

Rapaport, B. Z., and Hecht, R.: Psychosom. Med. Monograph IV, 1941.

Rogerson, C. H., Hardcastle, D. H., and Duguid, K.: Guy's Hosp. Rep., *85:* 289, 1935.

Schatia, V.: Psychosom. Med., *3:* 157, 1941.

Strauss, E. B.: Guy's Hosp. Rep., *85:* 309, 1935.

Chapter XVI

The Central Nervous System

Anxiety resulting from mental conflict may affect the central nervous system itself just as it affects other systems of the body. Insomnia, weakness and faintness, vertigo, numbness and tingling of the extremities, ringing in the ears, various ocular and visual phenomena, headaches including a large component of the disorder migraine, and even a certain element of the syndrome of epilepsy are some of the results of such anxiety.

INSOMNIA

Man's best escape from the stresses of life is provided by sleep—and the rest and recuperation which it affords. But sleep—and getting enough of it—is not a simple problem. Insomnia is a frequently encountered symptom. A victim of this disorder may state that he has trouble going to sleep, sleeps only a short time, and then awakens early. Or he may awaken frequently during the night, toss about restlessly, have disturbing dreams, and awaken unrefreshed and too fatigued to do his work.

The amount of sleep needed by each person varies. Some people get along on five to six hours nightly but they sleep soundly and awake refreshed. Most people never sleep so well for the first night or two upon changing arrangements, such as a different bed, or sleeping in a Pullman car, or sleeping where there are unfamiliar noises. But, of course, we are not referring to such conditions when speaking of chronic insomnia.

Insomnia and Anxiety. It is always important to inquire about sleep in taking a medical history. *Sleeplessness* is not just a symptom to be met with sedatives. Rather it is an indication of anxiety within the individual and the proper approach to the problem is to try to discover the cause of the anxiety. Unless sleeplessness is caused by pain, organic lesions of the central nervous system or advanced systemic organic disease, it may be considered a neurotic symptom and as such deserves the same careful attention as other symptoms due to emotional conflict. As with other neurotic symptoms people frequently make a fetish of their sleeplessness and surround it with all kinds of exaggerated importance. Every physician is familiar with the patient who insists "that he has not slept a wink" and yet the nurse reports that he has had a fairly good night. Some physicians are unwise enough to set traps for such patients and confront them with evidence to prove that they are mistaken. This is never a satisfactory approach to a neurotic symptom. It only increases the patient's unconscious determination to make the most of the illness, and he will seek another outlet for his anxiety. The proper way to approach the symptom is to listen attentively to the description of the horrors of the night but not to be too concerned and hence by this very attitude help the patient place the symptom in its proper perspective. Then an effort to understand the personality of the patient, in its relation to the life situation, may suggest a solution of the conflict and thus allay the sleeplessness.

Insomnia Not an Isolated Symptom. Many of our readers are familiar with an acute anxiety situation which will disturb sleep, such as concern over a sick child, an important pending business deal, the physician's very sick patient, the lawyer's important case. The anxiety here is a more rational anxiety, however, than we see in people suffering from chronic insomnia. In the case of chronic insomnia the patient may insist that he does not worry or that he has no problems. But it is the job of the physician to reveal to the patient the problem which is causing him anxiety. This anxiety, often borne of infantile insecurity, may be the result of misunderstanding in the management of sleep during early childhood. The child who is unable to sleep because of anxiety may be disciplined for being "bad," whereupon the insomnia is increased. He feels insecure as a result of the unfriendliness around him, as well as from his own hostility. Then, in adult life, although the same individual may have every outward reason to feel secure, he cannot sleep because he is inwardly prepared through his residue of experience (unconscious) to expect catastrophe.

Treatment. Lack of inner peace and security may cause enough tension to require psychotherapy and even psychoanalysis. But sometimes a few simple suggestions will help to encourage sleep.

1. Try to relax for at least one hour before bedtime with quiet music or an unexciting, easily read book.

2. Avoid too much physical activity just before bedtime. Plan to have tooth-brushing, bathing or other toilet duties done an hour before bedtime in order to avoid being "waked up" too much in case drowsiness comes.

3. Resting quietly in bed is better than turning and twisting with annoyance because sleep does not come. Sleep must be wooed, not fought.

4. All sleep is to some degree restless. The quiet period without motion during sleep averages twelve minutes. Hence waking at intervals does not necessarily mean a "bad night's sleep."

5. Just as the neurotic person fears to exert himself when he feels tired lest he do himself harm, so the person who sleeps with difficulty may look forward with apprehension to the activities of the following day if he has less than his usual allotment of sleep. Try not to make an issue of sleeplessness.

6. To be resigned to the disturbance in the sleep function—to accept it and neither fight it nor fear its consequences—may be a great help.

7. If seemingly insoluble problems tend to keep you awake, seek good counsel and start on the road to a solution.

8. Remember that rest alone will repair, to a certain extent, the effects of fatigue. To be satisfied with rest, without demanding the anesthesia of unconsciousness, requires fortitude, but this in itself is often an important step in overcoming insomnia.

It must be said that insomnia rarely occurs as an isolated symptom. It may be the most troublesome symptom but there are always other symptoms of emotional origin. The following case illustrates this point.

Case 46.   Insomnia

History and Symptoms.   A single professional woman came to her physician because of insomnia and crying spells. She reported difficulty in going to sleep, restless tossing, and early awakening. She could not at first give any reason for these symptoms. Inquiry into her life history revealed that she was the youngest in a family of three with an older brother and sister, both married. The father had been an ineffectual business man and the mother a kind but colorless woman with "few definite ideas about life." As a result the patient had entered into professional work which she had followed with a moderate amount of interest until her illness began. At 19 she had been infatuated with a man but the affair did not last long. She had had dates and was fairly popular with men but she never seemed eager to marry and have a home and family of her own. The result was that she felt she was no longer young and had failed to find what she hoped for in life. When we asked what she hoped for, she replied, "I'm ashamed to say I don't know. That sounds ridiculous because in my work I have to see that people have a plan of living that brings satisfaction. But I guess I never thought of that for myself."

LIFE SITUATION

We urged her to try to state what she wanted to get from life. She said, "Well, I suppose I wanted to be more important to someone than I am at present. I feel I'm only a cog in a machine, a rather impersonal machine at that. I thought professional women got a lot of glory and attention but all I seem to get is responsibility. Probably what I want is a husband and home of my own and my own children. Then at least I can feel that my efforts are invested in something permanent." She then made the often-heard complaint that she had never met a man whom she could love. We asked her, "Have you ever thought specifically about marriage and living a day-to-day life with any of the men you have known?" She admitted that she had not placed her ideas of love upon any one man but still had in the back of her mind the idea that the man who would awaken her to the idea of marriage was yet to come and would have something special to recommend him. He would be unusually handsome or unusually rich or otherwise be apart from the ordinary men she had met. We said, "It looks as if you needed to be shaken out of an adolescent dream state. You have already passed men by who could make you happy and it is time you looked around you and began to take an interest in your available chances of happiness before it is too late. You have been anxious, as if pursued by something, and that something has been *time*. You have been unable to relax and rest, as if there was some important thing you should be doing or thinking about. There is! But if you turn your attention to your emotional needs for physical love, home and family you will find that you can relax and rest."

TREATMENT APPROACH

As we said, insomnia is a signal of anxiety or distress but the cause may be unconscious. We must make the patient aware of his problem and set him consciously at work upon it. We saw our patient five times at weekly intervals. A male friend who had been mildly interested in her for some time began to be more responsive to her as soon as she began to realize what they could mean to each other. She was hesitant at first about the "niceness" of physical love-making with "just anybody." We pointed out, "Some degree of physical love-making is accepted in every community. You, like every other girl, must be willing to give your affection to some man in your community. To save it for a movie hero is not good judgment since there are only a few of them and most of them stay in Hollywood. Your friend is not just anybody. He is a respectable, well-thought-of man and you must respect him." This was followed by some discussion of love-making and sexual values which she had not received in her home, and upon which she had not informed herself. The result was that she came to be less self-centered and more able to interest herself in other people. She stopped crying and began to sleep better, and eventually made a successful marriage.

SUMMARY

We see from this case (and it holds true for others) how thoroughly we must enter into the life situation in order to elicit the cause of anxiety. Sedatives may occasionally be given the first few nights until the life problem is known and thrown into relief. But as we begin to understand the emotional background of the sleeplessness and set the patient to work remedying the situation we see an improvement in the insomnia.

WEAKNESS AND FAINTNESS
[See also Vertigo, p. 470]

We often hear these two symptoms spoken of in one breath. "I feel so weak and faint," the patient states. While they may be symptoms of physical disease, they are also frequently present in emotionally unstable individuals and are part of the neurosis. Fainting is apparently due to cerebral anemia as a result of a sudden autonomic imbalance, the emotional stimulus for which may be a frightening or an unpleasant sight. The autonomic action results in flight through unconsciousness. It is well known that fainting occurs not infrequently in nurses and medical students in the first part of their course when they do dissections, watch operations or postmortem examinations. But it is also a common occurrence in every walk of life in individuals who are emotionally unstable or who have not had the proper conditioning to blood, injury, filth and other unpleasant facts of life.

Significance of the Symptoms. Aside from the fainting which occurs in obvious physical disease and the once-or-twice-in-a-lifetime fainting of the average person, a history of "fainting spells" requires careful study. Many cases are found to be instances of *petit mal* and require the special management of the epileptic. Others are probably close to *malingering*. These "weak spells" or "fainting spells" are often used by self-centered people as a club over other people in the environment. They sit down or lie down, throw the head back, close the eyes, and thus many an argument is won. If it happens, and it often does, that they have been told about "a weak heart," they put their hand to the region of the heart as they throw back their head and close their eyes and thus, as the central character of the drama, they achieve an almost invincible position. These people never actually become unconscious. They are emotionally immature and so sensitive that if anything is said or done to hurt their feelings or if they are threatened with loss of love, attention or prestige, they feel the inner sensory discomfort of *anxiety*. They may be enraged but lack the ability to express this rage directly. The pain or rage is shunted into the autonomic nervous system; possibly they feel a little palpitation, breathlessness, or perhaps only the mild discomfort of anxiety which ordinary individuals go through every day but which these people stand so poorly; and they announce that a "weak spell" or a "fainting attack" is coming, go through the motions described and usually get the situation changed to their satisfaction.

The Mechanism of Syncope.   In a valuable study of syncope, Romano and Engel follow Alexander in differentiating between conversion reaction and vegetative neurotic symptoms (p. 64). Classifying their patients with syncope into two groups, they pointed out that in vasodepressor syncope the loss of consciousness is preceded by rather striking clinical manifestations, including pallor, sweating, sighing respirations, hypotension and sometimes bradycardia, while in hysterical fainting consciousness is lost without any demonstrable changes in circulation or respiration.

While the similarities are rather superficial both conditions are psychogenic, that is to say, they are caused by chronic repressed or, at least, unrelieved emotional tension. The mechanisms involved, however, are fundamentally different, both psychodynamically and physiologically. The conversion symptom is an attempt to relieve an emotional tension in a symbolic way; it is a symbolic expression with a definite emotional content. This mechanism is restricted to voluntary neuromuscular or sensory perceptive systems whose function it is to express and relieve emotions. A vegetative neurosis consists of a psychogenic dysfunction of a vegetative organ which is not under control of the voluntary neuromuscular system. The vegetative symptom is not a substitute expression of the emotion, but its normal physiological concomitant.

VASODEPRESSOR SYNCOPE.   In the application of this concept to fainting, Romano and Engel cited a patient with vasodepressor syncope in whom emotional experiences were accompanied by certain changes in the circulatory system which led eventually to loss of consciousness. These physiological changes were clearly demonstrable in the form of pallor, sweating, changes in respiration and pulse, and falling blood pressure leading finally to cerebral anemia and marked distortion of the electrical activity of the brain. The physiological mechanism suggested flight. The concomitant emotional experience appeared to be that of anxiety overwhelming the ego and preventing other compromise compensatory defenses.

Vasodepressor syncope could be initiated by a great variety of stimuli such as venous puncture, facing threatening situations, and so forth. Indeed it is common upon first exposure to a new and threatening situation.

HYSTERICAL FAINTING.   Romano and Engel contrasted fainting of hysterical patients in which there is a notable lack of change in respiration, circulatory dynamics and electrical activity of the brain during periods of unconsciousness. In other words, the absence of any alterations of electrical activity of the brain in these hysterical patients clearly distinguished them from the fainting which results from cerebral anemia. The specific hysterical structure of the neurosis manifests itself by the symptom of fainting as an attempt to express repressed sexuality in a symbolic manner.

Case 47.   Hysterical Fainting

A white girl of 19 complained of frequent fainting spells which had been occurring about once a month for the past year under various circumstances of "crowds, excitement, overwork, heat, et cetera." The patient fainted while relating the history and we observed that there were no circulatory changes. She simply rolled her eyes and slumped in her chair.

Previous health had been good, except for rather severe dysmenorrhea, and she thought that more fainting spells occurred about the time of the period.

Physical examination showed a healthy appearing girl with no evidence of organic disease. Routine laboratory studies were also normal.

LIFE SITUATION

The patient and an older sister and brother were brought up very strictly. Before she could go out on a date the father would give her a lecture about sex. When the patient was about 11 the brother became delinquent, later was apprehended for rape, and committed to a penal institution. With the background of her strict upbringing and this lamentable experience, the patient eschewed all thought of sexual matters and led a very narrow and prudish existence.

About the time that she was graduating from high school, and "excitment ran high," she developed the first fainting attack. She had known for some time that her parents were troubled but didn't know quite what about and forbore to speak of it, but about this time learned that her sister's husband had left because of her "fast" behavior and the sister had returned home. Now the patient expected more trouble.

One night "after having had her hair done" she was reading a book and the chapter closed with a woman falling off a cliff and at this point the patient fell out of her chair in a faint. Dreams followed that she was "falling or running away from something" and in her discussions it seemed very clear that her fainting was her response to sexual temptation, the danger of "a moral fall."

Treatment.   Bringing this material into the open, encouraging her to talk about her brother and his sexual defections, her sister's behavior, and her father's early admonitions regarding the dangers of sexual transgressions, together with better instruction in these matters, brought about considerable improvement so that one year later she was able to report that she had been free of attacks for a period of more than six months. In addition she was better adjusted socially and found more pleasure in the company of men.

HEADACHE

Headache is probably one of the most common symptoms confronting physicians in their daily practice. It has been estimated to be present in 50 per cent of patients, being exceeded in frequency only by constipation. Both symptoms are often regarded in the same way, namely as an inherent part of the body pattern, and the person takes it for granted that no relief can be obtained. It is true that some headaches are very refractory to treatment. The causative factor is difficult to locate and a therapeutic program that is not aimed at the causative factor is unlikely to bring relief.

Etiology.   Headache occurs both as a result of physical disease and in association with emotional disorders. Among the well-known physical causes are organic brain lesions, vascular disorders and toxic factors—for example, brain tumor, meningeal irritation, hypertension and uremia.

Most chronic headaches that are not migrainous or posttraumatic are "functional" and here psychic factors are all-important. Nor for that matter can psychic factors be disregarded in the first two groups. These will be discussed. Among the alleged causes which, in many instances, have only the remotest relation to headache are constipation, eyestrain, focal infection, low blood pressure and "sinusitis."

These headaches may be located in the frontal region, in the occipital region, directly on top of the head, on either side, or "all over." They may be dull or sharp, constant or intermittent. They may appear at the time of some emotional stress or more often in the absence of surface anxiety.

CONSTIPATION.   Probably the most frequently assigned cause of headache is constipation and it is very obvious why this should be so. On the assumption that "obstruction or accumulation" leads to absorption of toxins from the gastrointestinal tract which may prove poisonous, and that a symptom of such poisoning is headache, a great many sufferers from headache are addicted to the laxative, enema or colonic irrigation habit. We cannot say that there is no such cause of headache but certainly it is overemphasized both by the laity and the medical profession and also exploited by drug houses from the standpoint of advertisements for laxative preparations and by institutes for colonic irrigations. Every physician has had the experience of observing patients who are constipated for many days and do not have headaches. They are also familiar with the headache victim whose headache disappears magically just as soon as the bowels move—too soon for a physiological mechanism to be responsible.

EYESTRAIN.   There was a period only a few years ago when the eyestrain cause of all kinds of illness enjoyed a great popularity in the medical profession. It gave way to the focal infection concept in medicine but is still frequently held to be responsible for headaches. Again, as in the case of constipation, we believe that it is possible for eyestrain to be responsible for headache but not nearly so frequently as people think. Hardly ever do patients present headache as a chief symptom that they have not had their eyes refracted and glasses recently changed. It is almost as rare to see a patient suffering from repeated headaches who has not recently been refracted as it is to see a patient with arthritis who has not had teeth or tonsils removed. But just as in the latter instance the arthritis is rarely benefited, so in the former instance the headache usually persists. The subject will be discussed at greater length later.

FOCAL INFECTION.   Any obscure illness is very apt to be blamed upon focal infection but fortunately the wave of enthusiasm for that concept of the cause of disease, which resulted in the removal of countless thousands of teeth and tonsils, is coming to a close. While the idea still enjoys a certain vogue in rheumatic disorders, it is no longer common for physicians to order tonsils removed or teeth extracted because of a headache.

SINUSITIS.   Physicians ought to know that sinusitis is not the commonest cause of headache. A great many patients refer to their headache as a "sinus headache" and indeed so common is this idea that patients habitually refer to the fact that their "sinus" is troubling them again, instead of saying, "I have a headache." First of all, to have a sinus headache one must have sinusitis. As discussed elsewhere, we have at last discovered that vasomotor rhinitis is not in itself sinusitis nor is a "postnasal drip" necessarily an indication of sinusitis. Again we must beware of a little thickening of the mucous membrane, so often reported by x-ray, as an indication that sinusitis is responsible for headache.

A genuine sinus headache is usually localized in one region, is periodic in character, occurring at intervals during certain times of the day, and usually is accompanied by localized tenderness. Even the so-called "vacuum headache" has these characteristics. Therefore, vague headache without the demonstration of definite sinusitis should call for a thorough psychosomatic study before it is definitely decided that it is of sinus origin.

LOW BLOOD PRESSURE. The concept of low blood pressure as a disease entity or a cause of symptoms almost takes precedence over high blood pressure, and the latter is acknowledged to be one of the commonest disorders of civilized life. When patients present ill-defined symptoms or an illness of obscure origin and the physician finds that the blood pressure is low, he is very apt to assign this as a cause, and from that point on the patient speaks of "my low blood pressure" in the same way that he speaks of a "sinus headache." But the relationship is just as indefinite. The truth of the matter is that in recent years we have come to understand that low blood pressure is often a sign of longevity and therefore, rather than being a sign of ill-health, it is an evidence of sound physical structure. Once again, a little bit of fact is responsible for a great deal of fiction. There are instances of true *essential hypotension* in which postural circulatory changes take place and here the circulatory disorder may undoubtedly be responsible for headaches. Again, there are rare instances of adrenal disease in which the blood pressure is unnaturally low and may be responsible for certain symptoms. But the majority of patients who suffer head discomfort and blame it upon low blood pressure are really attributing the headache to a cause which does not exist. The blood pressure may be low but it should be interpreted as an indication of probable longevity rather than as a sign of disease.

HEADACHE OF EMOTIONAL ORIGIN. Therefore, in the absence of definite organic disease which is known to produce headache, the physician should be aware that the common cause of "reflex headaches," so-called, is emotional stress, conscious or unconscious. The results of fitting glasses, treating the sinuses, irrigating the colon, etc., for headaches of psychic origin are only temporary if they give any relief at all, and the time has come for the physician to realize what the layman has known for a long time—namely, that there are many life situations which produce anxiety which, in turn, expresses itself as headache. This has been well enough recognized for the expression to have crept into the language that a vexatious wife is a "headache" to her husband, a difficult customer is a "headache" to the salesgirl, or the irate boss may be a "headache" to his employees.

Tension headaches are usually bilateral and may be accompanied by a variety of associated signs, including anxiety, nausea and vomiting. Frequency and duration are variable but in general are much greater than those of migraine headaches. Migraine and tension headaches may occur in the same person.

Mechanism of Headache.   From available data, including observations of patients undergoing surgical procedures on the head and subjected to mechanical stimulation of the intracranial contents, Wolff stated that there are six basic mechanisms of headache from intracranial sources:

1. Traction on the veins that pass to the venous sinuses from the surface of the brain and displacement of the great venous sinuses.

2. Traction on the middle meningeal arteries.

3. Traction on the large arteries at the base of the brain and their main branches.

4. Distention and dilatation of intracranial arteries.

5. Inflammation in or about any of the pain-sensitive structures of the head.

6. Direct pressure by tumors on the cranial and cervical nerves containing many pain-afferent fibers from the head.

The cranium, the brain itself, the parenchyma of the brain, most of the dura and the pia-arachnoid, the ependymal lining of the ventricles and the choroid plexuses appear to be insensitive.

INTRACRANIAL PRESSURE.   Headache associated with altered intracranial pressure, high or low, is due to traction on pain-sensitive structures. Brain-tumor headaches arise from local traction upon adjacent sensitive structures, or from distant traction by extensive displacement of the brain. The histamine headache is a function of dilatation and stretching of cerebral arteries and surrounding tissues; the rise in intracranial pulsations in this situation has been demonstrated, together with the fact that the headache can be abolished by raising the intracranial pressure. Similarly, in headache induced by typhoid vaccine, an increase in arterial pulsations has been recorded and if intracranial pressure is purposely raised, a decrease is accompanied by abatement of the pain. Probably headaches associated with acute infections, sepsis, et cetera, are attributable to the same mechanism.

ARTERIAL PULSATION.   The soft tissues covering the skull, particularly the extracranial arteries, are pain-sensitive. It is from distention of cranial arteries, chiefly though not exclusively the external carotid, that migraine arises, and procedures that constrict these arteries and reduce their amplitude of pulsation will diminish or terminate the headache. The headache associated with hypertension seems to be on a similar basis, bearing no direct relation to the level of blood pressure, and susceptible to influence by agents that decrease the amplitude of pulsations of the cranial arteries. Here it is the contractile tone of the arteries which is of major importance; distention and headache occur in the hypertensive subject if this contractile state is impaired. Wolff and associates point out that even during headache-free phases a person subject to vascular headaches exhibits significantly greater variation in the contractile state of certain parts of the cranial vascular tree than does a person not subject to headaches.

MUSCULAR CONTRACTIONS.   *Tension headaches,* says Wolff, together with those on a vascular basis, constitute 90 per cent of the headache problem. These headaches may be psychogenic; they may arise from factors setting up contractions in various muscles of the scalp and neck, experienced most conspicuously as posterior headache or a "band-like" sensation. Such muscular contractions can be recorded electromyographically. The posttraumatic headache, too, is usually on a muscular basis. In the last analysis, no headache is imaginary: Emotions are quite capable of producing true headache, by their repercussions in the muscles or vessels from which the painful sensations arise.

Cautions in Diagnosis. Generalized and bizarre headaches, such as the feeling of pressure on the top of the head and the "tight band" around the head, are usually regarded as of psychic origin but Friedman and associates uttered a word of warning against making a diagnosis of psychogenic headache purely on the basis of the patient's description of the distribution and character of the pain. They illustrated this by the following case.

"A white female nurse, age 22 years, had been suffering from headaches for two months. These were described as a feeling of pressure throughout the head or in one or another part of it. They were occasionally accompanied by nausea or even vomiting and were usually relieved by aspirin. Two days before entry into the hospital, the headache grew worse, and the patient felt tired and listless. During the recent severe headaches, the patient screamed at times, was emotionally upset and even seemed confused but if she was spoken to she could always be roused and brought into contact. When the history was taken it was learned that she was dissatisfied with her present job, and that she had left her previous, congenial one just before the onset of her headaches. She lived with her family and was under considerable emotional tension, both because she disliked her stepfather and because the other members of the family disapproved of her fiancé.

"Physical and neurologic examinations were negative except for questionable blurring of the disk margins. Roentgenograms of the skull and lumbar puncture did not reveal any abnormality. An electroencephalogram was diffusely abnormal, more on the left than on the right. Since visual-field studies showed enlargement of the blind spots, a pneumoencephalogram was attempted, but the ventricles failed to fill. A ventriculogram then revealed dilatation of the entire ventricular system, and at operation a *medulloblastoma* was removed from the left cerebellar hemisphere."

Posttraumatic Headache. Symptoms unrelated to the physical injury often persist after head injury and many such patients continue to be misunderstood and badly handled. Ross and McNaughton pointed out that every head injury involves trauma, both physical and psychic. The physical effects are exerted on the meninges and the brain. Meningeal contusion and meningeal adhesions may be directly responsible for a localized type of headache mediated largely through the nerve supply to the dura from the fifth nerve. This may clear up spontaneously if there are no other factors in operation but the headache may persist for emotional reasons.

Many of the localized headaches appear to wax and wane with the presence and absence of fatigue and emotional stress, suggesting a relationship to cerebral functioning rather than to meningeal adhesions. Other effects include some intellectual impairment and some emotional instability with severe injuries, and at least temporarily after less severe injuries. These factors are interlinked with the psychic effects of the trauma, the previous personality of the individual and the situational factors in operation after the injury, to produce an emotional disturbance which may result in any of the symptoms of headache, dizziness, fatigability, irritability, lack of concentration and other mental symptoms so commonly present in psychoneurotic patients.

MECHANISM.   Simons and Wolff stated that between one third and one half of all persons who injure their heads sufficiently to warrant hospitalization develop chronic posttraumatic headaches. They studied 63 such patients, all of whom were known to have no epidural, subdural, subarachnoid or parenchymatous hemorrhage at the time of observation. The vast majority of patients with posttraumatic headaches that persist or recur for long periods of time after head injury have no such intracranial abnormalities to explain their headaches. Utilizing the electroencephalogram as an indication of muscle potential, they concluded that such headaches result from sustained contraction of the skeletal muscles of the head and neck associated with the occurrence of sustained resentment, anxiety, frustration, tension and fear, and are sometimes augmented by noxious stimuli arising from abnormal healing and scar formation within these extracranial soft structures of the head and neck. In many instances the amount of muscle contraction is minimal but it is probably the basis of complaint because it is sustained and because of an abnormal preoccupation with the head.

They concluded that, as to the basic pathophysiological mechanisms and symptomatology, chronic headaches which follow trauma closely resemble other headaches which accompany and follow stress and untoward life situations but which are unrelated to head trauma.

Kozol reported a detailed study of 101 civilians with acute head injuries. His method was a statistical analysis of fifty symptoms based on personality traits before and after the injury. Correlations were made with the nature and estimated severity of the acute cerebral trauma and with various potentially complicating factors, such as associated bodily injuries and various possible sources of psychological stress (litigation, occupation, and financial and marital difficulties).

A good portion of the posttraumatic psychiatric symptoms appeared in the patients with previous psychoneurotic personalities. No close correlation was found between the severity of the acute injury to the brain and the severity of the sequelae. A high correlation was found between the sequelae and persistent complicated sociological factors, such as continuing compensation, pending litigation, occupational stresses and persistent associated bodily injuries, and the severity and persistence of psychiatric sequelae. The conclusion was drawn that given psychiatric sequelae cannot be ascribed to one particular cause or to any particular group of cases, because the etiological factors are specific for each case.

DIAGNOSIS.   After calling attention to the necessity for a study regarding the presence or absence of skull fracture, and of neurological findings, the duration of coma, the amount of blood in the spinal fluid, the treatment given, and special tests such as x-ray, electroencephalogram, and psychological procedures such as the Rorschach method, Ross and McNaughton emphasized the study of situational factors as well as the previous personality background.

How was the patient's life situation altered by the accident and what other environmental circumstances are present which may be relevant? Does he fear the continuation of impaired mental power? Does he feel a threat to his earning power? Does he feel that he is deserving of pension or compensations? Are there any legal complications? Are unpleasant duties and responsibilities avoided because of the symptoms? If military service is involved what is the individual's attitude to the service and to his duties? Are there any concomitant reasons for anxiety or personality conflict? Was the individual working under an intolerable strain before the accident? These are questions which must be asked subtly, through indirect and tactful discussions, following up whatever leads are offered. They cannot be asked by direct query. When the proper approach is used, however, it may indicate what the patient's real "headache" is at the time of examination apart from his predisposition or the physical effects of the injury.

TREATMENT.   Treatment should consider the whole person, and prophylaxis to avoid the psychic concomitants is the best guarantee against the development of posttraumatic symptoms.

The treatment of the patient who has already developed posttraumatic headache and dizziness and is seen some weeks after the injury, begins with the thorough investigation already outlined. This is the first step needed in order to reassure the patient and in order to understand the personal situation which needs attention. The mere ventilation of the emotional problems may contribute to a cure, although generally further psychotherapy and situational therapy are needed, as well as palliative drug therapy.

According to Ross and McNaughton a measure offering greatest promise, especially for the compensation case, is "occupational therapy merging into therapeutic occupation" (Denny-Brown). "If the individual who has reverted to a child-like dependent attitude as a result of the accident, demanding a financial recompense for a real loss of personality security, can be persuaded to learn again how to become a mature and independent adult earning his own way, both he and the institution from which he would have obtained his pension will benefit. Pension claimants are rarely satisfied with their awards, and this resentment, together with the hope of further compensation, serves to aggravate the symptoms. In contrast with this it should be possible to fit injured individuals into employment which suits them and which reestablishes their self-respect and sense of security. How much better, both psychotherapeutically and financially, if compensation and pension boards would devote to rehabilitation the funds now going into partial disability pensions. Both the brain-injured individual and the psychoneurotic, as well as the patient with a little of both, could benefit from a reeducation program helping them to make the best use of their resources. Surely it would be more just to the injured war veteran or the handicapped industrial worker to establish the principle that he deserves a secure job and not a dole."

Case 48.   Headache of Emotional Origin

History and Symptoms.   A young farmer complained of severe headaches which were situated generally over the entire cranium. They had been present for about a year's time and had been unresponsive to drug therapy and dietary changes.

He was the youngest of five children, having two older brothers and two older sisters, all married. The *father*, also a farmer, had considered himself a very religious man. He had attended church regularly, prayed with fervor, and taught Sunday school, but at home he had been a tyrant who rarely spoke to his wife and when he spoke to his children it was only to reprove them. He had died of pneumonia two years prior to our seeing the patient. The *mother*, equally devoted to religion, was just as incapable of practicing its precepts in her daily life. She, like the father, was never affectionate with the children, never praised them, never took their interests seriously. She seemed to feel that if through scolding, threats or cajolery she could get our patient to church, all would be well. He had completed high school and had been working on the farm for his mother ever since, but his dissatisfaction with life was growing and his headaches were making it almost impossible for him to carry on.

LIFE SITUATION

Physically and neurologically he showed no sign of organic disease. He was seen twice a week over a prolonged period. He soon made clear his hostility toward his mother and father for their unsympathetic attitudes. He was particularly angry because they pretended to be so good, "talking about the love of God, the need for man to pattern his life after the tolerance of Christ, and preaching the need of love of one's fellow man." He added, "If they had been that cold and cruel and unfeeling toward others without acting in the name of Christianity I might have stood it. But the hypocrisy of it all, which they could not seem to see, nearly drove me mad. When father used to come home from prayer meeting and start scolding me for some minor or imaginary offense it used to hurt me and sometimes I would cry to myself. But since he has died and mother goes on the same way I can't cry. I only suffer and hate and get these intolerable headaches."

Social Adjustment.   His social adjustment was poor because all women seemed to him as his mother and sisters had been, i. e., "critical, fault-finding, and wanting something all the time and having nothing to give." Nevertheless he had a conscious longing for a woman's love, although he had masturbation fantasies in which he was cruel to women. He had so much guilt and anxiety about these fantasies that he could speak about them only with great difficulty. We said to him, "Since you feel that women have been cruel and indifferent to you it is natural that you think of retaliation. This retaliation happens to be combined with your sexual feelings and fantasies but do not be distressed too much by this. Speak of it freely and you will see that some separation will take place between your ideas of love and your fantasies of hate."

Expression of Hostility.   He despised the farm and hated going to church and finally got the courage to discuss these attitudes with his mother. She tried to make him feel ashamed but because of his discussion of these matters in an uncritical atmosphere he had gained courage and would not let himself be dissuaded by her. The result was that finally she rented the farm and he got a job in the city. He liked this better, and for the first time his headaches were less troublesome. In the first few weeks of treatment his headaches were so bad that while talking about his parents and their injustices to him he would hold his head in his hands, sway from side to side, and beg to be taken to the hospital and have some operation done upon him, "any operation. . . There must be something in there, a brain tumor or something. My hatred for things that have happened to me is intense but it can't be producing all this." We urged him to be patient and keep up the struggle.

Marriage. After leaving the farm he suffered from loneliness for which he sought relief in feminine companionship. These friendships always ended disastrously because he always expected the girl to be kind beyond reasonable possibilities. He wanted her to be a normal, active, friendly girl and yet make up to him in affection all that his mother had failed to give him. He could not bear to have her ask anything in the way of a favor from him and he was very sensitive to the slightest trace of disinterest in him. We said to him, "Remember, you have been a deprived person both as a child and as a young man. While you feel that you have missed a great deal and have much coming to you in the way of affection and regard, you must recognize that it cannot be all one-sided. Any girl expects from you a cheerful demeanor and some consideration of her desires. If you can forget yourself a little and think of the girl you will be rewarded by her gratitude."

He finally saw the point of this discussion and at the end of about two years met a girl whom he wanted to marry. By this time his headaches had entirely disappeared and he was reasonably happy at his work. He married and in the two years since then he has been symptom-free and happy.

MIGRAINE

There is a variety of headache which comes in attacks, often periodically, is usually one-sided (hemicrania), and is frequently accompanied by one or more of the following phenomena: scotomas or other visual disturbances, nausea and vomiting, constipation or diarrhea, urine retention or frequency of urination, and general or one-sided chilliness, numbness and pallor. The attack is often preceded by some kind of an "aura" and may be followed by fatigue and depression, although again the contrary may occur—the patient may be lively and energetic once the attack is over.

Clinical Features. Migraine has been called a familial headache, thus indicating the hereditary factor. In a clinical study of 2000 cases of headache Friedman and associates found a history of migraine in the family in 65 per cent of the patients studied whereas in tension headaches there was a family history in 40 per cent. Migraine has also been called the "sensory type of epilepsy," indicating that the two conditions are related. Migraine attacks in women frequently occur just before the onset of menstruation and often cease after the menopause. The attacks may occur as often as two or three times a week or as infrequently as once a year. Usually no definite interval between attacks is noted. The condition is most common in persons between the ages of 15 and 35. A visual *aura* may precede the attack; the eyes may feel hot and painful and the lids begin to droop with a feeling of heaviness. There are sensations of flashing lights and zig-zag bright lines, contraction of the visual fields, and other visual disturbances. Dizziness and ringing in the ears, strange odors and taste disturbances may also occur. Lippman described patients who have hallucinations associated with migraine attacks, for example, that the entire body, or certain parts of the body, are distorted in size and shape. Dizziness and soreness of the scalp may be present, accompanied by a sensation of "pins and needles" in the extremities. Once the head pain of migraine has developed any stimulation such as slamming of the door, noises from the street, or glaring lights will increase the pain. In at least one third of the cases of migraine psychic disturbances are common. These are anxiety, drowsiness and confusion, sometimes amounting to disorientation.

Mechanism.   The headache is thought to be due to spasmodic contraction, followed by dilatation, of the smooth musculature of the cerebral blood vessels. These vascular spasms in turn apparently cause ischemia and edema, which irritate the brain and its centers. The stimulation of these centers disturbs other systems, particularly those under the control of the vagus nerve.

In the course of aviation medicine experiments, Engel and associates have made some observations about a migraine-like syndrome complicating decompression sickness. They describe the scintillating scotomas, the focal neurological signs, and the headaches, which emphasize the similarity between this syndrome and clinical migraine and suggest that the mechanisms are similar. Their studies confirm the observations of Wolff on the mechanism of the neurological prodromes of migraine and suggest the identity of the two. The characteristics of the neurological disturbances suggest that they originate in the cerebral cortex and probably result from spasm of cerebral arteries. Moreover, the authors discovered a high incidence of migraine-like headaches in the subjects who were susceptible to this decompression syndrome, indicating that a predisposition to this particular type of vascular reaction is an important factor. They accept the interpretation that the scotomas and other neurological symptoms result from cortical ischemia due to spasm of intracranial arteries, but insist that the headaches result from dilatation of pain-sensitive cranial arteries. The headache was not associated with any changes in the electroencephalogram; this is consistent with experience of others in the study of clinical migraine.

The clinical and electroencephalographic findings in a case of migraine with severe and repeated preheadache focal neurologic phenomena are presented by Engel et al. Psychological data on the patient revealed many of the attacks to have occurred in a setting of unexpressed anger. The case is unusual in the severity and frequency of the focal neurological disturbances. The electroencephalographic findings during the attack were consistent with severe focal brain damage. However, follow-up showed a normal record clearly indicating the reversibility of the underlying process. The lack of permanent damage in spite of many attacks made it improbable that major vascular thrombosis took place at any time.

The hypothesis that vasospasm of sufficient degree to produce ischemia can occur in the cerebral arteries has often been challenged. It has been suggested that the transient focal symptoms of the encephalopathy of chronic hypertension are due to emboli or some other organic occlusion of the cerebral artery or arterioles. In the patient described by the authors it is difficult to conceive that this would be so. The lack of residual effects after many attacks favored the vasospastic hypothesis.

Personality Features.   The personality pattern most commonly seen consists of characteristics of inflexibility and shyness in childhood, giving rise to adult perfectionism, rigidity, resentment, ambitiousness and efficiency—in short, a constitutional predisposition to sustained emotional states. Apparently physiological mechanisms can be set in motion by psychic stress related to the personality structure of the patient with migraine. In a review (Weiss) of 24 patients studied from a psychosomatic standpoint we were impressed with the features that they shared in common: a *compulsive personality*, an inability to express hostile impulses adequately, a high incidence of various degrees of impotence among the men and frigidity in the women, and the patient's willingness to blame his headache upon the bowel, the sinuses, or "something he *et.*" To the last we usually answer "No, it is probably something you *met*," but because of this association to the gastrointestinal tract and the willingness of the patient to blame the headache upon a disturbance in bowel function he usually becomes addicted to the laxative or enema habit while, for the same reasons, his physician endorses the allergic approach.

The claim that migraine is an allergic disease has been based on the facts that (1) migraine is found in many patients with hay fever or asthma (in itself not very conclusive evidence), (2) some observers have found that a large proportion of patients with migraine have positive skin reactions to some allergen, (3) some observers have cured migraine by prescribing a restricted diet, (4) recurring sudden unexplained attacks are typical of other manifestations of allergy and (5) some observers have found eosinophilia in several patients with migraine. In a detailed analysis of a series of 191 asthmatics and 50 controls Schwartz found no significant evidence that would link migraine with any form of allergy and concluded that, although in an occasional patient migraine might be due to an allergy, such patients are relatively rare.

Emotional Immaturity.   In a study by Touraine and Draper of 50 migrainous patients it was suggested that there exists a characteristic constitutional type in which the skull shows acromegaloid trends, the intelligence is outstanding, but the emotional make-up is retarded in development. They observed that the headache was characteristically repeated in the same pattern for each patient and recurred in similar circumstances. Situations necessitating the individual to stand alone, such as loss of home protection or the assumption of adult responsibilities, marked the beginning of the headaches. Headaches were observed to come through the maternal line with the factor of unconscious imitation of the mother important in causation. Thus an effort must be made to differentiate factors of *true heredity* and *pseudoheredity*. Touraine and Draper found that there was an emotional attachment to the mother which could not be resolved. This resulted in retarding the process of emotional maturation so that arrest occurred at some point short of mature psychosexual adjustment. They concluded that the migraine attack was a syndrome comparable to any neurosis and the fact that migraine responded to such a variety of treatments spoke in favor of a psychic etiology. They felt that the psychological approach offered the most in research and therapy.

Relation to Hypertension.   Gardner, Mountain and Hines observed that migraine occurs very frequently in association with hypertension. Their study, conducted at the Mayo Clinic, indicated that migraine occurred approximately five times more frequently among patients with hypertension than in a control group without hypertension. This suggests a common factor in the pathogenesis of the two conditions. It is well known that vasoconstriction plays an important role in producing an attack of migraine as it does in the production of hypertension. The study also indicated that the association of migraine and hypertension is intimately concerned with *heredity* factors common to both conditions. They suggest that the common denominator in the two conditions may be influenced by genetic factors which particularly concern the inheritance of a certain type of personality. Once more we would call attention to the fact of pseudoheredity (unconscious imitation dating from childhood) which conceivably could operate in migraine but hardly in hypertension.

They refer to the study of migrainous patients by H. G. Wolff, who emphasized that the patient with migraine often demonstrates unusual ambition, is meticulous and exacting, and frequently proves himself to be a hard driver with the ability to accomplish much in a short time. These are also the characteristics of the personality noted in many patients suffering from hypertension.

Psychoanalytic Observations.   Fromm-Reichmann treated 8 patients with migraine by intensive psychotherapy. Of these, 5 were cured, 2 were improved, and 1 remained uninfluenced. She found that they were all people who had a marked hostility, of which they were not consciously aware, for some person to whom they were closely attached. Realizing that many ordinary headaches are also a conversion of anger or hatred, Dr. Fromm-Reichmann asked herself why the ambivalence of feeling (conscious devotion and unconscious hostility) is so intense in the migraine patient, or in other words, why it is so necessary to repress the negative feelings. The question of why the head is chosen as an area for expressing the hostility also interested her.

Unconscious Hostility.   She thought the answer to the first question lay in the fact that so often the migraine patient comes from a conventional family with strong solidarity and strong family pride. Aggression against each other is strongly forbidden. If one member dares to express hostility against another he is punished by exclusion and thus loses the protection of the family in the struggle of life. The fear of such a punishment is enough to keep him in line and keep his hostilities repressed. Then when anger is aroused and cannot express itself adequately either by words or direct action the individual takes it out upon himself, so to speak, in an attack of migraine. He punishes himself for the destruction he would like to visit upon another. Why the head is chosen as the organ to "take the punishment" seemed to be on the basis of rivalry with the intellectuality of the person to whom the sufferer is attached. It is as though in his impotent rage he could "dash his brains" against a solid wall. We submit, from previous discussion, that identification as well as rivalry may play a part in the choice of the head as a site for the expression of this form of "body language."

Rorschach Tests.   A careful study of migraine by means of the Rorschach method, using control groups (Ross and McNaughton), fails to confirm the clinical finding of repressed rage but does corroborate the personality features, namely: persistence toward success, difficulty in sexual adjustment, perfectionism, conventionality, intolerance, and in general, obsessive-compulsive features. They found that these personality features are associated with migraine to a greater degree than would be accounted for by chance.

Treatment Suggestions. In addition to medical treatment, psychotherapy is essential. At times intensive psychotherapy and even psy choanalysis may be necessary, usually because of other personality features as well as headaches, but most patients will have to be taken care of by the general physician and the following simple rules may prove helpful if the patient can be taught to make use of them:

1. This is not a perfect world. Families and friends, too, have their failings. Perfection is rarely attained, so be satisfied with less.

2. Tolerance makes understanding the other fellow easier. It sets an attainable standard.

3. Do not be a slave to the clock. Work at your own pace; do as much as you can. Trying to meet too many deadlines only creates tension.

4. You cannot please everybody, so stop trying. Popularity comes by giving your friends and family a chance to love you for yourself, not for your best performance.

5. Be efficient, yes. But not to the extent that perfection becomes a burden.

6. Speak up if you want to. You cannot please everybody, and honesty and directness break down barriers, make friendships easier.

7. Approve of yourself. You are as good as the next fellow.

8. Stop being so critical of your negative feelings. Everyone is ambivalent at times, so do not worry so much about loving and hating.

9. Stop feeling so guilty. We are all human beings and we all make errors. Give a little and you will get a lot—maybe even a reduction of the pain in your head.

Case 49. Migraine, Thought to Be Allergic; Good Response to Psychotherapy

A Jewess of 28 was raised in an orthodox home where, however, in her own words, religion was applied with a light hand. She married a man who observed the orthodox tenets of his religion with an almost fanatical zeal. Although migraine headaches antedated the marriage they now became very severe and occurred quite regularly on Saturdays.

The patient came from a family that was highly intellectual, but quite psychopathic. She considered herself scholastically the black sheep, although she was really a very intelligent girl, self-educated, and had accomplished a great deal for herself. The headaches were attributed to "sinus trouble."

Death of Mother. The mother died of bronchial asthma about the time that the patient's headaches began. The patient stated that she had a "sense of relief" because the mother had been so ill with asthma. Then the father remarried a rather ignorant woman (the patient's own words) in sharp contrast to the patient's own mother, and apparently this had something to do with the patient's determination to get married herself.

A fear of developing asthma because of the mother's illness was accompanied by a great fear of cancer, a real cancerophobia. Just before we saw her, she had had an anxiety attack and since then she had been nervous, weak and depressed.

Allergy Tests. She had been studied by allergists who, because of the occurrence of the headache on Saturdays, suggested that something in the orthodox food rituals might be related to the attacks. So she was subjected to skin tests and to a number of elimination diets which, however, failed to help her.

Husband's Fanaticism.   Much of her conversation had to do with her husband. She said that his whole life was religion; that his fanatical traits were especially marked on Saturday, the sabbath day; that he rushed her to get ready for that day and that she didn't liked to be rushed. There must not be a spot of dust for the holy sabbath. On one occasion he spoke to her about the fact that he couldn't love a woman who didn't see eye to eye with him on his religion. She resented this, saying, "His love of religion is enslaving me. If love is based on ritualistic observance, he can keep it. He says he can only love me if I give up my rebellious ways. I want to worship in my own way. He forces his religion on me and he won't compromise."

Sexual Frigidity.   In addition to that fact, just when she was so irritated and fatigued by preparation for the Sabbath, it was invariably on Friday nights that he asked for sexual intercourse. There is a special preparation for intercourse among those who observe the orthodox tenets: The woman has to immerse herself completely in a tub reserved for that purpose. She very much resented this preparation. She was frigid in intercourse, failed to obtain any satisfaction, and regularly on the night or the morning following she developed her attack of migraine. Before this was called to her attention she herself observed that when she was away for the summer, she didn't have migraine; in fact, she noted, "When I am away from home, I don't get migraine on Saturdays." When we pointed out her inability to express hostility directly and hence the mechanism of body language she replied that "hers was very eloquent."

She spent the summer away from Philadelphia. On her return, after having been free of migraine, she became irritable and depressed, complained of a heavy head, spoke about the boredom of facing another winter, said that she felt alone even when her husband was at home.

Improvement.   Finally, with our persuasion she decided to get herself some employment. We suggested that she try to find something that would fall in with her husband's interests. She got a job teaching, and derived a great deal of satisfaction from it. Her migraine improved during this period. The anxiety of the cancerophobia came up again. We discussed that with her. She said, "Yes, people sympathize with the headache, but not with anxiety. Even my husband walks around on tip-toe when I have my headache."

SUMMARY

A young married woman with typical migraine, thought to be allergic, failed to respond to the usual medical and dietary measures but obtained considerable relief from brief psychotherapy which permitted her to achieve a better personal and social adjustment.

EPILEPSY

In discussing symptom pictures related to the nervous system we must include the problem of epilepsy, which seems closely related to migraine. We approach the subject of epilepsy with less certainty than some of the other psychosomatic entities, being aware of how little is known of its real etiology and how resistant it may be to treatment. We agree with Lennox and Markham that emotional perturbations may accentuate but do not initiate epilepsy. However, our chief reason for including it is to bring to the attention of the physician the necessity for treating the personality problems of the patient who has seizures as well as restricting his activities and giving him drugs. The social personality problem of the epileptic is often overlooked. Only the seizures are treated and the personality that has to live and try to work out a destiny with such a handicap is ignored.

Predisposition.   The most fundamental factor in seizures is a predisposition in the nature of a cerebral dysrhythmia which can be demonstrated in *brain waves* measured by electroencephalographic tracings. Brain damage, physicochemical disorders in the body fluids, and emotional disturbances play their individual role in producing unconsciousness and the muscular activity of the seizure. From our own experience and from references to the literature it would seem that a certain number of patients with convulsive seizures respond well to minor psychotherapy; a few have been benefited by major psychotherapy; and in others even intensive psychotherapy has failed to break up the convulsive mechanism even though a greater emotional equilibrium has been achieved.

The discussion of the treatment of epilepsy has been divided into three phases by Lennox. He speaks of the physical, the pharmacological and the psychological-social fronts.

Treatment. PHYSICAL TREATMENT. On the physical front Lennox stresses a commonsense regularity of life without being either too dependent upon or too careless of rules. He believes that both physical and mental activity are indicated since activity seems to function as an antagonist of seizures. The greatest benefit is derived from activities which combine muscular exercise, intellectual interest and rest. He makes the point that anxious parents, whose minds are filled with visions of accidents of bodily injury to epileptic children, should consider the small chance of an attack occurring when the child is in a dangerous position and the large chance of invalidism and psychological damage as a result of oversolicitude and overprotection. The patient should eat the diet of the rest of the family. Plenty of rest and adequate elimination are, of course, indicated.

DRUG TREATMENT. Lennox warns that some patients are not helped by medicine no matter how much is taken and that sedative medication which stops seizures but slows up the body and mind to too great a degree is a failure. Likewise he suggests that an effective drug should produce some composure of the abnormal waves of the electroencephalographic record as well as stopping seizures. Drugs are only palliative; it is doubtful if they ever act as a cure in themselves.

SOCIAL-PSYCHOLOGICAL TREATMENT. The social-psychological front is important. The very diagnosis of epilepsy is in itself a shock to the patient and his family, who have usually hoped that the condition was only a "fainting spell" or the result of a digestive disturbance. A diagnosis of a condition which, with all its handicaps, may persist throughout a lifetime is news which is difficult to break to a patient or family. But once it has been proved, it is better to face the situation than to take the attitude that it may disappear at any time. One's life work has to be shaped around the condition, so it is much better to know the whole truth. The physician may emphasize to the patient that the seizures are not a threat to life and that various treatments are available but that time may be needed to find the best regimen for him. He can be reassured that while life with seizures has real difficulties one can still be happy and useful. Any feeling of shame or inferiority on the part of the family regarding epileptics must be dealt with, in order that the patient has at least the support of his family in meeting some of the inevitable prejudices in the world outside the home. *Neither the family nor the patient should be led to hope that seizures will disappear with puberty, marriage, motherhood, or any other life epoch.* The patient should be frankly told (not at one consultation, of course) some of the problems associated with the illness and prejudices that he may meet; and his life should be so ordered that he may be most useful to himself and to society. In other words, while some social and psychological protection to the epileptic may be given, he should, in so far as possible, assume the obligations and responsibilities of the other members of the family. This applies to children and adults alike.

Lennox and Markham suggest that the physician speak to patient and family in words such as these: "Epilepsy is not a mysterious disease and certainly is no disgrace. Simple epilepsy, like diabetes, is a metabolic disorder. It is perhaps, an enigma, but not a stigma. It does not tend to get worse with time. There are effective medicaments. The mind is rarely affected. A child should continue schooling, and the adult should work. Activity is an antagonist of seizures. Marriage and children are not necessarily precluded. Given social acceptance, the great majority of patients can lead normal lives."

About 10 per cent of epileptics who are outside of institutions become too dull mentally to be employable. About 10 per cent have difficult personalities, being stubborn, irritable, suspicious and opinionated. Other physical disabilities may complicate the problem. Altogether perhaps a third of adult epileptics are not proper subjects for training or regular employment. The remaining two thirds can give a good account of themselves if each case is considered individually.

Marriage in Epilepsy. A frequent question which may be asked of the physician is in regard to the marriage of those suffering from seizures. Records of the brain waves by means of the encephalograph show that many people have cerebral dysrhythmia who never have seizures. The person with cerebral dysrhythmia and seizures should take pain to marry a person who registers normal brain waves. Such a marriage reduces the chances of having a child subject to seizures.

In other words in epilepsy there is a tendency to hereditary transmission. This varies from person to person, and if the family history is not already too heavily weighted with psychopathic individuals or other epileptics and if he or she marries a person registering normal brain waves on the encephalographic tracing, the chances of having an epileptic offspring are not great. In fact two dysrhythmic individuals, even though seizure-free, might be more likely to produce an epileptic offspring than the union of an epileptic and a normal person. Sufferers from migraine are greater potential "carriers" of epilepsy than is commonly recognized.

Lennox provides further information on this subject in a letter to the Journal of the American Medical Association, answering an author who felt that the only hope of eliminating epilepsy is by birth control among epileptic adults. "Brain wave studies indicate that for every epileptic patient there are probably twenty or more nonepileptic patients who nevertheless are carriers of this or an allied disorder. Therefore, childlessness of all persons with epilepsy would eliminate only 5 per cent of epilepsy. Prohibitions applied to a person with epilepsy apply with equal force to one-half of his relatives and to something like 10 per cent of the whole population. Again the probability of having affected progeny depends in part on whether the person whom the epileptic person marries carries a predisposition to epilepsy. The marriage of two normal carriers of this disorder is more dangerous than the marriage of an epileptic person with a noncarrier. Logically brain wave tracings of both partners to a marriage should be secured if the physician is to offer specific advice to an individual. Even so he should consider the possibility suggested by unpublished observations that unusual, so-called 'abnormal' frequency of waves may be associated with high attainment or genius. Many implications of electroencephalography are as yet unexplored."

The psychological help to the person suffering from seizures may vary from an occasional friendly talk to intensive psychotherapy. The following case is illustrative.

Case 50.   Epilepsy

History and Symptoms.   A man of 39 was first seen in a psychiatric hospital where he arrived in *status epilepticus* following a series of convulsions. When he became conscious he was eager to relate his history. He was a friendly, good-looking man, appearing younger than his years, who had suffered many hardships. His mother had died when he was one year old and his father was a shiftless alcoholic who had left him to be cared for in a series of foster homes and by distant relatives who did not want him. He was ambitious to have an education but found it difficult to apply himself. Very often money saved for his education would be spent on a pleasure trip instead.

LIFE SITUATION

Marriage.   His first seizure occurred at the age of 22. At times there were as many as ten to twelve in twenty-four hours. At other times he might go for a number of days without them. He lost many jobs and began to be seclusive. Then he met a girl who fell in love with him. She thought that what he needed was a woman's love and care and they were married. But he was unable to appreciate the friendship and love of this warm-hearted person who worked and most of the time supported him. When we first saw him he was 29 and unemployed. He seemed anxious to receive help from psychotherapy. In spite of his apparent eagerness to cooperate it was evident, in the therapeutic relationship, that he wanted all the help given *to* him.

Psychotherapy.   When we asked him to write an autobiography he put this off for weeks although he had nothing else to do. However, he volunteered, "My seizures are a punishment for my laziness and my disinterest in other human beings." He knew from experience that if he would speak to someone during the aura preceding the attack he could often prevent a seizure. In spite of this he would ignore the aura and lapse off into unconsciousness. We said to him, "We know you have had a deprived childhood and have missed the personal interest, friendship, and guidance of capable and loving parents but you have a good wife and we all want to help you. If you are ambitious and want to enjoy the prestige and pleasure of occupying a place of usefulness in the world you must stop being sorry for yourself and start doing something for the people around you." As a result of emphasizing this point of view and showing him exactly how he could please his wife and his physician, he became more alert and cheerful.

Employment.   He obtained work in an office as a draftsman. We made a contact with his employer, who agreed to be patient, and he held this job for eight months. He had an occasional seizure at work but most of them came at night. Aside from being late to work in the morning following such a seizure he did tolerably well. He was at first elated at having the job but frequently lapsed into his old attitude that people did not appreciate his efforts. He deplored his meager education and complained that the job had no future. We would tell him, "Happiness and usefulness in this world do not depend entirely upon education, large salary, or high position. You could have those things in greater degree than you have now and still not be satisfied. You must learn to appreciate what you have." Then for another period he would be satisfied.

He was still ambitious to learn more, especially in the mechanical world. We pointed out the risks in this field and the greater intolerance of employers, but he insisted that he must try it. Finally he lost his draftsman's job and then felt that he must try engineering. His wife succeeded in getting him placed but in his third week he had an attack of petit mal in the engineering school and was dismissed. Then he obtained a job in a chain restaurant—work with which he was already familiar from years before. By application to work his wife had been able to save a little money and, with a friend who knew the restaurant business, she planned to open a little restaurant of their own where his occasional seizures would not bring up the constant fear of dismissal.

Results of Psychotherapy.   In this case we treated the emotional problems of the epileptic and his wife. We did not abolish the seizures but we felt that by combating despondency and a tendency to withdrawal in the patient we did succeed in reducing their number. We "kept him going," so to speak, by encouragement, by helping him to work out his plans, and by urging him to show greater friendliness and more appreciation for what he had.

DELIRIUM

Delirium refers to the mental symptoms associated with somatic disease. It may be gradual in onset or appear suddenly as a psychotic episode in a patient with advanced physical or metabolic disorder. Often it is associated with drug intoxication, febrile states, and advanced cardiac and renal diseases.

Generally the term is used to cover grossly disturbed behavior arising under the circumstances indicated above but Romano and Engel think that the term should apply to a much larger group of patients in whom the symptoms may appear very insidiously and are not so striking. After calling attention to the various noxious stimuli that bring about delirium, Romano emphasized that the most important variable is the nature of the personality structure which is reacting to the stimulus. Patients who are experiencing considerable anxiety in connection with their physical illness; patients who through language difficulties or superstition are apt to misinterpret events connected with the illness; patients of advanced age, with preexisting cerebral vascular disease; and patients of limited intellectual endowment: these three types are the ones apt to succumb to delirium.

Symptoms.   The early signs of an impending delirium are: inability to sleep; increased frequency of frightening dreams and nightmares; irritability; occasional misinterpretations of people, objects, shadows and noises; loss of appetite; and increased motor restlessness. Recognition of the primary disturbance, that is, the disturbance in consciousness, which can be tested by having the patient subtract serially, may aid in early diagnosis. At this stage, treatment may be successful in avoiding the development of the full-fledged delirium.

Electroencephalographic Study.   Studies by Engel and Romano of 53 patients with delirium of varying cause, intensity and duration revealed E.E.G. abnormalities in all patients who had disturbances in consciousness. These changes were found to be reversible to the extent to which the clinical delirium was reversible. Psychological data showed a direct correlation between the electrical abnormality and the disturbance of consciousness but there was less correlation with the more personal aspects of behavior, namely, the character and expression of anxiety, the content of thought, and the nature of sense deceptions. "The mere presence of abnormal brain waves in the electroencephalogram of a person with disturbances of behavior does not establish a relation between the two."

Treatment. The underlying physical or chemical disorder must be treated first. Adequate food and fluid intake should be maintained. Sleep may be obtained by use of the continuous tub bath at neutral temperatures, but most hospitals are not equipped for this procedure, and there is need to use a noncumulative, nontoxic chemical sedative such as paraldehyde or chloral hydrate. A low bed rather than sideboards is a good precautionary measure to prevent injury. The room should be kept well lighted at night to avoid shadows and misinterpretations, and tactful attendance and explanation of procedures to patients may aid considerably in avoiding further anxiety.

Although general hospitals should have facilities to care for such cases, most do not, and it may be necessary to transfer such a patient to a psychiatric hospital.

ORGANIC BRAIN DISEASE SIMULATING NEUROSIS

The situation which so many doctors fear—of missing an organic lesion and labeling the patient a neurotic—may actually occur. The problem sometimes happens in connection with *brain tumor*. The diagnosis of intracranial tumors is, of course, not difficult if the typical triad of headache, vomiting and papilledema is present. Unfortunately, this combination is usually a late rather than an early manifestation of brain tumors. Obviously, if the patient is to obtain the maximum benefit of neurosurgical skill, it is necessary to diagnose these lesions early but this is all too often extremely difficult, if not impossible. Early diagnosis is difficult when the chief symptoms seem to be psychiatric, when psychiatric symptoms that develop later obscure the true nature of the disease, or when a brain tumor incidentally develops in a person with neurotic symptoms. This is especially true in the absence of papilledema and roentgenographic abnormalities of the skull.

A review by Soniat of the records of 128 patients with proved intracranial neoplasms seen at the Ochsner Clinic found that approximately half exhibited symptoms on admission that could be considered "psychiatric."

Although tumors of the frontal lobe are commonly considered to be associated with psychiatric symptoms with greater frequency than are other types of intracranial neoplasms, Soniat points out that such symptoms are associated with tumors of the temporal lobe just as often. Tumors of the frontal lobe anterior to the motor areas often produce subtle peculiarities in the patient's personality that are insidious in onset. Other psychiatric manifestations, produced by frontal lobe tumors, appear gradually; these include impairment of memory (perhaps at first considered as absentmindedness but later becoming a more obvious and serious memory defect); difficulty in concentration; a flattening of the affect coupled with a growing apathy regarding domestic and commercial affairs; carelessness in personal appearance; and use of obscene and facetious speech.

Neoplastic lesions of the temporal lobe are notorious for causing hallucinations, which may be visual, olfactory or gustatory. Gustatory hallucinations consist in peculiar tastes, and olfactory hallucinations are peculiar odors that are usually described as unpleasant and likened to the odor of burning tar, asphalt, crude oil, gas or cooking cabbage. These types of hallucinations may be associated with dreamy states and uncinate fits. In such attacks, things seem unreal and distorted to the patient; sometimes strange things seem familiar and at other times patients describe the feeling as if one has been in a dream. The dreamy state may be followed by a generalized epileptiform convulsion. Of course, tumors of the temporal lobe may cause aphasia.

THE EMOTIONAL PROBLEMS OF CEREBRAL VASCULAR DISEASE

The emotions play an important part in circulatory disorders. The heart is the focal point for anxiety and it has been shown that functional disorders and even coronary occlusion may be precipitated by emotionally disturbing events. Does this apply to the brain? When we caution a friend about to get angry, "Look out for your blood pressure," we are hinting that a stroke may occur, and patients with high blood pressure as well as many others who suffer from headaches and dizziness worry about this, too.

Psychosomatic studies suggest that these popular ideas have some basis in fact and that vascular "accidents" in the brain as well as in the heart may be precipitated by emotional stress—that they are not so accidental after all.

Then there are the emotional problems which follow a "stroke" which are well known but inadequately treated. Apparently physicians become so absorbed in the physical features of the case that they neglect the emotional factors. We must become more aware of this important phase of rehabilitation.

Even more important to our health and economy is the question of the mental changes due to cerebral vascular disease. Psychosis associated with arteriosclerosis is one of the leading problems in psychiatry. The intensity of the psychosis is not necessarily correlated with the amount of organic damage, so that factors other than the amount of cerebral arteriosclerosis enter into the problems of the cause and treatment of this large group of mentally ill people. Life situations and emotionally disturbing events must be taken into consideration.

The Emotions and the Brain Circulation. There can be little question that the emotions affect the circulation to the brain. In vasodepressor syncope the obvious psychological factors and the striking clinical manifestations offer conclusive evidence that the two are related. The pallor, sweating, changes in respiration and pulse, falling blood pressure and marked distortion of the electrical activity of the brain which follow upon venous puncture, or some other threatening situation, attest to this relationship.

But another problem in circulatory dynamics which is of even greater significance from the standpoint of our subject has to do with the question of cerebral vascular spasm. The question of whether emotional factors are related to cerebral vascular disease depends to a certain extent upon the question of whether cerebral vascular spasm occurs.

Seidenberg and Ecker believe that intense emotion may cause cerebral arterial spasm and that this spasm in turn may be responsible for a "stroke." In a report of 6 patients under the age of 50 without gross pathologic lesions the authors demonstrated by means of angiograms that the intracranial portion of the internal carotid artery was affected by spasm. An interesting piece of experimental evidence is provided by Byrom, who observed the behavior of cerebral vessels in the rat by direct observation through windows inserted in the skull. The rats were made hypertensive by excising one kidney and constricting the opposite renal artery. The arterial spasm that was observed was related to hypertensive encephalopathy and could be abolished by lowering the blood pressure.

Migraine, of course, is a topic that comes to mind in this connection and a study by Engel and associates, already discussed (p. 454), is interesting in this regard.

Both of Engel's patients repeatedly developed transient focal neurological symptoms, presumably due to vasospasm, in a setting in which anger was the dominant emotion but either it was not expressed or guilt was felt when it was expressed. Both patients presented themselves as passive, compliant and restrained people who avoided trouble at any cost, but their dreams betrayed their aggressive and sadistic fantasies. The cerebral vasospasm apparently was related to the undischarged or incompletely discharged rage.

The authors speculate as to whether other cases of "stroke" may not also be initiated by vasospasm in psychologically stressful situations. Hypertensive encephalopathy and subarachnoid hemorrhage, apparently precipitated by emotional stress, have also been described (Weiss).

Ecker and associates believe that they have demonstrated vascular spasm by means of arteriograms and consider this spasm as significant in the pathogenesis of cerebral stroke. They state that in the general run of more than 500 angiographic cases, spasm was demonstrable in less than 19 per cent of the cases. On the other hand, in the patients with strokes (including various types of nontraumatic intracranial hemorrhage and cerebral edema or softening) spasm was demonstrable in approximately 90 per cent of the cases. In additional papers, they report in some detail the emotional factors that seem to precipitate the cerebral vascular accidents. In one study of 6 patients under the age of 50 without gross pathogenic lesions, Seidenberg and Ecker call attention to the problem of cerebral vascular disorders in young people and report in some detail the antecedent severe emotional disturbances.

In another report Ecker presents 20 patients with cerebral vascular disorders. In 13 cases there was nontraumatic intracranial hemorrhage and in 8 cases hemiparesis that was clearly organic. In 13 of these cases he found long-standing personality difficulty preceding the stroke and in 15 special emotional stress which immediately preceded the stroke. In 8 cases both factors were present. Angiograms technically suitable for the study of spasm of cerebral arteries were available in 15 cases and in all of these there was an excessive tendency to arterial contraction. Ecker feels that this spastic tendency may be one of the bodily expressions of the emotional disturbance, and that ischemia resulting from excessive arterial contraction contributes to the pathological changes in the brain and in its blood vessels.

"Little Strokes."   A few words must be said about "little strokes" so frequently discussed by Alvarez. No doubt, this is a useful designation and certainly refers to a common disorder. Alvarez refers to the frequent onset of a "little stroke" with a bad dizzy spell, followed by ear noises and a sense of insecurity. Later the story may be brought out of aging suddenly, a change in personality, moral deterioration, a loss of business judgment, insomnia, self-centeredness and that the patient has lost weight, no longer is well groomed, has become irascible and hard to handle. Now all of this is undoubtedly true and calls attention to an important clinical problem, but we would like to caution that just as the neurotic patient is frequently castigated with the term "constitutional inadequacy" which permits the physician to feel better about his inability to help the patient with his functional problems, so there is the danger of giving a physical label to the patient who has had an anxiety attack which often begins with a dizzy spell, followed by ear noises and a sense of insecurity, and often is followed by a limitation of activities. It is easy to call this a "little stroke" instead of taking the trouble to search for the unconscious mental conflict which stands behind the anxiety attack. In a sense it satisfies the bewildered patient to be told that he has had a stroke but at the same time it burdens him with the feeling that he has suffered irreparable damage and that a second stroke of greater severity and perhaps a fatal third stroke await him.

Case 51.   The Fear of Stroke

We would like to suggest that a great many people are disabled by the idea of stroke and that this is an important clinical problem. For example, a white woman, 62, was admitted to our hospital after taking barbiturate in an attempt at suicide.

Within a short time (1937–39) the patient had lost her mother, father and husband. She was 49, there were two children, and it was necessary for her to get a job. High blood pressure was discovered but, in spite of that, she worked very hard throughout the war years. Her son became a bomber pilot which, of course, gave her great concern. She did nothing about her blood pressure until 1944 since which time she had been under medical care.

The mother's death was due to cerebral embolism which occurred postoperatively (there had been high blood pressure in the mother's family). The mother had been a happy and cheerful person in her younger days but became depressed at the menopause and had hallucinations. The patient was 25 at the time and living at home. She, of course, was very much concerned about her mother.

In November 1952 the patient had an attack which affected her speech and caused left-sided weakness. This began to clear almost immediately and after two weeks of rest she remained pretty well until the summer of 1953. Then her employer, a man of 70, who was very exacting in his demands, had a stroke. The patient, greatly concerned, was preoccupied with this problem, and visited her physician who said, "You were lucky the first time but you can't go walking around with a blood pressure like this or something will have to give." She feared a stroke and becoming a burden to her children, became depressed, had trouble sleeping, and finally attempted to end her life.

The past history indicated that she had been frigid in her marriage to an unsuccessful lawyer, that she had been depressed for a time after the children were born, and also somewhat depressed after a partial hysterectomy in 1935 which had been followed by pulmonary embolism.

SUMMARY

A woman with hypertension had a cerebral vascular accident, from which she made a good recovery. Personality study revealed compulsive characteristics and depression. A physician's statement reinforced anxiety regarding stroke and precipitated mental depression. Family history was positive for hypertension and cerebral vascular disease as well as for psychopathology.

Family Reactions to Hemiplegia. When the immediate concern as to whether the patient will live has subsided, the problem of rehabilitation comes up. Important problems are bound to arise within the family group. The stroke often occurs in a person who has been very active and productive and is suddenly completely disabled. He feels useless and, unfortunately, the family often adds to this feeling. They become too sympathetic and may try too hard to help; to the hemiplegic patient they often seem to nag with their importunities to help. Questions are repeated because the patient may be slow to answer and this is annoying to the patient, or it may be to make the questioner understood when the patient cannot talk, even though he can understand. As time goes on the family becomes impatient with the patient's emotional lability or his rigidity, that is, his unwillingness to accept change or his distress from the slightest change in his surroundings or activities. It is necessary to be patient, to speak slowly and quietly in asking questions or making requests and not to expect quick answers. When the patient has learned to use his arm or leg, calling the attention of visitors to the fact will often induce self-consciousness and clumsiness again.

The hemiplegic patient should not be allowed to tyrannize the home. Tapering off with sympathy, attention and helpfulness and expecting the patient to stand on his own two feet are, of course, important considerations.

Psychosis and Cerebral Arteriosclerosis. The most important part of this discussion is the problem of psychosis associated with arteriosclerosis which, because of its tremendous incidence, is becoming one of the leading problems in psychiatry. Over a twenty-year period, annual hospital admissions for this disorder have risen tenfold, until today it is estimated that patients suffering from hardening of the arteries of the brain comprise the second largest group of mentally ill, second in number only to the schizophrenics. As to the cost of this ailment, some 200 million dollars a year in public funds are spent on custodial care for its victims.

Since the symptoms are familiar to all physicians and, in part, have been referred to in the discussion of "little strokes," we will not discuss them further except to say that so often the physician assumes, once he notes evidence of arteriosclerosis, that all of the patient's difficulties are directly attributable to the irreversible structural change, and this may be an oversimplification which operates to the disadvantage of the patient. Careful studies are necessary to ascertain the degree of organic change but, in addition, it is important to realize that the intensity of the emotional disorder is not necessarily correlated with the amount of organic damage. This has been repeatedly demonstrated and need not be gone into here.

In Clow's survey of 100 patients suffering from cerebral arteriosclerosis with psychosis at the New York Hospital severe emotional precipitants were noticed in 76. Drug toxicity sufficient to produce psychotic symptoms was present in 37. Treatment was both physical and psychiatric. Psychotherapy included stimulation of new interests in life, broader personal contacts, continued reassurance and occupational therapy. Under this regimen it became evident that by no means were all of these cases hopeless. Eleven patients recovered, 12 were much improved, 31 improved somewhat, and following therapy 49 were able to leave the hospital and return to their homes.

Fortunately we can end this discussion with the hopeful note that if we take other factors into consideration in regard to this problem of psychosis with arteriosclerosis, many of these patients can be helped. It is true here as elsewhere in the domain of psychosomatic medicine, that multiple factors enter into the cause of disease and disorder and hence must be sought for, and that multiple factors, including psychotherapy, are necessary in treatment and rehabilitation.

References

Alvarez, W. C.: The Neuroses, W. B. Saunders Co., Philadelphia, 1951, p. 194.
Byrom, F. B.: Lancet, *2:* 201, 1954.
Clow, H. F.: Am. J. Psychiat., *97:* 16, 1940.
Ecker, A.: Ann. Int. Med., *40:* 49, 1954.
Ecker, A., and Riemenschneider, P. A.: Neurology, *3:* 495, 1953.
Engel, G. L., Ferris, E. B., and Romano, J.: Am. J. M.Sc., *209:* 650, 1945.
Engel, G. L., Hamburger, W. W., Reiser, M., and Plunkett, J.: Psychosom. Med., *15:* 344, 1953.
Engel, G. L., and Romano, J.: Arch. Neurol. & Psychiat., *51:* 356, 1944.
Engel, G. L., Webb, J. P., Ferris, E. B., Romano, J., Ryder, H., and Blankenhorn, M. A.: War Medicine, *5:* 304, 1944.
Friedman, A. P., Brenner, C., and Merritt, H. H.: J.A.M.A., *132:* 489, 1946.
Friedman, A. P., von Storch, T. J. C., and Merritt, H. H.: Neurology, *4:* 773, 1954.
Fromm-Reichmann, F.: Psychoanalyt. Rev., *24:* 26, 1937.
Gardner, J. W., Mountain, G. E., and Hines, E. A.: Am. J. M.Sc., *200:* 50, 1940.
Kozol, H. L.: Arch. Neurol. Psychiat., *56:* 245, 1946.
Lennox, W. G.: (*a*) Science and Seizures. p. 109. Harper & Bros., New York, 1941; (*b*) Letter: J.A.M.A., *117:* 1806, 1941.
Lennox, W. G., and Markham, C. H.: J.A.M.A., *152:* 1688, 1953.
Lippman, C. W.: J. Nerv. & Ment. Dis., *116:* 346, 1952.
Romano, J.: Bull. New England M.Soc., *4:* 64, 1942.
Romano, J., and Engel, G. L.: M. Clin. North America, *28:* 629, 1944.
Romano, J., and Engel, G. L.: Psychosom. Med., *7:* 3, 1945.
Ross, W. D., and McNaughton, F. L.: Canad. M.A.J., *53:* 12, 1945.
Ross, W. D., and McNaughton, F. L.: Psychosom. Med., *7:* 73, 1945.
Schwartz, M. J.: J. Allergy, *23:* 426, 1952.
Seidenberg, R., and Ecker, A.: Psychosom. Med., *16:* 374, 1954.
Simons, D. J., and Wolff, H. G.: Psychosom. Med., *8:* 227, 1946.
Soniat, T. L. L.: Bull. Ochsner Clin., *10:* 4, 1951.
Touraine, T. A., and Draper, G.: J. Nerv. & Ment. Dis., *80:* 1, 1934.

Weiss, E.: Bull. N. Y. Acad. Med., *23:* 604, 1947.
Weiss, E.: Psychosom. Med., *2:* 249, 1940.
Wolff, H. G.: Arch. Neurol. & Psychiat., *37:* 895, 1937.
Wolff, H. G.: Lecture, Institute of Living, March 20, 1946.
Wolff, H. G.: Headache and Other Head Pain. Oxford University Press, New York, 1948.
Wolff, H. G.: Tunis, M. M., and Goodell, H.: Arch. Int. Med., *92:* 478, 1953.

Chapter XVII

Disorders of the Ear and Eye

DISORDERS OF THE EAR

The advent of antibiotics has changed the practice of otolaryngology. Davison says that most patients now need good differential diagnosis, instruction in hygiene, psychotherapy and medication rather than surgery. Of 1000 patients examined by him almost 20 per cent had psychosomatic complaints. He comments that such patients are regarded as nuisances by otolaryngologists interested solely in surgery. Davison emphasizes that the complaints of these patients must be taken seriously.

Dizziness and Vertigo

Vertigo is a symptom. The term "dizziness" is often used synonymously, as are the terms "giddy" or "light-headed," to describe sensations which vary from the slightest sensation of confusion to the most intense vertigo. Vertigo may vary in degree from a fleeting sensation of rotation, barely perceptible to the patient, to a sensation of violent rotation by a force so strong that the victim is immediately thrown to the ground. Consequently, when a patient complains of dizziness the physician must secure an accurate description of the sensations which the patient has experienced, a detailed statement of associated symptoms and definite information about conditions which predispose to or precipitate the symptom described as "dizziness," before he can evaluate its significance.

Differentiating Vertigo and Syncope. Patients commonly confuse vertigo with syncopal states of varying degrees and refer to all such sensations by the terms "dizzy" or "giddy." Distinction must be made between the two symptoms, because vertigo implies a disturbance of equilibrium, syncope a transient cerebral anemia. The diagnosis of the symptom of vertigo requires a sensation of rotation which is not present in cerebral anemia. Hypersensitivity of the carotid sinuses or petit mal epilepsy may be confused with vertigo by the patient.

Nystagmus and the past pointing reaction are almost constant accompaniments of vertigo, and nausea or vomiting or both may be present in severe attacks.

Menière's Syndrome. Menière's symptom complex is a condition of unknown cause characterized by recurring attacks of vertigo, nausea and vomiting, associated with tinnitus and deafness of the perceptive type.

Fowler and Zeckel studied 23 patients with Menière's disease from a psychosomatic standpoint and observed that clumping of red blood cells and sluggish flow in small blood vessels were pronounced in the conjunctival vessels shortly before and after Menière attacks. They believe that the same changes occur in the blood supply to the inner ear bringing about labyrinthine hydrops. Clinical and experimental work with intravenous injections of procaine assisted them in arriving at these conclusions. Observing conjunctival changes of a similar nature after experimental psychic stimuli they conclude that the effect of psychogenic factors seems to involve slowing and arresting of the small blood vessel circulation within the labyrinth on an adrenergic pattern. They believe that psychotherapy may reverse the course of the disease in early stages. In advanced Menière's disease they suggest that medical treatment and surgery will have to be continued but that in a large percentage of cases psychotherapy will be necessary in addition.

The term "pseudo-Menière's disease" has been used to indicate instances of severe recurring vertigo of unknown causation in which evidence of cochlear dysfunction is not exhibited. An infinite variety of treatments has been advocated for this condition, such as limitation of salt and fluids, and the Furstenberg regimen, which consists of a diet entirely free of sodium with the substitution of ammonium chloride to maintain the chloride level in the body. Nicotinic acid and thiamine hydrochloride have been tried, just as they have been in almost every obscure disease, but without striking results. Therapy with histamine is said at times to produce immediate relief of the attack of vertigo. Intracranial division of the acoustic nerve or its vestibular fibers has been recommended but destructive labyrinthotomy has largely replaced hemisection of the eighth nerve. Very little attention has been paid to emotional factors in the so-called pseudo-Menière's disease.

Relation to Anxiety States. Vertigo, ringing in the ears, and numbness and tingling of the extremities are phenomena which often result from psychic stress and usually occur together. The early symptoms of anxiety are usually expressed through the cardiovascular, respiratory, gastrointestinal and genitourinary systems. Only as the emotional illness progresses does it include symptoms referable to the central nervous system itself. So little is this understood that when psychosomatic disease has affected the nervous system, giving symptoms such as the above, some rare condition is usually thought of to explain them. Among these are Menière's disease, labyrinthitis, hypoglycemia, brain tumor and peripheral neuritis. Careful neurological examination will rule out disease of the nervous system. A patient often fails to receive a satisfactory diagnosis even though the physician finds the neurological examination negative. The physician continues to think that "there must be neurological disease somewhere." This means either that he does not believe emotion can produce symptoms referable to the nervous system or that he does not trust his findings. Psychological study is necessary, as well as tests aimed at exclusion of organic disease, to prepare the way for a psychotherapeutic program.

Case 52.   Vertigo

History and Symptoms.   A woman of 55 with a moderate elevation of blood pressure and pronounced symptoms of cardiac neurosis suffered an attack of severe vertigo. She was thoroughly studied at the hospital and no evidence of organic disease other than moderate elevation of blood pressure was found. The study included a complete neurological survey.

As one of us was leaving her room after the last interview, a casual comment seemed to have more bearing on the vertigo than all of the examinations just completed. In the course of the conversation, she said, "You have much to live for (meaning the profession of medicine), while I have nothing."

LIFE SITUATION

She had always aspired to a career in medicine, encouraged by a dominating mother who directed her own ambitions to the daughter. Instead, she married a man whom she idealized as a perfect person, "not primarily interested in woman as a sexual object," only to find that he made constant sexual demands. She never attained sexual gratification, but had five children in rapid succession. She devoted herself to her children (now grown). Following the death of her mother from heart disease, she developed a mild depressive reaction from which she had not recovered. The discovery of the hypertension permitted her to focus her anxiety upon her heart and the fear of death from a "stroke."

With psychotherapy, she was able to recognize and express the hostility against her husband, but had more difficulty with her guilt-laden wishes against her mother. It was with great difficulty that she was able to see her mother's domination and her own need for her mother's love, which had determined her pattern of submission, the development of unconscious wishes for her mother's death to relieve herself of this burden, and the ensuing guilt, which increased her own need to act the dutiful daughter. Then, from this identification, she punished herself with her mother's symptoms of heart disease, especially after anything that she considered self-indulgence or ostentation. After the "heart pain" there was a secondary depression associated with feelings of helplessness and inadequacy.

During the course of treatment her depression diminished and she was able to engage in more activities, such as a class in music appreciation, from which she derived great pleasure. The atmosphere at home improved. Then of her own accord she suggested diminishing the frequency of her visits to the psychiatrist, and immediately after this had the attack of severe vertigo that resulted in the hospital study. We thought of the symptom as representing symbolically her fear that she might not be able to maintain her balance without supportive therapy, but perhaps on a deeper level it had to do with fear of "falling" in a sexual sense.

Psychological Aspects of Deafness.   Psychological difficulties are fairly common among deaf persons. If a person is healthy and well adjusted prior to deafness he often accepts his deprivation and makes a good adjustment. On the other hand, if there are neurotic or psychotic trends before the onset of deafness these influence the patient's reaction to the disorder. Paranoid trends occur; mild suspicion and "having to know what others might say about him" is common. Zeckel discusses these problems as seen among the deaf and hard of hearing at a deafness clinic.

After the fenestration operation, psychological improvement frequently follows the improvement in hearing. Unfortunately, good results following this operation frequently do not last, and the patient is apt to become worse psychologically as hearing is lost again.

A hearing aid may be of tremendous psychological importance, since it makes communication possible and encourages socializing, but hearing aids are often refused, partly because they are an admission of incurable illness and the patient wishes to suppress the knowledge of his handicap from himself and others.

Physical symptoms such as tinnitus and vertigo may add to the feelings of insecurity and further accentuate neurotic trends.

OCULAR AND VISUAL DISTURBANCES

It has been said that the ophthalmologist is in a position to see a great many symptoms that are due to emotional conflict. The eye is an organ of orientation but it is also the receptor of stimuli that satisfy many needs. Much that is forbidden can be taken in by way of the eye. The eye is most important in learning the secrets of sex, and if sex has been too strongly tabooed during the childhood period the unconscious needs of the adult may determine a functional disturbance in the organ whereby he comes in contact with so much that is forbidden. Moreover, the eye not only absorbs pleasurable stimuli; magic and erotic power are supposed to emanate from the eye so that there are additional reasons why, in the unconscious, the organ is closely related to sexuality. Persons so disposed, who have seen something which they consider improper, may react with squinting, blepharospasm, watering of the eyes or hysterical blindness. As Freud expressed it in one of his early papers, "If the sexual component-instinct which makes use of sight—the sexual 'lust of the eye'— has drawn down upon itself, through its exorbitant demands, some retaliatory measure from the side of the ego-instincts, so that the ideas which represent the content of its strivings are subjected to repression and withheld from consciousness, the general relation of the eye and the faculty of vision to the ego and the consciousness is radically disturbed." Or, as he later states in the same paper, it is as if an accusing voice had uplifted itself within the person concerned, saying, "Because you have chosen to use your organ of sight for evil indulgence of the senses, it serves you quite right if you can see nothing at all now," thus giving its sanction to the outcome of the process. Any threat to the safety of the eyes in such persons may result in serious anxiety.

Anxiety and the Eyes. In certain anxiety states there may be bizarre complaints related to the eyes and vision. Vision is blurred, electric lights appear to have a ring around them, they are divided into sections, or they appear as if the light were being looked at through a screen. Others complain of pain or itching in the eyeballs in the absence of organic disease. "Tubular fields," tunnel or shaft vision is a common symptom. The treatment of these bizarre sensations is treatment of the underlying neurosis, which is usually a severe one. These sensations in the eyes or symptoms related to vision are similar to vertigo and paresthesia. Usually they represent late symptoms in a severe anxiety state although they are not generally thought of as symptoms of anxiety. Too often the physician thinks only of ocular or central nervous system disease, overlooking the possibility of a psychogenic disorder.

Hysterical blindness is a common symptom, occurring in one or both eyes or in various fields of each eye. Many cases have been "cured" by hypnotism or the profound suggestion of electrical treatments. Such "cures" are usually only temporary, however, because the underlying neurosis has not been modified. Real psychotherapy, in which the patient participates intellectually and emotionally, is necessary if we are to do more than temporarily abolish the symptom.

Asthenopia.   Rutherford defines asthenopia as "a syndrome in which the visual discomforts that attend prolonged close work are accompanied by feelings of fatigue and reflex manifestations remote from the eye. It can be classed as a psychoneurosis because of its mechanism and symptomatology. The term 'eyestrain' may be reserved for those cases in which visual discomforts are brought on by prolonged close work, are limited to the eyes, and promptly disappear when close work is discontinued." *Hence, the wise ophthalmologist recognizes that the patient with asthenopia needs a change in his outlook upon life rather than a change of his lenses.* Even when a headache has been attributed to "eyestrain" and actually cured by fitting glasses, it does not necessarily prove that the headache was due to a minor error in refraction. The elements of suggestion and transference must be evaluated.

Night-blindness.   Night-blindness is a disturbance of light perception which results in difficulty and occasionally an inability to adapt the vision to faint illumination. In a study of 52 soldiers with this disorder Wittkower and associates found no ocular cause for the night-blindness and in particular could find no indication of vitamin A deficiency as an etiological factor. However, "nervous" habits—nail-biting; speech disorders; food-fussiness; morbid fears, such as excessive fear of darkness and fear of injury, especially to the eyes; conflicts over aggressiveness; and abnormal prying interests—were commonly seen, and long antedated the onset of the disorder.

Forty-three patients had definite evidence of neurosis; the chief characteristic was a lifelong history of overdependence. Stressing the importance of sexual conflict in the early development of these patients, Wittkower thinks that it is not surprising that the blindness is limited to the night when we consider that night is predominantly the time for sexual expression and darkness is the best ally of the criminal aggressor. In other words, if the sexual curiosity of childhood centers in the eyes and has to do especially with trying to see in the darkness and the conflict is repressed because it is forbidden, then it is conceivable that under the stimulus of seeing in the dark, symptoms will occur.

Miners' Nystagmus.   In a study based on incapacity among miners, Halliday discussed, among other conditions, miners' nystagmus. This type of oscillation, found only among miners, was regarded as a disease and was sometimes associated with such symptoms as movement of objects, headache, giddiness and night-blindness. Inasmuch as it was a compensable condition, when its incidence increased a committee was appointed to study the disorder. The committee concluded that deficient illumination was the essential factor. Again the incidence rose. Culpin had already suggested that it was a psychoneurosis and Halliday called attention to the fact that, although insufficient illumination was held to be responsible for the disorder, the incidence increased ten-fold during the period when the physical environment generally was undergoing a progressive improvement as regards lighting, ventilation and hygiene. He concluded that miners' nystagmus is mainly, if not entirely, a psychoneurotic disorder with symptomatology centering on the eyes, the symptoms being fixed on the visual organs as a result of such psychological factors as suggestion, "knowledge," compensation and fear of blindness.

Incidentally, this is one of a series of observations which form the background for a sociodynamic approach to psychosomatic problems. Halliday has published a book on this subject.

Central Angiospastic Retinopathy. Just as general physicians became more aware of the psychosomatic concept as a result of medical experiences in World War II, so was ophthalmology influenced. Harrington commented that the precision of diagnostic and therapeutic procedures available to ophthalmology has led to a conspicious neglect of psychic factors in ocular disease. He feels that prolonged but reversible psychological disturbance can eventually give rise to irreversible organic disease in the eye just as in other body systems. Among other conditions he discussed central angiospastic retinopathy. This clinical entity begins acutely as a grayish edema of the macula which may vary from the faintest haziness with loss of foveal reflex to a disciform, sharply outlined, flat, serous detachment of the macula. As the edema subsides, a redistribution of retinal pigment gives a mottled and irregular appearance to the macular area. Frequently there are numerous discrete, punctate yellowish dots around the fovea. The pigmentary disturbance is followed by a gradual loss of substance in the fovea and the development of a sharply outlined, punched-out, slightly irregular and usually minute hole in the macula. Visual disturbance in the stage of edema is usually pronounced. This may be followed in the end stages by complete or partial restoration of central vision.

At the same time that Harrington was making his observations Zeligs reported on this condition among navy personnel and marines. He concluded that spasm of retinal blood vessels is induced by emotional factors. In discussing Harrington's paper, Zeligs stated that the ophthalmologist cannot treat such patients merely by asking them to abstain from smoking or by prescribing some antispasmodic drug, but rather they should be given the opportunity of psychotherapy.

In a study of 23 consecutive patients with circulatory disturbances in the central retina Nichollis classified 6 as having central angiospastic retinopathy. Emotional stress played an important role and treatment was most effective in the younger age group, in whom the disease was of short duration, arteriolosclerosis less pronounced and angiospasm associated with anxiety the most prominent feature.

Glaucoma. Attacks of primary glaucoma have been precipitated by emotional upsets. Schoenberg cited cases in which the attack seemed to be connected with accidents or with the death of a member of the patient's family, worry over ill health, or financial losses. Inman has referred to primary glaucoma as an organ neurosis and proposed the term "angioneurotic edema of the anterior eye."

Certain it is, stated Harrington, that there are many aspects of glaucoma which cannot be explained by the old mechanical theories of aqueous drainage. "More and more evidence is being accumulated to show the close relationship between the intraocular vascular circulation, the secretion of intraocular fluid and the autonomic nervous system. The susceptibility of the autonomic nervous system to emotional shock is well known."

In a study from the Chicago Institute for Psychoanalysis of 36 glaucoma cases, Piers found in 24 of them a close connection between glaucoma attacks and specific emotional events to which these individuals were especially sensitive. In 9 cases the original attack was precipitated by witnessing an accident which resulted in injury or death to someone with whom the patient had intense emotional ties. In the majority of the other cases, where such acutely traumatic upsets did not occur, there nevertheless were found chronic emotional conflicts involving the patient and one or more of his dependents.

A forty-four-year-old woman who had had an operation for glaucoma on one eye was studied psychoanalytically. A daily chart of the eye tension was kept; later biweekly readings of the ocular tension were made. From the beginning of the psychoanalysis it was obvious that the patient was laboring under intense anxiety. A relation was found between ocular tension and emotional tension; the ocular pressure rose whenever aggressive, hostile feelings with the concomitant anxiety were intensified and fell during periods of relative freedom from anxiety.

Treatment.   Among the few ophthalmologists who understand the ocular neuroses, the best advice regarding their management comes from Derby: "A diagnosis of neurosis is not hard to arrive at, but once it has been made one should be prepared to spend some time on the patient or, if not, to send the patient to someone else who will. One must gain the patient's confidence or no results will be obtained; a hasty, superficial examination will not inspire confidence. Once one is sure of the diagnosis, I think that the best procedure is to put all the cards on the table, tell the patient frankly what is the matter, and explain to the best of one's ability and as simply as possible how the trouble developed. Pain, as is well known, can become a habit; and as we all use our eyes constantly for one thing or another during our waking hours, the habit pain repeats itself frequently. . . . Most people can grasp the fact that the use of the eyes should be a subconscious function, that it is only when we are conscious of them that we suffer from discomfort, and that the only way to get rid of this discomfort, is to get the eyes back to the subconscious level. To do this depends largely on the patient's own effort. He should use the eyes, not rest them, and disregard discomfort; when the eyes feel especially uncomfortable they should be used. Such discipline will almost always effect a cure if the patient has confidence in his physician and has what is vulgarly termed 'guts.' I freely confess that in earlier days I supported these measures sometimes with prism exercises, sometimes with graduated reading (Dyer's method). Now I rarely use either but depend solely on the mental effect of a careful explanation of the trouble. It is far more dangerous to tell a patient to rest a healthy pair of eyes than to induce him to use them. Many a sensitive patient has been made hypersensitive by the prescription of rest and dark glasses; the potential psychoneurotic becomes an actual one. Our aim in this, as in other fields of medicine, should be prevention, and we can nip many a beginning neurosis in the bud."

CHANGING LENSES.   We refer here again to Derby: "There is entirely too much changing of lenses a fraction of a diopter or a few degrees of axis among us, and naturally so, because it is the path of least resistance. I believe that we ophthalmologists should take more pride in not prescribing glasses and in changing a minimum of glasses, than in the number of prescriptions we issue."

References

Ear:

Davison, F. W.: J.A.M.A., *160:* 105, 1956.
Fowler, E., Jr., and Zeckel, A.: J.A.M.A., *148:* 1265, 1952.
Furstenberg, A. C.: Ann. Otol., Rhin. & Laryng., *43:* 1035, 1934.
Zeckel, A.: J. Nerv. & Ment. Dis., *112:* 322, 1950.

Eye:

Culpin, M.: Recent Advances in the Psychoneuroses. J. A. Churchill, London, p. 193, 1931.
Derby, G. S.: J.A.M.A., *95:* 913, 1930.
Freud, S.: Collected Papers. Vol. II, p. 110, Hogarth Press, London, 1924.
Halliday, J. L.: Psychosom. Med., *5:* 71, 1943.
Halliday, J. L.: Psychosocial Medicine. W. W. Norton and Co., New York, 1948.
Harrington, D. O.: J.A.M.A., *133:* 669, 1947.
Inman, W.: Lancet, *2:* 118, 1929.
Nichollis, J. V. V.: Am. J. Ophth., *35:* 1737, 1952.
Piers: Ten-Year Report, Institute for Psychoanalysis, Chicago, p. 32, 1932–1942.
Rutherford, C. W.: J.A.M.A., *99:* 284, 1932.
Schoenberg, M.: Arch. Ophth., *23:* 76, 1940.
Wittkower, E. D., Rodger, T. F., et. al.: Brit. M.J., *2:* 671, 1941.
Zeligs, M. A.: Psychosom. Med., *9:* 110, 1947.

Chapter XVIII

Skin Disorders and Allergies

PSYCHOSOMATIC ASPECTS OF SKIN DISORDERS

Recent years have witnessed an increasing interest in the relation of the emotions to disorders of the skin. The skin, like the eye, is an organ of expression. Both the eye and the skin, including the hair, are said to sparkle and "glow" with vitality or to be dull and lifeless. The skin, like the eye, is important as a point of contact between the inner and outer worlds.

Blushing, pallor and sweating are well known skin phenomena which express behavior such as excitement, embarrassment, shame, fear and anger. But beyond these very obvious reactions we are interested to know whether definite skin lesions may also express behavior; in other words, whether emotional factors may be responsible for more permanent changes in the skin.

Attitude of Dermatologists. The general opinion of dermatologists in this regard is exactly similar to the attitude toward psychosomatic problems encountered among other specialists and general physicians as well. This has been discussed elsewhere. It is well expressed by Sulzberger in his book, "Dermatologic Allergy," wherein he states that there is no proof for "nervousness" as causal in the production of a dermatosis. "In our material, we have gained the impression that these occasional instances of 'nervousness' were (1) purely coincidental, (2) concomitant (*i.e.,* psychoneurologic disturbances caused by the same factor or factors which produced the dermatologic manifestation), or (3) clearly the entirely comprehensible result of and the normal reaction to the dermatosis and its 'maddening' itching, loss of sleep, and continuous worry about disfigurement, about the future, about economic and other personal and related conditions." Continuing, Sulzberger points out that "the older designations of neurodermite, neurodermatitis, angioneurotic edema, etc., have nothing to do with the present meaning attached to the words 'nervous,' 'neurogenic,' 'neurotic,' etc."

CONCEPT OF MULTIPLE CAUSATION. Stokes, on the other hand, has stood in the forefront of the dermatologists who accept psychosomatic influences in the etiology of skin disorders. He and Beerman have this to say on the subject.

"One might almost say that until relatively recently only self-infliction, recognizable by the bizarre and unclassifiable physical outlines of the lesion, was admitted to the field of the psychogenous in diseases of the skin. There is also recognizable in medicine in general, a disposition to think in terms of sole causes rather than complex interacting factors. This sole-cause attitude of mind has perhaps an admirable cutting edge in exposing the etiology of a relatively unknown group of ailments; but it must give place ultimately to a viewpoint which recognizes multiple causation and interrelations as equally fundamental with, if not more fundamental than the single isolated cause. The psyche rarely appears in dermatoses as a sole cause, and for that reason has met with more difficulty in acceptance, perhaps, than have fungi, body cells, and so forth."

With this viewpoint of *multiple* causation in regard to psychosomatic skin disorders, as well as other psychosomatic conditions, we are in complete agreement.

Neurodermatitis. A large amount of the case material of the dermatologist is made up of the "eczema-neurodermatitis" group of disorders. Often they are difficult problems, refractory to treatment. The question of multiple etiological factors, acting in complementary fashion, is important in regard to them.

In connection with the controversy of "nervous eczema versus contact dermatitis," we cite very briefly a case that is now old in the literature but which has some keen and critical comment that is still pertinent.

Rattner reported the case of a young man who two weeks after his marriage developed an acute dermatitis on his face and neck and the upper half of the body. He had a psychoneurosis and anxiety state. The dermatitis was assumed to be neurogenous. It was subsequently shown that this acute dermatitis was excited by perfumed cosmetics which his wife used.

For sixteen years this patient had had recurrent attacks of eczema, all of which were considered to be seborrheic dermatitis. Then, superimposed on this seborrheic habitus, the acute dermatitis was found to be a sensitization dermatitis. The importance, if any, of the neurogenous component, Rattner went on to say, could be estimated only by inference, whereas positive patch tests were tangible evidence that the irritant was at fault.

We had some correspondence with Dr. Rattner about this case and he said that the diagnosis of neurogenous dermatitis was made by a dermatologist in another city, only after a thorough search for irritants had failed. Another capable dermatologist concurred in the diagnosis. The patient then consulted a neuropsychiatrist who agreed that there was a psychoneurosis, but felt that the dermatitis was a thing apart.

We shall not give further details of the correspondence, except to say that the patient eventually got himself into the predicament of going to a psychiatrist for treatment of his skin and to a dermatologist to look after his psychological disturbance!

"Nervous Eczema." Dr. Pusey commented about the foregoing

case: "We are witnessing an intense agitation of the subject of nervous eczema. Dr. Rattner's case illustrates the pitfalls into which we are apt to get in following this lead. Here is a case which seemed made to order for the diagnosis of eczema of nervous origin. The sexual element is exaggerated, the psychic factors are all there, including, as is usually found in such cases, a readiness of the patient to accept the emotional origin of his trouble. The background is perfect and it takes but a few bold strokes of the sympathetic artist to give a striking picture of a neurogenous or psychogenous eczema. But what do the unsentimental facts show when they are worked out? The patient is sensitized to perfume and that is what is exciting his attacks. Many similar cases of nervous or other systemic origin which have vanished into thin air when they are traced down to their local irritations must occur to everyone with a large experience in skin disease.

"The insistence on the importance of nervous factors as a cause of eczema and many other dermatoses is a backward step into the old maze of conjecture, out of which we have been trying to find our way for more than a century. Each revival of the conjecture gives us a new set of terms, but the idea remains the same. Forty years ago they were treating neurasthenia by cutting off prepuces, correcting defects of vision and removing other actual or imaginary causes of reflex irritation to cure eczema. Then they called them 'eczemas of reflex nervous origin.' Now we are psychoanalyzing them and calling them psychogenous and neurogenous eczemas. The words are new, but it is the same old tune. The ideas are remnants of the old hippocratic humoral pathology which has obfuscated our views for twenty-five years."

"Multiple Factors."   To continue with Pusey, "One of the chief businesses of dermatology since it has been able in the last hundred years to study more accurately the physical and chemical facts of pathology has been to show in respect to one disease after another that these diatheses are broken reeds, extremely tempting and appealing in one way or another, according to the predilections of the individuals, but in the end broken reeds. When the diathesists are confronted with a case which they would have of a nervous origin but in which there has been demonstrated an external cause which excites the eruption and without which the eruption would not exist, they are wont to take refuge [and now it will be recognized why we are quoting this in such detail] in the explanation that the irritant is actually one of the causes, and that their theory still holds good because there are emotional or both factors in the case which may be contributory.

"That sort of reasoning," he states, "is begging the question. The same facts apply to every pathologic condition of specific origin that can be conceived. A longer list of predisposing causes can be offered for tuberculosis. One could even get up a list of respectable causes for scabies. But these predisposing facts in themselves are not the cause of the disease. You may emphasize them and elaborate them. You may indulge in all kinds of intellectual and physical gymnastics, but they alone are impotent; without the definite, specific cause, disease does not occur. And it may be added in the case of irritant dermatitides, without the discovery of the cause, treatment is likely to be ineffective."

PSYCHOSOMATIC APPROACH.   We will not carry the discussion further, because we have demonstrated Pusey's point of view and the point of view of a great many dermatologists today. For the sake of discussion let us take a case of fungus infection of the feet reported by Harris. This is a condition that is often complicated by an allergic reaction.

A virile-appearing, handsome, twenty-four-year-old marine had spent 210 days in naval hospitals during a two-year period of service, most of this time because of recurrent fungus infection. Personality study revealed a severe anxiety neurosis manifested by a great many psychosomatic complaints, very low self-esteem, and an unmistakable feminine trend in job preference. When the data were discussed with him he admitted bisexuality. Apparently the stress of constant stimulation and threat of exposure kept him in a state of anxiety. He was given sufficient insight to understand the mechanism of his trouble: homosexuality —anxiety state—excessive sweating of hands and feet—inability to cure the fungus infection in the presence of constant moisture.

This case of course cannot serve as an example for a complete presentation of the controversial problem because no one would contend that there is a specific relationship between this patient's personality and the fungus infection. And yet this is truly a psychosomatic problem from the standpoint that psychic and physical factors act in a complementary fashion to produce the disorder and that only by the utilization of psychological as well as physiological techniques can we understand the illness. But of course the real problem in regard to psychosomatic medicine is whether there is a specific relationship between the personality and the skin disorder, and the dermatologist wants to know whether psychogenic influences can be responsible for an actual dermatosis. The following case is intended to illustrate, not prove, this proposition.

Case 53.   *Neurodermatitis; Good Response to Psychotherapy*

History and Symptoms.   A woman of 50 had typical neurodermatitis behind the ears and the back of the neck, sometimes extending to the arms. In addition she suffered from asthma, migraine and hypertension. The migraine had begun in adolescence, the asthma and skin trouble had been present for perhaps fifteen years, and hypertension had been discovered in the last several years. In the beginning the migraine had been associated with menstruation which was irregular and painful. During high school she had suffered from "anemia" and had to give up school in her third year because of "fatigue." She had been free of headaches in the last several years. (She related that her physician had said "either they would wear me out or I would wear them out.") But the migraine apparently was replaced by the other difficulties. The patient had given up many of her household and social activities because she was "too nervous." She slept poorly and blamed it on the irritation of the skin. She had been studied in many excellent clinics and the diagnosis of neurodermatitis was well established. Allergy studies and elimination diets had not proved helpful.

LIFE SITUATION

The patient had been brought up in a small midwestern town by wealthy parents. The father was a benevolent tyrant, the mother a neurotic and overprotective person. The patient was married at 27 to an inadequate man who never made a satisfactory living. She had known him for four years but had to wait until her older sister married before she could marry. Then her marriage was disturbed by the mother's final illness and the mother's death took place a short time afterwards. The patient had had three pregnancies but only one child, a daughter now married and living in another city.

The patient had always been frigid and in the last several years the husband had become completely impotent and there was a great deal of resentment on the part of the patient. She thought that her husband was unfaithful and in an off-guard moment blurted out that "she hated him."

After about ten years of marriage the father died and a great deal of trouble arose in the settlement of the estate. There was a quarrel between two brothers who have not spoken since and the patient played a buffer role between them, her sympathy being with the younger brother, who suffered from a heart ailment. She felt that he was cheated out of his fair share of the estate. Because they were a close-knit family living in a small community she was constantly reminded of and humiliated by the family quarrel.

Treatment Not Directed to Skin.   She became aware of the fact that her feelings had much to do with her illness and that she had retired into herself, nursing the family problems. Attention was directed to the life situation rather than just to the skin, the asthma, or the high blood pressure. In fact nothing was done as far as the skin was concerned (it was largely ignored) while attention was centered on the main life problems of resentment against an inadequate husband, the highly charged tension of the family schism, the retirement from life's activities, preoccupation with symptoms and the attendant neglect of personal appearance.

Improvement.   As she learned to express her feelings and saw her problems in a somewhat different light, her attitude changed both toward her illness and toward the family situation. She was encouraged "to carry on in spite of symptoms." This meant doing more work, such as needlework and cooking (which incidentally kept her hands busy so that she bothered her skin less). It also meant going out more socially "in spite of the appearance of the skin." Her improvement was reflected in all aspects of her personality. She became more reassured, lost twenty pounds of her excessive weight, "spruced herself up as she came out of her shell," and took up many of her former life activities.

The clearing of the skin coincided with the other improvements and a checkup two years later found her in good shape even though she had returned to her former environment.

SUMMARY

A middle-aged woman with typical neurodermatitis presented additional features to establish a psychosomatic diagnosis. Dermatologic and allergic treatments failed to help her. Treating the personality, rather than the skin, seemed to account for marked improvement.

Acne.   Not only is the manipulation of the skin in acne an important aspect of the emotional disturbance but the relation of the psyche to the disturbance itself has been hinted at from time immemorial. The very fact that the disorder is so prevalent in adolescence suggests that it is related to the active psychosexual development during this period. A retardation of the emotional and psychosexual development seems to be related to the onset of acne and also to its persistence beyond the span of life usually allotted to puberty.

The vulgar explanations that are often given regarding the occurrence of acne in youngsters and the common belief that marriage is a cure for acne vulgaris are further indications of this line of thought. Clinical experience suggests that females with acne, who also have menstrual disturbances, undergo an improvement in the appearance of the skin as the menses become more regular. As in many of the other problems that we have been considering it seems probable that both endocrine and psychological factors are important in this condition.

Case 54.   Severe Acne—Improvement with Psychotherapy

A white girl of 25 was first seen early in 1946.

History and Symptoms.   Her face was badly scarred from severe acne of five or six years' duration. She had had numerous treatments, including x-ray. Fatigue was pronounced, the menses were regular but painful, and for about three or four years she had suffered from vasomotor rhinitis.

The family history was negative except for two younger siblings who also had acne, one quite severely.

Physical Examination.   The general physical examination disclosed no evidence of organic disease and routine laboratory studies were within normal limits.

LIFE SITUATION

The patient was raised in a small community. After graduating from high school she obtained a secretarial position in which she had remained until very recently. About the age 20 she had an offer of marriage from a young man with whom she had kept company for about a year but she felt that she was not ready for marriage, "that she was needed at home." Shortly afterwards the young man married and the acne became worse about this time. Her life was rather dull and monotonous and she restricted her social activities more and more because of the facial eruption.

Quite unexpectedly her employer, who was many years older than she, began to make advances with the plea that his wife was ill. She discouraged his attentions but was obviously excited by them. She was in a great conflict about whether to continue with her job but finally resigned and left home to consult a physician in another city. There she lived with relatives and for a time felt greatly relieved but the episode with her employer recurred in her thoughts repeatedly. She expressed great resentment toward him, obviously because he had turned to her only "because his wife was ill."

Sexual Conflicts.   With great reluctance, after many interviews, she stated that she had indulged in masturbation as a child, felt terribly guilty about it, and confessed to her clergyman at the time of a revival meeting. He explained how common the practice was and that there was no sin attached to it but she could not relieve her guilt and sought him out again and again to repeat over and over the story of her "bodily abuse." She had the erroneous idea that one could develop venereal disease in this fashion; secretly she had Wassermann tests on numerous occasions and now desired another.

Social Activities.   Now she went through the same situation in regard to making friends. Her attitude was that if her face would only heal she would have more confidence in making friends but again we said to her, "No, you must not wait for your face to heal, you must go out and make friends in spite of your acne. You will find that they do not care and as you establish more friendships, getting your interests out instead of in, we think your skin will undergo further improvement."

Gradually she made friends, extended the range of her social activities, and at the same time gratefully acknowledged that her face was considerably better.

SUMMARY

A young woman with severe acne of the face was involved in sexual conflicts carrying much guilt. As she overcame these conflicts and gained confidence in herself, her skin cleared although no local or systemic medical treatments were used. Followed to the present, her skin has remained clear, and her work adjustment satisfactory.

Urticaria.   Urticaria is a disorder in which allergic factors are at times clearly recognizable but at other times obscure. It is the puzzling, chronic cases to which "multiple causation with important psychic component" applies.

Wittkower notes that none of his 35 chronic urticarial patients had histories of allergy. This is in accord with the idea that acute urticaria is usually allergic but that chronic cases are not. Two-thirds of his patients stated that they had missed parental affection as children. This attitude was occasionally justified, but often ill-founded and due to their excessive needs. As children, one-half of these patients reacted aggres-sively to frustrating situations, and the other half reacted submissively. This basic pattern appeared to be carried forth into adult life, in that the first group tended toward being aggressive persons who, in effect, demanded attention and love, while the submissive group continued in a passive way, ingratiating and humble. Wittkower concluded that actual or imaginary loss of love preceded the onset of most of the attacks of urticaria. The subject will be referred to again in the section on allergy (p. 489).

Pruritus.   On the basis of extensive experience with patients pre-senting disorders of the skin, Wittkower, a psychiatrist, and Russell, a dermatologist, discuss emotional factors in skin disease. They find that patients fall into two major groups, namely, those who complain of abnor-mal skin sensations and those who display abnormal skin manifestations. There is also a small group, psychiatrically ill, who believe that their skin is diseased when it is not. The authors regard the skin, interposed between the inner and outer world and in contact with both, as an organ of emotional expression as well as of perception. By means of repression, the individual may divorce skin sensations from the emo-tional content. Scratching is an aggressive act; it also serves for the removal of something unpleasant, whether real, fantasied or figurative. Hostility that cannot be expressed overtly may become self-directed.

Pruritus Vulvae and Pruritus Ani.   Individuals suffering from pru-ritus vulvae and pruritus ani are representative of the group who com-plain of abnormal skin sensations. In married women, pruritus vulvae suggests something amiss, something about their genitals that is repug-nant or dangerous to them. Superficially, these patients can be classified as the "shouldn'ts" (those who feel guilty over an illicit affair or thoughts of one), the "won'ts" (those who feel duty bound to cohabit with a man whom they loathe), and the "can'ts" (those who are denied sexual gratification or fertility). Pruritus ani shows a striking connec-tion with the so-called anal personality and the patients involved present immature forms of sexual gratification. In the authors' experience, all female patients were frigid, and disorders of sexual function were com-mon in the males.

Pruritus ani is also regarded by many other dermatologists as having a strong psychogenic component. Macalpine made a systematic study of 64 cases of pruritus ani and found the proportion of males to females to be about 2:1. Depressive and paranoid trends were common and 13 patients were classified as prepsychotic with 3 actually psychotic. For the most part, the psychopathology suggests a hypochondriacal syndrome with specific content. No distinct personality type could be established. Macalpine regards the structure of the syndrome as different from that of the psychoneuroses. By the absence of overt anxiety it can be sep-arated from anxiety hysteria and by the absence of true obsessions from obsessive-compulsive neurosis. She found that its origin can be traced to a reactivation in adult life of infantile fantasies about procreation centering around the anal function, which precedes genital interest and the knowledge of sex. She also finds that the syndrome responds to psychotherapy and that in many cases just a few psychotherapeutic sessions could abolish symptoms of long duration. Response to psychotherapy depended most on whether the depressive or paranoid trends were predominant; depressive patients had a better prognosis.

Hostility and Skin Disorders. Both Menninger and Ackerman have cited cases of dermatitis in which there was a great deal of repressed hostility in addition to the sexual component. The skin lesions not only served a sexual purpose but also served as a punishment for the hatred which the patient had held toward a parent. In a study of self-mutilation and self-imposed injuries inflicted upon the skin, Menninger discovered that quite regularly the unconscious motive for such attacks depended upon (*a*) impulses relating to the expression of otherwise inexpressible hostility toward someone or something in the environment, (*b*) impulses relating to the punishing of self in response to the sense of guilt which such hostility engendered, and (*c*) the erotic capitalization of the suffering in a masochistic way. In addition, of course, there are the obvious conscious motives of secondary gain, such as the sympathy and attention which the patient obtains.

In a discussion of seborrheic dermatitis Wittkower has this to say: "Whereas the effort syndrome patient is predominantly concerned with problems of honor, morality and religiosity, the peptic ulcer patient preoccupied with bread-and-butter problems, the patient suffering from colitis with cleanliness and tidiness, difficulties in social contacts are the most prominent feature in seborrheics. It looks as if the seborrheic patient not only feels ostracized because of his skin affection but also is prone to develop his skin affection because he feels—and has always felt—ostracized. Whatever the psychological and physiological dynamics of the disorder may be, the malady disturbs his social relationships still further and relegates him in many cases to the position of a pariah. Though outwardly protesting against this state of affairs and actually suffering through it, the seborrheic may inwardly accept the affliction as being well deserved."

Necessity for Psychotherapy. Saul made some observations regarding pruritus ani during psychoanalysis. One young man complained of attacks of pruritus ani which occurred regularly when he was in the company of older men who were personally interested in him. The patient's association showed clearly that passive and homosexual wishes were aroused by these situations. He occasionally indulged in anal masturbation and stated that he used the pruritus as an excuse for this indulgence. His pruritus was sometimes relieved by a satisfactory defecation, which likewise may give much sensual satisfaction. French, in a communication to Saul, told of a woman patient who similarly had a strong desire for anal gratification by inserting the finger in the anus at the time of scratching. Her pruritus was cured by helping her to achieve a greater capacity for genital satisfaction.

Thus it would seem that, in addition to physical causes, pruritus ani may represent a perversion of sexual desire, that is, an itching for satisfaction which cannot be achieved in genital sexuality. The treatment, of course, is not so simple as to advise sexual intercourse, but consists of an attempt to remove the inhibitions to the normal flow of sexual energy through the genital channels. This may occur from superficial psychotherapy but it usually requires many psychotherapeutic sessions at the hands of a skilled therapist.

Many other psychosomatic considerations apply to skin disorders, for example, the psychological material concerning the asthma-prurigo syndrome which has already been discussed under Bronchial Asthma in Chapter XV. Additional references will be found in the section on Allergy.

NECESSITY FOR PHYSICAL STUDIES.   Nor must we forget, as Sulzberger has pointed out on many occasions, that we must be very skeptical about accepting the coincidence of emotional factors and symptoms as a proved casual relationship. For example, a spinster of 47 who had had her uterus removed and then began to itch and scratch was referred by her physician as a case of "nervous itching." There were many aspects of her life situation, besides the fact that she was a spinster of 47 and had just lost her uterus, to suggest a background for nervousness, but the appearance of the skin indicated the necessity for further physical study and after a prolonged search one of our colleagues found unmistakable evidence of scabies.

THE RELATIONS BETWEEN THE EMOTIONS AND ALLERGY

Allergy and psychosomatic medicine have much in common. The allergic population and the neurotic population are so large that they must overlap. Therefore, if for no other reason, these disorders exist together in many people.

There are additional reasons why allergists and physicians interested in psychosomatic medicine should be concerned with one another's problems. Applied in an empirical way for many years, both subjects were established on a firmer scientific footing about the time of World War I and both saw a more complete integration into general medicine during World War II. Utilized to some extent by many practitioners, both subjects have become a part of the understanding of all physicians. There is no type of practice in which the principles of both disciplines are not involved. In order to accomplish the necessary integration, increased facilities must be established in medical education for undergraduates and graduates. But there is a negative aspect. Both subjects have been exploited by irregular practitioners when orthodox medicine has disdained to endorse them, and both have potentialities for doing harm as well as good.

In addition to these aspects which they have in common, there is an intimate relation between them. Psychosomatic medicine would seem to have a special application to allergy. It has long been recognized that emotional factors enter into problems of allergy but up until recently we have lacked any exact methods of measuring these effects. This is one of the problems with which Abramson concerned himself in a detailed discussion of the subject.

It is generally admitted that there is a high incidence of neurosis among allergic individuals, so high indeed that we must pay particular attention to the personality of allergic patients to see whether we cannot find psychic factors that are fundamentally important in the background of the illness and also important from the standpoint of precipitating attacks. Impressed by psychological factors, Mitchell and his associates studied 600 consecutive cases of the common allergic disorders seen in private practice and commented that those who fail to give skin reactions when tested allergically are also the ones who present multiple complaints (in addition to the allergic symptoms), whereas the patients with positive skin reactions to allergic substances ordinarily do not have such a variety of complaints and respond more readily to treatment. Upon analysis the negative skin reaction and multiple complaint group show definite evidence of psychological maladjustment.

The Psychosomatic Point of View.   As previously stated, a person gets sick for a variety of reasons, physical and psychic. In other words, it is usually not one thing that determines illness, but rather multiple factors acting together. As Halliday points out, in our approach to illness we must think:

1. What kind of *person* are we dealing with? (inherited and acquired characteristics, physical and psychological).
2. What has he *met?* (germs, allergens, or emotionally disturbing events).
3. What has *happened?* (the physiological mechanism or pathogenesis of the disorder).

For example, allergic responses occur when a prepared organism, possessing certain physical and psychological characteristics, meets certain elements, physiological and psychological. In some allergic disorders a single preponderant factor may be largely responsible, as for example in pollen hay fever. In others, such as asthma, there are frequently multiple interrelated factors, allergens and psychic disturbances, which act in a complementary fashion to produce the disorder.

The Common Cold.   In an article devoted to the subject of emotions and allergy, Saul suggests a hypothesis as to the mechanism of emotional factors in hay fever and in allergy in general. Attention has been called to his observations upon common colds in patients who were being treated by psychoanalysis (p. 421). Colds occurred in situations in which the patients suffered intensification and frustration of passive receptive wishes, usually with a prominent oral component, that is, in which the wishes for love, attention, care and help from others were represented in the dreams and associations largely in the form of being taken to dinner, receiving gifts of candy, and otherwise being fed. These colds sometimes disappeared dramatically with insight into these situations or with alleviation of the frustration. This suggested that these colds were not primarily infectious, but that they were perhaps allergic, related to the coryza of hay fever. Saul has repeatedly observed the occurrence of colds in patients when their analyses had to be temporarily interrupted, for example by the absence of the analyst for a week or so. He has also observed that colds occurred regularly in several patients who were very passive, dependent persons, when they forced themselves to do sustained work. In this regard they approximate the hay fever mechanism.

Hay Fever.   Wilson introduces the subject of structural and instinctual conflicts in cases of hay fever by suggesting that "man's assumption of the upright position was the beginning of greater utilization of the visual and auditory sensibilities and a lessening of olfactory perceptions. This produced a corresponding increase in the visual and auditory acuity, accompanied by a diminution in olfactory sensitivity. It is a well-established fact that primitive vertebrates rely primarily upon olfactory perception for the maintenance of existence and as the stimulus for reproduction. Danger, food, and sexual stimulation are all perceived by the olfactory centers before perception takes place in either the optical or auditory spheres."

PERSONALITY STUDY.   He then reports a psychoanalytic study of 7 cases of hay fever (5 female and 2 male patients). The material presented by these patients during psychoanalysis led him to the assumption that the psychological component of the hay fever symptom is a result of unsuccessful olfactory repression. Probably the first and most important factor in determining this unsatisfactory repression is that of unsatisfied, thwarted and inhibited sexual curiosity. The failure or refusal of parental figures to enlighten and instruct the child who is attempting to satisfy and master his sexual curiosity leads to a displacement and an increase in preoccupation with other bodily functions— particularly elimination. This function is intimately associated with odors: breath, perspiration, urine and feces. When parents and other persons in authority place a strict taboo upon the sexual curiosity, while at the same time they encourage the child to become preoccupied with the excretory functions, this displacement readily occurs.

PARENT-CHILD RELATIONSHIPS.   The mothers of his patients were all sexually inhibited women, who had themselves been reared and brought up according to strict, mid-Victorian patterns including a strict taboo of anything sexual. The fathers of these allergic patients maintained complete aloofness to their children's curiosity along sexual lines. Wilson does not infer that children reared in such an environment are predestined to hay fever. The parent-child relationship that he has indicated is fairly common, both for children who develop other types of neuroses as well as for children who make fairly satisfactory psychological adjustments. What he does try to demonstrate is that these patients were reared in an atmosphere that was conducive to the repression of sexual curiosity and at the same time encouraged the indulgence of olfactory perception.

DISPLACEMENT OF SEXUAL INTEREST.   A study of the material collected during psychoanalysis of 7 patients convinced him that the psychological component in hay fever is based upon a displacement of sexual curiosity from the visual to the olfactory sphere. When this occurs the eyes and nose (the organs of sexual curiosity) assume the character of sexually stimulated genitals with congestion and increased mucous secretion. This results in a diminution of both olfactory and optic sensitivity.

INTERACTION OF PSYCHIC AND PHYSICAL FACTORS.   Wilson concludes that analysis of unconscious material makes it possible to hypothesize the specific psychological factors in patients suffering from hay fever. The interplay between these inner conflicts, attempts at their solution, and the external agents (specific pollen allergens) which precipitated the actual hay fever attack remains unknown. Patients who, as a result of their psychosexual development, have substituted olfactory for visual sexual curiosity may, because of this, become more sensitive to pollens. Olfactory curiosity that has never been relieved may be considered to be a constant irritant to the mucous membrane of the nose. An added irritation from an external agency such as pollen may produce an attack. Certainly there are cases in which the local sensitivity alone, in the absence of psychological stimulation, may be sufficient to precipitate an attack. It is possible that sometimes, when the psychological stimulation is increased by the mobilization of repressed sexual tension, this alone may suffice to produce an attack of rhinitis. This would explain the resistance to pollens that was obtained by patients who had undergone analysis. When the genital inhibitions and the chronic psychological stimulus were eliminated the pollen irritation could no longer precipitate an attack.

In an experimental study of hay fever, Holmes, Treuting and Wolff tried to find evidence of summative effects of life situations, emotional reactions, attitudes and mixed ragweed pollen to the experimental production of the hay fever syndrome.

The nasal mucous membranes were observed directly through a nasal speculum and simultaneous information concerning life situation and emotional reactions was obtained. Subjects were observed in a room containing a known concentration of mixed ragweed pollen. The authors discovered that the intensity of hay fever coryza is enhanced if the nasal mucous membranes are assaulted by pollen in a setting of conflict and anxiety. They concluded that the character of the mucous membrane response in the hay fever syndrome appears to depend not only on the intensity of the nasal hyperfunction produced by the exposure of "sensitive" individuals to pollen, but on the magnitude and duration of the hyperemia, hypersecretion and swelling in the nasal chambers provoked by other threats and assaults to bodily integrity. Of major importance among these etiologic factors is a life setting engendering conflict and anxiety.

Asthma.   More material dealing with emotions and allergy was provided by observations on psychoanalyzed asthma patients made by the same group working at the Chicago Institute of Psychoanalysis (French, *et al.*). This material was referred to in the discussion of bronchial asthma (p. 428). It will be recalled that the close attachment to the mother was the central feature. The asthma occurred regularly when this was suddenly threatened.

Urticaria.   Two young women, both with severe prolonged generalized urticaria, have been analyzed by Saul. In both of these cases the central feature was deprivation of parental, but primarily of maternal love in childhood, with consequent strong masochistic attachment to the father. In one case the mother died when the patient was two years old and the patient was exploited by the father. The stepmother received almost no love or regard from either of them. The other girl's parents overtly preferred the other children and treated her as the ugly duckling or Cinderella of the family. The attacks of generalized urticaria occurred regularly and exclusively when the first patient's longings for love were intensified and frustrated. The second patient had attacks under the same conditions. In these cases the longings for love were expressed in dreams largely in the form of wishes to be admired, to be beautiful and to have fine clothes. Both patients wanted to be dancers; the first acted in amateur theatricals and the second modeled for artists.

Exhibitionism. The evidence, though meager, suggests that where the wishes for love are in the form of exhibitionistic desires and related to the skin, and where there is a heightened skin eroticism, this operates as one determinant of the skin as a site for the symptom. Wilson's paper discussed the choice of the nose as the site of the symptom of hay fever as determined by repressed olfactory sexual curiosity. The hypothesis as to the site of the symptom in asthma, as described in the asthma study, is that the asthmatic attack replaces a cry, which is stimulated by the threatened loss of the mother's love or by the separation from her, but which is repressed. In the urticaria cases, weeping relieved the attacks and apparently could replace them, it being an alternative mode of expression for the feelings of frustration.

General Theory. This leads Saul to suggest a general theory as to the mechanism of emotional factors in allergy. In all these studies of symptoms of an allergic nature in which emotional factors were found to play a role, the central emotion related to the symptom was a strong longing for love, basically for the mother's. This suggests that intense, unsatisfied longing for love affects the individual's allergic sensitivity. This longing is of the infantile, dependent kind of the child for its mother. It further suggests as a hypothesis to be tested, that when this longing is especially intensified and frustrated or threatened with frustration, the allergic sensitivity is increased and the symptoms appear.

THE CHILD'S LONGING FOR THE PARENT. Of course such longings are important in everyone but they apparently bear a special relationship to allergic symptoms. The following excerpt is taken from Saul:

"The situation appears then to be as follows: The emotional factor which is important for the allergic symptoms in these particular cases is libidinal longing probaby basically of the nature of the child's for the mother. This longing must of course come to expression in specific ways and involving specific body sites in each case. The choice of these particular sites must be determined by specific psychological and biological factors. There is nothing mutually exclusive about these, for allergic individuals usually present symptoms in different organs at one time or another. The specific factors determining the site of the symptoms in the asthma cases are apparently: 1. The sudden threat to the attachment to the mother, and 2. the repression of the consequent tendency to cry out. Further study may reveal further specific elements. The specific factors in cases of the common cold of the type described above have not been worked out in detail but the evidence suggests that one of these is the frustration of the oral components of the longing. Wilson's paper has demonstrated the specific factors involved in localizing the libidinal longings in his hay fever cases to the nose, namely, the suppression of the olfactory sexual curiosity, which was found to express not an adult genital sexuality but an immature, dependent, demanding attitude. Not enough cases of urticaria have been studied to reveal the specific elements of the skin as the site for the symptom but the three analyzed cases all showed a relationship to the repressed longing which did not achieve genital sexual expression and which apparently resulted in a high degree of erotization of the skin (as seen in strong exhibitionistic tendencies). In all these allergic cases in which the emotions appear to play a role in the production of the symptoms, the central factor related to the symptoms was intense libidinal longing and certain specific factors involving the status of the longing. Its manner of frustration and mode of expression determined the bronchi, upper respiratory passages or skin as the particular sites for the symptoms."

PSYCHOLOGICAL AND ALLERGIC FACTORS.   To continue from Saul:

"The observation of the relationship of intense, repressed, frustrated longing to allergic sensitivity provides a theory which takes account of both the psychological factors and the pollen sensitivity, for according to this concept the one complements the other. The situation is this very simple one, that the emotional state leads to physiological changes which either 1. imitate the allergic symptoms, or 2. render the tissues more sensitive to allergens, or 3. do both; and conversely an individual who is allergically sensitive on presumably an entirely organic basis might conceivably through the very fact of this sensitivity more readily produce symptoms which are psychologically determined. For example, a patient may have seasonal attacks of hay fever due to pollen sensitivity, entirely apart from his emotional state. However, if his longings increase, his hay fever may become more severe. Further, if the repressed frustrated longing becomes sufficiently intense, then the symptoms may appear on this basis alone. An individual in whom certain tissues are constantly stimulated and sensitive because of his emotional state (like a congestion of the nose from a chronic tendency to cry for mother, or of the skin from a chronic tendency to blush) may well be more sensitive in these tissues to irritating allergens. Conversely, it is easily conceivable that an individual whose tissues are irritated by allergens will react more sensitively in these particular sites to emotional stimuli.

"It must not be forgotten in all these discussions that when we refer to psychogenic factors we do not mean certain intellectual ideas of the patient, but on the contrary, the emotions, which are powerful and eminently biological. The child's longing for the parent and its anxiety when left alone are deeply biological; they are concerned with the individual's very existence, and when such deep-seated emotions are aroused, they produce far-reaching biological changes."

PERSONALITY TRENDS.   Now the question arises: Are these various disorders related to one another and to the personality of the patient? Studies demonstrate that they have certain features in common which correspond to the clinical picture of a vegetative neurosis and meet the previously discussed criteria for a psychosomatic affection. In other words, there is a positive family history; evidence for childhood neurosis or psychosomatic disturbance; the personality structure of neurotic character; exacerbation at crucial life periods in connection with specific life situations; demonstration of specific behavior on exposure to a conflict situation, such as may occur in a medical interview; and improvement by the hyposensitization of psychotherapy or the avoidance of the trouble by avoiding a provocative situation. Although the work that has been done on the question of the specific relationship of personality to disease is impressive it cannot be regarded as conclusive. Nevertheless certain trends within the personality seem to favor certain disturbances.

In regard to this question Saul, in another paper, calls attention to the fact that it is the oral form of attachment to the mother—consisting of a mixture of impulses, desires and feelings which become interwoven with the sucking and later the eating mechanism—that enters into psychosomatic gastrointestinal problems, while other biological mechanisms and forms of attachment to the mother seem to be important in the allergies. These are the dermal and the respiratory. In other words, in many persons the form of attachment to the mother as seen in fantasies, dreams and real life is not, as in many instances of gastrointestinal disorders, strongly "oral," but consists rather in a desire for shelter. The longings are represented not by wishes to be fed and all that this can imply emotionally, but rather in wishes to be sheltered and protected. Such persons often gravitate to modes of life which gratify such tendencies. Perhaps it could be said that, given a choice, they would prefer snug housing to good food. Here, too, can be points of weakness and fixation, to form a physiological pathway for the attachment to the mother and become interwoven with powerful feelings and longings. When the relationship to the mother, with all of its significance to the child (and later in life, unconsciously to the adult) is threatened, or when a person is under stress, the longings for help or consolation are expressed in various combinations or forms in different persons: wanting to be fed, wanting to be carried or led, wanting to be snuggled and sheltered, and so on, reflecting the oral, ambulatory, dermal, respiratory and other mechanisms and forms of attachment to the mother. The impulses may be *gratified* by personal relationships, sexual or sublimated, which reestablish in some degree the relationship to the mother. The gratification may be *sublimated* (oral: eating and drinking; respiratory: talking and crying; dermal: baths and massage). The impulses may be *repressed* so that symptoms appear when the tension disturbs organ function. Of course oral as well as dermal and respiratory trends can exist in the same individual. But Saul states that it is the person in whom the dermal and/or respiratory mechanism has some weakness, or is a point of fixation, or in whom the attachment to the mother predominately takes these forms, who seems to be predisposed to skin and respiratory allergy.

He concludes, "The dermal and respiratory mechanisms, trends, and

relations to the mother are analogous to the oral ones. They are fundamental to an understanding of psychological functioning. Preliminary
observations strongly suggest that they play a role in the skin and
respiratory allergies similar to that of the oral ones in the gastrointestinal
disorders."

Cooperative Therapy.   In addition to the treatment aspects already discussed in the sections dealing with asthma, migraine, and so
forth, are the cooperative efforts of an allergist (Miller) and a psychotherapist (Baruch) who dealt with 22 patients, 7 of whom were children.
In all cases the history of classic allergic symptoms was confirmed by
positive skin reactions to various allergens. Recognizing that clinical
allergy must be practiced with constant awareness that psychogenic
factors influence physical results, the authors utilized both individual
and group psychotherapy in dealing with their patients. Repeatedly they
observed that the fluctuation of symptoms paralleled the degree of freedom with which a patient expressed his feelings and that the intellectual
appreciation of the dynamics involved was not important to the patient.
Marked improvement was observed in 19 of the 22 allergic patients.
Miller and Baruch feel that allergic symptoms express hostility, mask a
feeling of guilt or anxiety, and at the same time represent attempts to
gain sympathy.

Mitchell states "In at least one third of patients with perennial
asthma, the history, cutaneous tests and clinical trial with disguised
allergens fail to demonstrate specific hypersensitiveness and no physical
cause such as heart disease, emphysema, tumor, foreign body, or bron-
chiectasis can be found. There remain then those difficult cases of asthma
in which the condition fails to fit the allergic pattern and is classified as
'intrinsic.' Since personality factors are often of major significance in
many nonseasonal allergic disorders, a good history is essential. When
the patient is permitted to tell his story in his own way, pertinent
diagnostic data are obtained, but of greater importance is the therapeutic
effect of such free expression. Moreover, if the physician is more than
a kindly attentive listener and carefully abstracts the feeling and the
emotional content from the patient's statements, calmly reflecting these
back to him, a dynamic process is initiated which allows further discussion of deep emotional feelings and significant personal problems. . . .
Thus, relating the history becomes a profound psychotherapeutic experience where, with the aid of the interviewer's skill, problems are
faced and worked through to a satisfactory solution."

Conclusions.   The allergic and the neurotic populations are so
large that they must overlap. If for no other reason, therefore, these
disorders will exist in the same individual. But in addition, personality
studies suggest a more intimate connection—a specific relatonship between neurotic character structure and allergic disorder—possibly representing parallel manifestation of the same basic fault, the one dis-
charging on the level of psychic representation through thoughts and
feelings and the other on the physiological level by means of disturbances
in organ functioning.

Psychosomatic study of an allergic problem, therefore, utilizes separate techniques, psychological and physiological, applied simultaneously; and diagnosis must be established not only by exclusion or evaluation of physical factors but with additional positive evidence of personality disorder meeting certain psychosomatic postulates. This will demonstrate that in a given case physical and psychological factors act in a complementary fashion to produce the disorder; in one instance specific physical factors may predominate, in another instance specific emotional factors. The latter seem to be determined by certain trends within the personality, for just as oral attachments seem to determine gastrointestinal disorders so do respiratory and dermal attachments (to the mother) apparently determine respiratory and dermal allergic manifestations (Saul).

The allergic disorders seem to fall for the most part into the group of organ neuroses that can be termed vegetative (Alexander), representing early and profound deviations of personality development. What role the constitution may play cannot be determined, since no methods are available to delimit constitutional and acquired factors. One can, however, evaluate physical and psychological factors, and proper management depends on such evaluation. Then psychotherapy plus the allergic approach will mean better treatment for the individual with an allergic disorder.

References

Abramson, H. A.: Psychosomatics and the Allergic Patient. Bruce Publishing Co., St. Paul, 1948.

Ackerman, N. W.: Psychosom. Med., *1:* 366, 1939.

French, T. M.: Psychosom. Med. Monograph IV, 1941.

Halliday, J. L.: Brit. J. M. Psychol., *19:* 367, 1943.

Harris, H. J.: Psychosom. Med., *6:* 336, 1944.

Holmes, T. H., Treuting, T., and Wolff, H. G.: Psychosom. Med., *13:* 71, 1951.

Macalpin, I.: Psychosom. Med., *15:* 499, 1953.

Menninger, K. A.: Man Against Himself. P. 359. Harcourt, Brace & Co., New York, 1938.

Miller, H., and Baruch, D. W.: The Practice of Psychosomatic Medicine as Illustrated in Allergy. McGraw-Hill Book Co., Inc., New York, 1956.

Mitchell, J. H.: J.A.M.A., *140:* 15, 1949.

Mitchell, J. H., Curran, A., and Myers, R.: Psychosom. Med., *184:* 191, 1947.

Rattner, H.: J.A.M.A., *99:* 1934, 1932.

Saul, L. J.: (*a*) Psychoanalyt. Quart., *7:* 336, 1938; (*b*) Psychosom. Med., *3:* 66, 1941.

Saul, L. J:. Psychosom. Med., *3:* 66, 1941.

Saul, L. J.: The Nervous Child, *5:* 332, 1946.

Stokes, J. H., and Beerman, H.: Psychosom. Med., *2:* 438, 1940.

Sulzberger, M. B.: Dermatologic Allergy. Charles C Thomas, Springfield, Ill., 1940.

Sulzberger, M. B.: J.A.M.A., *136:* 156, 1948.

Wilson, G. W.: Psychosom. Med., *3:* 51, 1941.

Wittkower, E. D.: Bull. Menninger Clinic, *2:* 148, 1947.

Wittkower, E.: Psychosom. Med., *15:* 116, 1953.

Wittkower, E., and Russell B.: Emotional Factors in Skin Disease. Paul B. Hoeber, Inc., New York, 1953.

Chapter XIX

General Surgery and Dentistry

PSYCHIATRIC PROBLEMS OF GENERAL SURGERY

Psychiatric problems of surgical illness have been mentioned many times in this book. Our attention was first called to this important problem many years ago by the following case:

A young woman at the age of 19 had her first attack of pain in the right lower quadrant. At 20 the appendix was removed. Six months later she had a pelvic operation because of painful menstruation. At 26 she had her third operation for abdominal adhesions. For the next four years she complained more or less constantly and was in bed for considerable periods because of the pain in the right side. Stricture of the right ureter was suspected but not proved and finally, after a great deal of hospital investigation, a fourth operation was performed in the belief that there was disease of the large bowel, but all organs were found normal.

Here, then, was a patient who had been incapacitated for many years and who during this period of time had been repeatedly subjected to searching physical investigations and many abdominal operations. What the many physicians attending her had not discovered, or did not know the significance of, was that this long illness began shortly after the fourth of her five sisters married and this patient thought that she would in all likelihood remain a spinster and would then endure a life of drudgery and comparative loneliness. Meek and submissive, unattractive and unintelligent, she unconsciously turned to illness when she found it impossible to compete with her sister's superiority. Further personality studies disclosed her very immature emotional development and confirmed the opinion that the sister's marriage had precipitated an invalid reaction in this psychoneurotic individual.

Chronic Invalidism.   A great many chronic invalids with multiple surgical scars upon the abdomen have begun their invalid career in this way, that is, with the simple removal of a so-called "chronic appendix." Fortunately the problem is not encountered as frequently as twenty years ago. It was then that operations for pain in the right lower quadrant of the abdomen were frequently done for "chronic appendicitis," and the pathologist, we may say, played into the surgeon's hands by reporting involutional changes in terms of disease. Please do not think that we are accusing the surgeon of a deliberate deception; quite the contrary, he was deceived by his organic training into thinking that he could cut out of the body a pain that had its origin in the emotional life. We are not going to discuss whether there is such a thing as "chronic appendicitis," but we certainly know that it is not nearly so common as was once believed.

The problem has much to do with frigidity, as discussed by Ruesch and his associates in a monograph devoted to a study of chronic disease and psychological invalidism. The life histories of the frigid women in their series resembled each other closely. They were characterized by a high rate of marriages, marriages at an early age, greater than average divorce rate, and a large number of medical experiences and operations. There was a great lack of love and security in childhood. Marriage often served the purpose of breaking away from home at an early age, in a search for security and love, and to prove that they were grown-up people.

The Abuse of Surgery.   One of the most frequent syndromes encountered in Ruesch's patients was that of the patient with a history of many abdominal operations. The case is cited of the girl who marries early and soon afterwards develops abdominal pain, which is followed by appendectomy. At short intervals other abdominal operations follow; finally ovaries, tubes and uterus are removed. The castration effect of the loss of the uterus is often a great blow from which a woman may find it impossible to recover. Unfortunately attention to the emotional life usually comes only after irreparable damage has been done (p. 311).

One or more major operations occurred in more than 65 per cent of frigid women contrasted with about 40 per cent in nonfrigid women.

This is one of the problems discussed by Karl Menninger in his well known paper "Polysurgery and Polysurgical Addiction," in which he showed that many deeper emotional needs can be temporarily satisfied by a surgical procedure. By submitting to surgery the patient avoids facing something that he fears more than surgery. This may be marriage or divorce or even a visit to a psychiatrist. At times, as already mentioned, an unconscious desire for punishment, arising from a sense of guilt, is being satisfied. Sometimes having an operation represents the act of an indecisive patient who places himself under the care of a strong, paternal figure who takes vigorous action and, in that connection, we must not forget that the cooperation of a masochistic patient who is willing and even eager to be operated upon and a surgeon who is willing and eager to operate represents a combination that can result in near-evisceration. One of the dangers in polysurgical addiction is to the surgeon himself when he is unwittingly drawn into the patient's plan. Just as the surgeon makes certain that his patient is investigated from a cardiovascular-renal standpoint, so must he make certain that the patient is psychologically equipped for surgery or is psychologically prepared for surgery.

Surgery for most people has an overlay of fantasy containing aspects of awe and mystery that are as deep as any that must have surrounded human sacrifice. They are similar to the fantasies of war and battle. Some are conscious and some unconscious. They go as follows: "They will hurt me and I can't endure it. I will crack up—go crazy under the pain, and never get back to normal. The anesthetic won't work. I'll still feel pain. I'll talk when under the anesthetic and reveal secrets I couldn't bear to have known. Perhaps I won't wake up from the anesthetic. If I do I'll be changed and deformed."

Next come fantasies which bring more rewarding albeit neurotic solutions to problems. "I insist upon an operation to cut my pain away. The operation will bring me attention and sympathy. It will soften my unfriendly husband. It will bring my alienated children to my side. It will bring me a rest and the sympathy of friends and also of my critics and enemies. It will make me an object of interest. The operation will vindicate me and show that something is wrong and that I am not as neurotic as they say."

Finally some patients feel that the operation will change their sex. This is a deep complex but occasionally it exists, and should be given due consideration when patients are too eager for certain operations. As we have pointed out elsewhere, some people aren't satisfied with their sex, males as well as females, and the impression that surgery will change them to be more nearly what they want to be is a definite wish existing in the unconscious.

Apprehension about surgical operations needs to be dealt with patiently, and if anxiety is too great operations should be postponed until the anxiety is dealt with. Some patients have become suicidal postoperatively and also developed full-blown psychoses as a result of their anxiety. This seems especially true in heart surgery (p. 219). It must be kept in mind that the patient's anxiety is not necessarily correlated with the severity of the case. Intense anxiety may be present for the simplest surgical procedure. Here one must be especially patient. The surgeon himself is generally the person who is best able to explain and reassure.

Emotional Disorders in Surgical Patients. The relationship of emotional problems to surgical illness has been carefully studied by Zwerling, Titchener and associates at the University of Cincinnati in a survey of 200 representative surgical patients. They applied their data to the following hypotheses: (1) Emotional disorders exist in a significant proportion of surgical patients; (2) emotional factors are related to the etiology and pathogenesis of some surgical disease, and to the formation of some symptoms which bring patients to the attention of surgeons; (3) emotional factors are related to the course of surgical patients during hospitalization, including response to conservative therapy, to anesthesia, to surgery and to postoperative care; (4) emotional factors are related to the adjustments made by surgical patients after their discharge from the hospital. As noted in Figure 11 there is an extraordinarily high incidence of mental disorder among surgical patients, indicating the need for close liaison between the surgical and psychiatric staffs of a general hospital. Since World War II it has become increasingly clear that close liaison is necessary between the departments of medicine and psychiatry and this study by the Cincinnati group indicates that the same is true in regard to psychiatry and the department of surgery and the surgical specialties. The occasional request for psychiatric consultation for a grossly disturbed patient is obviously inadequate. The services of psychiatry are essential to the surgical department.

INCIDENCE OF MENTAL AND EMOTIONAL ILLNESS.   The fact that the incidence of mental disorder among surgical patients (Fig. 11) seems to

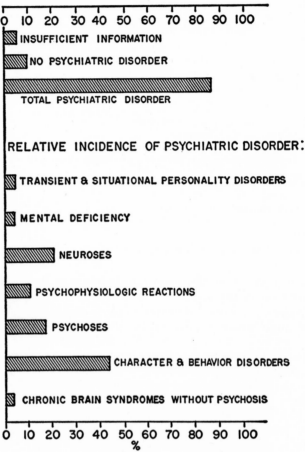

Figure 11.   Incidence of psychiatric disorder in surgical patients. (From Titchener et al., J.A.M.A., vol. 160, 1956.)

be much higher than in the total population was accounted for on the basis that these patients, representing the group usually seen in the wards of a large city hospital, were drawn from the lowest socio-economic strata of the community. Secondly, the onset of a surgical illness and the admission to the hospital may cause severe stresses, particularly in a population with marginal financial means, and finally the surgical illness itself, in many instances, seems to represent an eventuality growing out of the psychiatric disorder. In 48.5 per cent of the patients there was a significant relationship between the surgical status of the patient at the time of presentation to the surgeon for treatment and emotional disorder.

DELAY IN SEEKING SURGICAL CARE. The problem of delay in seeking surgical care was developed in a separate paper (Titchener, et al.). The incidence of delay in the series of patients studied amounted to 31 per cent of the total. The psychological causes are shown in Table 4 and result from conscious and unconscious psychological factors that are in operation before, during and after the patient's recognition of a sign or symptom which would ordinarily take him to a physician. It will be noted from the table that ignorance of the significance of a symptom plays a very small part while unconscious or unreality factors play a

Table 4. Psychological Causes of Delay in Seeking Surgical Treatment

	%
Fear of punishment from surgical treatment	26.0
Fear of death in surgical treatment	15.3
Reaction formation or overcompensation to dependent needs	13.7
Shame; wish to avoid exposure, being seen, or revelation of attitudes or parts of body unacceptable to the self	13.0
Suicidal wishes or resignation to fatal outcome	9.2
Iatrogenic causes	6.9
Ignorance of significance of symptoms	4.6
Secondary gain or the histrionic gesture as cause of delay	3.8
Other causes	7.6

From Titchener et al.: J.A.M.A., *160:* 1187, 1956.

large part in delay. Fear of pain or mutilation may be far in excess of that appropriate to the operation. This is the same mechanism which often keeps people away from dentists. Fear of death as a cause of delay in seeking surgical care is based on the mechanism of deep-seated guilt feelings in conflict with unaccepted hostile impulses toward significant persons. Here the hostility may be so intense that people unconsciously feel the need for ultimate retaliation, that is, death, so that the actual risks of surgery are exaggerated and anxiety may be greatly intensified. Again, denial based on overcompensation to dependent needs may play an important role in delay in seeking surgical help. Such people commonly interpret illness as a sign of weakness and may deny the existence of the illness and the need for help. People who highly value virility, toughness and independence frequently are overcompensating for the opposite traits of weakness, passivity and dependency, and since they cannot admit to these characteristics they deny illness which to them is evidence of weakness (Weiss et al.). Still another important group feel shame and the wish to avoid exposure. Illness in the genital area and shame about sexual impulses have to do with this cause for delay in seeking help. Depression with resignation to fatal outcome, often with suicidal wishes, plays a part in delaying surgical care. Iatrogenic factors enter in many subtle ways to interfere with the normal processes of diagnosis and treatment.

Titchener et al. emphasize that medical education for the public must recognize that people resist diagnosis and treatment not because they are ignorant of medical signs or symptoms but because maladapted and neurotic behavior results in irrational procrastination.

PSYCHOSIS IN SURGICAL PATIENTS.   Commenting upon the incidence of psychosis in certain surgical patients the same authors found that it was present in 22 per cent of their 200 surgical patients and that the psychoses observed represented nearly the whole range and variety of known syndromes. An acute brain syndrome or delirium was often the first sign of impending relapse in the general medical condition of the patients. A delirium was frequently the first sign of continuing mental deterioration, leading in elderly patients to a chronic brain syndrome or some lesser defect in mentation. These findings indicate the need for early recognition and prompt treatment of even the subtle signs of delirium.

Aging patients who lost the closeness and support of family, friends or visitors developed an organic psychosis in response to the stress of illness and surgery more often than those who retained close family contacts.

Elderly men and women immobilized for treatment of hip fractures were prone to mental deterioration, in contrast to patients with hip fracture who were allowed early ambulation. A similar liability to psychotic break appeared among elderly patients undergoing amputation of an extremity.

Psychotic *depressive reactions* represented the major functional psychosis occurring in their series of patients after admission to the hospital. The majority of these reactions occurred in cancer patients. The psychosis became manifest in cancer patients when the commonly found inner sense of abandonment and guilt isolation was reinforced by realistic factors in their environment. It is postulated that impotent rage and ensuing guilt against the environment because of actual or marginal awareness of the cancer may enhance the development of the depressive reaction. The authors suggest that treatment methods and the physician's attitude toward cancer tend to enhance the oft observed abandonment and isolation which cancer patients experience. Their need for closeness, support and continuity of contact with others should be considered in the planning of their care within the hospital milieu.

The authors do not admit either the existence of such a separate etiology entity or the usefulness of "postoperative psychosis" as a diagnostic term. The psychoses which they observed have no circumscribed form distinguishing them from other psychoses.

PSYCHOSIS AND RECUMBENCY.   Getting a sick man out of bed is generally recognized as an important part of symptomatic and supportive treatment for a number of disorders. We are largely indebted to surgeons for demonstrating that early ambulation has remarkable physical and psychological advantages for a patient.

In considering psychological benefits of the method, we are accustomed to think in terms of improvement in morale. But sometimes moving a patient from bed to chair or making him walk about does much more for his state of mind than provide a simple boost in spirits. Many physicians have noticed that mental deterioration is prevented, or at least reduced, when an elderly hemiplegic is put in a chair early in the course of his disease. Eye surgeons in particular have recommended immediate ambulation for patients who develop psychotic disturbances after operations for glaucoma or cataract.

It may be that the improvement noted in delirious or aged persons when they are placed in an upright position consists in restoring the patient to a position that is biologically and psychologically more nearly normal.

Plastic Surgery. While the correction of nasal deformity (rhinoplasty) is not the only kind of plastic surgery, it is one of the most frequent operations performed. Deformities vary from real disfigurement to minor irregularities that are hardly noticeable but about which the patient may be greatly concerned. Psychiatric study of such patients shows mild neurotic reaction at one extreme, and overt schizophrenia with delusions and hallucinations at the other. Linn and Goldman studied a group of such patients and found them shy and seclusive and suffering from social anxiety. They would often develop peculiar mannerisms to avoid having the nose looked at and many were severely inhibited in their school, social and work life. After operation the patient is often elated and soon inferiority feelings may be replaced by self-confidence. Friends and acquaintances may not realize just what has happened but find a change in appearance which they attribute to a "new hair-do," or find the smile more pleasant, etc. Many patients are precipitated into marriage, often with unfortunate results. Previously ineffective people find themselves in situations to which they cannot adjust.

Probably of great importance in respect to nasal surgery is the fact that the nose is an organ with secondary sexual characteristics. Deformities may not become noticeable until puberty when a period of rapid nasal development occurs. Thus it is that psychological disturbances having to do with the nose begin about this time. Since concern about physical appearance is more normal in a female than in the male, rhinoplasty is apt to be more successful in women. Younger people are more easily satisfied than older ones. Courses in charm schools and reducing clinics may give patients a superficial self-confidence which melts away when they meet difficult situations, and rhinoplasty and the correction of deformity often act in the same way. It is a good rule to assume that all patients who come for plastic surgery are in need of psychiatric evaluation, and they should be warned that the achievement obtained through plastic surgery may impose new psychological burdens. Plastic surgery can make an important contribution to social development but it should not be done or attempted without the benefit of psychological studies.

So far as the cosmetic surgeon is concerned Cohen warned that he must have a perfect technique and a stout heart. He must learn when to say no to patients and he must learn when to refuse to attempt further correction. Very often people who blame lack of success on their nasal imperfection are the people who will never be satisfied. This, of course, is true because nasal imperfection, which may be very slight, is not the real cause of their so-called "failure." People seeking secondary correction especially are the ones who blame their troubles on their faulty nasal contour. No branch of surgery necessitates a closer working relationship between surgeons and psychiatrists.

Emotional Problems of Cancer.   Cancer propaganda is both good and bad. The chief hope of reducing the high cancer death rate depends on treating the disease in its first stages. Wide publicity has been given to the symptoms and signs of cancer to encourage the public to seek medical advice early. Most physicians believe that the importance of making America cancer-conscious outweighs the disadvantages of producing cancerphobia.

REACTIONS TO BREAST CANCER.   Renneker and Cutler found that depression is a frequent reaction following mastectomy. In this study by an analyst and surgeon, breasts were found to have two major psychological meanings to women: a particular sexual significance and a symbol of motherhood. The primary emotional reaction of a woman with breast cancer is not fear of death but fear of losing her badge of femininity. Loss of the breast during the menopausal period increases the problem of adjustment. The greatest psychic trauma from cancer and amputation of the breast occurs during the preclimacteric and climacteric periods and varies in proportion to the patient's youth and degree of feminine achievement (sexuality, husband and children). In a neurotic woman, mutilation of the breast intensifies an underlying neurosis.

The physician should be constantly aware of normal and abnormal reactions in the breast cancer patient as well as of the important role the patient's husband plays in his wife's postoperative adjustment. Preoperative psychic sensitivity on the part of the surgeon will pay dividends in patient cooperation and shorten a severe postoperative emotional reaction: every woman in the authors' series on discovering a lump in her breast associated it with cancer and the prospect of mutilation and possible death. All the women with breast cancer were sooner or later anxious about possible death. This development of anxiety should be anticipated, looked for and utilized therapeutically. "Ideally, the surgeon should ask in the very beginning of the first interview, during the history taking—and before the physical examination—whether or not the patient has been worried about the possibility of cancer." The patient should be prepared for biopsy and potential mastectomy and should be acquainted with realistic facts concerning cancer in general, her cancer, biopsy, convalescence, postoperative treatment and prognosis.

SHOULD THE PATIENT KNOW THE TRUTH?   Fitts and Ravdin sent questionnaires to 444 physicians to find out what they tell patients with cancer. Seventy per cent of the physicians either always tell or usually tell. Most dermatologists, who treat cancer with a more favorable prognosis, tell patients that they have cancer. Most physicians treating visceral cancer usually do not tell. A century ago Oliver Wendell Holmes said "Your patient has no more right to all the truth you know than he has to all the medicine in your saddle bags. . . . For it is a terrible thing to take away hope, even earthly hope, from a fellow creature." On the other hand, Renneker and Cutler stated that all of a group of 50 patients with cancer of the breast actually knew they had cancer even if not told by their physicians.

This problem is by no means a simple one and in attempt to answer it Meyer asks, "What patients? and What truth?" He asserts, as Holmes did, that there is no general dictum or prescription for this troubled aspect of the communication between physician and patient. "What is good medicine for the one may prove catastrophic for another, and indeed the only rule whereby the doctor may be wisely guided is for him to know the facts, know his patient, and know himself." In this thoughtful and well-written essay Meyer indicates that there can be no set policy, "for a policy implies uniformity and uniformity is a distillate of indolence and insensitivity having no place in the practice of medicine." After indicating the difficulty of separating what is true and what is false Meyer adds that this does not relieve the physician of his moral responsibility. "On the contrary, the difficulties that arise from the immense complexity of the phenomena do not diminish, but rather increase the moral responsibility of the physician, and one of my objects has been to describe the facts through which the nature of that moral responsibility is determined.

"Far older than the precept, 'the truth, the whole truth, and nothing but the truth,' is another that originates within our profession that has always been the guide of the best physicians, and, if I may venture a prophecy, will always remain so: so far as possible, 'Do no harm.' You can do harm by the process that is quaintly called telling the truth. You can do harm by lying. In your relations with patients you will inevitably do much harm, and this will be by no means confined to your strictly medical blunders. It will also arise from what you say and what you fail to say. But try to do as little harm as possible, not only in treatment with drugs, or with the knife, but also in treatment with words, with the expression of your sentiments and emotions. Try at all times to act upon the patient so as to modify his sentiments to his own advantage, and remember that, to this end, nothing is more effective than arousing in him the belief that you are concerned wholeheartedly and exclusively for his welfare."

PSYCHOSOMATIC ASPECTS OF DENTISTRY

Of all branches of medicine, dentistry has perhaps been the one most separated from the psyche. The word "dental" has come to be associated with the idea of "mechanical"; fillings, extractions, dentures, appliances and devices. It is the purpose of this discussion to point out that we cannot divorce a man from his teeth. In other words, not everything dental is synonymous with "mechanical." The cliché "the very idea of going to the dentist stops the toothache" is an indication that psychosomatic influences enter into dental practice.

Poor oral hygiene is not limited to people in the lower income brackets who cannot afford dentistry; it occurs as well in the middle and upper income brackets, for the reason that the patient is afraid to go to the dentist—he is afraid of being hurt. Many people have great anxiety about physical pain, and while they are very ashamed of it, they can do nothing about it. The idea of being stuck with a needle for a blood count or a Wassermann test fills them with dread. After being hurt by a dentist's drill they have great difficulty in returning for treatment.

Another reason for avoiding the dentist is that the loss of teeth may have a greater significance than just the association of pain or discomfort. Losing a tooth, according to an old adage, means "losing a friend," but it also means, in the unconscious thinking of many people, loss of strength and loss of virility. Of course, there is the conscious idea of the effect on the appearance, but quite aside from the notion of a possible alteration in the appearance is the idea that the wearing of dentures is a sign of old age. This is true not only of women, but of many men. It is one of the reasons that many chronic illnesses of psychosomatic origin can be traced to a dental operation, or the fitting of dentures and the failure of the patient to adjust to them.

Dental Problems of Childhood.   A partial answer to this problem is for the parent and the dentist to cooperate in persuading children to regard dental treatment as sensible and necessary and something with a minimum of discomfort, rather than as an ordeal. Many adults exaggerate how painful a visit to the dentist can be so that the child comes to fear the dentist's office as a modern torture chamber.

Adults should therefore avoid conveying to the child the idea that a visit to the dentist is going to be painful, and visits should be started before painful procedures have to be carried out. This gives the dentist and the child an opportunity to get acquainted and enables the child to find out that the visit can be fun rather than torture. If early in the life of the child parents do their part and the dentist does his, there will be less neglect of dental hygiene because of fear.

Once the child is in the dentist's office he should not be babied by either mother or dentist. Often the child will sit in the chair and be content to be alone with the dentist, and the mother can remain in the waiting room. It is bad practice for the mother to hover about inquiring if her child is being hurt. Suggestion may work in subtle ways and if the parent and dentist assume the child will behave like an adult he will often do so, whereas if they expect him to be afraid and to refuse to cooperate he may also readily do this. If a child refuses to cooperate it is not wise to use force unless a real emergency exists, for the combination of force and pain will cause him to dread the next occasion all the more and be the means of establishing an attitude which in later life means dental neglect.

THUMBSUCKING.   While this subject is discussed in more detail elsewhere (p. 23) it has special significance for the dentist and especially the orthodontist because of the problem of deformity. The orthodontist feels that malocclusion must be avoided at all costs but, with Binger, we must ask ourselves if malocclusion of the personality is not more serious than malocclusion of the teeth. The need to get solace and comfort from sucking is the most powerful craving of early life and when it persists into later childhood it means that this symptom is answering a bodily need that is imperative. If it is met with forcible restraint (for example, by the use of mechanical devices or worse yet by shame and ridicule) the craving simply seeks another outlet which may be more serious so far as the developing personality is concerned than a continuation of the practice of thumbsucking.

Korner and Reider observed psychologically 3 patients whose thumbsucking was disrupted by means of a dental device. They discovered that it is impossible to understand either the meaning of the sucking to each child or his response to the appliance without prolonged individual study. Aside from their highly individual reactions, all of the children showed activation of hostility and guilt reactions. Parenthetically, they noted that the appliance failed to stop thumb or tongue sucking in these 3 children; instead, it focused the child's attention on thumbsucking.

Relation of Dentistry to Emotional Aspects of Surgery. Just as in childhood the dentist is feared, so does the opposite situation sometimes exist in the adult patient. He may be all too amenable to the idea of losing his teeth. Indeed, he may derive a certain perverse satisfaction from having teeth extracted. As Menninger states, these are the people addicted to *polysurgery*. As may be imagined, they are psychoneurotic. When they have some physical discomfort, having heard of illnesses being cured by the removal of "foci of infection," they become their own diagnosticians and often conclude that a tooth or several teeth should be removed. Like the patient who wants his tonsils or appendix removed, they usually manage to get the operation done.

There are some powerful unconscious impulses at work in these people that cause them to be so persistently illogical. First, the idea of a "focus of infection" makes them feel that they harbor something "unclean." The idea that "toxins" (impurities) are being discharged from an "unclean" (infected) area and entering the blood stream causes them anxiety. Their whole attitude is one of "Out with it!" as soon as possible and they will not rest until the tooth, the appendix, or even the gallbladder is out. Often the patient is assisted in his desire by a dentist or a physician who is not certain of the advisability of the operation, but feels that "it will do no harm." That it will do harm has been demonstrated by numerous case reports of confirmed invalidism.

Another unconscious motive in this sacrifice of organs is to help get rid of a sense of guilt. This sense of guilt usually dates back to childhood and resides in the unconscious mental life, so that such patients do not realize that they are trying to assuage guilt when they periodically suffer the pain and make the sacrifice of having something removed, be it from the mouth, abdomen or pelvis.

Case 55.   *Emotional Aspects of Extractions*

A man of 44 complained of pain in the left chest which he suspected was due to heart disease. At first he said that his trouble had begun a year ago following an indiscretion in eating. At that time he had consulted a gastroenterologist, who explained his trouble as due to a spastic colon and treated him on this basis. Later when he developed pains in the left chest he was referred to a cardiologist, who told him that he did not have heart disease. But the patient saw a report which was sent to his physician and this stated that "he should be watched because of a family history of heart disease." This was sufficient to reinforce his suspicion of heart disease. His physician told him that his trouble was "all in the head," which annoyed him, and that he "probably ought to see a psychiatrist," which annoyed him further.

In reviewing his history it was noted that chest pains had really begun many years ago at the time of a business crisis. Then during a period of several years he had worked very hard, eaten irregularly and smoked a lot, and he felt that this was the real basis of his gastrointestinal disturbance. In the background of his trouble was long-standing difficulty with his wife who was not "sympathetic" and advised him only to "stay away from doctors."

Finally, at the suggestion of his physician, six teeth were extracted. He felt "nervous" for a long time afterward and became very angry that the teeth were removed and at the necessity for wearing a bridge. He blamed the dentist for unnecessary surgery and was very vindictive toward him. He continued to regard the denture as a foreign body. (He could not get used to it, and "felt burned up every morning" when he put the bridge in his mouth.) Moreover it served to remind him of the fact that his father had died of heart trouble not a long time after the son had urged him to have some dental extractions. We allowed him to talk over this situation on more than one occasion until his guilt was somewhat mitigated.

We satisfied him as to the absence of organic disease; showed him the relationship between his life situation and his symptoms, particularly his identification with his father and his hostility for the dentist; and urged him to adopt his prosthesis as a part of himself. On this basis he made considerable improvement.

Personality of the Dentist

Everyone has a personality and an unconscious; the dentist and surgeon are no exception. The following material applies to the general surgeon and surgical specialist as well as to the dentist. Lyons explains that the psychiatrist listens to complaints of patients, absorbs their hostilities and aggressions, and puts up with their infantile demands. With many psychiatrists this is made easier because in their training they have gained insight into their own emotional needs and can look upon those of the patient more realistically. No one has full insight into his own emotional problems. The dentist and surgeon are subjected to many of the same attitudes, feelings, hostilities and demands as is the psychiatrist, but are not usually trained to recognize or handle them as objectively. It is much more difficult to remain emotionally neutral to the emotional fluctuations of the patient. The dentist is also engaged in an occupation in which he actually inflicts pain or discomfort on the patient. This can be difficult for the dentist as well as for the patient. If the dentist has an unconscious emotional conflict about his own aggression and hostility (as most of us do), then the infliction of pain on others may be accompanied with guilt and self-reproach. Such a dentist may reach the end of the day depressed, fatigued and uncomfortable, as a result of his own unconscious feeling about the necessary instrumentation and infliction of even unavoidable pain. This is simply one of the occupational hazards of being a dentist.

The dentist is also exposed to the reactions of his patients who may present open or concealed hostility to his procedures thereby adding more to the dentist's own problems. We are all familiar with our own personal reactions to openly hostile, critical or demanding people. Hostility begets hostility in any interpersonal relationship. Few of us are well enough integrated and composed to withstand constant criticism, sarcastic comment, or the over-reaction to pain for most of the day.

The dentist has another problem. Good dental care requires periodic check-ups. Thus the dentist must develop and keep a good interpersonal relationship between the patient and himself. This entails an acquired or at least an intuitive knowledge of personality types so that he can adapt himself to the situation and handle it in the way best suited to the needs of the patient. The patient's neurosis can even be used as an aid in the prophylaxis which is necessary as time goes on.

Personality of the Patient

Several basic personality types as outlined by Tarachow will be described in an effort to indicate the large variety of emotional reactions seen in different people. The list is by no means conclusive and it must be emphasized that the following traits are present, in varying degrees, in normal as well as neurotic persons. Also many individuals will have traits from more than one of the character types. Personality is the complicated result of inherited characteristics conditioned to a changing, dynamic environment.

The Narcissist. This trend, more or less observed in everyone, derives its name from the youth in Greek mythology who, staring into the pool, fell in love with his own reflected image. These individuals are characterized by self-love, and a great need for love from others, coupled with mistrust. They are the exhibitionists who seek gratification frequently in the choice of professions—one in which they are constantly before the public. They live on praise, love and importance—vanity is their main characteristic. They form attachments to people who admire them and who are willing to be their audience.

At the same time they are mistrustful and in constant need of love and reassurance. In severe forms these attitudes may assume psychotic proportions in being suspicious of everyone's motives or feeling everyone is out to cheat them. These persons are mistrustful in business and marriage and are often extremely jealous. They have no real interest in others unless others are exactly like themselves or will serve them as an audience.

The dentist will find it helpful to understand the values which motivate such individuals. These include vanity, egocentricity, selfishness, and the need for love and admiration. Their mistrust and hostility may be difficult to handle. They have no respect for someone they can intimidate. In dealing with them the dentist should be as proud about his work as the patient is about himself.

Narcissism, or self-love, to a certain degree is a normal emotion in us all and understanding this can be very helpful in the proper handling of patients. It accounts for some of the worry of patients about the results of dental procedures that will affect their looks.

The Compulsive. The compulsive personality is recognized by his rigidity and inflexibility in character and behavior. Emotional reactions are repressed, giving an appearance of well controlled equanimity. He is neat, well mannered, obsequious, and everything must be done just so. Ceremonials are common; clothing must be arranged, put on and taken off in a certain manner. His whole life is governed by a set of rigid, orderly laws. Everything is scheduled and pigeonholed. Any deviation from this orderly schedule makes him annoyed and anxious. These people are extremely moralistic, stubborn and unyielding, and change their minds with great difficulty. This discipline unluckily is not only applied to themselves but to as many others as they can involve. Wives and children come under their stern attempt to rule, and the dentist is no exception.

However, with a proper understanding of this type of personality the dentist can frequently work out a harmonious relationship with such persons. He can appeal to their inherent emphasis on orderliness, cleanliness and propriety, and make good use of these characteristics from the standpoint of prophylaxis. He can foresee their need to involve him in their orderly system and make the necessary adjustments to forestall anxiety and resentment on their part. At least there will be little disturbance on the dentist's part because of missed or late appointments since another aspect of the compulsive personality is punctuality.

The Hysteric.   The hysterics are the romantic type to whom everything is related to getting love, or who are preoccupied with sexual fantasy. They fall in and out of love easily, and not infrequently with their dentists, doctors, ministers or teachers. This ability to effect a rapid positive attachment is common in this personality type and must be watched for and handled diplomatically by the doctor. Many dentists and surgical specialists have had experiences in which professional skills were not totally responsible for the gracious thanks, seductive looks and undying devotion of the grateful patient.

The wish for love in this type is usually unconscious and if an explanation were made it would be met by violent objection. This is because the person is so guilty about his unconscious needs that he could never admit them to himself. These wishes, however, find expression in various symptoms, attitudes and behavior.

Since the mouth is so important in the emotional development of the individual, it stands to reason that it should be a common area for psychosomatic complaints in the hysteric type. This must be considered by the dentist when careful examination reveals no evidence of organic disease yet the patient persists in his complaints of intractable pains, and the like.

Furthermore, because of the frustrated wish for love in the hysteric type the dentist must be on his guard in handling these patients. It is this type who accuse doctors of rape, attempted seduction, or who circulate stories about the "doctor getting fresh with me." Actually their wish for love might be so strong that their fantasies involve intimacies with the doctor. These may be so real that the patient will interpret innocent remarks, accidental contacts, or instrumentation as a sexual advance. This is especially so where general anesthesia is used and the wish can be granted in a dream so vivid that the patient may actually believe she has been assaulted. It is, of course, good insurance to have a nurse or assistant present whenever such a person is being treated, or whenever a general anesthesia is used on anyone.

The Masochist.   The masochist enjoys hurting or depreciating himself and actually gets pleasure out of pain. He always assumes the blame, he feels inferior, and is soft-spoken and gentle. Open attack or any form of overt aggression to others is incomprehensible to him. All his anger is unconsciously taken out on himself. He has a strong sense of obligation and comes early to his appointments. The "hard luck guy" falls in this group. He is the one who is always getting frustrated, who never attains his ambitions, or with whom something always goes wrong just at the last moment. Careful observation, however, usually reveals he is the one who frustrates himself because his own guilt makes success or aggression intolerable.

In handling this type the dentist will find most success in a direct appeal to the sense of obligation and duty. These people are usually extremely cooperative especially in painful procedures, as this fits in with their need to suffer. Pathological extremes, when recognized, should be referred for psychiatric help, as "accident prone" people and suicides are high in this group.

The Borderline Psychotic. This type is difficult to describe specifically as there are many types of borderline psychoses. Broadly speaking, this is the group who are so overwhelmed by their conflicts that they begin to lose contact with reality. Their attitudes and symptoms are interesting. Some may be mystics or fanatics. Others may deny the fact that dentists can help them. Another group may become so preoccupied with their bodies that they become obsessed with false ideas about hair, skin, teeth or gastrointestinal tract. These individuals may spend a great deal of their time looking in mirrors and using mouth washes.

The dentist should evaluate each of these individually. If their worry be bad breath, telling them not to worry or reassuring them about it will be of no avail. Their internal problems have become so great that it is necessary for them to believe their breath is bad. Only skilled psychiatric treatment at this stage will he helpful.

Other common dental problems in badly disturbed patients are those resulting from poor oral hygiene. The patient's withdrawal from reality makes any regular oral hygiene unlikely so that caries, gingivitis, pyorrhea and Vincent's disease are not uncommon in psychotic individuals.

There are also numerous instances of *hypochondriacal preoccupations* pertaining to the oral region. These individuals are not psychotic, as their hold on reality is secure except for the particular preoccupation. Tarachow reports a case of a patient who went from one dentist to another insisting that he had a tooth cavity which needed filling. No one was able to find a cavity. This preoccupation developed shortly before the man was to be married, and psychiatric study revealed that his complaint was a symptomatic reflection of his fear of being sexually inadequate in his approaching marriage. He was looking for help to bolster his fears. The repair of the defective tooth really meant a repair of his defective masculinity.

Patients like this are probably seen frequently. They are unnecessarily seeking dental treatment just as the individual with functional gastric complaints seeks help from the internist. It is an easy temptation for a dentist to unwittingly play up to the requests of these mentally ill patients. Any doctor should have both the personal and scientific approach to his patient so that he can deal with him in the most effective as well as the most human fashion. Without sympathy and understanding it is very easy to mishandle neurotic patients. A neurotic patient will often besiege his dentist with complaints, demands and needs for assurance. A good practitioner should have the personal qualities which make it easy for him to handle and understand such an individual. However, under the constant impact of such extreme demands it is only human to get annoyed and react like an exasperated parent to a demanding child.

Bruxism (Clamping and Grinding Habits). The treatment of periodontal disease is based on the control and elimination of factors causing the periodontal breakdown. An important factor in the etiology of this condition is the habit of clamping and grinding of the teeth (bruxism).

For the successful treatment of periodontal disease, clamping or grinding must be recognized and controlled. It must be remembered that these habits frequently are a manifestation of inner tension in the individual and that the grinding is frequently an outward manifestation of inhibited rage or frustration. In some cases the individual may be helped by reeducation and making him aware of the habit, with the aim in view of having him inhibit it by conscious control. When the grinding is nocturnal the handling becomes much more difficult. Sometimes instruction to sleep on the back will be helpful, or the addition of a small pillow to the nape of the neck. However, this treatment is only symptomatic and does not get at the cause—the unconscious feelings which manifest themselves in the grinding. In most of these cases concurrent treatment by a psychiatrist will be the quickest and most effective way of bringing the problem under control.

Some psychogenic organic symptoms, such as tremor or blushing, are the direct expression of emotion or conflict, while others are only their indirect results. Structural damage to teeth as a result of grinding is an example of the latter.

A case, which Saul reports, was a young man with strong oral trends who complained that his teeth and the left side of his jaw pained him, although the dentist found no oral pathosis. As his oral aggression was discussed, he stated that his dentist had told him his teeth showed 25 more years of wear than they normally should and that it was due to nocturnal grinding.

As treatment continued, his teeth and jaw, especially the left side of his maxilla, were constantly sore and he found himself grinding or clamping even during the day. Repeated dental examination failed to find organic pathosis, and a rubber mouth guard failed to relieve his symptoms.

After two months of treatment he suddenly admitted what he had so long denied—that his show of strength and superiority was a denial to himself and the world of inner weakness due to his marked dependent needs. The insight touched him deeply, especially the realization of his hostility when his dependent needs were frustrated.

At the next visit he reported with great astonishment that within an hour after his past interview he noted a marked relief of pain in his teeth and jaw; six hours later he was able to eat comfortably and his ache was gone. It disappeared completely that evening, and he continued symptom-free with no trace of pain.

Cancerphobia. The mouth is a common location for patients to suspect cancer. Zaidens states that this fear occurs most frequently in the middle age group, and in women more than in men. In the majority of cases, the patients are prompted to seek advice because of popular cancer propaganda, cancer in the family, or death in the family caused by cancer. What they really want is reassurance from an authority. Fear of death is the underlying mechanism.

Glossodynia. This condition usually refers to painful or burning tongue and the adjacent tissue, without any objective findings. Patients interpret these sensations as symptoms of cancer. The sex ratio and age level are the same as in cancerphobia. Psychiatric investigation reveals sexual conflict, frigidity, and maladjustment prior to menopause, with increase in anxiety at the approach of menopause, which represents a major threat to their sense of self-esteem as women. Glossodynia occurs in women who are preoccupied with fear of death and fear of cancer in the mouth—the organ which sustains life through eating.

Psychological Preparation for Surgical Operations

It is necessary for the dental surgeon, just as it is for the general surgeon, to be on guard with neurotic patients lest he play into their hands by performing useless operations. If it were just useless, it would not be so bad, but it adds to the misery of the patient and eventually results in criticism and trouble for the surgeon. Both the general surgeon and the dental surgeon must learn that there is such a thing as psychological preparation for operations, just as there is a physical preparation. Surgeons are always so careful to prepare their patients physically for operations. They would not think of performing a major operation without knowing that the cardiovascular-renal system had been surveyed, but they almost never give any consideration to the personality of the patient: how much anxiety is present, and what the effects of a surgical experience may be as far as the personality is concerned. We recently had in the hospital ward an elderly woman who had a huge enlargement of the thyroid gland, which was removed because it was pressing upon the trachea. She had had discomfort, but not severe dyspnea. The anatomic problem loomed large in the clinical picture, but the patient was very apprehensive before the operation and after the operation she became frankly psychotic. As it turned out, we wonder whether perhaps she would not have been better off with the lump in her neck. Similar instances occur in dental surgery.

An attractive single woman of 30 years complained of fatigue, nervousness and constipation. She had had the same symptoms at 17 and her physician had said that the illness was due to focal infection and he ordered all of the upper teeth extracted. This was during the period when the theory of "focal infection" was so enthusiastically endorsed by the profession that the removal of teeth and tonsils proceeded at a prodigious rate. Every obscure illness was held to be due to focal infection.

If we could pile together the teeth and tonsils that have been unnecessarily removed from patients with illnesses of emotional origin, we would have an imposing monument to an era of overcredulity in regard to a significant American contribution to medicine—the theory of focal infection. What sins we have committed in its name!

The removal of the upper teeth in this young woman, despite the fact that a very satisfactory denture replaced them, was a circumstance that affected her whole life, coloring her reactions in all of her personal contacts. She became extremely sensitive about her mouth and thought that everybody was looking at it and making remarks about it. She developed marked feelings of inferiority. These feelings interfered with her position and with her marriage. It is impossible to conclude that it was unnecessary to remove her teeth, but from her description of them it seems probable that it was a radical and unwise procedure. Nor do we wish to contend that her sense of inferiority was entirely determined by this circumstance. Undoubtedly, she had some such feelings to begin with, but the surgical operation added to her problem and burdened her whole life.

Many pains about the head, face and neck are wrongly assumed to be due to dental pathosis. Teeth are extracted or sinuses operated upon, when a careful analysis of the pain would show that atypical neuralgia due to "focal conflict" rather than "focal infection" is present. A study of the life situation rather than a search for "foci of infection" is the proper approach.

For many reasons it is advisable to proceed cautiously in the case of the patient who is eager to have a surgical operation, either general or dental. The mouth is an area around which a great deal of interest and pleasure are centered during infancy and childhood. Likewise, it is an area around which fantasies of hostility are likely to occur. The child identifies himself with the animal who attacks and destroys with the mouth. He thinks of himself as doing likewise, and then has guilt and anxiety over his destructive thoughts. These fantasies often remain buried in the unconscious mind of the adult and then come to the surface when psychological conflicts arise.

The Mouth and Personality Structure

The mouth is the earliest and most important organ of aggression in animal evolution. Hart tells us that "even the lowly insect has multiple mandibles that seize his prey and demolish it in a thoroughly hand-to-mouth fashion. The first cranial nerve to be myelinized is the trigeminal or fifth, which supplies the jaw and mouth and teeth. The oral zone is the first in the infant to become sensitive to pain and touch. Man has not become less aggressive in the course of evolution, he has only substituted speech for the gnashing of his teeth. Hence, though his jaw recedes in importance, his oral zone is still an organ that is so destructive that the wild mouthings of Hitler could send millions of men into battle and death. Malicious gossip is far more deadly a weapon than an actual bite with the teeth—even from the man who, according to the recent papers, refused to pay the dentist for his denture and bit the dentist in his rage."

Binger pointed out that the mouth, quite aside from its utilitarian attributes is, psychologically speaking, directly or symbolically related to the major human instincts and passions: to self-preservation, to cognition, to love and sexual mating, to hate and the desire to injure or kill. From the standpoint of psychopathology this is of the greatest importance. Since the mouth represents the organ for the expression of certain instinctual cravings it is charged with a high psychological potential. Therefore, when operations are performed on this area reactions occur which may seem irrational and bizarre to those who look upon the mouth simply as an organ for taking in food. The human infant puts everything in its mouth. In other words, it tests out its environment in this fashion, and the sucking impulse, which appears at birth and continues long past weaning, is an important method of deriving emotional satisfaction. In addition to chewing there survives in man a tearing and biting impulse. Again to quote Binger, "Darwin pointed out that in states of rage, the teeth are not only clenched and ground together, but the corners of the upper lip are drawn back and the teeth bared—which he thought remarkable, considering how seldom they are used by men in fighting. This attribute of the human mouth is now largely transferred to its verbal offerings. We speak of 'sharp' words, 'biting' wit, or 'mordant' humor . . . Other functions, gustatory and olfactory, properly belonging to the mouth, may be conferred on our utterances which are described as 'bitter,' 'sweet,' 'acid,' 'pungent'—even 'foul.' "

Nor should the mouth as an organ of love be forgotten. Love, genetically, is closely related to sucking and swallowing. A doting mother, cooing over an infant, says: "I could just eat you up." Such terms of endearment as "sweetheart" and "honey" indicate that the object of our affections is conceived of as a dainty morsel. Binger goes on, "In any case the lips and tongue and buccal mucosa are highly erogenous zones and throughout life retain an important pleasure-giving function.

"Suppressed, controlled and redirected though they may be, these atavistic traits, that is, these impulses to use the mouth for purposes of attack, for example, remain in all of us, and can be easily revived. For our personalities are built up of archeological layers and our earlier experiences and tendencies have left in us living, through perhaps dormant traces, not merely dead bones and pot shards. These traces possess a dynamism which affects our health, our relationships and our destiny."

Binger refers to the menopause as a period of life when dental operations are apt to promote unexpected reactions. A woman often feels that a denture is the last straw in her already wounded vanity and self-esteem. Depressions, long periods of invalidism, and even attempts at suicide may be preceded by dental operations.

Commenting that the fatigue state is often the result of heavy emotional expenditures, Ryan states that persons who tire easily may be suffering not from the results of dental foci but from emotional toxemia. He advises dentists to keep this in mind in making diagnoses and planning treatment. He does not suggest that the dentist assume the role of the psychiatrist before he passes judgment on a pulpless tooth. Nor does he recommend that in any situation the dentist attempt to function as a psychiatrist. *To have the psychosomatic point of view is not the same as attempting to practice psychiatry.* Just as physicians and surgeons are urged to think in psychosomatic terms and to integrate this point of view with other treatment methods, so should the same situation prevail for dentists. "Psychosomatics," Ryan states, "is an adjunct to dental diagnosis and practice, not a substitution for other procedures."

Thus we see that the work of the dentist may have a significance far beyond the superficial, purely mechanical ideas that are usually associated with dental procedures. If the dentist becomes a little more aware of the structure of the personality, in the same way that he is now aware of the structures in the mouth, he may avoid many unfortunate occurrences. The teeth can no more be divorced from the personality of the patient, so far as psychosomatic medicine is concerned, than can any other part of the body.

References

Binger, C.: Ann. Dentistry, *4:* 175, 1946.
Cohen, S.: Personal communication, 1956.
Fitts, W. T., Jr., and Ravdin, I. S.: J.A.M.A., *153:* 901, 1953.
Hart, H. H., in Landa, J. S.: The Dynamics of Psychosomatic Dentistry. Dental Publishing Co., Inc., Brooklyn, N. Y., 1953.
Korner, A. F., and Reider, N.: The Angle Orthodontist, *25:* 23, 1955.
Linn, L., and Goldman, I. B.: Psychosom. Med., *11:* 307, 1949.
Menninger, K.: Psychoanalyt. Quart., *3:* 173, 1934.
Meyer, B. C.: J. Mt. Sinai Hosp., *20:* 344, 1945.
Renneker, R., and Cutler, M.: J.A.M.A., *148:* 833, 1952.
Ruesch, J., et al.: Chronic Disease and Psychological Invalidism. Psychosom. Med. Monograph. Paul B. Hoeber, Inc., New York, 1946, p. 126.
Ryan, E. J.: Psychobiologic Foundations in Dentistry. Charles C Thomas, Springfield, Ill., 1946.
Tarachow, S.: N. Y. J. Dent., *16:*189, 1946.
Titchener, J. L.: J.A.M.A., *160:* 1187, 1956.
Titchener, J. L., et al.: Surg., Gynec. and Obst., *102:* 59, 1956.
Weiss, E., Dlin, B., Rollin, H. R., Fischer, H. K., and Bepler, C. R.: Arch. Int. Med., *99:* 628, 1957.
Zaidens, S. H.: N. Y. J. Dent., *24:* 218, 1954.
Zwerling, I., et al.: Am. J. Psychiat., *112:* 270, 1955.

Chapter XX

Arthritis and Orthopedic Problems

CHRONIC ARTHRITIS

Chronic arthritis is perhaps the oldest of all known diseases. Harbin, in Champion's book, states, "The word 'cripple' is derived from the Anglo-Saxon word, 'creep.' The word 'dwarf,' used sometimes in referring to a cripple, is closely akin to the Sanskrit word 'Dhvaras,' meaning 'evil one incarnate.' Convinced that the cripple embodied an evil spirit of ill omen to the community, that he would never be an asset to their armies, and that he was likely to become a social burden, our forefathers ostracised him, sacrificed him to their gods, or abandoned him in his infancy. The Romans later, however, made the first recorded provision to care for cripples. Pope Gregory, in 590 A. D., included them in his classifications of infirm and destitute to be supported by public funds. However, it was not until 1832 in Munich that the first institution, the Royal Bavarian School and Home for Crippled Children, was established; in the United States the first institution was the Hospital for the Ruptured and Crippled which was opened in New York City in 1863."

Focal Infection.   Rheumatism, the term that is generally used in lay circles, includes all forms of aches and pains in the muscles and joints, as well as arthritis. Fortunately, "focal infection," which has been so exploited as the cause of chronic rheumatism, has been generally abandoned. European medicine never paid so much attention to the idea. Consequently, Europeans did not sacrifice quite so many teeth or tonsils on the altar of this concept. It was because medicine felt so helpless in dealing with this disease and because there was often such obvious indication of an infection that the concept of focal infection was so eagerly grasped. One almost never saw an arthritic who had not lost his teeth and his tonsils, and had various other areas in his body attacked on the presumption that infection flourished there. Fortunately, that is not so true today. But even when medicine was attacking arthritics most vigorously from the standpoint of removing their "foci of infection," it recognized at the same time that there were other factors of importance in the disease.

Polypharmacy.   There is hardly any therapeutic process in medicine that has not been utilized in the treatment of arthritis. All kinds

Page 515

of drugs have been used. Gold said, "I know of few subjects in therapeutics which seem to be in a more unsettled and unsatisfactory state than the treatment of arthritis. It does not seem possible to chart the progress in this field by other than a horizontal line with repeated spikes representing new therapeutic ventures. The rise of the spike represents the 'passive faith' which is so common a reaction to new agents or procedures and the fall of the peak represents 'aggressive skepticism.' In few therapeutic fields do we find such sharp contrasts of views concerning matters which should be matters of fact. One arthritis specialist working with a new compound reports dramatic results and another complete failure." As an editorial concerning the treatment of arthritis stated, ". . . almost any form of treatment seems to produce about 20 per cent of claimed cures or arrest of cases, 30 per cent of improvement and 50 per cent of failure."

Because of the difficulties in dealing with arthritis, such patients are exploited by quacks and irregular practitioners. One has only to witness, for example, the countless thousands of people who visit shrines and faith healers. Most of these people are suffering from some form of chronic arthritis. Many magical shrines are famed for the piles of crutches that have been thrown away by cripples, who, for the moment, consider themselves cured but most of whom have to buy more crutches after they get home.

Social Implications of Chronic Arthritis. Most chronic arthritis is something quite apart from the crippling of one joint by a specific infectious agent. The end result of chronic arthritis is apt to be much more serious in the degree of crippling. The two great types are rheumatoid, or arthritis deformans, also referred to as chronic infectious arthritis, and osteoarthritis, the chronic hypertrophic variety. These are the common forms of chronic arthritis that are responsible for so much disability, and because they are so widespread and so frequent, especially among the poor, they enter very importantly into the problems of unemployment and dependency. In fact, one may well say that the interrelation of chronic disease and social dependency is nowhere better illustrated than in chronic arthritis. Chronic arthritis makes for social dependency and social dependency adds to the problem of chronic arthritis.

Clinical Features. Rheumatoid arthritis often resembles an infectious disease. That is to say, it frequently begins with fairly acute manifestations—redness, swelling of the joints and fever, and other constitutional symptoms that frequently accompany an infectious disease. It may begin acutely and then gradually subside only to recur. Or it may begin insidiously and run a progressive course, both forms leading to considerable destruction of the joints and, hence, crippling. It is a disease which frequently attacks the small joints first and the larger joints may follow. Eventualy the disease may be so crippling that the patient becomes bedridden, or confined to a chair. Rheumatoid arthritis is quite common in the younger age groups, whereas osteoarthritis is a disease of the older age groups. Of the two, rheumatoid arthritis is less well understood from the standpoint of etiology and less amenable to treatment.

Sociological Factors.   Cobb, Bauer, and Whiting, in an effort to
throw light on this subject, studied 50 patients with typical rheumatoid
arthritis from a social and psychological point of view and concluded
that there was a significant relationship between life stress and the
arthritis in over 60 per cent of the patients (Chart 5). Their study was
conducted by means of life charts one of which is reproduced here (Chart
6) and which shows the chronological relation between different events
in the patient's life. The severity of the arthritis is indicated in black in
the middle column of Chart 6. Thus one can tell roughly how often the
environmental burdens occurred at the time of the onset of the arthritis

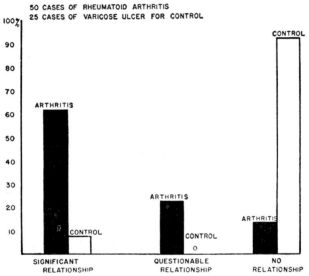

Chart 5.   Temporal relationship between the environmental stress and the onset or
exacerbations of rheumatoid arthritis. It will be noted that a significant relationship was
encountered in a large number of the arthritic patients and rarely in the control group
(patients with varicose ulcers). (Cobb, Bauer and Whiting: J.A.M.A., *113:* 668, 1939.)

or in relation to an exacerbation of the arthritis. The authors state that
in some instances the patient himself emphasized this relationship in
telling his own story. They do not regard this method of study as psychological in any deep sense but rather as a sociological approach. They
comment, "This study was undertaken in order to determine whether
or not there existed a temporal relationship between environmental
stress and the onset or exacerbations of rheumatoid arthritis. It was
thought that, by employing a relatively simple method such as the
Meyer life charts, the synchronism between social and medical events
might become apparent if it existed. Examination of the life charts
reveals that such relationships are demonstrable, whereas they might
have been overlooked had they been recorded in the conventional medical record. Our failure to elicit similar temporal relationships in the
control series adds to the probability that such relationships represent
more than coincidences. Certainly the results obtained from this rela-

tively simple study suggest that more detailed psychologic studies should be made. A statistical analysis of more detailed studies on a large series of cases, correlated with the many other factors, should make it possible to evaluate more correctly the exact etiologic role of such environmental and psychic factors in rheumatoid arthritis. Irrespective of the results obtained a better definition of the host of this chronic disease and the many environmental factors (social and otherwise) with which he has to contend will result." (Chart 6).

CASE #13 ♀		HOSPITAL–#264864	DATE : 1936	
Year	Medical Data	Arthritis	Social Data	Age
			BORN IN ITALY	
1898			ADOPTED IN FAMILY OF 11 CHILDREN	1
1902			NOT VERY HAPPY	5
1907			SCHOOL	10
1909			CAME TO UNITED STATES · SCHOOL	12
1913			MARRIED · LIVED WITH MOTHER	16
1914			OWN HOME · FIRST CHILD BORN	17
1915			SECOND CHILD BORN · HUSBAND OUT OF WORK	18
1916	ARTHRITIS OF ANKLE FOLLOWING THIRD PREGNANCY		THIRD CHILD BORN · UP IN 1½ DAYS · MOVED · LITTLE WORK FOR HUSBAND	19
1917			MOVED FROM DAMP HOUSE · HUSBAND WORKED OCCASIONALLY	20
1918	ARTHRITIS WRIST & KNEES		SECOND CHILD DIED · FOURTH CHILD BORN · "NOT WELL"	21
1919	HOSPITALIZED			22
1920	REMISSION		FIFTH CHILD BORN	23
1921	EXACERBATION·REMISSION		SIXTH CHILD BORN	24
1922	EXACERBATION			25
1923	WRIST OPERATION		FOURTH CHILD DIED	26
1924	HOSPITALIZED · SEVERE EXACERBATION		HUSBAND ILL WITH TUBERCULOSIS	27
1925			HUSBAND IN TB SANATORIUM · SEVENTH CHILD BORN · UP IN 3 DAYS	28
1926	IMPROVING		HUSBAND WENT TO COLORADO · RELIEVED	29
1927			MOTHER'S AID RECEIVED · NOT SO WORRIED	30
1928			HUSBAND IN COLORADO · LIVING EASIER	31
1929			''	32
1930			''	33
1931			''	34
1932			''	35
1933			''	36
1934	EXACERBATION · HOSPITALIZED		MOTHER'S AID STOPPED · 1 SON WORKING · COULDN'T KEEP 5 CHILDREN ON $13.00 A WEEK	37
1935			ON PUBLIC WELFARE · NO FUEL · SON OUT OF WORK	38
1936	MARKED MALAISE AND FATIGUE		NOT ENOUGH FOOD AND FUEL · DESPERATELY WORRIED AND VERY TIRED	39

Chart 6.   Life chart of arthritic patient. (After Cobb, Bauer and Whiting: J.A.M.A., *113:* 668, 1939.)

Those authors conclude that "Environmental stress, especially poverty, grief, and family worry, seem to bear more than a chance relationship to the onset and exacerbations of rheumatoid arthritis. The relative importance of these factors in the etiology of rheumatoid arthritis can be established only by a much more detailed psychiatric study on a large group of such patients."

The Social Worker and Arthritis.   Speaking of the care of the patient with rheumatoid arthritis, Margolis states that the physician who would assume full responsibility for treating such patients must be an internist in the fullest sense of the word, combining psychotherapy with physical measures. Moreover, the psychotherapy will have to be based on more than intuition; at least the rudiments of psychodynamics must be understood. In addition, the medical social worker occupies an important role in treatment. He defines that role as follows: "By discovering the causes of blocking to the acceptance of recommendations for medical care and eliminating them, the case worker may really start the patient on his course. Discussions that allow the patient to vent his hostility reduce emotional tension that might otherwise be going into diseased joints. For the reticent, sensitive patient, the worker may serve as a liaison, helping the patient through the trying experiences of meeting and talking with the doctor. The worker also helps the patient express his fears about his disease and its effect on his future plans. She offers constructive help as the individual becomes ready to move ahead step by step when his physical activity is increased, when he becomes capable of leaving for short walks, when he is allowed resumption of employment, which may mean the return to an old job or taking on a new one, in which case still further emotional adjustments may be required.

"There are also the problems of family adjustments. The patient often needs help in his interpersonal relations with his family, and the latter, in their reactions to the patient and his illness. Inadequate and perhaps unable to face the situation, and confused by the illness and its burdens, the family may wreck all plans for the patient's rehabilitation unless they have the guidance and help of a skilled social worker.

"These and many other aspects of the medical social worker's job must be integrated within the framework of the therapeutic problem as a cooperative venture in which the worker utilizes the physician's medical recommendations and in which they pool their psychologic understanding to bring about the best results attainable.

"Although the medical social worker carries the major responsibility for giving social case work help to the arthritic patient who is under the care of the hospital or clinic, community social workers also have a large and fertile field for constructive help in this problem. In many communities they are the only ones available for such help, especially when they are serving arthritic clients not under the care of a hospital but rather receiving medical supervision from a private physician.

"The fact that many patients with rheumatoid arthritis come from the lower income groups must mean a large prevalence of arthritic clients in the case loads of community agencies. Therefore, not only medical but community social workers as well should be informed about what medical science has to offer to the arthritic patient."

Commenting upon the role of the social worker Schless shows that the case work method utilizes the patient's conscious feelings about the illness but is based on an understanding of the unconscious motivation for behavior. "Accepting the difference between herself and the psychiatrist, the social case worker shares with the patient that difference and confines the scope of her helpfulness within the limit of the realistic services she offers."

Emotional Factors.   Jelliffe, a pioneer in psychosomatic medicine, was one of the first to call attention to the importance of the psychic factor in arthritis. It is gradually being recognized that the emotions have something to do with the disease but what part they play is not understood. The prevailing view is that if a person develops such a painful and crippling disease, it is no wonder that he is nervous. The opposite point of view would be that the cart is placed before the horse in this attitude—that arthritis is largely due to a response to certain strong emotional influences which arise within the individual and influence the function of the joints. Then there are those who traverse the middle road and feel that it is neither wholly one nor the other, but that many factors are at work of which the psychic factor is only one—sometimes important, sometimes not, and sometimes missing altogether. This is our belief.

Personality Studies.   In a detailed study of selected cases of rheumatoid arthritis, Thomas found that in many cases "the rule was to find that for years the patient had been neurotic, then an unusually severe conflict developed, and in the midst of this struggle arthritis appeared. The sexual adjustment of most of the patients was inadequate; the women usually thought sex disgusting, and many were so reticent that it was impossible to obtain any details."

Johnson, Shapiro, and Alexander in a preliminary report of the psychodynamic findings in 33 patients with rheumatoid arthritis found impressive similarities in the nuclear conflict situations and in the general personality structure of the women patients, of whom there were 29.

In adolescence many were of the athletic, tomboy type, but in adult life showed a strong control over their emotional expression. (Halliday also stressed this tendency to control and self-restriction.) They manifested the so-called masculine protest reaction with a rejection of the feminine role. Often they had passive and compliant husbands. In addition to a rejection of the feminine functions the patients showed an excessive masochistic need to serve others, which acted as a discharge for hostility and a denial of their own dependency.

The general psychodynamic background is a chronic, inhibited, hostile aggression relieved by discharge through these personality trends.

While the precipitating factors of the disease covered a wide range of events, analysis of what these events meant to the patient provided certain formulations:

1. Circumstances which increase the unconscious rebellion and resentment against men.
2. Events which tend to increase hostility and guilt feelings.
3. An intensified masculine protest reaction as a defense against fear of sexual attack.

The same authors conclude that the majority of these patients learned to discharge hostility through masculine competition, physical activity, and serving, and also through domination of the family. When these methods of discharge are interrupted the increased muscle tonus resulting from the inhibited aggression and defense against it apparently precipitates the arthritis. But, they continue, this constellation of psychodynamic factors is found so commonly in patients who do not suffer from arthritis that additional etiological factors, still unknown, must be postulated. They suggest that these factors are probably somatic: inherited, traumatic or infectious. They found that their patients improved as they became better able to receive help in analysis.

Essentially similar material was derived by Ludwig in a study of 8 patients with rheumatoid arthritis, 7 of whom were women. Ludwig does not imply that emotional factors alone operate in the causation of rheumatoid arthritis. However, all of these patients showed high degrees of emotional immaturity present long before the onset of the disease. Both the onset and subsequent exacerbations seemed to be related, at times in a predictable fashion, with emotional events implying loss of security. "It must be emphasized that the personality pattern described in these patients is not specific for rheumatoid arthritis." Very similar patterns have been observed by the author and by others in individuals suffering from ulcerative colitis, bronchial asthma, and so on. However, in this group, as well as in the patients with other psychosomatic disorders, the abnormal personality pattern could be demonstrated to have been present for many years before the onset, and in each instance the onset appeared to have been precipitated by some profound emotional shock, often in the nature of loss of support. One such shock was the "Anniversay Reaction" (p. 104).

THERAPEUTIC IMPLICATIONS. Ludwig recommends that one should look for and evaluate emotional disturbances associated with the onset or exacerbations in each case. Since loss of security and underlying dependency of many of these patients appear to be significant, the physician should provide or restore as much security as possible in the treatment situation. This can be done by interest in the patient as a human being, and by allowing and encouraging him to air his problems. It is vital for such a patient to have one person who is his doctor and in charge of the case in order to interpret the opinions of the others and to advise the patient with authority. "Some patients with rheumatoid arthritis need the added care of a psychiatrist, but most of these cases can be treated by the internist who understands and is willing to take the time to practice the art of medicine."

In the work that is now being done on the rehabilitation of the rheumatoid arthritic cripple, Lowman, Lee and Rusk find that certain personality traits, such as refractoriness of deep-seated dependency and passivity, are the most restrictive factors in accomplishing rehabilitation.

RORSCHACH STUDIES. Rorschach studies on male arthritics by Cleveland and Fisher showed many of the pathological features usually seen in the psychotic personality, including contamination and confabulatory responses, color naming, and extensive poor form level. In line with studies regarding other vegetative disorders (such as asthma and ulcerative colitis), there is also some evidence indicating that it is unusual for rheumatoid arthritis and schizophrenia to be present simultaneously in the same individual.

Osteoarthritis

Current theories regard the causes of osteoarthritis as senescence and trauma, and the fact that no obvious psychosomatic changes in glandular secretion or muscle contraction are demonstrable to explain the development of bony overgrowth makes it seem difficult to establish a relation of life situation and emotion to this disorder.

Irvine decided to get a brief life story on a number of cases of systemic osteoarthritis with special reference to childhood emotional trauma, early neurotic traits, circumstances associated with the onset of the arthritis, and evidences of emotional disturbances during the course of the disease. In the investigation of 50 cases, an opportunity was also found to observe whether there was a parallelism of emotional disturbance and progression or arrest of the organic disease.

Irvine found that noxious emotions, especially fear, anxiety and grief, of unusual severity and duration, are important in the genesis and persistence of activity of systemic osteoarthritis. Widespread, progressive and persistently painful osteoarthritis as well as many lesser lesions (such as Heberden's nodes) were found to have a background of severe emotional trauma shortly prior to the onset of the arthritis, often in a psychic field sensitized by trauma in early life.

When the emotional state improved in such cases, the arthritis became less painful and progression of bony overgrowth ceased. The severity of the emotional disturbance and that of the activity of the arthritis were usually parallel. Thus, Irvine would erase the artificial distinction between "articular" and so-called "nonarticular" categories of musculoskeletal disease.

Nonarthritic Rheumatism ("Fibrositis")

A common problem in the practice of medicine is the patient who complains of aches and pains in muscles and joints, who is "achy and stiff," but has no arthritis and does not develop it. Fatigue and sometimes slight fever are prominent symptoms. Physical examination and laboratory studies are usually negative. Many difficulties in diagnosis arise. Attention is often focused on the slight rise in temperature and the patient undergoes repeated studies from the standpoint of obscure infection. In addition to "fibrositis" and early arthritis, rheumatic fever and chronic brucellosis are frequently thought of. In the course of the many physical and laboratory studies slight deviations from normal are found and additional diagnoses add to the patient's concern. Endocrine dysfunction, low blood pressure, anemia and neurocirculatory asthenia are frequently mentioned in the histories of these patients, and if the subject is a woman and near middle age the climacteric is almost certain to be held responsible. The patient thinks of herself as a burden to her family and imagines that she will lead a wheelchair existence from arthritis or become seriously disabled by some other organic disease. Urged to rest and subjected to many medical and physical treatments, she leads a restricted life and becomes more and more of an invalid. This story continues, sometimes for years, often with prolonged periods of hospital observation and sanatorium care.

These observations are based (Weiss, 1955) on a study of 93 patients, all but 10 of whom were women and most of them married. Thirty of the patients had slight fever, usually less than 100° F. Low back pain of a nagging character was a frequent association, and atypical neuralgias of the face, shoulder region and leg were often associated with the body aches and pains. Headaches were frequent and were usually blamed upon "sinus infection," so that the patient sometimes referred to his "sinus" rather than to the headache. "Focal infection" was often held responsible for the neuralgic pains and pelvic abnormalities were incriminated for pain in the back.

Diagnostic Problems. When a patient with generalized aches and pains, and perhaps fatigue, presents no evidence of arthritis or of any other organic disease as determined by physical examination and laboratory studies, and when there are evidences of neurosis as determined by personality study, there is not much question about the diagnosis; one can speak of psychogenic rheumatism or, better yet, designate the exact type of neurotic difficulty, and explain the illness to the patient on the basis of tension of emotional origin which will not permit him to relax, and thus "wears him out."

When slight fever is added to the above clinical picture, difficulties enter. Because attention is apt to be focused on the temperature elevation, the physician frequently requests that the patient keep a written record of the temperature, and the idea of an obscure infection occupies the attention of both patient and physician.

"FIBROSITIS" AND BRUCELLOSIS. Diagnosis presents two major problems, namely, (1) what is referred to as "primary fibrositis," and (2) chronic brucellosis. There are capable observers who believe that neither exists. We regard "primary fibrositis" as just another and less satisfactory name for psychogenic rheumatism, a term which, in itself, is open to certain objections. But it at least points in the direction of the chief etiologic factor, even though it does not define that factor adequately. Graham, writing of the "fibrositis syndrome," states that the term fibrositis suggests an inflammatory origin but that it has not been established that inflammation is concerned in its pathogenesis. The term has become a catch-basket for many varieties of nonarticular rheumatism. Graham thinks that it is important for the physician to obtain a better understanding of this condition so that we can have a more fundamental treatment than "teeth, tonsils and aspirin." He, of course, is speaking of primary fibrositis, not the secondary fibrositis which certainly occurs in association with various forms of arthritis and also as a result of strain or injury, exposure, occupation, posture and the like.

In our experience it has been very difficult to help these patients as long as the question of *chronic brucellosis* beclouds the issue. Unless there is suggestive history and high or rising agglutination titer, in the absence of the organism (which is so seldom found) one had better not raise the issue of chronic brucellosis or at any rate should settle it promptly and meanwhile study the patient from the standpoint of emotional conflict. If then one can reasonably exclude organic disease by history, physical examination, and laboratory study and find positive evidence from a personality standpoint of significant emotional conflict, one must explain to the patient that there is no disease and that the symptoms are of emotional origin.

Psychological Symptoms.   Our study, utilizing the simultaneous application of physiological and psychological techniques, proved the presence of psychopathology rather than tissue pathology. Psychological symptoms most frequently encountered were poor sleep and poor sexual adjustment, and a marital conflict was the most frequent underlying problem. Significant emotional conflicts were found which were apparently responsible for the fatigue, but the special feature associated with muscular aches and pains was the presence of chronic resentment of which the patient was usually totally unaware.

Psychodynamics.   The muscles serve as a means of defense and attack in the struggle for existence; thus internal tension is most easily relieved by muscular action. When the external expression of aggression in the form of muscular action is inhibited by repressing forces, then muscular tension may result which is felt by the individual as pain and limitation of movement and is often erroneously interpreted by the examining physician as fibrositis or muscular rheumatism. When we say to these people that their aches and pains and fatigue are due to the fact that they are always in a state of tension, that they do not know how to relax, even at night, and that because their muscles are taut they are crying out in protest with aches and pains, it makes sense to them and provides a stepping-stone for them to begin to talk about their emotional problems.

Instead of calling this psychogenic rheumatism, fibrositis, or even muscular rheumatism, the most suitable diagnostic term, as Flind and Barber point out, is the psychiatric diagnosis applicable to each case because it is the psychopathology which is chiefly responsible for the syndrome and it is by means of psychotherapy that we can deal with these patients most effectively.

Previous Studies.   Halliday deserves credit for opening up the whole subject of the psychosomatic aspects of rheumatism in his studies on the insured population of Scotland. In a survey of 1000 consecutive cases he found that 15 per cent were certified with a diagnosis of rheumatism and of this group 70 per cent were nonarthritic and were usually referred to as cases of fibrositis. Occurring mostly in males having dangerous occupations, rheumatism was found to be a major cause of incapacitating sickness.

Boland and Corr found psychogenic rheumatism to be the most frequent cause of disability in 450 consecutive cases diagnosed as arthritis or allied organic conditions in an army general hospital. Approximately one third of the patients in the entire series were considered incapacitated because of psychic difficulty. The sedimentation rate was normal in all cases and in one third of the cases there was a history of invalidism or semi-invalidism from rheumatism in one or more members of the immediate family.

An outstanding characteristic in their patients with psychogenic backache was persistence of disability in spite of prolonged bed rest,

They emphasize this feature of the disability when they cite the patient with advanced active rheumatoid spondylitis who was found pushing another with pure psychogenic backache to the post exchange in a wheelchair.

Treatment Hints. Instead of cautioning rest and more rest, which only permits these people to "stew in their own juices," we recommend that they "carry on in spite of symptoms" and this they will often be able to do once they have divorced their pain from the fear of arthritis, heart disease, cancer, or what not. Once neurotic pain is divorced from a fear of organic disease, it is remarkable how rapidly it will disappear or diminish. As soon as possible we try to get them away from injections of vitamins and hormones, from sedatives and even physiotherapy, or if some of these measures are continued we make it clear to them that they are being used in a supplementary capacity and that the cure lies in emotional reeducation. Halliday has called attention to physiotherapy and fixation of symptoms in his insured patients and we see the same thing in private and hospital practice. It is of course sometimes necessary to make certain concessions to the previous organic miseducation which the patient has had. We cannot go too quickly in changing our approach from disease to disorder, from the idea of doing something for the patient to having him do something for himself, from education along physical lines to the necessity for emotional growth. The essence of psychotherapy, which should be a part of the equipment of every physician, is not to go faster than the patient is prepared to go.

When patients are tense, taut and uncommunicative, they will often begin to talk when they are put at ease and muscular relaxation occurs; of course, the reverse is equally true, that when patients can be encouraged to talk their muscle tension often diminishes.

Chronic resentment—smoldering discontent—is the special emotional problem in these patients, and it is one that had best be approached indirectly. One must avoid the crude suggestion that the patient is angry at someone near and dear to him or for whom he is expected to have filial respect. That problem can be approached by gradually making the patient aware of the discontent and chronic aggravation in his life as we study his day-to-day existence and note how his tension increases finally to the point where symptoms appear. We must let the patient see that he is suffering not from disease of body or mind but rather from a disorder of his feelings.

In connection with *physical medicine* one more word ought to be said, and that is on the problem of belts, braces and supports. So often we find these patients wearing sacro-iliac or abdominal supports when what they need is *inner* support. Instead of trying to bolster them up with a crutch what we ought to do is try to develop their inner emotional security so that they will not have to lean on supports or braces, or for that matter on their physician.

ORTHOPEDIC PROBLEMS

It took the medical experiences of World War II to persuade us that the emotions enter importantly into orthopedic problems. Heretofore the specialty of orthopedics had been just about as divorced from psychological considerations as dentistry. Statistics showed that disorders of the musculoskeletal system ranked high among the psychosomatic problems in military medicine.

The Low Back Problem.   The problem of the patient with low back pain has been with the medical profession since our first great ancestor pulled himself from the four-footed to the upright position. The low back takes all the strain. It is one of our points of least resistance. It is like the poor—it is always with us. And very much like the poor, it is apt to be shoved away into a corner so that we will not be bothered by seeing it. Thus Stimson, who saw how frequently low back pain was an incapacitating factor in the British Army, as it was in the American Army, refers to the fact that it is also a common problem in civilian medicine.

Working at New York's Presbyterian Hospital, Stimson saw the problem as follows: "If the patient had a proved orthopedic lesion such as a spondylolisthesis, a protrusion of the nucleus pulposus, or a compression fracture, he fitted well into the orthopedic or fracture clinic. But if he had a pain in the back with negative x-rays for these orthopedic lesions, medicine didn't want him, arthritis didn't want him, and he certainly didn't fit into the fracture or orthopedic clinics. There really was no place for him. This procedure of handling patients with low back pain did not seem right. As far as the patient was concerned, he or she still had a pain in the back, and no one seemed to be doing very much about it. At best, these patients were sent down to the physical therapy department for diathermy and massage three times a week, *ad infinitum.*"

THE LOW BACK CLINIC.   On the basis of the above observations a combined clinic for the handling of low back pain was set up. The personnel of the clinic consisted of a physician, a neurosurgeon, a member of the physical medicine department, a psychiatrist, a rheumatologist, and three members from the fracture service. Gaston reported the working classification of 300 cases from this clinic as follows:

Posture	60
Osteoarthritis	57
Acute low back	30
Congenital anomalies	27
Neuropsychiatric	26
Miscellaneous	23
Myositis	18
No back diagnosis	14
Rheumatoid arthritis	13
Diagnosis deferred	10
Herniated discs	9
Coccygodynia	5
Compression fractures	3
Scoliosis	2
Gluteal bursitis	2

He reports that the largest single group in the neuropsychiatric category was the returning servicemen.

Commenting further on this material Stimson states, "The posture group consists quite largely of women who have borne one or more children, who have very weak abdominal muscles, and who have low backache at the end of the day. We find that we can do a great deal for this group, thanks to the cooperation of our physical medicine specialist, who is present at every session of the clinic. Exercise, proper beds, et cetera, have done wonders, and these patients are already among our most grateful."

Nor should we forget that the syndrome of low back pain and fatigue is often an expression of emotional conflict which frequently occurs in association with pelvic preoccupation on the part of both patient and doctor. Tired women with nagging or even "excruciating" pain in the back, who are overconcerned about some slight pelvic abnormality and who are eager to have it corrected surgically, should be suspect from a psychosomatic standpoint and caution should be exercised before permitting an operation.

From observation of a group of patients with low back pain Brown and his associates, in a study from the Massachusetts General Hospital, derived criteria about the patients' attitudes toward their symptoms and treatment and their reaction to illness that are indicators of the presence of complicating psychological factors. These criteria are based on the following six characteristics, which are readily observable if the patient is encouraged to discuss his condition:

1. History of the present illness that is vague because of confused chronology and because of the introduction of material apparently having nothing to do with the injury and symptoms.

2. Expression of either open or veiled resentment to and criticism of the doctors and ancillary personnel because of alleged mismanagement or neglect.

3. Dramatic descriptions of the symptoms and of the patient's reactions to them.

4. Difficulty in localization and description of pain and other symptoms.

5. Failure of the usual forms of treatment to give significant relief from pain.

6. Accompanying neurotic symptoms.

TREATING PATIENTS RATHER THAN X-RAYS. In these days when we are seeing so many patients whose backs have been operated upon in an effort to relieve them of pain in much the same way that abdominal exploratory operations formerly were done, that is, in a vain effort to remove a pain from the body that actually resides in the spirit of the individual, it is well to remember that no area of the body lends itself to such misinterpretation of x-rays as does the low back area. Chamberlain cautions as follows: "A great many variations, and deviations from the so-called *normal,* are visualized by x-ray films, and are quite meaningless from the standpoint of the etiology of the patient's pain. To ascribe a patient's low back symptoms to an enlarged transverse process of a fifth lumbar vertebra, or to some hypertrophic spurs and fringes at some of the joint margins, is to jump to an unwarranted conclusion. Careful studies have shown that many of these positive x-ray findings are very poorly correlated, or not correlated at all, with the presence or absence of low back pain."

Stimson also comments on this subject: "Some of the arthritic patients come in with x-rays which show marked osteoarthritic spurs, lists, and scoliosis. (We are learning not to treat x-rays, but patients.) A nice woman, of about fifty-two years, came into the clinic. She said she had had a little pain in her back for the past four months. She had one of the most appalling x-rays of an osteoarthritic spine that I have ever seen, but she had only this mild backache over a short period of her life. Other patients have a great series of symptoms, and x-rays which show only mild changes. We are finding that we can relieve the osteoarthritics, especially in the older age groups, with proper fitting girdles."

She concludes that patients whose workups are negative and whose x-rays are essentially negative present the real problem but with the help of a physician, a psychiatrist and the physical medicine expert most people can be helped.

Painful, Stiff Shoulder. The common complaint of pain and stiffness in the shoulder often presents a difficult diagnostic and therapeutic problem. Few physicians recognize that emotional factors enter into this type of musculoskeletal disability. In a study of 300 patients seen in psychosomatic consultation Lorenz and Musser found that 20 per cent complained of this syndrome. The authors feel that in the presence of excessive muscular tension, whether due to emotional stress or another cause, the minor effort of daily muscular activity may be sufficient to produce injury. With few exceptions, pain and stiffness in the shoulder area occurred in a setting which was emotionally stressful for the patient.

It is noteworthy in this regard that demonstration of aberrant calcification in roentgenograms of the shoulder seemed to have no bearing on the severity of symptoms, physical findings or degree of disability in this group of patients.

Working with the "myofascial pain syndrome" Long, specializing in rehabilitation at the Henry Ford Hospital of Detroit, finds more and more psychogenic causation in such disorders as tension headaches, the trapezius syndrome, the scapulohumeral syndrome, and the scalenus anticus syndrome in his approach to the problem of "fibrositis."

Intractable Pain Syndromes. In a psychosomatic study of 80 patients whose activities were limited either by absence or disease of an extremity and/or chronic intractable pain, Kapp and Rosenbaum noted that 51 patients had some type of chronic, severe, intractable pain and of these 17 had phantom limb pain. Many had had a variety of neurosurgical procedures without obtaining relief.

PHANTOM LIMB. The initial emphasis of the study dealt with the postamputation phenomenon of phantom limb. Here the concept of a pain body-image describes the specificity of the site of pain in the limb (phantom or real) where the pain does not seem to be related directly to the current injury. Rather, it appears to be associated with pain experienced in the past by the patient or by a person with whom the patient has identified. Such previous pain and the injury associated with it are invested intensely with emotional significance for the patient. At times the type and local area of the pain appear to resemble an hysterical conversion symptom. Other workers agree that phantom limb is a consequence of the proprioceptive body-image which every individual develops in childhood.

INTRACTABLE PAIN.   Kapp and Rosenbaum write, "Every person has a 'pain memory' which is gradually built up by the painful experiences suffered and witnessed by the individual since early childhood. There are certain individuals who re-suffer previous pains in an effort to relieve some current interpersonal difficulty. Such pains represent a neurotic manifestation. They are sometimes associated with demonstrable auto-nomic nervous system discharges which accompanied the original pain, and become part of the neurotic symptomatology. Trivial injuries or disease often are the precipitating factors in the initiation of such neu-rotic pain and trophic reactions. We found that a majority of our patients with phantom limb pain and minor causalgia had such reactions.

"A number of patients were observed who developed chronic in-tractable pain syndromes after industrial accidents. They were bitter, hostile, mistrusting people with whom the therapist had to establish a warm positive relationship before relief could be expected. This we attempted to do in a controlled hospital environment by gratifying the patients' frustrated dependency. Only then could therapy be directed toward resolving the intense hostility intimately attached to the painful syndrome."

The Accident Habit.   Among the causes of disability in this country accidents rank first and in addition are an important cause of deaths.

Dunbar made a systematic study of patients admitted to a large hospital in an effort to determine the role that emotional factors play in illness and decided to use fracture patients for a control, thinking that they would represent the most "normal" group that could be found in the hospital. She was surprised to find that they were far from "normal" so far as emotional factors were concerned and that, indeed, it was this aspect of their personality that had to do with the accident. Dunbar found that others had been working on this problem and that many authorities were agreed that the majority of accidents are linked to the personalities of the victims. She tells of a public utility company which operated a large fleet of trucks and became seriously alarmed at the rate of accidents. After a futile effort to determine the cause they fell back upon the simple expedient of shifting men with bad accident records from the driver's seat to other work. In this way they reduced their accident rate to about one fifth of what it had been, so far as the trucks were concerned, but they found that these same men, instead of smashing up their vehicles, were injuring themselves at work or at home.

The National Research Council, which had made a study of this company as well as of three others, reported that the automobile accidents and personal injuries of more than 2000 drivers tended to accumulate side by side.

Tillman and Hobbs made a study of the psychiatric and social back-grounds of the accident-prone automobile driver. Dealing chiefly with taxi drivers, they discovered that the high-accident group showed a marked intolerance for, and aggression against, any authority, and that this behavior dated from early childhood. The origin of the aggression was found in an unstable home background and showed up in the antisocial behavior in the individual's life history. Analyzing 96 drivers from the general population who had had four or more accidents and comparing them with a control group of accident-free drivers, they found that 66 per cent of the high-accident group were known to social and law enforcement agencies as compared with only 9 per cent of the control group. Commenting upon the question of the selection of drivers by personnel managers, they stated that safe driving depends more on judgment, caution and consideration of the possible errors of others, than upon reaction time and binocular vision. They added that any intelligent personnel manager could learn to take the kind of life history that is necessary to detect the unstable person who is prone to accidents.

PERSONALITY STUDY. Dunbar found that the hospital group with accident-proneness are generally impulsive people who concentrate upon daily pleasures with little interest in long-term goals. While their illness rate is below that of the general population their accident rate is high. They are usualy extremely resentful of authority, often on an unconscious level, and an unusually large proportion of them had neurotic traits in childhood. These traits often expressed themselves in the form of walking and talking in their sleep, in persistent lying, stealing and truancy. Later these tendencies disappeared, apparently replaced by the accident habit. The decisiveness of the accident-prone person is part of a drive for independence and self-reliance in a situation of the moment rather than as a part of a planned career or program. Dunbar finds that when this personality pattern is set beside those of other groups of the population, it turns out to match precisely that of the juvenile delinquent and the adult criminal. "The behavior characteristic of the persistent breaker of laws is virtually identical with that of the persistent breaker of bones right up to the point where the one commits a crime and the other has an accident." One group carries the early record of lying, stealing and truancy into a broader field and becomes a criminal, while the other begins to hurt himself instead of the community.

Treatment for patients with the accident habit involves a deep understanding of all the factors which enter into their accident-proneness. The following case illustrates the many factors that may enter into a "purposeful" accident, determined by unconscious motivation.

Case 56.   A Purposeful Accident

History and Symptoms.   A very obese, hypochondriacal, middle-aged, white woman had been obsessed for several years with the idea that she had cancer of the throat and despite the reassurance of many physicians who had studied her carefully, she continued to believe that "there must be some physical basis for the pain and burning sensation in the back of the throat." She also had a great fear of infection, was meticulously clean about her home, and was forever washing her hands. She was very insistent about having something done for her throat and she herself would make topical application of irritating solutions until, on many occasions, bleeding occurred. Even this did not satisfy her need for suffering so that she finally succeeded in persuading a dentist to remove her perfectly good teeth. She encountered less difficulty in sacrificing her tonsils. Both operations gave temporary relief but the symptoms returned worse than ever.

LIFE SITUATION

She was so fixated upon her physical symptoms that it was impossible to accomplish more than the most superficial investigation of her life situation. The only digression she would make from a discussion of her physical symptoms was to upbraid her local physician for fancied mistreatment and insulting behavior. He had sent her for a general diagnostic survey but continued to supervise her care. She spent a great deal of time criticizing him for a lack of interest in her condition and for the "contemptuous way" in which he treated her. Nevertheless, it was obvious that underneath the surface hostility there was a very positive attachment to her physician which was indicated by her continuing under his care and by such statements as: "she had great faith in his scientific ability; on occasions he had been very kind to her; and her children and her husband were devoted to him."

She was a very religious person and went to church every morning seeking help for her illness. We had refused to help her to decide whether to leave her local physician, and so on one occasion when she felt that she had been more than ordinarily mistreated by him, she went to church to seek help in making a decision on two related questions: first, whether finally to quit her physician and seek another and secondly, whether for financial reasons it would be better to give up a health insurance policy which provided nursing service in case of a confining illness. She had carried this costly policy for a long time without realizing benefits and now her funds were low.

On the particular morning in question she prayed for help in making these two decisions. As she left church she noted that it had been raining and while ordinarily, because of her overweight, she took special precautions in descending stairs, "she was not as careful as she should have been" and on reaching the third of three steps, slipped on a wet spot, fell and fractured the left ankle. As she explained on the telephone the next day, "she got her answer quicker than she thought." She seemed in a cheerful frame of mind as she told with evident satisfaction, that her physician had immediately responded to the call after this accident.

COMMENT

Aside from the purposefulness of the accident the marked ambivalence for her local physician was the striking feature of this case. Just as many neurotic people take up much time in criticism of some member of the family, just so did this woman express herself toward her physician. On the surface she was markedly hostile and yet she continued under his care and obviously held him in great respect and even with some evidence of underlying affection. He found the patient a very disturbing factor in his practice and confessed that when it was necessary to see her, "it made a wreck out of him." When the psychological background of this relationship was explained to him, he found matters a little easier, but needless to say, was pleased when the patient finally made up her mind to place herself under the care of an older physician who had "taken care of her in childhood." However, to conclude the story related above, once the fracture had healed, she was back once more with her old throat complaint and criticism of her local physician.

The ambivalent relationship to her physician, so excessive in this particular instance, is a very important element in the doctor-patient relationship, as yet not understood in general medicine.

PSYCHOSOMATIC ASPECTS OF PHYSICAL MEDICINE

There is great need for psychosomatic study in physical medicine. Many problems exist to which such studies might contribute valuable information.

What are the elements of the physician-patient relationship that enter into these problems, and can they be evaluated? Is the ordinary positive relationship between patient and physician (or attendant) heightened by the factor of actual physical manipulation? What are the feelings of warmth, security and protection that may be created and which in many instances seem to support the patient by reminding him of an earlier relationship to a parent or protective figure? On the reverse side of this picture is the question of physical therapy giving too much gratification so that the patient unconsciously may be encouraged to hold on to an illness. Here is an important aspect of the subject that needs illumination, when it is found, for example, that the patient tends to utilize the treatment as a substitute for making an adjustment to real life. What personal elements enter into the question of massage? Are there certain personalities in which massage works and others in which it does not? It would seem likely that there may be elements in the personality structure that find massage "too stimulating," rather than relaxing.

Spas.   What are the elements of suggestion that enter into spa treatment? If they were properly evaluated would it not help us in the development of spas in the United States? It has always been suspected that this motivating force entered into spa treatment and it may even be that with our determination to advance scientific medicine in the United States there has been a neglect in the development of spas. European spas were always looked upon with some suspicion by the American medical profession. If we could evaluate this factor and utilize it scientifically would it not help us in the spa development which is occurring in this country?

What we must do is try to decide how much benefit may be due to physical therapy and how much to emotional factors. Perhaps we have reached the point where we can apply fairly precise measurements to both.

Physical Relationships.   There is another important aspect of the problem and that is the question of the relationships between general physicians, including psychiatrists, and specialists in physical medicine. One group has looked upon the other with suspicion. The general physician or the psychiatrist has noted that patients treated in commercial institutions for the application of physical therapy have been influenced by suggestions that were harmful; for example, the state of the circulation, the pulse, the condition of the blood pressure ("too high" or "too low"), the question of bowel function ("autointoxication"), the matter of muscle tone, and so forth. Specialists in physical medicine, influenced by their training in organic disease and by methods of physical measurement, have perhaps not been fully informed regarding the principles of psychodynamics which permit scientific applications of psychotherapy. Certainly many specialists in physical medicine have been reluctant to accept patients with psychological ills, apparently because they do not wish to "contaminate" their specialty by applying it for purely suggestive purposes. Studies of the kind that we have in mind might go a long way toward resolving these problems.

Still another question in this connection is whether physical therapy and psychotherapy are incompatible in the same patient (in psychosomatic affections). For example, if a muscle group is painful and this discomfort is on the basis of spasm resulting from tension, is there more than one way of relieving this tension? Can the methods be applied at the same time or are they mutually exclusive? The psychiatrist may feel that emotional factors are responsible for the tension and that the only way to make the patient face the necessity for discussing these emotional factors is to approach the problem from a purely psychological standpoint. He may feel that if a physical name is given to the affection ("fibrositis," for example) and he allows the patient to undergo physical therapy it may "fix the neurosis" and make it impossible for the patient to appreciate that psychological forces are responsible. The physical therapist often feels that because it is simple to apply physical measures to get relief from muscular tension that there is no point in doing more. Perhaps these problems could be settled by a cooperative study.

Practical Suggestions. Watkins and Finesinger attempt to answer some of these questions in a discussion of the psychiatric aspects of physical medicine. They caution against prolonging passive procedures, such as massage and hydrotherapy, and recommend that the patient take up exercises and more active procedures, such as occupational therapy. In planning occupational therapy they encourage the patient to work independently as soon as possible.

These authors call special attention to the necessity for avoiding unnecessary physical contacts such as patting the patient or holding his hand. Such gestures suggest a social situation and tend to change the professional relationship. They also give some good advice about what to say and what not to say in dealing with the patient in a physical medicine relationship. They avoid probing for information, avoid giving the patients lectures on physiology as well as psychology, avoid making promises that cannot be kept. They try to use reassurance in moderation. Wisely the authors recognize that the therapist often praises the patient to relieve his own insecurity or because he does not know what else to do. Consequently they try to avoid flattering patients. Nor (and this is a good point for medicine in general) do they respond when patients attempt to flatter them. They prefer to have a relationship with a patient characterized by attitudes of earnestness, honesty and cooperation in working toward alleviating the patient's suffering.

References

Boland, E. W., and Corr, W. P.: J.A.M.A., *123:* 805, 1943.

Brown, T., Nemiah, J. C., Barr, J. S., and Barry, H.: New England J. Med., *251:* 123, 1954.

Chamberlain, W. E.: Personal communication, May, 1946.

Champion, W. M.: Medical Information for Social Workers. Wm. Wood & Co., Baltimore, 1938. Chapter by Harbin, M., p. 347.

Cleveland, S. E., and Fisher, S.: Psychosom. Med., *16:* 327, 1954.

Cobb, S., Bauer, W., and Whiting, I.: J.A.M.A., *113:* 668, 1939.

Dunbar, H. F.: Mind and Body, Psychosomatic Medicine, Random House, New York, p. 98, 1947.

Dunbar, H. F.: Ann. Int. Med., *14:* 839, 1940.

Flind, J., and Barber, H. S.: Quart. J. Med., *14:* 57, 1945.

Gaston, S. R.: Personal communication, October, 1947.

Gold, H.: Weekly Roster, Phila., Sept. 20, 1941. Quoted from New York State J. Med., *41:* 688, 1941.

Graham, W.: Bull. Rheumat. Dis., *3:* 33, 1953.

Halliday, J. L.: Ann. Int. Med., *15:* 666, 1941.
Halliday, J.: Brit. M. J.: *1:*213 and 264, 1937.
Irvine, J. H.: Am. Soc. Research Psychosom. Problems, Atlantic City, May 3, 1947.
Jelliffe, S. E.: Tr. Am. Neurol. Assoc., 1923, p. 419.
Johnson, A., Shapiro, L. B., and Alexander, F.: Psychosom. Med., *9:* 1295, 1947.
Kapp, F. T., and Rosenbaum, M.: Personal communication, Sept., 1947.
Lowman, E. W., Lee, P. R., and Rusk, H. A.: J.A.M.A., *158:* 1335, 1955.
Long, C., II: Henry Ford Hosp. Med. Bull., Dec., 1955, pp. 189–192.
Lorenz, T. H., and Musser, M. J.: Ann. Int. Med., *37:* 1232, 1952.
Ludwig, A. O.: Bull. Rheumat. Dis., *2:* 15, 1952.
Lyons, J. W., Jr.: Penna. M. J., *16:* 9, 1949.
Margolis, H. M.: The Family, *25:* 331, 1945.
Schless, B. G.: The Family, *25:* 331, 1945.
Stimson, B. B.: Psychosom. Med., *9:* 210, 1947.
Thomas, G. W.: Am. J. Psychiat., *93:* 693, 1936.
Tillmann, W. A., and Hobbs, J. E.: Am. J. Psychiat., *106:* 321, 1949.
Watkins, A. L., and Finesinger, J. E.: J.A.M.A., *135:* 1050, 1947.
Weiss, E.: M. Clin. North America, *39:* 601, 1955.

Index

Page numbers in *italic* type refer to case material.

Blood pressure, low, 196
  essential, 447
  headache due to, 447
Blushing, physiological explanation, 58
  psychological explanation, 59
Body language. See also *Organ language.*
  explaining to patients, 85
Borderline psychotic, 509
Bowels. See *Intestines.*
Brain, circulation, emotions and, 464
  disease, organic, simulating neurosis, 463
  tumor, simulating neurosis, 463
  visceral, 62
Breaking point in emotional illness, 11
Breast cancer, reactions to, 502
Breast feeding, 386
Breath, shortness of. See *Dyspnea.*
Breathing. See also *Respiration.*
  effect of emotions on, 415
Brief psychotherapy in diabetes mellitus, 337
Broken homes, significance in psychosomatic diagnosis, 100
Bronchial asthma, 428. See also *Asthma.*
Brucellosis, chronic, vs. fibrositis syndrome or psychogenic rheumatism, 320
  fibrositis and, 523
  vs. neurocirculatory asthenia, 203, 204
Bruxism, 92, 510

CANCER, emotional problems of, 502
Cancerphobia, 511
Cannon theory of emotions, 58
Cardiac. See also *Heart.*
Cardiac neurosis, 182, *195*
  as symptom of hypertension, 234
  drugs in, 192
  electrocardiograms in, 185
  emotional disturbance preceding, 183
  erect philosophy in, 192
  explaining illness to patient, 193
  history in, importance, 191
  pain of, angina pectoris and, 184
  physical examination in, importance, 191
  practical suggestions, 195
  precipitating factors, 182
  predisposition to, 191
  prophylaxis, 191
  psychotherapy, 192
    organ language in, 194
  symptoms, 183
  treatment, 191
  vs. neurocirculatory asthenia, 197, 198, 204
Cardiospasm, 285, *288*
  clinical picture, 286
  etiology, 285

Cardiospasm, personality study in, 287
  treatment problems, 288
Cardiovascular system, 181–224
  essential hypertension, 225–53. See also *Blood pressure, high.*
Career, family attitudes about, inconsistent, 129
  marriage and, conflict in mucous colitis, *274*
  social work as, 124
Career women, neurosis in, 117
Carrier of neurosis, parent as, 18
Case illustration in history-taking, 86
Case work, social, psychosomatic concept in, 122
Casual remarks as diagnostic aids, 105
Catharsis, mental, in expressive therapy, 162
Central angiospastic retinopathy, 475
Central nervous system, 440–69
Cerebral arteriosclerosis, psychosis and, 467
Cerebral vascular disease, emotional problems of, 464
Cerebral vascular spasm, 465
Changes of life, psychosomatic significance, 375
Character disorder in coronary occlusion, 213
Chemical hibernation, 153
Chest, oppression in, organ language in, 85
Childhood. See *Children.*
Childless couples, significance in psychosomatic diagnosis, 101
Child-parent relationship, repetition in psychotherapy, 119
Children, advice to have, 136
  asthma in, personality structure, 429
  curiosity about sex, 29
  dental problems of, 504
  diabetic, psychological problems in, 336
  effect of menstruation on, 357
  hostility expressed through bowel and bladder, 25
  interests of, conflict with aging, 147
  longing for parent, in allergy, 490
  medical history of, in psychosomatic diagnosis, 97
  neurosis, evidences for, 74
  problems of, 32
  sex education, 98
  toilet training, 24
  ulcerative colitis in, 281
  unconscious hate for, 19
Chlorpromazine in psychotherapy, 152
Christian Science, 155
Chronic appendicitis, 495
Chronic invalidism. See *Invalidism.*
Chronologic development of life history, 84
Chvostek sign in cardiac neurosis, 188

Somatic component of anxiety, 20
Somatic disease with emotional factors vs. vegetative neurosis, 260
Spas, value of, 532
Spasm, vascular, cerebral, 465
Special psychotherapeutic procedures, 149–78
Special service histories, 80
Specialists, relationship to general physicians, 532
Specialties, medical, special applications of psychosomatic medicine to, 179–534
Specificity in organ neurosis. See under *Organ neurosis.*
Sphincter control, emotional control and, relation, 403
Spinal puncture, effect in anxiety with hyperventilation, *421*
Spinsters, emotional deprivation in, 142
Spondylitis vs. cardiac neurosis, 187
Spontaneous abortion, 384
Spontaneous hypoglycemia. See *Hypoglycemia.*
Standardized histories, criticism of, 79
Sterility, 387
  functional, mechanisms in, 388
    psychology of, 389
  in female, 387
  personality survey, 390
  reactions to, in female, 393
  treatment, 392
Stomach, in digestive disturbances, 256
  reaction, to ACTH, 292
    to cortisone, 292
    to pilocarpine, 292
    to pituitrin, 292
  secretion, action of stress on, 293
Stress, 60
  action on gastric secretion, 293
  arthritis related to, 517
  life, importance in diabetes mellitus, 334
  psychological, in coronary occlusion, 213
  renal blood flow during, experimental observations, 227
  response to, in man, 61
Stroke, 465
  fear of, *466*
  little, 466
Structural alteration, relation to psychological disturbances, 6
Succinylcholine in electroshock therapy, 48
Suggestion, in psychotherapy, 154
  posthypnotic, 154
Suicide, in aged, 147
  tendency in manic depressive reactions, 47
Superstitions, over menstruation, 356
  power of, in anxiety with hypertension, *421*

Suppressive therapy, 149, 150
Surgery, abuse of, 496
  cardiac, 219
  emotional aspects, relation to dentistry, 505
  fantasies about, 496, 497
  general, and dentistry, 495–514
    psychiatric problems, 495
  gynecological, 394
  peptic ulcer and, 299
  plastic, 501
Surgical care, delay in seeking, 499
Surgical operations, psychological preparation for, 511
Surgical patients, emotional disorders in, 497
  psychosis in, 500
Sustenance, emotional, food instead of, 346
Symbolism of symptoms, 85
Sympathectomy in hypertension, 242, 243
Symptom formation, correlation with life situation, 88, 89
  psychosomatic, 67
Symptoms, meaning of, 119
  needed by patient, removal of, 168
  psychosomatic, of hypertension, 230
  symbolism of, 85
Syncope, mechanism of, 444
  vasodepressor, 444, 464
  vs. vertigo, 470
Syndrome, adaptation, 60
  asthma-eczema-prurigo, 429
  effort, 183, 184, 197, 416
  fibrositis, 319
  intractable pain, 528
  irritable colon. See *Mucous colitis.*
  Menière's, 470
  menopausal, 375
  postgastrectomy, psychiatric aspects, 300
  postural, 201
System review, 90
Systemic dyspepsia, 258

TABOOS, menstrual, 356
Talk, allowing patient to, 83
Talking with patients, 82
Tantrums, 30
  management of, 31
Tasting life and food in anorexia nervosa, *330*
Teeth, clamping and grinding, 510
  extraction of, emotional aspects, *505*
  in system review, 91
Temperature chart phobia, 388
Tension, during rest, in coronary occlusion, 217
  gradually mounting, in coronary occlusion, 213, *214*
  premenstrual. See *Premenstrual tension.*